The AVMA: 150 years of education, science, and service

ISBN 978-1-882691-41-8

_table of
contents_

Preface

Ceci n'est pas un livre d'histoire.

(with apologies to René Magritte)

This is not a history book.

Kurt Matushek

In the preface to his 1963 book "The American Veterinary Profession," which chronicles the development of the veterinary profession in the United States from the mid-1800s to the mid-1900s, J.F. Smithcors writes that the book "represents the distillation of several thousand volumes—by conservative estimate, somewhere between one and two million pages of material" and laments that the "best part of six years' research and writing—one year of it full-time—has been inadequate to achieve the consistency and balance a work like this should have."

In the years since Dr. Smithcors' book was published, the amount of written material related to the veterinary profession in general and the American Veterinary Medical Association in particular has only grown. So, when the AVMA staff first started talking about celebrating the Association's 150th anniversary in 2013, it quickly became clear that we had neither the time nor the resources to devote to a history project of that scope.

The book you hold, therefore, is not a definitive history of the AVMA. And, is not meant to be. That's not to say that there isn't history in it. Actually there's quite a lot, including many interesting and, I hope, entertaining stories of the formation of the AVMA, its growth over the years, and the individuals who helped shape it.

What this book does represent is a celebration of the AVMA and all it has accomplished for its members and the veterinary profession during its first 150 years. Written from eight unique perspectives, it focuses on what have come to be called the core competencies of the AVMA: the annual convention and scientific journals and the AVMA's roles in advocating for the veterinary profession and improving veterinary education. The USVMA was formed during the first annual meeting of the Association in response to a perceived need to elevate the visibility and standing of the veterinary profession, and education was one of the topics of discussion during that meeting. The *JAVMA* was originally published as a way to provide a lasting record of papers presented during the annual meetings. Other chapters focus on the volunteers who have been such an important part of the governance of the Association, the professional staff who have supported the Association's efforts throughout the years, and the partners who help advance the Association's goals.

I hope that you enjoy these stories of the AVMA and that you see this book not just as a look back at the history of the Association but also as a foundation from which we can look forward to the next 150 years. Of course, if you happen to have the next five or six years free, that definitive history of the AVMA still awaits.

ACKNOWLEDGMENTS

Much gratitude goes to all of the AVMA staff members who had a role in the conception, writing, editing, and design of this book. The writers, of course, are identified with their chapters. I am extremely grateful for, and impressed by, all the work they put in, while keeping up with their usual job duties. Thanks also go to the AVMA Design Services Department—Cheryl Atkins, design services manager; Sarah Jurecka, new media specialist and senior designer; and Michele Morin, production designer—who are responsible for the design and layout and to Diane Fagen, AVMA librarian, who assisted in tracking down historical materials. Without all these individuals, this book would not have been possible. The book is printed on Sappi 100lb McCoy Silk, generously provided by Sappi Fine Paper and Bulkley Dunton, an xpedx company.

Growth of a profession

Greg Cima

When Dr. Ival A. Merchant entered veterinary college in 1920, friends and family reacted as though he were studying to design stagecoaches.

"Many people, including my family, thought I was stupid because they thought veterinary medicine was a dying profession due to the advent of automotive power," he told the *Journal of the American Veterinary Medical Association* in 1963. "This idea must have influenced many young men those days, because classes were really small. There were 16 in our class."

Dr. Merchant, who received his veterinary degree in 1924 at Colorado State University, made the comments as he retired as dean of the Iowa State University College of Veterinary Medicine. The nation's veterinary profession, initially built on horse medicine, would decline and recover between the time he entered one college and retired

from another. At the start of 1963, veterinarians in the U.S.—including more than 15,600 AVMA members—were caring for ever-increasing livestock and pet populations, inspecting meat, controlling disease, improving public health, and conducting research.

Dr. Merchant's retirement year coincided with the 100th anniversary of the formation of the American Veterinary Medical Association, which had grown during that century from a gathering of several dozen men, mostly foreign-educated veterinarians, self-educated horse care providers, and physicians. Nearing on the 150th anniversary, it had grown to about 84,000 doctors, including more than 10,000 board-certified specialists in 22 AVMA-recognized specialty organizations, representing 41 specialties. Companion animal care is now the largest sector within veterinary medicine.

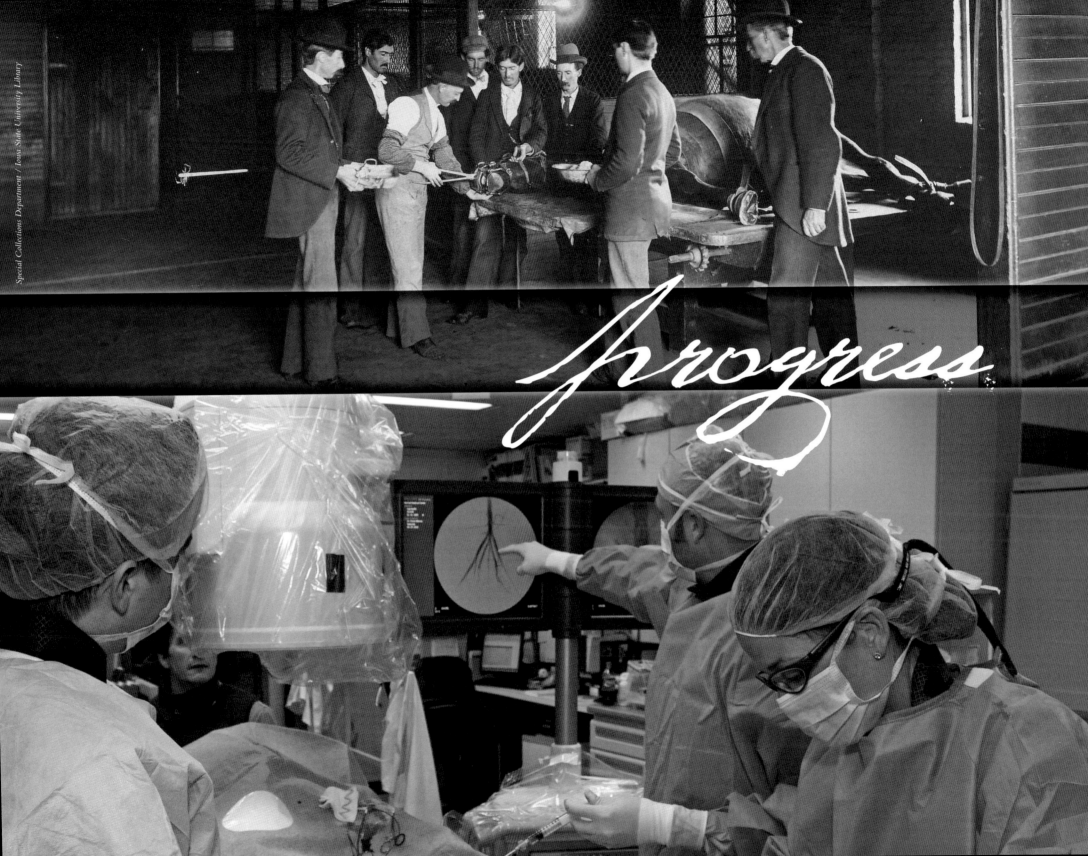

Progress

UNITED DURING THE CIVIL WAR

Dr. Harry A. Gorman, who was AVMA president in 1976, reflected at the time on veterinary medicine's "dark ages" during the nation's founding 200 years earlier.

"The few animal practitioners in America were uneducated or, at best, self-educated. Most people believed prompt dispatch of a suffering animal was more economical and certainly more merciful than consulting a professional. Although early veterinarians, mostly trained in Europe, recommended rational innovations to improve livestock conditions, they were generally ignored," Dr. Gorman said.

In a 1934 *JAVMA* article, Dr. Joseph M. Arburua wrote that ignorant farriers and cow leeches preceded veterinarians in the 1700s, and books on veterinary care were expensive and rare. During the mid-1800s, few educated animal pathologists were available, and, at any given time, likely 10 or fewer graduates of foreign colleges and physicians provided qualified animal care.

"Many of the depraved, drunken, and disreputable horse traders, anvil artists, and livery stable parasites, whose principal qualifications were greed and dishonesty, decided to call themselves farriers and veterinary surgeons, often assuming that title overnight. Many of them inherited their desire and so-called attainments from their fathers, men like themselves, and felt thus well qualified to prey upon the public," Dr. Arburua wrote.

The public paid such men to cure ailments such as "wolf in the tail," "chest founder," and "moon eyes."

Dr. Robert Jennings taught veterinary courses to students at medical colleges in Philadelphia starting in 1846, and in 1850, when he was 26 years old, he promoted creation of a veterinary college in the city, according to Dr. J. Fred Smithcors in his 1963 book, "The American Veterinary Profession." Dr. Jennings secured $40,000 for the Veterinary College of Philadelphia, which was chartered in 1852 but failed to open multiple times. Dr. Jennings later wrote that graduates of European veterinary schools thought the project was premature, and he said no young men of education and respectability would "engage in a profession of so low a standing."

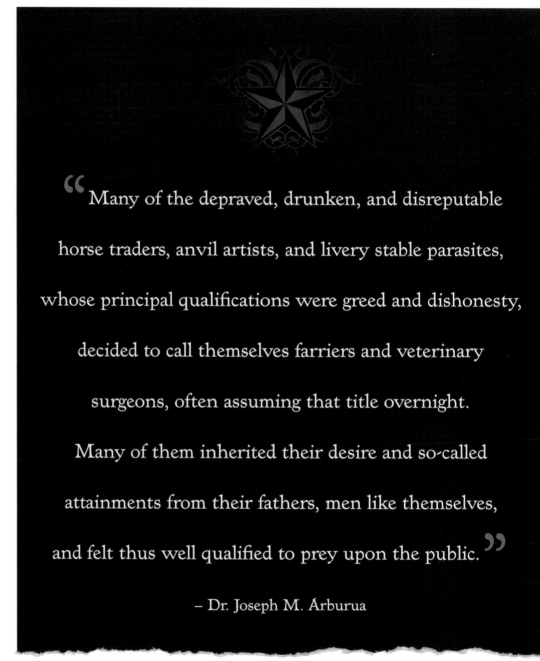

"Many of the depraved, drunken, and disreputable horse traders, anvil artists, and livery stable parasites, whose principal qualifications were greed and dishonesty, decided to call themselves farriers and veterinary surgeons, often assuming that title overnight. Many of them inherited their desire and so-called attainments from their fathers, men like themselves, and felt thus well qualified to prey upon the public."

– Dr. Joseph M. Arburua

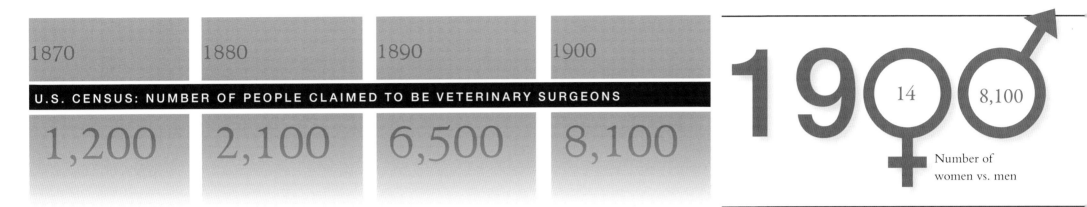

U.S. CENSUS: NUMBER OF PEOPLE CLAIMED TO BE VETERINARY SURGEONS

1870	1880	1890	1900
1,200	2,100	6,500	8,100

1900

14   8,100

Number of women vs. men

Dr. Jennings further wrote, as recounted by Dr. Smithcors, that he remained undaunted, and he sought to unite the veterinary profession. In 1854, he helped found the American Veterinary Association in Philadelphia, with members mostly from Pennsylvania, New Jersey, and Delaware and the objective of elevating the veterinary art. Its members would become the chief sponsors of the organizational meeting for the United States Veterinary Medical Association, now the AVMA.

In 1863—the third year of the Civil War—the American Veterinary Association's leaders voted to meet in June in New York City with colleagues who were interested in removing the nation's veterinary profession from the grasp of uneducated men. "The American Veterinary Profession" cites the profession's deplorable condition at the time as the reason veterinarians were kept from providing their services to U.S. Army horses.

The two-day meeting was attended by a "small, intensely serious group of veterinarians, veterinary medical practitioners, and physicians," Dr. Everett B. Miller wrote in the December 1988 issue of the American Veterinary History Society bulletin "Veterinary Heritage." The USVMA had 39 founding members: 13 in New York, nine in New Jersey, eight in Massachusetts, six in Pennsylvania, and one each in Delaware, Maine, and Ohio.

The first USVMA president was a London graduate who practiced in Boston; the secretary was a Toulouse, France, graduate who practiced in New York; and the treasurer was self-educated and practiced in New York.

The founding members agreed to admit, after oral examination, any "veterinary practitioner" or student of three years' standing in the profession who had documents and testimonials related to their qualifications, Dr. Smithcors wrote. By contrast, admission in 1913 required graduation from a school with at least a three-year program and references from two active members.

Proceedings from the USVMA's first decade note political squabbles, accusations of "quackery" and records tampering, and expulsion of some founding members, according to "The American Veterinary Profession." Recruitment nearly matched losses, and, in those 10 years, the Association had in effect gained one member. The USVMA gained about 25 percent more members in 1875, when 11 were admitted.

One of the expelled officers was Dr. Jennings, then a practitioner in New Jersey, who was ejected in 1866. Some have claimed that he had intended to form the USVMA to help him develop and become director of a veterinary college in Philadelphia, according to a 1976 *JAVMA* article by Dr. Arthur Freeman, then AVMA editor-in-chief.

At the time the profession formed a national organization, the country's few full-time veterinary practitioners worked among "a multitude of farriers, shoeing smiths, local 'experts,' and part-time healers," Dr. Miller wrote. Apathy toward the newly founded USVMA would challenge the organization's survival, as would horsemen, wagoneers, farriers, physicians, and others who enjoyed income from horse care.

The book "Evolution of the Veterinary Art" states that, in the late 1800s, men with no medical education continued calling themselves "veterinarians" and giving a false impression of the veterinary profession. It also states that the U.S. Army had "no veterinary service deserving of the name before the Civil War, and commissions were not granted before World War I."

Dr. George C. Christensen, while dean of the Iowa State University College of Veterinary Medicine from 1963-1965, wrote in a chapter of "The American Veterinary Profession" that Civil War–era veterinary schools had been primitive, lacking in trained educators, and primarily located in livery stables or similar structures in large cities. The profession's early leaders made "no little accomplishment" in convincing legislators and the public that scientific veterinary institutions were needed.

Yet, by 1879, Dr. Alexandre F. Liautard, editor of the *American Veterinary Review* (which would become *JAVMA* in 1915) wrote an editorial that praised the veterinary profession for its great progress since before the USVMA's founding, when only one or two educated veterinarians might be found in a large city and domestic animals were attended by "ignorant men, many of them unable to read or write and entirely unfit for the calling they were following." The profession, with help from the Journal, had identified contagious diseases of horses, cattle, sheep, and swine. Veterinary sanitarians were called to action, cattle commissioners were appointed, agriculture societies began calling on veterinary surgeons to deliver addresses, and the federal government was replacing farriers and horse doctors with veterinary surgeons.

U.S. census archives indicate about 1,200 people claimed to be veterinary surgeons in 1870, and the number rose to 2,100 by 1880. The latter number tripled in the next 10 years, reaching almost 6,500 by 1890. Those figures don't indicate how many of the respondents were college-educated. In fact, the AVMA's last surviving nongraduate veterinarian, Thomas Bland of Waterbury, Conn., had been admitted to the USVMA in 1887, according to his obituary in *JAVMA*. He died in December 1933.

AVMA leaders who attended a meeting in March 1887 unanimously passed a resolution that veterinary colleges should adopt uniform matriculation examinations, veterinary education of at least three six-month terms, and graduation examinations by a common examining board. Three years of veterinary education would become required for membership starting in 1893.

The need for equine veterinarians increased during the 1870s and 1880s, when the U.S. horse population grew by about 45 percent every 10 years, according to an 1891 article in *American Veterinary Review*. The horse population was nearly 15 million at that time.

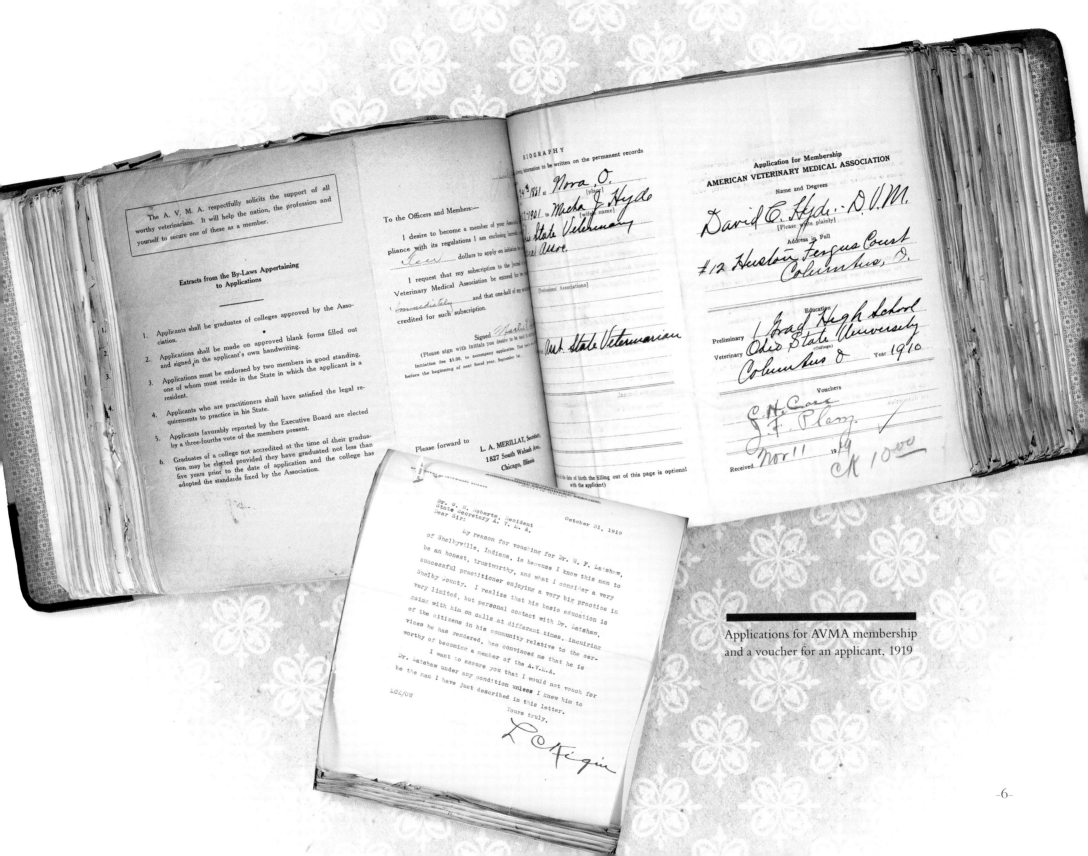

Applications for AVMA membership
and a voucher for an applicant, 1919

-6-

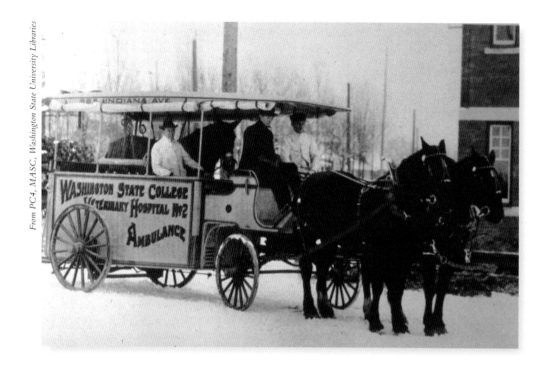

From PC4, MASC, Washington State University Libraries

The USVMA became the AVMA in September 1898. Association President Daniel E. Salmon noted in a speech at the annual meeting that the profession, meeting that year in Omaha, Neb., had grown to include representatives throughout the country and that changing the name aligned with the Association's growth. At the time, the American Public Health Association was cited as an example of an organization that had successfully embraced members throughout North America.

The veterinary profession had established itself beyond just horse medicine, even though horse care remained a large part of the profession and its reputation. Dr. Salmon noted in his 1898 speech that veterinarians' progress in meat inspection allowed people to buy meat with assurance that it didn't come from "an animal diseased, injured, or otherwise unfit to furnish wholesome food."

WAR, DEPRESSION, AND CARS

About 8,100 men and 14 women claimed to be veterinary surgeons at the time of the 1900 U.S. census, although those figures include many individuals without formal training. The AVMA had nearly 400 members and accredited 19 schools.

The nation's first college-trained female veterinarian, Dr. Mignon Nicholson, graduated in 1903 from McKillip Veterinary College in Chicago, according to *JAVMA* archives.

Practitioners' time at work, by species

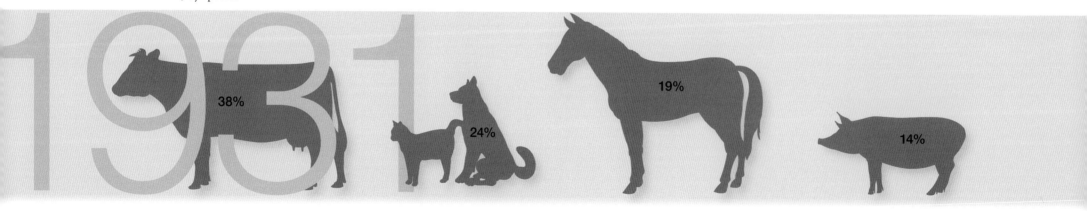

38%   24%   19%   14%

Dr. Elinor McGrath graduated from Chicago Veterinary College in 1910 and went on to become the AVMA's first female member. She and Dr. Florence Kimball, who graduated from Cornell University the same year, became small animal practitioners.

The AVMA had grown to include 1,650 members by its 50th anniversary in 1913, but the expansion would stall because of war and the expanded use of automobiles (at least one *American Veterinary Review* article from earlier in the century expressed concern that people were giving up horses for bicycles). The number of veterinary college graduates crashed from 867 in 1918 to 214 in 1919, the first year after World War I. Dr. Christensen wrote that demand for soldiers during the U.S. involvement in the war caused a decline in graduates that continued after the war, and, by 1925, the number of new graduates was lower than the number of veterinarians who died each year.

"Most of the veterinary colleges had average enrollments too small to make class work either effective or economic. The very best of them did not boast of being adequately supplied in material, equipment, or staff," Dr. Christensen wrote.

Even though needs in agriculture pushed enrollment back up to nearly 800 by 1928, the Great Depression would soon make college unaffordable for many students and animal care an unjustifiable expense for many livestock owners.

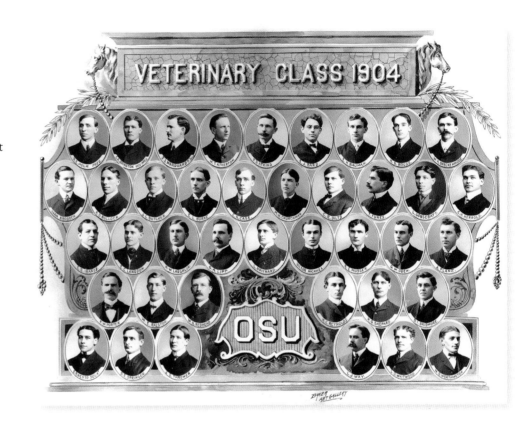

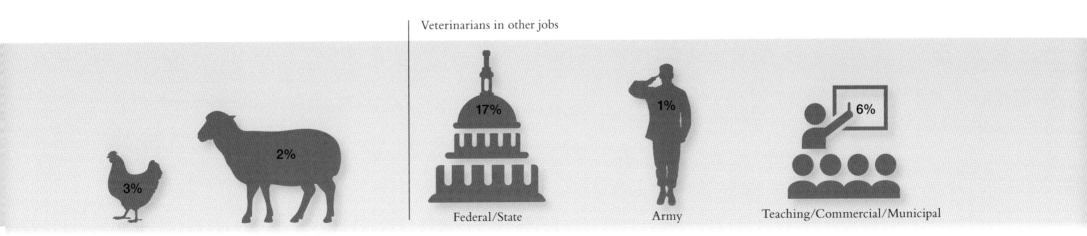

Veterinarians in other jobs

3%

2%

17% Federal/State

1% Army

6% Teaching/Commercial/Municipal

The veterinary profession also remained an almost entirely male-dominated field, and census figures indicate that many of the women who did graduate from veterinary college did not remain in the profession. Figures from the 1920 U.S. census indicate the country's veterinary surgeons included 13,493 men and only one woman.

In 1920, AVMA leaders indicated that of the nearly 13,500 veterinary surgeons in the country, only about 8,000 would have been considered eligible for membership and only about 4,100 had become members, *JAVMA* archives state. Transcripts from the AVMA Annual Meeting in August 1920 include descriptions of dropping membership applications, declining numbers of accredited veterinary colleges, and low numbers of new veterinary college graduates.

In addition, small animal practitioners were considering forming a separate association to compare ideas and discuss topics relevant to their area of practice. Small animal topics had been scarce during the AVMA meetings, and members debated whether such topics could be given a separate section at the meeting without hurting general practitioners.

Dr. Helen Richt Irwin, secretary of the AVMA meeting's section on small animals in 1937 and first woman to hold an office in the AVMA

During the 1920 meeting, the membership applications of the AVMA's first black members, Dr. R.V. Cannon and Dr. J.G. Slade, were approved by large majorities, according to a *JAVMA* article.

In the same year, AVMA President Charles A. Cary urged that veterinary schools focus less on horse anatomy and more on studies of other animal species, improved husbandry, and improved facilities, "The American Veterinary Profession" states.

By 1930, the population of veterinary surgeons listed in the census would fall to about 11,900, almost the same number as in 1910. Only 11 were women.

That year, the nation's 13 AVMA-accredited schools produced about 190 graduates, down from 20 schools with 410 graduates a decade earlier.

An AVMA Committee on Education survey of 608 practitioners showed that, in 1931, about 38 percent of the veterinarians' time was devoted to cattle, 24 percent to small animals, 19 percent to horses, 14 percent to swine, 3 percent to poultry, and 2 percent to sheep, according to "The American Veterinary Profession." About 17 percent of veterinarians in the U.S. had federal or state jobs, 1 percent worked for the Army, and 2 percent each held teaching, commercial, or municipal jobs. About 2,800 of U.S. veterinary practitioners had not graduated from veterinary college.

Rural practice was floundering in the mid-1930s, while small animal medicine was developing rapidly, according to a 1935 editorial in the monthly publication Veterinary Medicine. The latter's practitioners constructed elegant hospitals as rural practice passed into the hands of charlatans.

"For two decades the Agricultural Extension program has fostered quackery in animal medicine. The results are apparent in the decline of veterinary medicine in its field simultaneously with the growth of clinical medicine in a field it has not reached—the pet-animal industry," the article stated.

The progress in pet care was helped by the 1933 founding of the American Animal Hospital Association, which focused on improving small animal medicine. The first issue of the journal Animal Hospital would be published in February 1965.

Editorials in Veterinary Medicine lamented the fact that the veterinary profession's knowledge of medicine was not being put to good use, observing that in 1934, hog cholera cost U.S. agriculture producers orders of magnitude more than it cost Canadian counterparts as a result. Veterinarians were not responsible for control of hog cholera in the U.S., where the disease resulted in losses of about $500,000 per million hogs, but were responsible for its control in Canada, where hog cholera resulted in losses of only about $175 per million animals.

"Veterinary medicine is a medical science, not an agricultural science. The handling of animal disease is a medical—a veterinary medical—problem," the editorial stated.

The AVMA advocated that congressional authorities stop federal extension service personnel and county agents from encroaching on veterinary medicine, and the Association indicated that county employees were illegally selling veterinary medicine. Veterinarians had abandoned practices because of this encroachment, and continued actions that undercut the profession would deprive agriculture of needed services, according to "The American Veterinary Profession."

In a 1938 speech to members, AVMA President Oscar V. Brumley indicated that the Association had grown in its 75 years to 4,700 members, who, in addition to the majority of members who lived in the U.S. and Canada, included a few in Asia, the Caribbean, Mexico, South America, Central America, and Europe. The profession was also prospering, and many communities had insufficient numbers of veterinarians. He also noted that veterinary medicine was in its infancy, and well-trained and -educated veterinarians would be needed as new fields of service emerged.

Dr. Brumley pointed out that, since the USVMA had been formed, the profession had established a veterinary education system, become indispensable to livestock owners, helped develop sanitary sciences, and started public health programs. Dr. John R. Mohler, chief of the Department of Agriculture's Bureau of Animal Industry, wrote for *JAVMA* that, among other developments, the veterinary profession had eradicated contagious pleuropneumonia in the U.S., prevented outbreaks of foot-and-mouth disease, nearly eradicated bovine tuberculosis in the country, reduced the incidence of brucellosis, discovered the virus responsible for hog cholera and developed the products needed to prevent the disease, aided development of a federal meat inspection service, developed treatments and sanitary products, discovered a remedy for hookworm in dogs, and advanced standards of veterinary education and practice.

A year later, AVMA President Henry D. Bergman would describe the AVMA as "the sole protection of every individual veterinarian in this country."

WAR RETURNS, VETERINARIANS RESPOND

Capt. R.W. Menges, a veterinarian in the U.S. Army, wrote to *JAVMA* in 1944 about his duties at a railhead in California, where he inspected rations and checked the sanitary condition of food shipped in trucks and boxcars and stored in warehouses. He was among veterinarians in the Army Veterinary Corps who worked during the Second World War to ensure sanitation and food safety, quality, and wholesomeness. Another issue of *JAVMA* indicated the Navy alone would need 1.1 billion pounds of food in 1942.

Dr. Christensen wrote that members of the Army Veterinary Corps also cared for communication pigeons, guard dogs, and research dogs. Specialized training programs let veterinarians continue their studies while in the service, and an expanding roster of veterinary colleges would serve them after the war. He noted that seven veterinary schools were founded in the U.S. between 1945 and 1948.

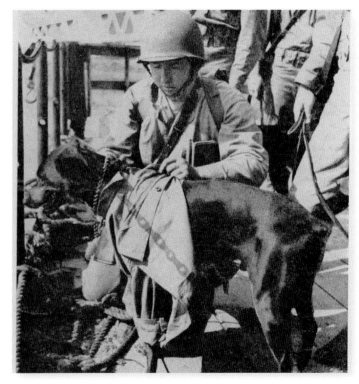

U.S. Marine Corps photo taken during World War II

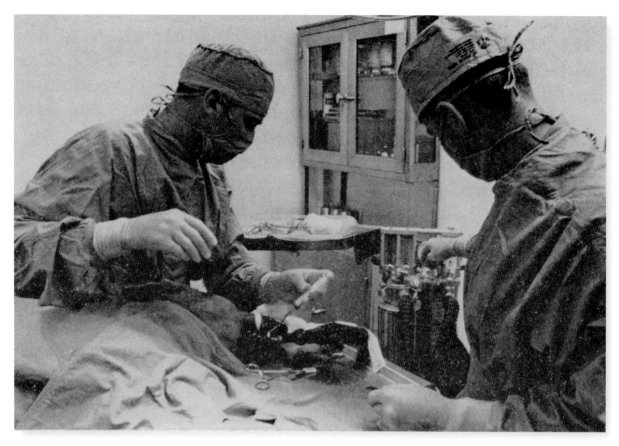

Veterinary care during
hostilities in Vietnam

Not all veterinarians' military service related to their medical training. Earlier in 1944, another *JAVMA* article indicated the Selective Service had limited occupational deferments for those younger than 26 years old, causing many veterinarians to receive draft orders.

"Because the needs of the Army Veterinary Corps for officer personnel have been met since the fall of 1943, by [Army Specialized Training Program] graduates, inducted veterinarians at present have no opportunity to obtain commissions and use their professional skills in the Army," the article states.

The article, however, included a statement from Lt. Col. G. Tinsley Garnett, who said doctors of veterinary medicine were considered as necessary for the nation's health and welfare, and local draft boards had been instructed to consider whether an individual's occupation was essential to a community.

JAVMA articles from 1942 include descriptions of duties for dogs in war, farm veterinarians' eligibility for additional gasoline rations, veterinarian participation in civilian defense organizations, defense measures for stockyards (such as air raid and poison gas protection), and limitations on production of x-ray equipment for sale to ensure the armed forces' needs would be met.

Articles from that year also indicate some people saw potential profits in veterinarians' service. A *JAVMA* editorial criticized the author of an article in the journal American Druggist who said many of the nation's veterinarians were involved in pet care or were serving in the Army, giving pharmacists opportunities to promote veterinary medicines among nonveterinarians.

"While to us the proposed drug-store quackery has the earmark of Hitler-Hirohito propaganda, we'll just call it a money-making scheme with a high potentiality for harm and of no merit," the editorial states.

After the end of the war and the Air Force's separation from the Army in 1947, the new military branch established a distinct veterinary corps. The Air Force Veterinary Corps was started in July 1949 with 150 officers on active duty; their duties included food inspection, medical care for animals, food and mess sanitation and nutrition, and attention to zoonotic disease.

During the Korean War, the Army trained veterinarians in biological and chemical warfare; the effects of radiation on humans, food, and animals; disease agents; nutrition; and food control. Veterinarians again worked in food safety duties, and *JAVMA* reported that a five-veterinarian Army Medical Service detachment received a Meritorious Unit Commendation for inspecting 69 million pounds of rations from March through September 1951.

In September 1965, the Department of Defense called for the Selective Service to furnish about 1,500 physicians, 350 dentists, and 100 veterinarians starting in January 1966 if sufficient numbers hadn't volunteered, a *JAVMA* article states. Another article from late 1968 stated that more than 1,000 dogs and about 100 veterinarians were being used by the U.S. Army in Vietnam.

Military dogs were used as scouts, sentries, and trackers in Vietnamese jungles and required treatment for a wide variety of maladies including skin problems, heatstroke, foot lacerations, kidney problems, and heart attacks, a 1970 *JAVMA* article states. Military veterinarian detachments examined each dog that arrived through Bien Hoa Air Base, and the dogs were held in 104 kennels. Veterinarians would each supervise medical operations for two or three platoons of dogs, as well as perform surgery on wounded dogs.

"Assigned to every infantry scout dog platoon in Vietnam is a veterinary technician. He is to the animal what a medic is to the foot soldier, and the dispensary in which he works is much the same as an outpatient clinic for soldiers," according to the article.

THE SLOW SHIFT IN GENDER DEMOGRAPHICS

Dr. Dorothy Segal told *JAVMA* in 2007 that, when she enrolled in preveterinary courses at Michigan State University in the 1930s, the veterinary college dean told her to "Go back to the kitchen." She was one of seven women in her class at the time, and one of two who graduated.

In 2007, about 75 percent of graduating veterinarians were women, and about 95 percent of retiring veterinarians were men. In 2009, women first outnumbered men employed in the U.S. veterinary profession.

Despite the dean's harsh words, Dr. Segal, 90 years old in 2007, said that she and the dean later became friends. Other women have also told of resistance to their entry to the veterinary profession.

Dr. Janet M. Willetts, who earned her veterinary degree at the Ontario Veterinary College in 1945, had initially attended Cornell University. But male students resisted the presence of women, and male students who corrected papers were accused of throwing away female students' papers, Dr. Willetts' sister Marjorie Maiden told *JAVMA* in 2006.

The women in U.S. veterinary schools were not alone.

An article published in 1941 in The Veterinary Record—and republished the next year as an abstract in *JAVMA*—indicated that the Society of Women Veterinary Surgeons, a division of the National Veterinary Medical Association of Great Britain and Ireland, had identified discrimination against women veterinarians by the National Registration for Employment.

cites reports that women were taking over what had been "almost entirely a man's occupation" by helping farmers maintain milk purity and increase meat production and by helping people who began raising poultry, pigs, and rabbits in yards because of food shortages.

The article indicates increasing numbers of women were becoming veterinarians prior to the Second World War. At the time of the article, women also were conducting veterinary research in England and colonial Africa.

In the U.S., the Women's Veterinary Association had its first meeting Aug. 18, 1947, in Cincinnati, and it became the Women's VMA in 1949. The group's first business meeting was attended by 16 veterinarians from the U.S., Brazil, Canada, and Cuba. A history from the Association for Women Veterinarians Foundation states that, at the time, the association had contacted 37 women who were members of the AVMA and had identified about 100 women as practicing veterinarians in North America.

"The group will represent women veterinarians throughout the Americas and has made extensive plans for promoting the interests of women students as well as graduates," *JAVMA* archives state.

A 1957 rejection letter from Iowa State University, as recounted in *JAVMA* 50 years later, indicated the university declined to enroll a woman because she could displace a man in the limited space available in the veterinary college. The letter stated in part that the university didn't think women would be physically able to handle the requirements of large animal clinics.

Meat inspection remained enough of a male-dominated field through the late 1960s that the April 1, 1967, issue of *JAVMA* included a profile of female veterinarians who performed such work for the USDA.

Yet, more than 300 female veterinarians were in practice in the U.S. and Canada in 1968, and 332 women were enrolled in veterinary colleges, according to figures presented at the July 1968 Women's VMA meeting. The AVMA was receiving about 500 letters monthly from girls in grade school and high school who wanted more informa-

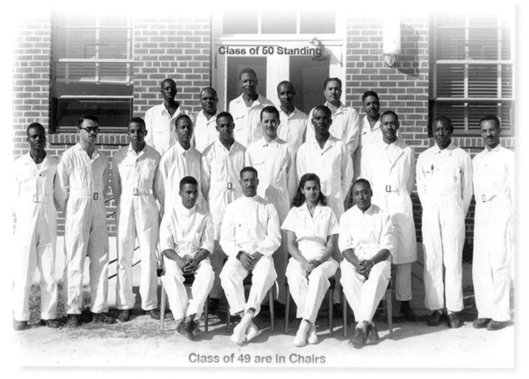

Class of 50 Standing

Class of 49 are in Chairs

One woman was a member of the 1949 and 1950 classes at the Tuskegee University School of Veterinary Medicine.

The group also had called for colleges to improve the prospects for students interested in small animal practice by offering specialized or postgraduate courses on small animal medicine. The article indicated that fellow veterinary students had voiced the opinion that they were encumbered by those who weren't interested in agricultural work.

In December 1942, another *JAVMA* article indicated that women veterinarians in Great Britain were serving their country through work on livestock, despite a misconception that women veterinarians wouldn't be needed, because their previous work had involved primarily pet care and the nation had declining pet populations. The article

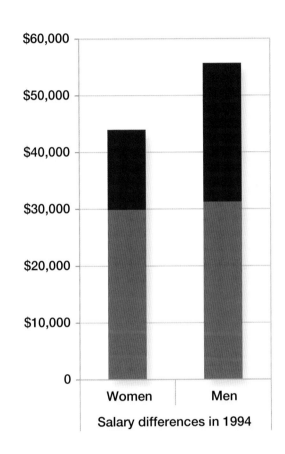

Salary differences in 1994

■ 6-10 years in practice

■ Starting salary

tion about the profession, and the Women's VMA had received about a thousand inquiries about veterinary medical careers so far that year.

"There is indeed a place for women in veterinary medicine," Dr. Jean R. Hagan, president of the Women's VMA at the time, said. "They are found in all fields of the profession."

The article indicated about 60 percent of female veterinarians were involved in private small animal practice.

JAVMA also published in May 1969 the article "Women DO practice veterinary medicine," which indicates most female veterinarians at the time were members of the AVMA, Women's Auxiliary to the AVMA, or both. About 150 were members of the Women's VMA.

A survey of women who graduated from veterinary colleges in 1973 showed that, of 83 respondents, 35 worked in small animal practice, 17 worked in general practice, nine were involved in research, six were in equine practice or an equine residency, and three were in a pathology internship, according to *JAVMA* archives from 1974. Of those women, 58 were in private practice and four were self-employed.

AVMA President-elect Harry J. Magrane said at the AVMA Annual Meeting in 1975 that women then made up about 5 percent of the profession, which had grown to more than 25,000 members, and about 25 percent of veterinary students, AVMA transcripts state. He said the Association needed to encourage more women to become involved in AVMA governance.

"When we review the AVMA official roster, we find there are no women veterinarians among our officers, on our Executive Board, councils, insurance trusts, Retirement Committee, or the Committee on Scientific Program, and only one woman among our 126 delegates and alternates in the House," Dr. Magrane said. "Therefore, I think we need a change here."

Dr. Magrane said black colleagues fared no better in AVMA governance, and the profession needed a concerted effort to elect qualified women and black veterinarians to leadership positions in local and state levels, where they could gain the experience needed to become leaders in AVMA.

"Certainly, to develop a profession that is representative of our whole society, we must quit dragging our feet and cut the barriers that make sect or color distinctions a factor in qualifications for organizational work," he said.

"We are the profession that understands and is involved in all steps of the animal food chain, making sure the animal-based food that reaches our tables is wholesome and safe. We are the profession whose researchers gave medicine its earliest clues to understanding the AIDS virus. We are the profession whose knowledge of zoonosis and epidemiology helps prevent the spread of disease, whether that be in populations human or animal. And, finally, of course, we are the profession that treats and protects the animals with which we share our planet by speaking for their needs and seeing that they are treated humanely."

– Dr. Mary Beth Leininger, president-elect's address
to the AVMA House of Delegates, 1996

But through 1976, the AVMA business session proceedings, which summarized the previous year's AVMA Annual Convention, include separate lines on attendance by "veterinarians" and "women." The 1977 proceedings instead referred to "veterinarians" and "spouses."

In 1978, attendees at the AVMA Annual Meeting received a greeting speech by the Auxiliary to the AVMA, the new name for the Women's Auxiliary. The organization changed its name and opened membership to all members of veterinarians' families.

The number of women training to become veterinarians rose sharply in comparison with the numbers of men. In fall 1985—10 years after Dr. Magrane's speech—women would outnumber men in veterinary colleges, according to *JAVMA*. By fall 2004, less than 30 years after the speech, the female-male ratio among U.S. veterinary college students had reversed, and women outnumbered men 3-1.

The percentage of U.S. veterinarians who were women tripled from 1980, when 9.5 percent were female, to 1994, when 28.7 percent were female, Dr. Gay Y. Miller wrote in a 1998 issue of *JAVMA*.

About 60 percent of veterinary graduates were women in the early 1990s. Mean starting salary for women in 1994 was $29,900, whereas mean starting salary for men was $31,300, Dr. Miller wrote. The compensation gap grew with years in practice. Women who had been in practice between 6 and 10 years earned $44,000, while men with comparable experience earned $55,700. While women's earnings remained about level through the next 20 years, men's average earnings grew to $73,200.

Study results published in *JAVMA* in 1999 would agree that women earned less than their male colleagues in veterinary medicine. The study by the company KPMG LLC on the market for veterinarians and veterinary medical services, which was commissioned by the AVMA, American Animal Hospital Association, and Association of American Veterinary Medical Colleges, also found that women worked fewer hours, owned proportionally fewer practices, and may have priced services below those of men.

Dr. Mary Beth Leininger would become the AVMA's first female president in 1996. In her speech to the House of Delegates, she described the diverse work by the veterinary profession:

"We are the profession that understands and is involved in all steps of the animal food chain, making sure the animal-based food that reaches our tables is wholesome and safe. We are the profession whose researchers gave medicine its earliest clues to understanding the AIDS virus. We are the profession whose knowledge of zoonosis and epidemiology helps prevent the spread of disease, whether that be in populations human or animal. And, finally, of course, we are the profession that treats and protects the animals with which we share our planet by speaking for their needs and seeing that they are treated humanely."

SPECIALIZATION AND CIVIL DEFENSE

The AVMA had more than 10,300 members in 1950, and the Association estimated about 15,000 veterinarians were practicing in the country. After decades of declining numbers of veterinarians and schools, the nation's veterinary profession was expanding. About 830 veterinarians would graduate from 15 AVMA-accredited schools, and four more schools would have classes starting in 1951 and 1952.

Veterinary medicine had become so broad that it needed specialized branches. AVMA immediate past president Dr. William M. Coffee made that statement in a September 1951 issue of *JAVMA*.

"When I review the new fields of opportunity in veterinary medicine that have developed since World War I, I feel that the surface has only been scratched," he said.

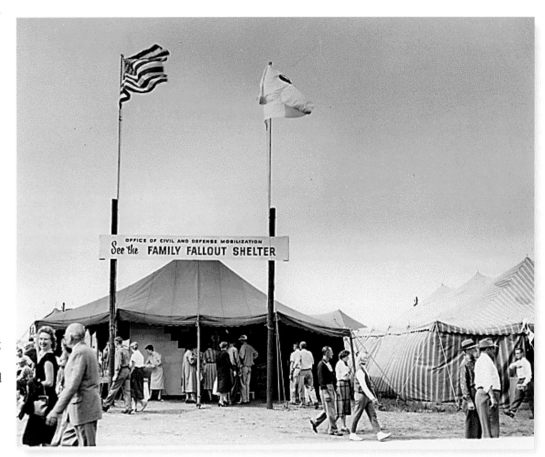

Veterinary specialties were first recognized by the AVMA that same year, starting with the American College of Veterinary Pathologists and the American Board of Veterinary Public Health.

By 2011, the 21 AVMA-recognized specialty boards and colleges would together have about 10,600 members, although the actual number of specialists would be smaller because some veterinarians belonged to multiple specialties. The largest of those specialty organizations, the American College of Veterinary Internal Medicine, had about 2,300 members, of whom more than 1,100 specialized in small animal internal medicine.

Speeches at AVMA meetings in the early 1950s also noted the need to organize the veterinary profession in defense of the nation as well as defend the profession and animal health from laypersons and humane organization members who would undercut veterinarians.

"The American Veterinary Profession" includes passages from Dr. William A. Hagan's presentation on the Cold War during the 1951 meeting that are reminiscent of present-day warnings about the risks of biological attacks by terrorists. Dr. Hagan said enemies armed with animal diseases could strike without using conventional warfare, and veterinarians needed to be vigilant against unusual diseases. An abstract in the AVMA convention program names foot-and-mouth disease and rinderpest as agents that could be used against U.S. livestock. The book notes another presentation on the need to prepare for the days following a nuclear attack, and the meeting program notes a session on "special weapons defense."

The 1952 AVMA Annual Meeting program includes information about presentations on pathologic abnormalities among a group of dogs exposed to radiation from an atomic explosion and veterinarians' role in identifying the results of biological warfare.

These speeches were delivered during a period when the USDA was losing veterinarians in its research agency. About half as many veterinarians

"We need to develop the more accurate idea that the veterinarian is an educated, well-rounded medical scientist whose services in some way touch the life of every man, woman, and child, and who is able and willing to assume a responsible role in society outside the narrow confines of his professional interests."

– Dr. Willis W. Armistead, president's address to the AVMA House of Delegates, 1958 worked for the Agricultural Research Service in 1954, when 1,375 worked for the agency, as did in 1940, Dr. Walter R. Krill, dean of the College of Veterinary Medicine at The Ohio State University, said in an AVMA statement to a Senate subcommittee. The number was below the minimum needed for national defense, he said, and the AVMA recommended a legislative change that would provide military deferment for veterinarians employed by the USDA.

And despite the increased employment of veterinarians and enrollment at schools, Dr. Abner H. Quin warned in 1955 that the profession needed to expand further. He said in an address as AVMA president that 1,000 counties in the U.S. and Canada had no veterinary services, and the veterinary profession needed to supply ample numbers of trained veterinarians "in all branches of veterinary service to the two great nations of America," according to a transcript in *JAVMA*.

"There are, in addition, many specific areas where veterinary service is too sparse to be economically practical," he said.

Dr. Quin indicated even more veterinarians would be needed to meet increasing needs in food production, as economists expected production of animal-source food would increase about a third within 20 years. States also needed to protect veterinarians and animals from "mercenary and unqualified charlatans" and dangerous pharmaceuticals and biologics by revising their state practice acts, some of which hadn't been updated in 60 years.

In 1958, Dr. Willis W. Armistead warned in his address as AVMA president that consolidation of small farms into large ones and vertical integration of agriculture would increase demand for specialists and decrease need for general practitioners, according to "The American Veterinary Profession." Veterinary college enrollment hadn't kept pace with overall university enrollment, and nearly all graduates wanted to enter private practice.

"We need to develop the more accurate idea that the veterinarian is an educated, well-rounded medical scientist whose services in some way touch the life of every man,

woman, and child, and who is able and willing to assume a responsible role in society outside the narrow confines of his professional interests," he said.

GEMINI, APOLLO, AND TERRESTRIAL MEDICINE

Veterinarians were among the scientists who developed the life-sustaining equipment needed to safely propel astronauts into space, including the first humans to walk on an extraterrestrial surface.

In 1960, 18 veterinarians in the Air Research and Development Command were working on "man's conquest of the vertical frontier," a *JAVMA* article states. They conduct-

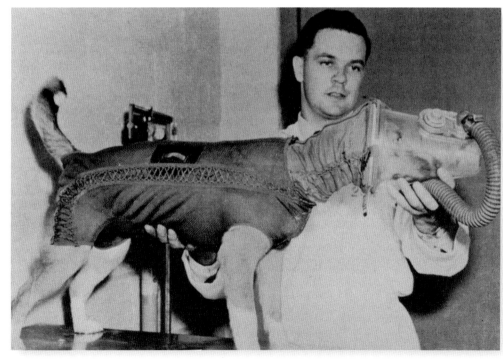

Capt. Keith Kraner, a veterinarian, holds a dog wearing a pressure suit and oxygen helmet.

ed human and animal tests on windblast, deceleration, high-altitude balloon flight, zero gravity conditions, isolation, and ejection seat and capsule physiology.

One of those veterinarians, Lt. Col. Albert A. Taylor, was chief of the ARDC biomedical division, where he guided research and development on problems of space exploration. Photos from the era that were published in *JAVMA* show veterinarians with the program examining test animals and studying a dog in a pressure suit and oxygen helmet.

The first chimpanzee astronaut, Ham, flew 115 miles from the Earth's surface aboard a Mercury capsule in January 1961. After the capsule and chimp were recovered from the Atlantic Ocean, Ham was examined by Maj. Richard E. Benson, an Air Force veterinarian. The 37-pound chimpanzee had been trained to pull levers and switches during the flight, and he was among 15,000 cats, dogs, mice, primates, rabbits, and rats to be involved in space-related research.

Veterinarians also worked in NASA's Manned Spacecraft Center in Houston during the Apollo missions of the late 1960s. They were among the scientists who planned and developed the precautionary practices and quarantine procedures for materials astronauts would bring back from the moon.

"Initially, investigations of the lunar material will determine the presence, if any, of living matter," a January 1968 *JAVMA* article states. "If such material is found, further studies will be conducted to try and identify it."

"Life is persistent, variable, and adaptable, and exists in every conceivable extreme of temperature and environment. Worms live in glaciers, bacteria in ammonia, and insects in hot springs and in oil. Fossil bacteria more than 3.1 billion years old have been discovered. The chemistry that has created life on Earth is conceivable elsewhere in space. In any event, scientists are preparing for it."

JAVMA articles also identify federal veterinarians who worked on space travel–related projects involving contamination prevention, food quality, sample assessment, radiation, virology, and pathology.

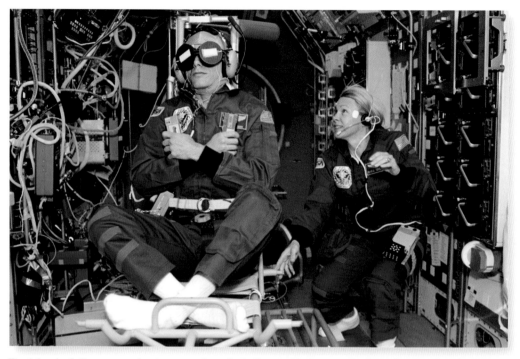

Dr. Martin J. Fettman spins in a rotating chair for medical research aboard space shuttle Columbia in 1993.

Dr. Martin J. Fettman became the first veterinarian in space when he flew aboard the shuttle Columbia in October 1993. He brought two AVMA flags on the flight. Dr. Richard M. Linnehan took four space flights and spent 58 days in space between 1996 and 2008.

Veterinary medicine's growth in terrestrial fields also continued during the 1960s.

An editorial published in *JAVMA* in 1961 indicated that the demand for veterinary services had risen dramatically since 1945, and expanding fields of specialization included public health, space medicine, and radiation research. Veterinarians were also a larger part of the U.S. population, increasing from 8.5 of every 100,000 people in 1946 to 11.6 by 1958.

A pet population census indicated that, in 1959, U.S. citizens owned about 25 million dogs, 27 million cats, 15 million parakeets, 6 million turtles, 100,000 monkeys, and 10,000 skunks, according to *JAVMA*. At least 55.6 percent of families owned at least one pet, and more than 20 percent of veterinarians were engaged in small animal practice.

But AVMA members surveyed at the 1960 AVMA Annual Convention were most committed to large animal medicine. Of those surveyed, 34 percent worked primarily or exclusively in large animal medicine, 18 percent worked in research or education, 17 percent worked mostly or exclusively in small animal medicine, 12 percent saw equal numbers of large and small animals, 8 percent worked in regulatory or inspection jobs, and 11 percent worked in other fields of the profession.

Veterinarians inspected about 20 billion pounds of meat and meat products annually and 35 million dairy animals, most of which were cows. They supervised and produced about $150 million worth of biological products and drugs, enforced trade regulations, conducted upward of 1,000 research projects on animal diseases at any given time, and trained thousands of undergraduates, veterinary students, and graduate students.

However, Dr. Mark L. Morris Sr., AVMA president-elect, said in 1961 that the profession had a public relations problem demonstrated "when one realizes that only one person out of three you meet on the street in any American city can tell you the answer to 'What is a veterinarian?'"

Despite that assessment of veterinary medicine's low profile, President John F. Kennedy praised the veterinary profession two years later for its "history of impressive contributions to the health and welfare of our nation." His comments were printed in the convention proceedings for the AVMA's 100th annual meeting.

"By establishing and maintaining a superior level of animal health in this country, doctors of veterinary medicine have enriched our knowledge in the biological sciences, deepened our understanding of the basic medical problems, accelerated scientific research, and benefited human health in many ways," President Kennedy said.

Increasingly, veterinarians were also better-educated than their peers from a generation earlier. Graduating veterinarians had spent an average of seven years in college, and about 4,000 veterinary students were enrolled in 18 institutions during the 1962-1963 academic year, according to a transcript of comments by Dr. W.T.S. Thorp, chair of the AVMA Joint Committee on Education, before a Senate subcommittee on labor and public welfare.

A statement from the AVMA included in the record noted that only 5 percent of U.S. veterinarians worked for the federal government. The U.S. Public Health Service and state and local public health departments together reported a shortage of 535 veterinarians, and a shortage of 400 USDA veterinarians was predicted over the next five years. Of the nation's 21,600 employed veterinarians, between 14,000 and 15,000 were in private practice.

Dr. Willis W. Armistead, wrote for *JAVMA* in 1966, while dean of the Michigan State University College of Veterinary Medicine, that the face of the veterinary profession had changed with the demise of "fire engine"–style large animal practice, growth in prevention and consultation services, increasing interest in research, the shift among many practices from large animal to small animal care, and an increasing shortage of veterinarians.

Research spending had tripled since 1960, he wrote. Consolidation of farms and the remaining farms' need for specialized, rather than generalized, care was contributing to declining income for large animal practitioners. Opposition to women in veterinary medicine was "dissolving rapidly." Exotic animal disease threats were increasing with international commerce. Coordination of teaching and research and increased interest in education techniques had improved veterinary instruction.

"Like the farmer who has just turned his truck from the country road onto the freeway, the veterinary profession is finding the new pace both bewildering and exhilarating. And, like the farmer, the profession may find a faster vehicle in order. But the trip ahead looks exciting and productive," he wrote. Dr. Armistead was AVMA president in 1957-1958.

The Student AVMA, initially called the National Conference of Student Chapters of the AVMA, was formed in 1969 by 34 delegates from 20 veterinary colleges. The organization started hosting annual conferences in 1971, and its members gained a voice— but no voting rights yet—in the AVMA House of Delegates in 1972. Over the next 40 years, the organization would grow to include more than 10,000 members.

The AVMA exceeded 20,000 members in 1969, ending the year with about 20,200. They included about 19,500 of the 26,000 U.S. veterinarians, 580 Canadian veterinarians, and 200 veterinarians from other countries. The AVMA membership would exceed 30,000 in 1978.

CHANGING EXPECTATIONS

Veterinarians had, by the mid-1970s, become more numerous, conspicuous, and involved in their communities than in prior decades, Dr. Arthur Freeman, then AVMA editor-in-chief, said in a 1974 *JAVMA* editorial.

"More than ever before, young people recognize veterinary medicine as one of the more exciting and diversified professions," he said. "Moreover, socially concerned citizens with a special interest in the health and welfare of the animals in our environment have developed an awareness of veterinarians and an interest in their activities."

The increased visibility of the profession was accompanied by increased vulnerability to criticism, including public and press focus on weaknesses rather than achievements, Dr. Freeman said. He said the tendency among some to view veterinarians as "potential villains and targets for censure rather than protectors of the flock and of the companion animal" was enhanced by an extraordinarily critical mood among consumers and resentments about rising service costs.

The editorial cited complaints sent to the AVMA by animal owners, an unflattering portrayal of veterinarians in Parade magazine, protests at the 1973 AVMA Annual Convention, and increasing professional liability insurance claims.

The editorial states that professional liability claims through the AVMA insurance program had increased over 10 years from about one claim for every 12 insured veterinarians to one claim for every seven.

"The animal-owning public obviously is becoming intolerant of anything short of flawless veterinary service," the editorial said.

Earlier in the decade, AVMA leaders had begun efforts to discourage discrimination within the profession.

The AVMA House of Delegates passed in July 1971 a resolution that called for the AVMA to send a statement to U.S. veterinary college deans about the importance of avoiding discrimination against members of minority groups during student selection. The AVMA was also to work with the presidents of the Tuskegee Alumni Association and the Women's Veterinary Medical Association to draft a list of colleges most likely to produce minority candidates qualified to enter veterinary colleges.

In 1975, AVMA President-elect Harry J. Magrane noted at a business session of the annual meeting that the AVMA had grown to include more than 25,000 members.

"Eighty percent of all veterinarians in the United States belong to the AVMA, and this makes our professional membership percentage the highest of any medical field," he said.

CAT CARE LAGS

Cats were virtually ignored by veterinarians in the first half of the 20th century, and they "were the last domestic animal to receive attention by veterinarians," Dr. Amy Lynn wrote in the November 2006 edition of the bulletin "Veterinary Heritage." But more cats were brought indoors when commercial clay litter was introduced in 1947 as

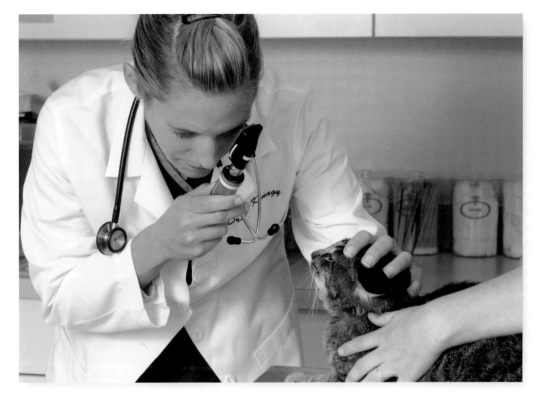

The American Association of Feline Practitioners was founded during the 1970 AVMA Annual Meeting in Las Vegas, and the organization's 1971 annual meeting included clinical and business presentations. By 1982, the organization would host its first extended continuing education meeting.

By the mid-1980s, the average cat was seen by a veterinarian 0.4 times yearly, whereas dogs visited veterinarians about 1.1 times yearly, according to AVMA statistics. The AVMA, Morris, and 9-Lives Cat Food were cosponsors of the first Cat Health Month in September 1986, and a public relations program was created to educate cat owners about their pets' needs. AVMA documents from the era indicate the program was timed to take advantage of the need for check-ups and vaccinations following the spring and summer peak breeding seasons as well as to fill a typically slow time in veterinary clinics.

The Academy of Feline Medicine was established in August 1990, and the AAFP sought feline practitioners' support as it pursued recognition by the AVMA's Advisory Board on Veterinary Specialties of a specialty in feline medicine, according to articles in the journal Feline Practice. The American Board of Veterinary Practitioners would add a Feline Practice specialty in 1995. That specialty had 80 diplomates in 2011, and the Canine & Feline Practice specialty had 469. About 32 percent of U.S. households owned cats, according to the 2007 U.S. Pet Ownership and Demographics Sourcebook.

an alternative to sand and wood ashes, and their increasing confinement in houses was connected with increased veterinary care.

In fact, the early American veterinary literature didn't consider cats to be an important veterinary species. The first edition of the American Veterinary Journal, published in 1855, reprinted a story told from the perspective of a man who, after hearing a group of noisy cats outside his home, rose from bed, loaded a shotgun, and shot and killed the cats' apparent leader.

Dr. Lynn's article noted that Dr. Louis J. Camuti opened the nation's first feline-only house call service in 1932 in New York City, and Dr. Robert L. Stansbury would open the first cat-only veterinary clinic 23 years later in Pasadena, Calif.

MEMBERS OUTNUMBER FOUNDERS BY 1,000-TO-1

After 121 years, the AVMA's membership had multiplied from 39 members to beyond 39,000 in 1984, topping 40,137 members by the end of the year. Although the profession's primary focus had shifted from equine care, the number of veterinarians in equine-exclusive practices alone surpassed 1,700. About 9,300 other veterinarians worked with all species of large animals or some mix of large and small animals.

At the time, the AVMA dedicated $76,000 toward studying the potential oversupply of veterinarians. Dr. Duane T. Albrecht noted during AVMA House of Delegates' 1983 business session, where he became AVMA president, that a previous report had projected a national surplus of 3,900 veterinarians by 1985. He urged deans and state

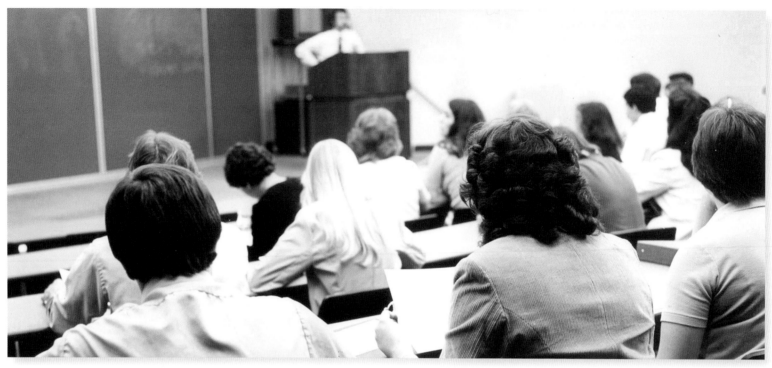

Veterinary students at Mississippi State University in the early 1980s

legislatures to address the supply of veterinarians and said veterinary students should be told of opportunities outside private practice.

Two years later, another AVMA president, Dr. Delano L. Proctor Jr., said veterinarians in small animal practice were challenged by increasing numbers of graduates, generally poor economic conditions, government-sponsored low-cost spay and neuter clinics, and an ability "to diagnose and treat far in excess of the average pet owners' ability to pay," Dr. Proctor said. These problems could be reduced, he said, with the help of business programs, newsletters, advertising, computerization, political action, and possibly use of third-party payment services.

As for food animal practice, Dr. Proctor said food animal veterinarians needed a financial reward structure that would compensate them for their professional competence and time, and veterinarians needed to understand the needs of the corporate farms that were replacing small family farms. He said animal health must be managed with emphasis on prevention and health maintenance, and the days of "therapeutic fire engine practice" were waning. Instead, veterinarians must relate to prevention, administration, communication, data processing, and business management.

"The future of food animal practice is dependent on the success of the livestock production industry," Dr. Proctor said. "The problems faced by the producers and their veterinarians are similar. They must be good at the biological aspect of their jobs, but they also must be good businessmen and good managers."

Dr. Proctor also indicated an in-house survey of 1984 graduates showed 77 percent expected to work in private practice, 13 percent planned to enter graduate studies, 7 percent would be self-employed, and 3 percent would seek jobs in government or industry. Of those graduates, about 85 percent would have education-related debt, and the mean debt was $20,000. The mean starting salary for graduates also was about $20,000.

In 1986 about 51 percent of AVMA members would work primarily or entirely in small animal practice, representing the majority of AVMA members for the first time.

The AVMA represented about 83 percent of all U.S. graduate veterinarians at the time of Dr. Proctor's speech, which he noted was a much higher ratio than that enjoyed by the American Medical Association or American Dental Association.

"It came to my attention that if we placed every veterinarian in the United States in one spot, we could only fill about half of one of our large football stadiums," Dr. Proctor said. "Gentlemen, we cannot afford to be divisive or to become polarized to the point that we fail to cooperate. Organized veterinary medicine needs the help of every veterinarian, and I feel that veterinarians need organized veterinary medicine. It is a fact that 40,000 voices can be heard when they are in concert."

Study results published in an August 1985 issue of *JAVMA* said at the time that the U.S. would likely have a surplus of private practice veterinarians through the year 2000. The projections indicated demand for veterinary services would grow during that time but

AVMA members, 1986

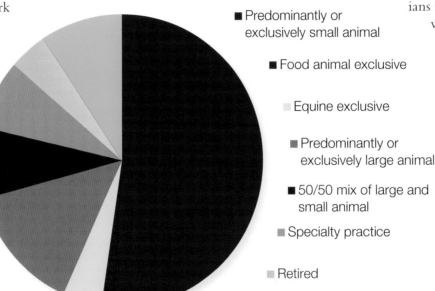

■ Predominantly or exclusively small animal

■ Food animal exclusive

■ Equine exclusive

■ Predominantly or exclusively large animal

■ 50/50 mix of large and small animal

■ Specialty practice

■ Retired

■ Other or unknown

be outstripped by 73 percent growth in the supply of veterinarians from 1980-2000. The surplus was also expected to hurt veterinarians' income.

The report, which was authored by J. Karl Wise, PhD, AVMA staff economist, and John Kushman, PhD, a professor of agricultural economics at the University of California-Davis, indicated that small animal veterinarians in New England could experience a mean 50 percent decline in the number of veterinary service visits from 1980-2000. The mean decline among veterinarians in the Rocky Mountain region could be 15 percent. Even if veterinary colleges were able to decrease their numbers of graduates 20 percent starting in 1990, pet visits per small animal veterinarian would still decline by 17 percent, and the demand for livestock services by 22 percent, they said.

"Declining ratios of demand to supply and declining veterinary incomes in private practice partially reflected a lower valuation of additional veterinarians to society," the study synopsis states in part. "At some point, additional veterinarians will be a poor investment for society if the need for private veterinary services is met."

A February 1986 article in *JAVMA* indicates that demand for small animal veterinary services and large animal services would likely grow by 31 percent and 23 percent, respectively, and the supply of private practice veterinarians would grow 73 percent during the same period. Also in 1986, the Minnesota VMA endorsed a proposed 20 percent reduction in the size of veterinary classes at the University of Minnesota in response to the projected oversupply of veterinarians. *JAVMA* archives from 1987 indicate officials with the university then proposed closing the entire veterinary college because of the perceived oversupply and the establishment of a veterinary school at the University of Wisconsin, which admitted its first class in 1983.

said. Some veterinarian shortages existed on the East Coast, and other areas had over-supplies, he said.

The AVMA would exceed 50,000 members in the first year of the next decade, an increase of about 10,000 members in six years. The pace would slow in the 1990s, as the AVMA would need seven more years to gain another 10,000 members.

BALANCING VETERINARIAN AND ANIMAL POPULATIONS

In 1991, President-elect Gerald L. Johnson said that the AVMA had, a few years earlier, indicated the U.S. had too many veterinarians, but he suggested that this was a misconception "based upon the perceived oversupply of some practitioners in some geographic areas."

"As a result, colleges of veterinary medicine were urged to reduce the number of students admitted each year," he said. "Students were discouraged from applying to the schools and colleges of veterinary medicine."

Yet, Dr. Johnson said the AVMA realized that the veterinary profession needed to increase the number of top students who chose to pursue careers in veterinary medicine. He called for creation of a national public education program aimed at educating grade school students on veterinarians' roles in animal welfare, food safety, and responsible pet ownership.

A year earlier, about 53 percent of members primarily or entirely worked in small animal practice, AVMA records state. About 7 percent worked in mixed animal practices, with an even split between large and small animal practice, and about 17 percent worked in livestock or equine practice. Only 4 percent exclusively provided equine care.

Those members were increasingly women, who by 1993 represented more than a quarter of U.S. veterinarians and nearly half the AVMA members who were less than 40 years old, according to proceedings from an AVMA business meeting.

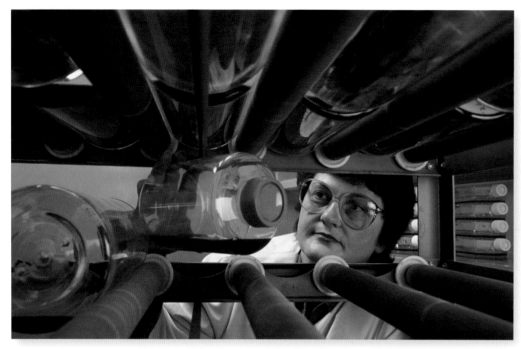

Dr. Janice Miller observes cultured cells infected with rhinotracheitis virus grown for an experimental vaccine.

In July 1987, President-elect Richard B. Fink scolded the "doubting Thomases" who felt that the U.S. had no oversupply of veterinary clinicians. He said in part that "as long as the starting salary for new graduates is $21,000 for 7.7 years of higher education, we have a crisis."

Yet the mean income of veterinarians in private clinical practice had risen 10 percent from 1985-1987, when the mean was about $47,000 annually, *JAVMA* articles state.

Tuition also increased about 75 percent between 1980 and 1988, and financing eight years of college was putting students into enough debt to consume about a quarter of their starting income, then AVMA President-elect Walter L. Martin Jr. (1988-1989)

The AVMA launched a series of initiatives during the 1990s both to help veterinarians make more money and to make sure they could find jobs.

Veterinary school graduates had a mean starting salary of about $31,000 in the mid-1990s, while physicians earned about $110,000 annually as medical interns, Dr. Sherbyn W. Ostrich, then AVMA president, said in one of a series of reports published after a 1996 AVMA symposium on economics. Other reports from the meeting expressed concern over whether all veterinarians would find work in their profession, but one noted that the situation was far less dire than a 1978 prediction that the nation would have 55,000 veterinarians and demand for only 42,000.

Dr. Janver D. Krehbiel said in his report that the numbers of applicants to veterinary colleges dropped from 7,200 in 1980 to 3,900 in 1989 but recovered to the 1980 level by 1996. While the nation's 22 veterinary schools had about 2,200 openings for students in 1977, the five colleges added by 1996 resulted in only 100 additional openings for students.

Women accounted for 70 percent of veterinary school applicants in 1996, Dr. Krehbiel wrote. Only 4.7 percent of applicants identified themselves as Hispanic, 2.9 percent as Asian or Pacific Islander, and 1.2 percent as black.

Dr. Krehbiel said the selection process for students wasn't easy, but it must be consistent, fair, and equitable.

"Recognizing the socioeconomic changes in agriculture and changes in societal expectations of our profession, we have shifted our recruitment efforts toward a more diverse student body. Our understanding of the role of companion animal medicine and the mental health of pet owners clearly justifies our shift from a primarily agricultural-oriented profession to a broadened allied health service capability, including the areas of food safety and environmental toxicology," he wrote.

Dr. John W. Albers said in his report that veterinary colleges reported high rates of job offers for graduates, and corporate practices had difficulty hiring enough veterinarians to staff clinics. But some cities had long lists of veterinarians available for work, and

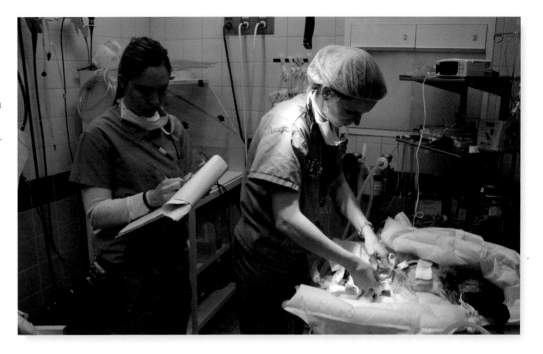

state license requirements and spouse employment limited some veterinarians' abilities to find work. He said economic pressures in companion animal practice were real, serious, and in need of attention by the profession.

Veterinary colleges also had responded to budget cuts with disproportionate reductions in food animal medical programs, Dr. James A. Jarrett said in his report. Many such colleges had secured state funding by promising to educate food animal veterinarians. He said the higher starting salaries given to food animal veterinarians than to companion animal veterinarians backed survey findings that more food animal veterinarians were needed.

The KPMG LLC study commissioned by the AVMA, American Animal Hospital Association, and Association of American Veterinary Medical Colleges indicated, in findings published in 1999, that veterinarians' income lagged behind those in similar medicine cal professions, hurting the ability to repay student loans or attract students. Women in the profession earned less than male colleagues.

But consumer spending on pets was robust, showing the potential for an increased demand for veterinary services.

The findings published in *JAVMA* indicated an excess of veterinarians was pushing down service prices and would likely cause stagnant income over the coming decade, even though expenses on veterinary services had increased about 7 percent annually since 1980 after adjusting for inflation.

The median net income in small animal practice appeared to increase about 16 percent from 1983-1995 after inflation, while mixed animal practice net income increased about 44 percent, the study authors concluded, on the basis of figures from AVMA Biennial Economic Surveys and the consumer price index. But median net income declined about 28 percent in large animal practice and 21 percent in equine practice during the same period. Increases in large animal practice expenses outpaced income, while both income and expenses declined in equine practice.

In the same year, AVMA figures indicated increasing numbers of veterinarians had pursued specialty training. Board-certified diplomates represented about 10 percent of AVMA members by January 1999. At the time, 36 distinct specialty areas were

identified in 20 recognized and provisionally recognized specialty organizations.

Veterinarians also had a lesser role in government during the 1990s than in prior decades, Dr. Mary Beth Leininger, as AVMA president, said in her 1996 address to the House of Delegates that year. The numbers of veterinarians working for the military had declined 50 percent since 1966, the numbers working in regulatory medicine had dropped 75 percent, and the number working in public health had dropped 80 percent, she said.

"If we are serious in our intent to reverse this trend and get more veterinarians in nonclinical practice careers, we must do better. We need to build on our successes like the congressional fellowship program and Aquavet and Envirovet and find other opportunities for members to gain experience in alternate career paths."

CONSOLIDATION AND ECONOMIC UNCERTAINTY

Veterinarians increasingly began working in group or corporate practices during the 2000s. Respondents to the AVMA Biennial Economic Survey indicated more than half of veterinarians in small animal–predominant or –exclusive practices had solo practices in 1999. By 2009, only 31 percent of companion animal–predominant and 21 percent of companion animal–exclusive practitioners worked alone.

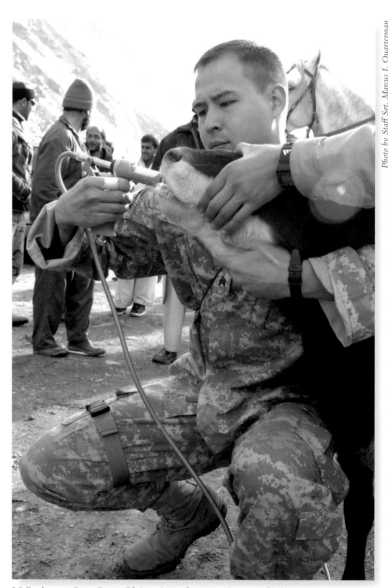

U.S. Army Sgt. Sam Chiu gives deworming medicine to a cow during a 2007 veterinary civic action program in Afghanistan.

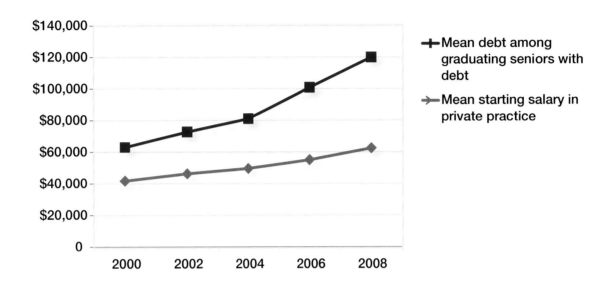

Among those exclusively in food animal practice, the percentage of those in solo practice decreased from 65 percent to 35 percent in the same period. In addition, the percentages of food animal–predominant and mixed animal practices with only one veterinarian each declined slightly during that time to about 40 percent in each category.

Only equine practice continued to have a majority in single-veterinarian practices, although the survey responses indicated the percentage of those in solo practice had declined from 63 percent to 57 percent.

While private practice veterinarians' income would rise about 5 percent annually during that 10-year period, educational debt would take an increasingly large bite out of their income.

In 2000, veterinary school graduates in private practice had a mean starting salary of about $42,000 annually, and those with debt had a mean debt of $63,000, according to figures from the AVMA Graduating Seniors Survey. The starting salary would increase to about $62,000 by 2008, but the mean debt to about $120,000, according to the survey.

The AVMA also continued examining the need for veterinarians, particularly in livestock production.

Study results published in 2006 indicated more veterinarians were needed in food production, but fewer veterinarians were interested in such careers. The Food Supply Veterinary Medicine Coalition Report stated that the vulnerability of animals and the public to disease, and concerns about the number of veterinarians available to protect against those diseases, could damage the profession.

The report concluded, in part, that emphasis in the veterinary profession on providing pet medicine at the expense of work on food animal medicine would cost opportunities for the profession's growth and endanger human and animal health. It stated:

"The profession must decide if it intends to largely relegate itself to the treatment and welfare of two species—dogs and cats—or if veterinary work intends to encompass other species. If a greater view and a wider role for the veterinary profession are envisioned, then there must be a strategic commitment to the welfare of all animals and to maintaining a safe and wholesome food supply for the USA and Canada. The leaders in academia, government, practice, and industry as well as those in the major professional associations will have to join forces to take the veterinary profession to the next stage in its evolution by boldly allocating resources to food supply veterinary medicine."

> " If there is not enough work for this veterinary profession, we haven't done a good job of creating the value and demand for our services. "
>
> – Dr. René A. Carlson, president-elect's address to the AVMA House of Delegates, 2011

and the country's remaining underserved areas might be unable to sustain veterinary practices.

"Continuing to increase the number of veterinarians interested in serving rural areas will not solve this problem. In fact, creating an 'over supply' of food supply veterinarians will lead to widespread unemployment or underemployment of food supply private practitioners and will have a significant detrimental effect on salaries for all veterinarians," the AABP reported.

Many veterinarians were hurt by the recession that started in 2008. A survey conducted in late 2008 indicated a third of veterinarians reported decreases in visits and a quarter had declining revenue, according to a *JAVMA* article. The National Commission on Veterinary Economic Issues reported 5 percent of practices polled had laid off veterinarians, and 16 percent were considering layoffs.

Salaries jumped for food animal–exclusive veterinarians from 2005-2007, when survey respondents indicated their mean income increased from $107,000 to $140,000. The median increased from $91,000 to $109,000, and food animal–exclusive veterinarians surpassed equine-exclusive practitioners to become the top-paid private practice veterinarians.

The mean salary for food animal–exclusive practice would decrease to $131,000 by 2009 but remain the highest in private practice.

By 2011, about 44,000 of the AVMA's 83,000 members worked exclusively in companion animal medicine. About 6,700 members also indicated they worked predominantly in companion animal practice, but the figures may overlap because the AVMA analysis allowed veterinarians to select multiple practice categories.

That year, the American Association of Bovine Practitioners published a report that said sufficient numbers of people were interested in careers in rural veterinary practice,

Information provided by the NCVEI in 2012 also indicated that the number of companion animal veterinarians increased by nearly 50 percent from 1996-1997 to 2006-2007, and pet ownership increased by about a third over the same period.

A survey of graduating veterinarians during 2011 indicated about 74 percent had received at least one job offer, down from 92 percent of graduates four years earlier.

Income among at least some specialty practices declined more sharply than did income at general clinics, according to a 2010 *JAVMA* article. A partner at a veterinary consulting firm indicated the loss could be connected with the cost of emergency and specialty procedures, and increased reluctance in general practices to refer cases rather than handling them in-house.

Through the recession and the years immediately following it, the veterinary profession also fought to keep procedures ranging from horse teeth floating to bovine embryo transfer defined as the practice of veterinary medicine. Farm organizations and some state legislators in particular fought to alter state veterinary practice acts to allow more people to provide more services, sometimes with the argument that insufficient numbers of veterinarians were available to perform the services. Of course, reducing veterinarians' income had the potential to exacerbate those problems.

The AVMA joined international veterinary associations in 2011 to celebrate World Veterinary Year. The year represented both the 250th anniversary of the founding of the world's first veterinary school in Lyon, France, and the year eradication was declared for rinderpest, the devastating disease that helped justify construction of the Lyon school, giving birth to the veterinary profession. Rinderpest was, after smallpox, only the second disease—and the first animal disease—to be declared eradicated worldwide.

Rinderpest, or cattle plague, was connected with wars and famines over the centuries, killing more than 200 million cattle in western Europe between 1711 and 1769.

In 2012, the AVMA was among several organizations with pending studies on the supply of veterinarians and the future demand for their services. And the Association was starting a new program to increase pet visits to veterinary clinics.

Dr. René A. Carlson, 2011-2012 AVMA president, said in a July 2011 speech before the AVMA House of Delegates that she had heard optimism that the future of veterinary medicine could offer—without decades of financial burden—careers with personal and financial reward, education that is the envy of the world, a respected AVMA that provides open leadership and member engagement, public understanding of veterinarians' level of education, and roles for veterinarians across health disciplines.

"This is a defining time for veterinary medicine and the AVMA," she said.

Dr. Carlson said the public needs to understand how veterinarians improve the health of animals, people, and the environment.

"There's got to be enough work for everyone. If there is not enough work for this veterinary profession, we haven't done a good job of creating the value and demand for our services," she said.

ENDURING DEDICATION TO KNOWLEDGE, HEALTH

The USVMA's first few members dedicated their organization to the "diffusion of true science and particularly the knowledge of veterinary medicine and surgery," as they said in the Association's first constitution.

Generations of veterinarians, including the first ones educated in U.S. veterinary schools, adapted and edited that mission to suit their expanding profession as they applied their skills to increasingly diverse scientific fields and public needs. Yet, those generations have maintained their Association's dedication to improving animal health and human understanding while broadening the Association's mission and objectives.

Today, the AVMA's mission is to "improve animal and human health and advance the veterinary medical profession." Its objective is to "advance the science and art of veterinary medicine, including its relationship to public health, biological science, and agriculture."

After 150 years, the Association's original and modern goals remain similar enough to nearly apply interchangeably between the 39 original members and 82,000 today. Both groups sought improved animal health, medical knowledge, and the ability of their members to prosper, along with the public they serve.

A call to service

2

Kurt Matushek

In 2012, the American Veterinary Medical Association boasted more than 84,000 members, including more than 80 percent of all veterinarians in the United States. Quite a change from the small group of men who came together in 1863 to form the United States Veterinary Medical Association, now the AVMA. Although many factors have contributed to the remarkable growth of the past 150 years, unquestionably one of the most important has been the dedication of the thousands of members who have volunteered their time in service to the Association. Understanding how the governance of the AVMA has changed over the years helps us not only learn about the history of the Association but also prepare for the future.

THE FIRST CONSTITUTION

The broad outlines of the events that led up to the formation of the USVMA are generally well-known. In March of 1863, Robert Jennings proposed during a meeting of the American Veterinary Association in Philadelphia that a convention of veterinary surgeons be called for the purposes of forming a national veterinary association. Although the idea of a national association had been around for several years, this time it elicited a more favorable response. Concerns were expressed, however, both that the qualifications for membership not be so rigid as to exclude all self-educated practitioners, leaving the proposed association to be dominated by graduates of the European colleges

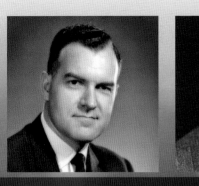
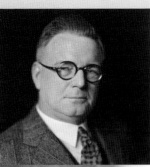
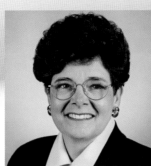
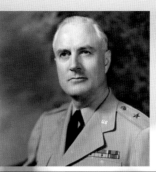
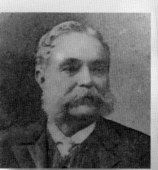
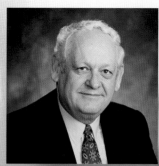

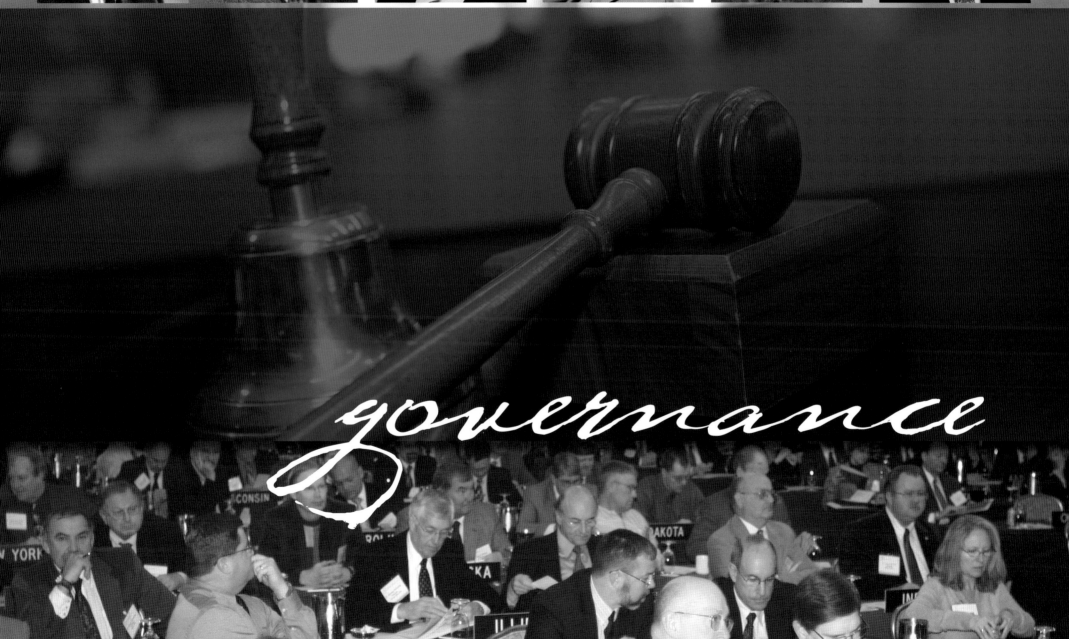

governance

of veterinary medicine, and that the qualifications not be so loose as to allow for the admission of quacks.

In April of 1863, the AVA again met to consider the proposal, passed a resolution that the meeting be held in June of that year, and appointed a local organizing committee. Notices of the meeting were published in The New York Times on June 7 and 8 that read "To Veterinary Surgeons. There will be a meeting of veterinary surgeons at the Astor House on the 9th of June, at 2 o'clock P.M. All interested in the advancement of veterinary science are invited to attend." The men met as scheduled at the Astor Hotel in New York City on June 9 and 10, 1863.

During the first day's meeting, a committee headed by Josiah Stickney was selected to draft a constitution and bylaws. The document was read during the next day's meeting and adopted, and new officers were elected. Josiah Stickney, a London graduate, was elected president; Alexandre Liautard, a graduate of Toulouse, was elected recording secretary; and A.S. Copeman, a self-educated practitioner, was elected treasurer.

According to notes from Robert Jennings from the organizational meeting, there was considerable discussion regarding the name of the new association, but no information is available on the details of those discussions. Most likely, "United States" was chosen, instead of "American" because an American Veterinary Association had been established in Philadelphia some years before. J.F. Smithcors, in his 1963 history "The American Veterinary Profession," points out, however, that the initial meeting was held during the Civil War and that this may have played a role in the naming of the association, in that "American" would have included the Confederate States of America. Smithcors cautions that this is only conjecture. Isaiah Michener of Pennsylvania later claimed the he was the one who suggested the name that was finally chosen.

According to Smithcors, the charter members of the USVMA consisted of 39 men from seven states. From various notes, it is apparent that others were present at the or-

CHARTER MEMBERS OF THE UNITED STATES VETERINARY MEDICAL ASSOCIATION

NEW YORK

W.H. Banister
C.H. Birney
Louis Brandt
John F. Budd
Charles Burden
John Busteed
A.S. Copeman
R.H. Curtis
A. Large
A. Liautard
W.T. McCoun
James Mulligan
E. Nostrand

W. Saunders
J.H. Stickney
E.F. Thayer
C.M. Wood
Robert Wood

PENNSYLVANIA

J.C. Essenwein
R. McClure
G. Mellor
I. Michener
E.H. Palmer

NEW JERSEY

A.C. Budd
T. Cooper
Jacob Dilts
J.C. Higgins
S. Humphrey
R. Jennings

W.R. Mankin
A. Philips
Jacob Philips
J.F. Walton

MAINE

E.F. Ripley

OHIO

G.W. Bowler

DELAWARE

W.A. Wisdom

MASSACHUSETTS

R. Farley
O.H. Flagg
James Penniman

Taken from "The American Veterinary Profession," by J.F. Smithcors

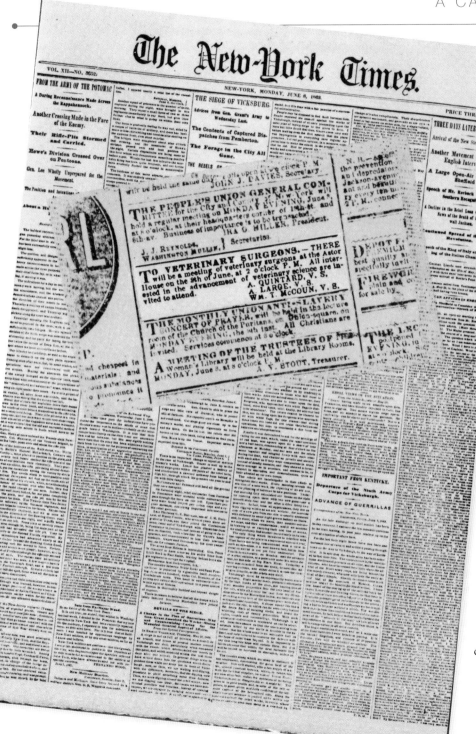

ganizational meeting. It is not clear why they were not included as charter members. In accordance with the new constitution and bylaws, a vice president was elected from each of the seven states represented among the charter members; the individuals selected were R.H. Curtis, W. Saunders, R. McClure, Robert Jennings, E.F. Ripley, G.W. Bowler, and W.A. Wisdom. In addition, W.T. McCoun, Robert Wood, Isaiah Michener, and J.F. Walton were selected as corresponding secretaries, and A. Large, E.F. Thayer, J.C. Essenwein, E.H. Palmer, Jacob Dilts, and C.M. Wood were elected as censors.

Two aspects of the original USVMA Constitution and Bylaws stand out. The first is that the members of the Comitia Minora were charged with examining applicants to determine whether they were qualified, before allowing them to become members of the Association. During the 1864 meeting, for example, P.J. Curran Penny and T.B. Raynor presented their credentials and were examined by the Board of Censors. Penny passed his examinations in anatomy (presented by A. Large), physiology (presented by E.F. Thayer), and the theory and practice of medicine (presented by C.M. Wood) and was accepted as a member, but Raynor apparently refused to answer any questions, claiming that he had a right to be a member because of his work in helping to organize the Association, and was refused. Although requiring prospective members to pass an examination seems strange today, it made sense at the time, when so many supposed practitioners were little more than charlatans and quacks, with no training and little knowledge of veterinary medicine.

The second interesting aspect of the original constitution and bylaws was that the president of the United States—Abraham Lincoln at the time of the organizational meeting—was an ex officio honorary member of the Association.

EARLY CHANGES

Remarkably, particularly given that the original constitution and bylaws were written in a single evening, relatively few changes were made to the organization of the USVMA during its early years, although a revision of the constitution was adopted in 1867. One change that year was the decision to select a single vice president rather than the multiple vice presidents from the states represented in the Association. William Wisdom, who had been serving as one of the vice presidents since the founding of the USVMA, was selected to fill that role.

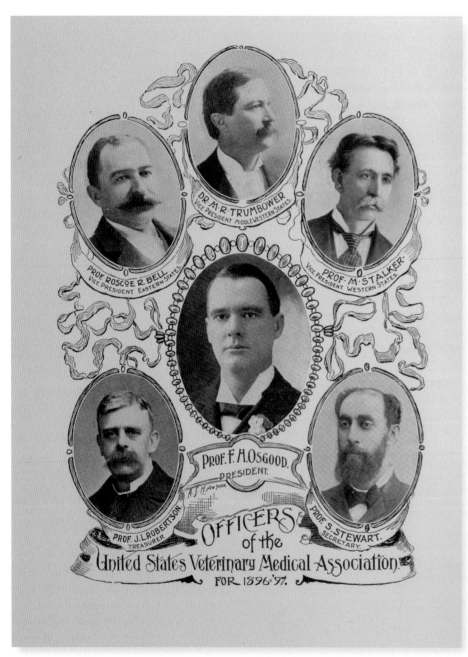

A page from the January 1897 issue of the *American Veterinary Review*

During the 1870 meeting, the officers of the previous year were re-elected, setting a precedent that lasted until about the mid-1890s. And, in 1884, the number of censors elected each year was increased from five to seven. This change was presumably in response to concerns that the USVMA did not, in fact, represent the veterinary profession in the entire country and that veterinarians in what were then the "Western" states were dissatisfied. One of the censors elected in 1884 was John Meyer Sr. of Cincinnati; another was W.J. Crowley of St. Louis.

A revised constitution, which had apparently been in preparation for some time, was adopted at the annual meeting in 1889. Two of the most important changes were the decisions to hold a single meeting each year, rather than the twice-yearly meetings that had been held up to that time, and to make the Board of Censors an appointed, rather than an elected, body.

A major step was taken in 1892 with the unanimous adoption of an amendment requiring that any future applicant for membership in the USVMA "shall be a graduate of a regularly organized and recognized veterinary school, which shall have a curriculum of at least three years, of six months each, specially devoted to the study of veterinary science, and whose corps of instructors shall contain at least four veterinarians." With the USVMA having become the accepted representative body of the veterinary profession in the United States, this change went a long way to helping establish a uniform standard for the education of veterinarians in the country.

The following year, Walter Williams, 1892-1893 USVMA president, noted that, for the first time in the history of the Association, many applicants were refused admittance. He explained that the new three-year educational requirement excluded from membership the graduates of many of the veterinary colleges operating at that time and extolled the Association's move to impose a higher educational standard.

In 1894, the USVMA decided to reinstate the earlier practice of electing multiple vice presidents, with representatives to be selected from the Eastern, Central, and Western segments of the profession.

A NEW NAME

In 1897, AVMA President Frederick Osgood, citing the close professional and economic union between veterinarians in the United States and their counterparts in Canada, suggested that the name of the Association be changed to the National Veterinary Association of North America. A.W. Clement introduced a resolution calling instead for adoption of the name American Veterinary Medical Association, which was tabled that year. The following year, however, a recommendation to adopt the AVMA name was unanimously accepted.

The change from USVMA to AVMA reflected, at least in part, the fact that the Association had extended its scope beyond the United States to include Canada. In further recognition of this, six Canadians joined the AVMA the year after the name change, more than doubling the Canadian membership, and Fred Torrance of Winnipeg was elected vice president. Also, the 1903 AVMA Annual Meeting was held in Ottawa, Ontario, and John G. Rutherford, 1908-1909 AVMA president, was from Canada.

INCORPORATION

As early as 1869, discussions were held on the benefits of incorporating the new Association. A committee was appointed that year to study the advisability of petitioning Congress for a charter of incorporation. Three years later, the committee reported that on the basis of legal advice it had received, pursuing a charter would be inadvisable.

It appears that several important figures in the Association objected to incorporating it, but their specific reasons for doing so have largely been lost. One argument that was advanced was that incorporating the Association would allow individuals to sue it. Without incorporation, however, individual officers of the Association could be, and were, sued over matters for which they themselves were not responsible. In addition, without incorporation, another group could potentially assume the Association's name, depriving the original group of the right to use its own name.

The matter of incorporation was discussed again in 1893 but was again tabled. The following year, C.P. Lyman reported that an act of incorporation for the USVMA had

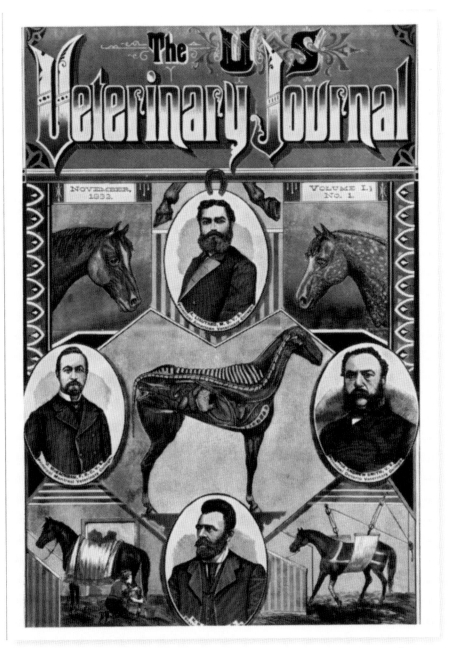

An early rival of the *American Veterinary Review,* the U.S. Veterinary Journal ceased publication after only two years.

been presented to Congress through Sen. Henry Cabot Lodge of Massachusetts, but the bill apparently died in committee.

The issue was apparently dropped after that until 1915, when the Executive Committee recommended that the Association pursue incorporation, with AVMA Secretary Nelson Mayo pointing out that establishment of a journal—which the Association had been without since 1881—required development of a definite business organization and that incorporation was needed to allow the Association to collect outstanding bills. The committee's recommendation was unanimously passed, and the Association was finally incorporated in 1917 under the laws of Illinois.

THE HOUSE OF DELEGATES

In 1882, a new journal, the United States Veterinary Journal, made its appearance. Although ostensibly edited by A.H. Baker, the co-founder of the Chicago Veterinary College, the real force behind the new journal apparently was T.E. Daniels, who had conceived the idea of organizing the veterinary profession in the United States, with his journal serving as the official organ.

Daniels' plan did have one strong point. His national association was to be governed by delegates chosen by the state veterinary medical associations, and Daniels had already been successful in getting state associations organized in Illinois, Indiana, Michigan, Missouri, New York (in competition with the existing state society), and Ohio. Daniels' plan did not come to fruition, however, and the United States Veterinary Journal ceased publication in 1884.

In 1897, F.H. Osgood discussed the undesirable aspects of electing the officers of the Association by a majority vote of those members present at the annual meeting, pointing out that members who wished to vote for the Association's officers had, in effect, to pay for the privilege, because of the costs associated with traveling to the convention and closing their practices while attending. Osgood suggested that voting rights be vested in delegates from the constituent associations, so that the will of the membership could not be subverted by members from the region where the meeting was held. Osgood's suggestion did not go forward at that time.

> "There really is no provision, legally, for a presiding officer, but, as I am in the habit of doing various and sundry odd jobs, I have taken it upon myself to call this meeting to order."
>
> – H. Preston Hoskins, AVMA secretary-editor, opening the inaugural meeting of the AVMA House of Representatives

Similarly, several changes in the structure and operation of the Association were discussed during the 50th anniversary meeting in 1913, including a recommendation for creation of a House of Delegates that would be the representative body of the constituent associations and would elect the officers of the Association. However, the recommendation was not adopted.

Nearly 20 years later, the AVMA Executive Board appointed a Special Committee on Affiliation of State and Provincial Associations with the AVMA to examine the relationship between the AVMA and the various state and provincial associations. During a meeting of the Executive Board in December 1930, the committee presented an outline of a plan for the board's consideration that included a recommendation to "Create a new body to be known as the 'House of Representatives' which shall transact the business of the Association heretofore transacted at the general business sessions, including receiving and acting upon recommendations of the Executive Board."

ing them. The presiding officer may direct the order in which communications shall be read.

CHAPTER 12. SPECIAL MEETINGS

At special meetings no other business, except such as shall have been specified in the requisition, and in the published call for the meeting, shall be transacted.

CHAPTER 13. ADMISSION OF MEMBERS

Article 1. When any Veterinary practitioner or Student of 3 years standing in the profession, applies for admission into this Association, the documents and testimonials relative to his professional qualifications shall be placed in the hands of the Secretary, who shall lay them before the Comitia Minora: whose duty it shall be to examine the same, and if they deem it expedient examine also the candidate and if they approve thereof, they shall grant him a certificate of fellowship.

Article 2. No person, immigrating from a foreign country, and claiming the right to practice Veterinary Medicine and Surgery shall be admitted a fellow of this Association by the Comitia Minora, unless he shall produce satisfactory testimonials of his professional qualifications.

Article 3. Every member shall sign the Constitution and the Bylaws.

Article 4. Every candidate, before signing the Bylaws and receiving his certificate of fellowship, shall be required by the Secretary to present the Treasurer's receipt for his initiation fee of Five Dollars, which shall be

appointed to the use of the Association; whereupon the Secretary shall present him with a copy of the Bylaws.

Article 5. No person shall be considered a member of this Association, until he has complied with the preceding article.

Article 6. Every member shall observe the code of medical ethics adopted by this Association and be answerable to the Comitia Minora, for breaches of the same.

Article 7. The following shall be the form of the Certificate of Fellowship

These are to certify that _____ is a fellow of the United States Veterinary Medical Association incorporated in the year of our Lord one thousand eight hundred and sixty three.

In testimony whereof, we have affixed our hands and the seal of the Association, this _____ day of _____ 18__

Censors   President   Secretary

CHAPTER 14. CONTRIBUTIONS AND ARREARS

Article 1. The Association, at the anniversary meeting, may assess such amount as shall meet the yearly expenses.

Article 2. The treasurer shall, from time to time, at the cost of the Association, collect the arrears of each member.

CHAPTER 15. HONORARY MEMBERS

Article 1. Any member may propose a candidate as an honorary member; the medical rank or station held by him shall be furnished in writing by the proposer, at or previous to the time of such proposal; the person so proposed shall be balloted for at a subsequent meeting. A majority of votes shall constitute him an honorary member.

Article 2. No more than three honorary members shall be elected annually.

Article 3. The honorary members may take part in debate but shall not be entitled to vote.

Article 4. The President of the United States, for the time being, shall be ex-officio, an honorary member.

The following shall be the form of diploma for honorary member:

This is to certify that we, the President, Vice-Presidents, and Fellows of the United States Veterinary Medical Association have received _____ as an honorary fellow of our Association and the said _____ is hereby authorized to claim and enjoy all the rights, privileges and honors belonging to the said fellowship.

In witness whereof, we have caused these presents to be signed by our President and Secretary and sealed by our common Seal, this day, _____ day of _____

President   Recording Secretary

Are we nine years too late?

Throughout the years, various authors have contended that the establishment of the United States Veterinary Medical Association in 1863 did not, in fact, represent the founding of a new organization and that the USVMA merely represented a reorganization of the American Veterinary Association, which had been founded in Philadelphia in 1854. This, of course, would mean that in 2013, the AVMA is actually 159, not 150, years old.

It is true that the American Veterinary Association was founded in Philadelphia on May 7, 1854, by Robert Jennings of New Jersey and Isaiah Michener of Pennsylvania. The newly formed association was quickly recognized by the Pennsylvania Society of Agriculture, an early sponsor of formal agricultural education in the country. During the society's September 1954 exhibition, the AVA was awarded a silver medal for its collection of anatomic and pathological specimens.

Most of the AVA's early members came from Pennsylvania, New Jersey, and Delaware. In 1859, Jennings and Michener began to consider how to expand the association beyond the boundaries of these three states, and during an April 1863 meeting of the AVA, plans were made to accomplish that goal. A resolution was passed that read: "Resolved, that the friends of veterinary science favorable to maintaining a national veterinary association for the advancement and diffusion of veterinary knowledge meet in convention in New York City, Tuesday, June 9, 1863, and be it further Resolved, that veterinary surgeons in all parts of the United States and all persons favorable to such an organization, be invited to attend the convention." The secretary was directed to invite practitioners from the adjacent states to the ninth annual meeting of the AVA at the Astor House in New York on June 9, 1863. One of the first pieces of business at this meeting was the reading of the minutes of the two previous meetings of the AVA.

It seems clear, however, that the original members of the USVMA themselves considered this to be a new organization. Jennings was chosen as the recording secretary for the organizational meeting of the USVMA, and in this capacity, he apparently entered the minutes of the two previous meetings of the AVA on the first pages of what would become the USVMA Minutes Book. Other members objected to this, and during the 1866 semiannual meeting of the USVMA, which Jennings apparently attended, it was moved and seconded "that some action be taken at the annual meeting, in regard to the late Secretary R. Jennings, he having introduced into the records, the minutes of two meetings, held in Philadelphia, dated March 1863, and prior to the existence of the USVMA…," according to J.F. Smithcors in his book "The American Veterinary Profession."

At the subsequent annual meeting, which Jennings did not attend, a committee was appointed to investigate the charges that Jennings had tampered with the Association's records. The committee "considered it a most unwarrantable act on the part of said R. Jennings, and in consequence thereof, they deem it but just to the members of this society, that he be expelled." It was further moved and carried "that the minutes inserted by R. Jennings be expunged from the records." Subsequently, the only record of those minutes was the following notation on the first two leaves of the USVMA Minutes Book: "Margin of leaves on which R. Jennings inserted minutes of meetings held in Philadelphia previous to the formation of the Association, and while acting as Secretary."

Jennings' expulsion was certainly not solely the result of his perceived mishandling of the minutes. He had a reputation as being a thorn in the side of the new Association and reportedly also was engaged in advertising and selling quack medicines. Nevertheless, his associates were not happy with how Jennings' expulsion was handled, and the situation likely added to the rift between the Philadelphia and New York members of the USVMA. How much of an effect this discord had on limiting the scope of the USVMA during those early years is not known, but it certainly tended to divide the loyalties of veterinarians in the Philadelphia area. For many years after its formation, the Keystone Veterinary Association, which met in Philadelphia, had a larger membership and greater meeting attendance than did the USVMA.

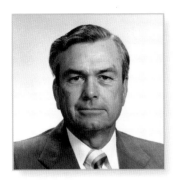

WILLIAM L. ANDERSON

1977–1978

Born and raised in Rockwall County, Texas, William Anderson received his veterinary degree from Texas A&M University in 1953. After a stint with the Air Force Veterinary Corps, he practiced in Rockwall County, and in 1958, co-founded a practice in the Dallas area. He served on the Texas Animal Health Commission from 1972-1976 and was considered a leader in programs for continuing education.

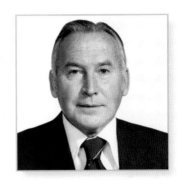

VERNON L. THARP

1978–1979

Following his graduation from The Ohio State University veterinary college in 1940, Vernon Tharp was a field veterinarian with the Bureau of Animal Industry. He returned to Ohio State in 1942 as an instructor in the Department of Veterinary Surgery and Clinics. He served as chair of the Department of Veterinary Medicine from 1961-1970, chair of the Department of Clinical Sciences from 1970-1971, and assistant dean of the college from 1972-1983. Dr. Tharp was formally honored by Ohio State in 1990 when the street in front of the veterinary hospital was named after him.

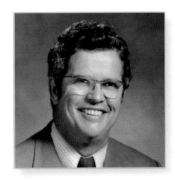

WILLIAM F. JACKSON

1979–1980

William Jackson received his veterinary degree from Michigan State University in 1947. He began his career at the University of Georgia but established a veterinary practice in Lakeland, Fla., in 1951. One of the founders of the American Board of Veterinary Practitioners, he was also a diplomate of the American College of Veterinary Surgeons and the American College of Veterinary Ophthalmologists. Dr. Jackson served as editor of the Journal of the American Animal Hospital Association from 1973-1981. In 1996, he was elected president of the World Small Animal Veterinary Association.

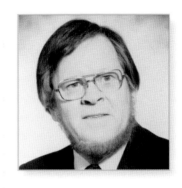

STANLEY M. ALDRICH

1980–1981

A 1950 veterinary graduate of Cornell University, Stanley Aldrich founded an animal hospital in West Babylon, N.Y., in 1951. For 10 years, he was a member of the New York State Board for Veterinary Medicine. In 1981, he was named New York State Veterinarian of the Year. He received the AVMA Award in 1983, and in 1991, was elected to the National Academies of Practice in recognition of his contributions to the veterinary profession.

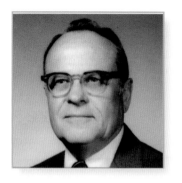

JACOB E. MOSIER

1981–1982

Jacob Mosier's career at Kansas State University spanned 47 years. After graduation, he joined the faculty of the KSU College of Veterinary Medicine as an instructor in the Department of Anatomy and the Department of Surgery and Medicine. He was an assistant professor at the University of Illinois–Urbana from 1949-1950, then returning to the KSU Department of Surgery and Medicine. Dr. Mosier served as head of the department from 1961-1981, and in 1985, became director of development for the college. He was a diplomate of the American College of Veterinary Internal Medicine.

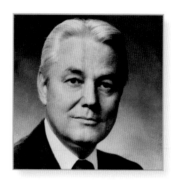

PAUL F. LANDIS

1982–1983

Paul Landis graduated from the University of Pennsylvania veterinary school in 1939 and worked in private small animal practice and for the Pennsylvania Bureau of Animal Industry before joining the Army Veterinary Corps in 1941. He established a private practice in Norfolk, Va., in 1946. As AVMA president, he focused on the challenge of government-subsidized veterinary services, the need to expand public relations, and support for the AVMA Political Action Committee. Dr. Landis played a crucial role in the creation of the Virginia-Maryland Regional College of Veterinary Medicine.

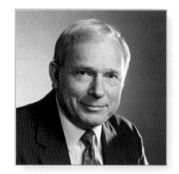

DUANE T. ALBRECHT

1983–1984

After graduating from the Iowa State University veterinary college in 1950 and interning at Angell Memorial Animal Hospital in Boston, Duane Albrecht took a position in small animal surgery at Iowa State. From 1952-1990, he was director of the Aspenwood Animal Hospital in Denver, the small animal practice he founded. In 1980, Dr. Albrecht was named Colorado's Veterinarian of the Year. He served for 10 years as secretary for the Colorado State Board of Veterinary Medicine.

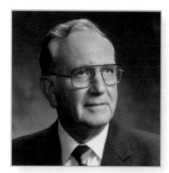

CHARLES R. RIGDON

1984–1985

A 1951 graduate of the University of Georgia, Charles Rigdon entered the Air Force Veterinary Corps after graduation. He served two years of military service, then began private practice in his hometown of Tifton, Ga. For 38 years, Dr. Rigdon owned DeKalb Animal Hospital, a small animal practice in Tucker, Ga., that he established in 1958. He served on the AVMA Executive Board from 1977-1983.

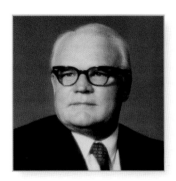

DELANO L. PROCTOR JR.

1985–1986

Delano Proctor received his veterinary degree from Cornell University in 1942 and served in the Army Remount Service from 1943-1946. In equine practice in Kentucky since 1946, Dr. Proctor was a diplomate of the American College of Veterinary Surgeons. He was elected president of the American Association of Equine Practitioners in 1969 and served on the AVMA Executive Board from 1979-1983.

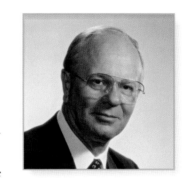

ALTON F. HOPKINS JR.

1986–1987

A Texas native, Alton Hopkins received his veterinary degree from Texas A&M University in 1956. After graduation, he spent five years in practice in Dallas and one year inspecting chicken farms for the Department of Agriculture, before establishing his own practice in Dallas in 1964. He served on the AVMA Executive Board from 1979-1985. One of Dr. Hopkins' proposals as AVMA president was to separate the "large animal practice" category of representation on several AVMA entities into categories for food animal practice and equine practice.

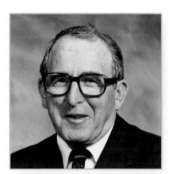

RICHARD B. FINK

1987–1988

From 1944-1946, Richard Fink was part of the Canine Corps in the Army Infantry. He received his veterinary degree from the University of Illinois in 1952 and practiced in the North Hollywood–Van Nuys area of California before establishing a practice in Whittier, Calif., in 1953. In 1988, Dr. Fink was knighted by the Royal Rosarians, ambassadors of good will from Portland, Ore., just before the second session of the House of Delegates held in conjunction with that year's AVMA meeting in Portland. He received the AVMA Award in 1995.

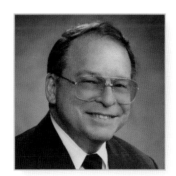

WALTER L. MARTIN JR.

1988–1989

After receiving his veterinary degree from Auburn University in 1953, Walter Martin entered small animal practice in Chattanooga, where he worked for the rest of his career. He served as AVMA treasurer from 1981-1987 and served in the AVMA House of Delegates from 1965-1973 and again from 1977-1980. He was one of the founders of the Animal Hospital Technology Program at Columbia State Community College in Tennessee, the first of its kind in the state.

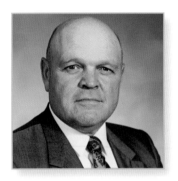

SAMUEL E. STRAHM

1989–1990

Immediately after graduating from the Kansas State University veterinary college in 1959, Samuel Strahm entered a mixed animal practice in Hominy and Pawhuska, Okla., where he worked for more than 30 years. He was chair of the National Board Examination Committee and president of the American Association of Veterinary State Boards, and he received the AVMA Award in 1985. In 1992, Dr. Strahm became chair of the AVMA Council on Governmental Affairs, which was instrumental in advancing the Association's legislative effort to legalize extralabel drug use in animals.

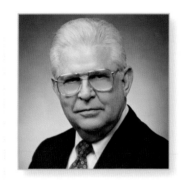

SHELTON PINKERTON

1990–1991

A 1954 graduate of Auburn University, Shelton Pinkerton practiced in Troy, Ala., before moving to Pensacola, Fla., in 1961. He served on the AVMA Executive Board from 1983-1989, and, in 1988, chaired the committee that selected the AVMA's first Congressional Science Fellow. In 1991, Dr. Pinkerton was elected vice president of the World Veterinary Association.

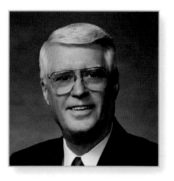

GERALD L. JOHNSON

1991–1992

After graduating from the University of Missouri-Columbia in 1956, Gerald Johnson practiced small animal medicine for 11 years in Independence, Mo. He then joined the professional services staff at Haver-Lockhart Laboratories, which later became Miles Inc., retiring in 1993. He was a member of the AVMA Executive Board from 1985-1988. On the board, he was a member of the task force that evolved into the Animal Agriculture Liaison Committee.

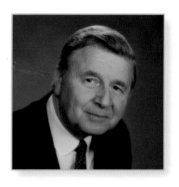

L. EVERETT MACOMBER

1992–1993

Born in Oakville, Wash., in 1937 and raised on a dairy farm, Everett Macomber received his veterinary degree in 1963 from Washington State University. Following graduation, he worked as a mixed animal practitioner in Centralia, Wash., for five years before restricting his practice to equine medicine. Dr. Macomber served in the AVMA House of Delegates from 1976-1984 and on the Executive Board from 1984-1990.

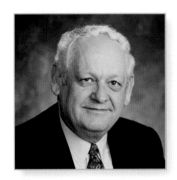

LEON H. RUSSELL

1993–1994

After receiving his veterinary degree from the University of Missouri-Columbia in 1956, Leon Russell received a master's degree in public health from Tulane University in 1958 and a doctorate from Texas A&M University in 1965. A diplomate of the American College of Veterinary Preventive Medicine, he has been a professor of veterinary public health, veterinary microbiology and immunology, and food science and technology at Texas A&M. He served on the AVMA Executive Board from 1985-1991. He was president of the World Veterinary Association from 2005-2008.

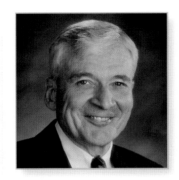

DAVID R. BARNETT

1994–1995

A native of Richland, Wash., David Barnett received his veterinary degree from Washington State University in 1957. After graduation, he worked in private practice in Salinas, Calif., for a year, and in 1959, he established a mixed animal practice in Colma, Calif. He served on the AVMA Executive Board from 1985-1991. Dr. Barnett was instrumental in the move to provide the Student AVMA a seat in the AVMA House of Delegates.

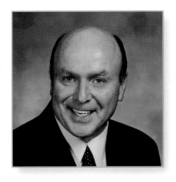

SHERBYN OSTRICH

1995–1996

A small animal practitioner, Sherbyn Ostrich received his veterinary degree from the University of Pennsylvania in 1963. During his presidency, Dr. Ostrich worked to implement new rules for funding of AVMA presidential campaigns and to change the process for selecting sites for the AVMA Annual Convention. He served on the AVMA Executive Board from 1987-1993, and, after completing his term as AVMA president, he accepted a position as executive director of the Pennsylvania Animal Health and Diagnostic Commission.

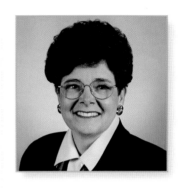

MARY BETH LEININGER

1996–1997

Mary Beth Leininger received her veterinary degree from Purdue University in 1967, and, for more than 25 years, co-owned Plymouth Veterinary Hospital in Plymouth, Mich. She was the first woman to serve as president of the AVMA. Following her term as president, Dr. Leininger worked as the director of professional affairs at Hill's Pet Nutrition for 10 years, then spent two years as project manager for the North American Veterinary Medical Education Consortium, a collaborative national initiative to improve veterinary education.

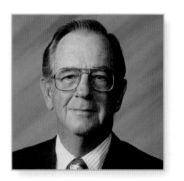

JOHN I. FREEMAN

1997–1998

Before his retirement in 1996, Dr. Freeman was thoroughly involved in public veterinary medicine, working as chief of the Environmental Epidemiology Section of the North Carolina Department of Environment, Health, and Natural Resources, and heading the Veterinary Public Health Branch of the Division of Epidemiology in the department for 16 years. He also served as an Epidemic Intelligence Service officer for the U.S. Public Health Service. Dr. Freeman received his veterinary degree from Oklahoma State University in 1964 and was a member of the AVMA Executive Board from 1989-1995.

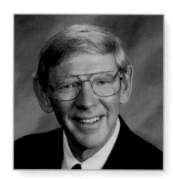

RICHARD C. SWANSON

1998–1999

Richard Swanson received his veterinary degree from Colorado State University in 1960. He originally entered private practice in the Denver area, but, in 1963, left to establish a general practice in Longmont, Colo., where he worked for the next 15 years. After a short stint as a food animal ambulatory clinician at Colorado State, Dr. Swanson opened a large animal practice in Longmont in 1989. He was a member of the AVMA Executive Board from 1988-1994.

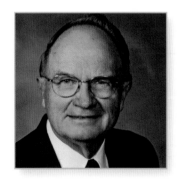

LEONARD F. SEDA

1999–2000

A food animal and companion animal practitioner, Leonard Seda received his veterinary degree from Iowa State University in 1956. After working in Hudson, Iowa, for a short time, he moved to Victor, Iowa, where he worked for the next 40 years. He served on the AVMA Executive Board from 1990-1996. In 2000, the AVMA Executive Board approved Dr. Seda's proposal to restructure the board districts to better reflect the distribution of the U.S. veterinary population, sending the plan to the AVMA House of Delegates for approval.

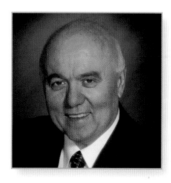

JAMES E. NAVE

2000–2001

Following his graduation from the University of Missouri-Columbia in 1968, James Nave served in the Army. After returning to civilian life, he moved to Las Vegas, where he opened multiple veterinary hospitals. During his presidency, Dr. Nave helped to create a mentoring program and worked to establish new AVMA Executive Board districts. He served on the Executive Board from 1991-1997 and co-founded the National Commission on Veterinary Economic Issues in 2000, serving as its first chair from 2000-2007. He also served as the AVMA director of international veterinary affairs and as North American councilor to the World Veterinary Association.

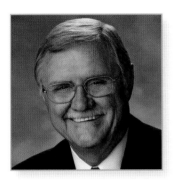

JAMES H. BRANDT

2001–2002

After graduating from Oklahoma State University veterinary college in 1964, James Brandt worked in small animal practice in Nokomis and Venice, Fla., from 1965-1997. He was elected AVMA president after serving 10 years in the House of Delegates. Dr. Brandt chaired the Architectural Design Committee that oversaw the redesign of the entrance, lobby area, and surrounding landscaping for the AVMA headquarters building in Schaumburg, Ill.

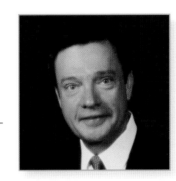

JOE M. HOWELL

2002–2003

A 1972 graduate of the Oklahoma State University veterinary college, Joe Howell grew up in rural Oklahoma and practiced veterinary medicine in Oklahoma City for his entire veterinary career. A part owner of Britton Road Veterinary Clinic, a small animal practice in Oklahoma City, he also owned an investment company. Before being elected to the AVMA presidency, Dr. Howell served on the Executive Board from 1997-2000.

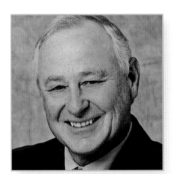

JACK O. WALTHER

2003–2004

Jack Walther was born and raised on a small ranch near Reno, Nev., and, after receiving his veterinary degree from the University of California-Davis in 1963, he returned to Reno to open an equine practice. He spent two years in the Army Veterinary Corps and the next 35 practicing small animal medicine, building three hospitals in the Reno area. Dr. Walther also served as an adjunct professor of veterinary medicine at the University of Nevada at Reno, where he helped to establish the preveterinary program there.

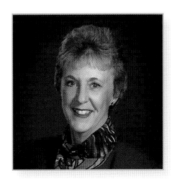

BONNIE V. BEAVER

2004–2005

Bonnie Beaver received her veterinary degree from the University of Minnesota in 1968 and has been involved in organized veterinary medicine her entire career. She was only the second woman to serve as AVMA president. A professor in the Department of Small Animal Medicine and Surgery at Texas A&M University, she was also a charter member of the American College of Veterinary Behaviorists. Dr. Beaver served on the AVMA Executive Board from 1997-2003. Establishing an Animal Welfare Division at the AVMA was a centerpiece of Dr. Beaver's presidency.

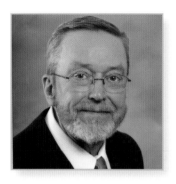

HENRY E. CHILDERS

2005–2006

A 1954 graduate of the Auburn University School of Veterinary Medicine, Henry Childers became owner and manager of a small animal practice in Cranston, R.I., in 1957. A diplomate of the American Board of Veterinary Practitioners, he also has taught at the Tufts University Cummings School of Veterinary Medicine. Dr. Childers served on the AVMA Executive Board from 1998-2004.

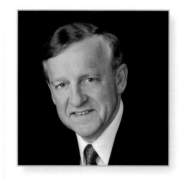

ROGER K. MAHR

2006–2007

Roger Mahr owned and operated a small animal practice in Geneva, Ill., for 31 years after receiving his veterinary degree in 1971 from Iowa State University. He was elected to the AVMA Executive Board in 1999, serving six years. As AVMA president, Dr. Mahr made the recommendation that led to the establishment of the One Health Initiative Task Force. This eventually led to the formation of the One Health Commission, which focuses on the connections between human, animal, and environmental health.

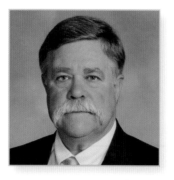

GREGORY S. HAMMER

2007–2008

After receiving his veterinary degree from Kansas State University in 1973, Gregory Hammer served two years as a veterinary medical officer in the Air Force before becoming a small animal–equine practitioner, eventually establishing Brenford Animal Hospital in Dover, Del. Dr. Hammer served in the AVMA House of Delegates from 1986-1999 and served on the Executive Board from 1999-2005.

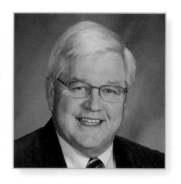

JAMES O. COOK

2008–2009

Shortly after earning his veterinary degree from Auburn University in 1976, James Cook started a mixed animal practice in Lebanon, Ky. Dr. Cook was a member of the AVMA House of Delegates from 1996-2001, when he was elected to the Executive Board, serving from 2001-2007. Dr. Cook was honored as Kentucky Veterinarian of the Year in 1988.

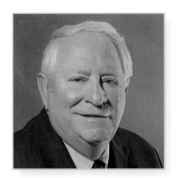

LARRY R. CORRY

2009–2010

Larry Corry received his veterinary degree from the University of Georgia in 1966, served two years in the Air Force Veterinary Corps, and then entered private practice, eventually becoming the owner of two small animal practices. He served on the AVMA Executive Board from 2002-2008 before being selected as AVMA president.

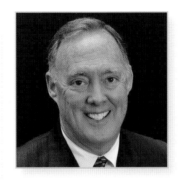

LARRY M. KORNEGAY

2010–2011

After graduating from the Texas A&M University College of Veterinary Medicine & Biomedical Sciences in 1971, Larry Kornegay went into companion animal practice in Houston. In 2003, he was elected to the AVMA Executive Board, serving for six years prior to his election as AVMA president. He has been active in organized veterinary medicine at the local, state, and national levels throughout his career, and has had a particular interest in increasing diversity in the veterinary profession.

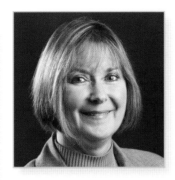

RENÉ A. CARLSON

2011–2012

A 1978 graduate of the University of Minnesota College of Veterinary Medicine, René Carlson served two terms as AVMA vice president (2004–2006) before her election as AVMA president. She was only the third woman to serve as AVMA president. She also served on the AVMA Council on Education. Dr. Carlson has been in small animal practice since graduation, opening the Animal Hospital of Chetek in 1996.

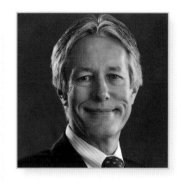

DOUGLAS G. ASPROS

2012–2013

Douglas Aspros has been a companion animal veterinarian and practice owner ever since his 1975 graduation from the Cornell University College of Veterinary Medicine. In 2006, Dr. Aspros was elected to the AVMA Executive Board. He has also served on the AVMA Council on Education, and, for five years, was director of the National Board of Veterinary Medical Examiners. Dr. Aspros also initiated the New York State Veterinary Medical Society's Leaders 2000, a program to engage and mentor young professionals to take on leadership roles in organized veterinary medicine.

Making it all work

Nick DeLuca

To keep up with the demands of its growing membership, the American Veterinary Medical Association—on suggestion from then AVMA President Robert A. Archibald—first began searching for a permanent home in 1916. Four years later, during the 1920 meeting in Columbus, Ohio, AVMA President Charles Cary, remarking on the fact that the Association had had three editors and four secretaries since 1915, declared that "In addition to an all-time Secretary and Editor, we need an all-time home for this double head and heart of the organization" to provide a sense of stability and definitiveness of purpose. The idea of a permanent location for the Association was approved, and the Executive Board was directed to investigate potential locations and costs.

In 1922, Dr. Horace Preston Hoskins, son of former United States Veterinary Medical Association President William Horace Hoskins, was appointed to the position of executive secretary/editor, becoming the first full-time staff member of the Association.

Shortly thereafter, the AVMA officially established its first headquarters when it leased office space in Detroit in the early part of 1923. Since moving into that first office, the AVMA headquarters has been relocated on five occasions—to three leased locations in Chicago and two AVMA-owned buildings in Schaumburg, Ill. In 2004, the AVMA also purchased a building in Washington, D.C., rather than continue renting space for the staff who work on Capitol Hill.

In mid-2012, the Association had 149 approved staff positions spread across 12 distinctive divisions—Office of the Executive Vice President, Animal Welfare, Communications, Convention and Meeting Planning, Education and Research, Finance and Business Services, Governmental Relations, Information Technology, Membership and Field Services, Publications, Scientific Activities, and Veterinary Economics—located at its offices in Schaumburg and Washington, D.C.

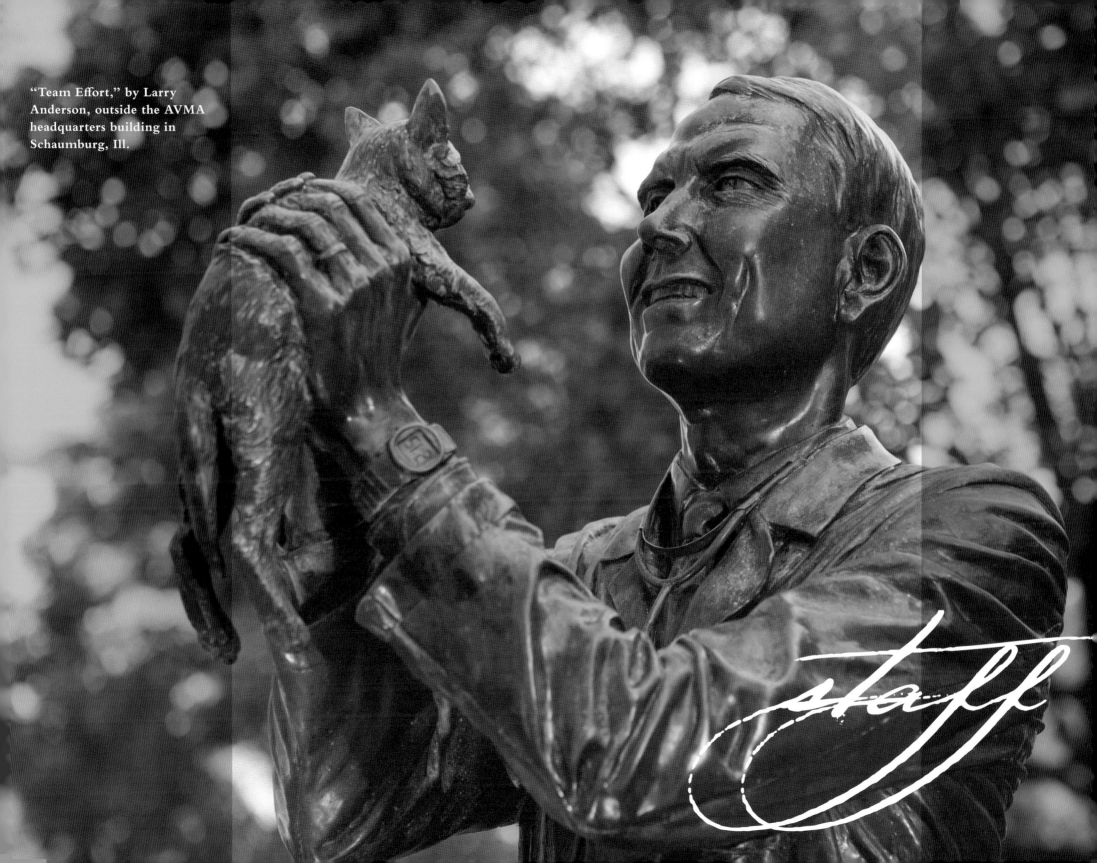

"Team Effort," by Larry Anderson, outside the AVMA headquarters building in Schaumburg, Ill.

staff

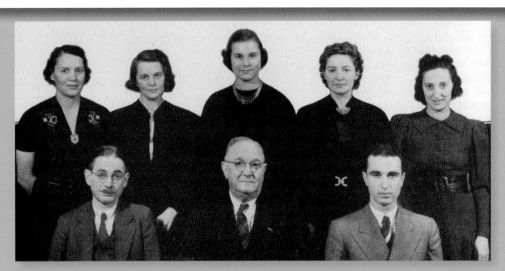

Staff of the 1939 AVMA Secretariat. Front row, left to right: Dr. H. Preston Hoskins, Dr. L.A. Merillat, Julius Shaffer; Back row, left to right: Ruth Anderson, Cecil Harris, Adele Ray, Wanda Landwehr, Jean Weinert

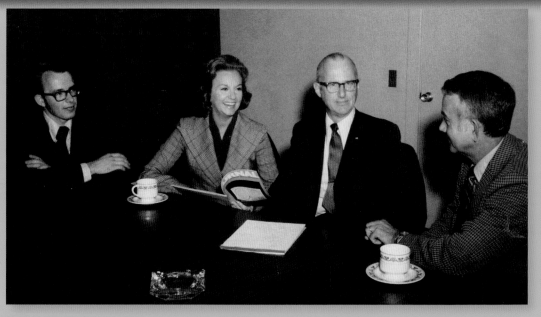

AVMA staff members Karl Kessler of the Public Information Division, Dr. D.A. Price, executive vice president; and Dr. W.M. Decker, assistant executive vice president, meet with actress Carmelita Pope.

THE DIVISIONS

OFFICE OF THE EXECUTIVE VICE PRESIDENT

The Office of the Executive Vice President provides administrative oversight for all divisions of the AVMA and is primary staff support to the Executive Board, Board of Governors, House of Delegates, House Advisory Committee, Judicial Council, Governance Performance Review Committee, and various task forces. The office also manages human resources, corporate relations, legal review, international affairs, and the Association staff.

ANIMAL WELFARE DIVISION

The Animal Welfare Division is charged with monitoring the science of human-animal interactions and assisting the AVMA in proactively addressing issues related to animal welfare and the human-animal bond. These issues come into play when animals are used for companionship, biomedical research, education, food and fiber production, work, recreation, and exhibition. The division interacts with a variety of stakeholders— including governmental and nongovernmental organizations (veterinary and nonveterinary), educators, industries that use or provide services for animals, the public, and the media.

Some of the division's main areas of concentration are strategic planning, with a focus on meeting the Association's animal welfare goals; environmental scanning and issue

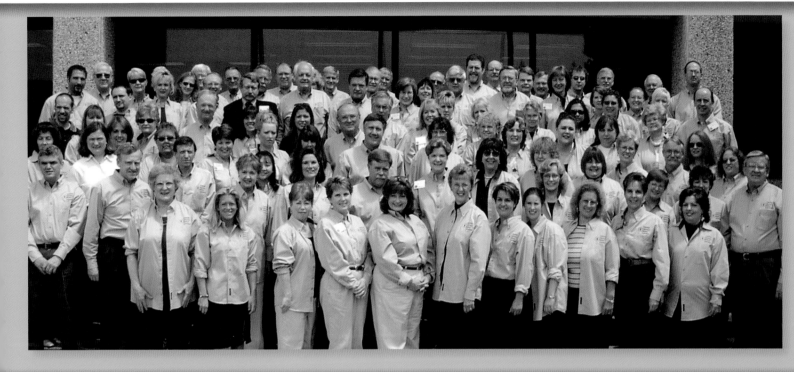

AVMA staff members pose outside of the Schaumburg, Ill., headquarters building in spring 2002.

identification; authoritative source development, including background information as well as documents setting industry guidelines and standards; scientific and regulatory review and advocacy regarding issue support on the local, state, and federal levels; interactions with foreign entities to help with development and implementation of international standards; and education for veterinary students, graduate veterinarians, veterinary staff, individuals in the animal-use industries, and the public.

ton, D.C. As a result, the division works closely with all other AVMA divisions, along with AVMA councils and committees, allied organizations, and sponsors, to help them develop and implement effective member service, marketing, and communications initiatives. The division oversees the creation and distribution of more than 20 websites, newsletters, and publications and has been at the forefront of the social networking movement within the veterinary community.

COMMUNICATIONS DIVISION

The Communications Division comprises six departments: Media Relations; State Legislative and Regulatory Affairs; Electronic Communications; Marketing; Professional and Public Affairs; and Public Affairs at the Governmental Relations office in Washing-

CONVENTION AND MEETING PLANNING DIVISION

The Convention and Meeting Planning Division is responsible for the planning and implementation of the AVMA Annual Convention, the annual AVMA Veterinary

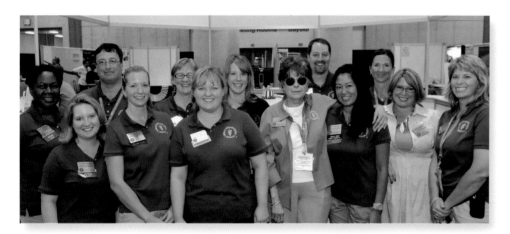

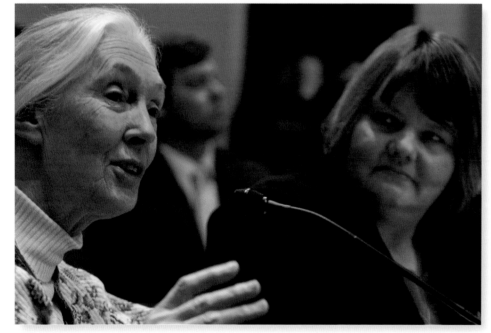

Top: AVMA staff take a break at the 2012 AVMA Annual Convention in San Diego. Bottom: Dr. Gail Golab (right), director of the AVMA Animal Welfare Division, listens to primatologist Jane Goodall speak on Capitol Hill before giving her own testimony on March 11, 2008, in support of the Captive Primate Safety Act.

Leadership Conference, and the meetings taking place in the AVMA headquarters conference center.

In regard to the AVMA Annual Convention educational program, the division works in tandem with the Convention Management and Program Committee to plan the opening session, more than 900 educational sessions, and a host of interactive labs. The division also plans and implements activities for the exhibit hall, convention registration and housing, and social and sporting events.

Additionally, the division manages the logistics for House of Delegates and Executive Board business meetings, luncheons, receptions, and other functions held immediately prior to the convention. The division acts as the liaison to the CMPC, the Veterinary Leadership Conference Planning Committee, and the Institutional Animal Care and Use Committee, which ensures that animals used on-site at the convention receive proper care and that safety regulations are met. The division supports those committees in planning the content of their respective meetings in an effort to meet the needs and expectations of members and attendees as well as to maintain the proper care and safety of animals used during the AVMA convention.

The division has overseen a tremendous growth in the AVMA Annual Convention, with overall attendance numbers for recent meetings exceeding 10,000.

EDUCATION AND RESEARCH DIVISION

The Education and Research Division provides staff support for two AVMA councils, seven committees, one task force, and two international working groups. These entities are responsible for accrediting veterinary colleges and veterinary technology programs, certifying the educational equivalence of foreign veterinary graduates, providing oversight for U.S. veterinary specialty organizations, and working collaboratively with international veterinary accrediting agencies and international veterinary specialty recognition entities. These entities are also responsible for developing policies on animal health research, advising the AVMA Executive Board on international veterinary affairs, working on issues of mutual concern with the Association of American Veterinary Medical Colleges and the National Association of Veterinary Technicians in

America, assessing AVMA Council on Education candidate qualifications, and developing a quality assurance plan for veterinary internships.

FINANCE AND BUSINESS SERVICES DIVISION

The Finance and Business Services Division is responsible for all the financial and accounting functions of the Association. In addition, the division provides financial support and accounting functions for the American Veterinary Medical Foundation. The division also oversees the operation of all investments and the Association's mailroom, negotiates and secures liabilities and other forms of Association insurance, and acquires equipment, furniture, and supplies. The division is also charged with overseeing the management and maintenance of the Schaumburg, Ill., headquarters and Washington, D.C., office.

GOVERNMENTAL RELATIONS DIVISION

Brig. Gen. James A. McCallam established the Association's first Washington, D.C., office in March 1953. Brig. Gen. McCallam performed double duty by serving as the first administrator for the Association's capital office while toiling on the Executive Board as president-elect. A telephone answering service was used to receive messages for the general when he was away from the Washington office dealing with other Association business.

The GRD advocates for the Association's policies and positions on federal legislative and regulatory issues that influence animal and human health and advance the veterinary profession. The GRD director and assistant directors are registered lobbyists who conduct visits to congressional members and their staff as needed to advance the AVMA's legislative agenda. The GRD provides staff support to the AVMA Political Action Committee Policy Board and the Legislative Advisory Committee as well as consultative support to other committees, councils, and task forces as requested.

The AVMA is an active member of several coalitions the GRD works with—the Agriculture Coalition, Small Business Coalition for Affordable Healthcare, and Pet Health Consortium—developed to allow small organizations to have a stronger, unified political voice while working collectively for or against legislation and regulations. In the GRD's grassroots network—the AVMA Congressional Advocacy Network—AVMA members serve as local links to veterinary medicine and the veterinary profession for legislators.

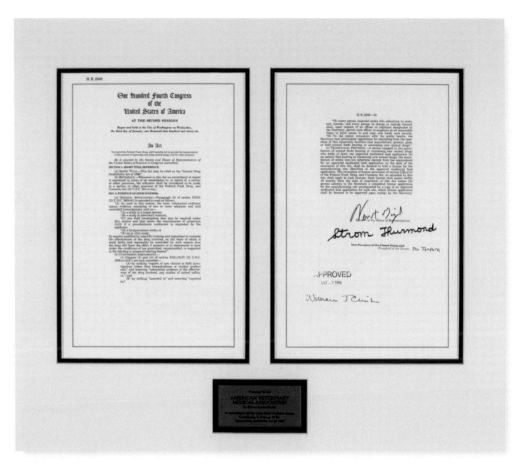

A copy of the 1996 Animal Drug Availability Act

The GRD also administers the AVMA Fellowship Program and the AVMA GRD Veterinary Student Externship Program.

INFORMATION TECHNOLOGY DIVISION

The role of the Information Technology Division is to provide the personnel and resources to actively support the daily operations of the AVMA headquarters and Washington, D.C., offices to ensure an efficient, stable, and secure infrastructure.

The division has a strong commitment to moving the organization forward with ongoing development projects involving new applications and new technologies. Members of the division continuously work to better understand the business needs of staff to help ensure that goals and objectives are met.

The IT staff manage the AVMA network—consisting of file storage, sharing servers, program servers, user rights, and email use. The division maintains network security, support for meeting technology needs, and oversight and support of communication devices.

The IT staff develops documentation, procedures, and guidelines for the use of software applications and trains staff in the use of hardware, desktop software, phones, and voice mail systems. The division also oversees the planning and coordination of activities relating to AVMA informational databases to ensure integrity of the data.

MEMBERSHIP AND FIELD SERVICES DIVISION

The AVMA Membership and Field Services Division has four core areas of responsibility for the AVMA: membership operations, veterinary career services, student programs, and the online resource MyVeterinarian.com, which enables animal owners to search for veterinary practices. The division has also developed a staff position and committee that focus on recent-graduate initiatives for the AVMA.

Membership operations include the collection of annual dues, efforts to retain current members, and recruitment of new members as well as management of the online membership directory, collection of member data, and providing of assistance for member concerns.

Career services include the online Veterinary Career Center, the AVMA Student Externship Locator, the Veterinary Practice Resource Center, and the Working Diagnosis. The division coordinates partnerships with 30 state veterinary medical associations, seven national associations, and 27 veterinary and technician schools to form the Veterinary Career Network. Membership staff are also available to answer career-related questions.

Student programs include visiting veterinary campuses on a yearly basis, working directly with the AVMA vice president to provide direct support to the Student AVMA and the 29 student chapters of the AVMA (32 student programs in all), and coordinating student externships, scholarships, and an annual meeting with faculty advisers and student officers.

PUBLICATIONS DIVISION

The Publications Division is the Association's most heavily staffed division. It may also lay claim to the title of oldest division, in that the earliest Association staff members were hired as both executive secretary for the Association and editor of its Journal.

The division has grown from that single editor position into a staff of 32. The purpose of the division is to publish peer-reviewed research of importance to the veterinary and biomedical professions, provide news and information relevant to veterinarians across all practice sectors, and inform veterinarians and the public as to the role of organized veterinary medicine in advancing the profession and promoting animal and human health and well-being.

The division looks to fulfill its mission by publishing the world's two most revered scientific veterinary journals—the *Journal of the American Veterinary Medical Association* and the *American Journal of Veterinary Research*—in both print and online formats. The *JAVMA* has been published since 1877 (originally as the *American Veterinary Review*) and is the oldest continuously published veterinary journal in the world. The *AJVR* has been published continuously since 1940; its focus is applied biomedical research with

As the years passed by, Dr. Liautard gradually tempered his role of good-natured gadfly, and in 1896 he sold an interest in the Review to Dr. Roscoe R. Bell. Then, as the calendar turned over to the 20th century, Dr. Liautard severed his financial interest in the Review and returned to France. Although Dr. Liautard retained the title of senior editor and still contributed periodically to the Review, Dr. Bell became in effect the sole editor and proprietor. Drs. Merillat and Campbell state of Dr. Bell's junior editorship that "there was an immediate improvement in the publication. He supplied a technique and finesse that the senior editor did not possess."

Nonetheless, over the next decade and a half, the fortunes of the Review would gradually dwindle. Although the quality of the Review steadily improved under Dr. Bell's stewardship, he died in 1908, at which time Dr. R.W. Ellis, an associate editor of the Journal, purchased the remaining interest for $2,500. It appears that Dr. Ellis was a perfectly able editor of the Review (although still a junior editor in title under Dr. Liautard), but, even so, was unable to turn around the financial decline of the Journal, which Drs. Merillat and Campbell describe at this time as "moribund." Without the generous support of veterinary book publishers and colleges, the Review "would have failed as so many American veterinary publications have done." Finally, in 1915, the AVMA purchased the rights to the Journal— for the same $2,500 that Dr. Ellis had paid for it seven years earlier.

THE REVIEW BECOMES THE JAVMA

In 1914, the AVMA Executive Committee resolved "to take such measures as may be necessary to establish an official organ of the association to be known as the *Journal of the American Veterinary Medical Association*." Hence came the purchase the next year of the rights to the *American Veterinary Review* and the changing of its name to something more familiar to today's readers.

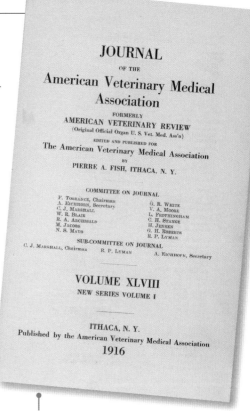

First page of the first issue of the *Journal of the American Veterinary Medical Association*

In 1996, work from the International Exhibition on Animals in Art began appearing on the cover of the *JAVMA*.

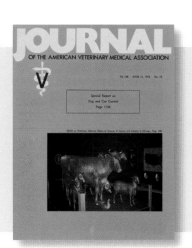 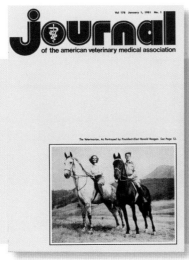 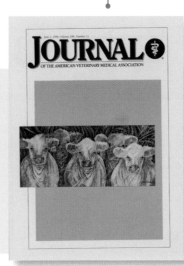 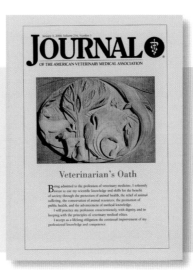 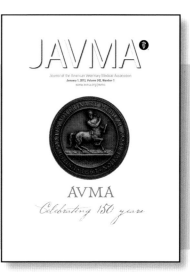

In those early years with its new name, however, the Journal lacked the clear direction it had benefited from in previous incarnations. This is apparent from the way the Journal was used at the time, according to Drs. Merillat and Campbell: "[The *JAVMA*] was little more than an installment publication of the proceedings of the AVMA, in lieu of the annual bound volumes."

It should be noted that one of the main reasons the Journal had been acquired was indeed for it to serve as a repository for the proceedings of the meetings, and, in fact, the early volumes of the *JAVMA* did contain considerably more scientific reports and other pertinent material than did the Review in its declining years. But, clearly, there was a common sentiment that the Journal was not being used to its greatest potential.

Maybe the rotating editorship had something to do with that. Initially, in 1915, Dr. Pierre A. Fish was appointed editor, but in 1918, he left the Journal to enter military service. Dr. William H. Dalrymple succeeded Dr. Fish, then promptly relinquished the post because of failing health, and Dr. John R. Mohler took over the position in 1919. In 1920, President C.A. Cary put it thus: "Our frequent and sudden changes of Secretary and Editor have given us no stability or definitiveness of purpose." Then, in 1923, the offices of secretary and editor were combined, and Dr. H. Preston Hoskins was tabbed to fill the position. He did so until 1939, finally bringing some stability to the helm of the Journal.

The *JAVMA* then entered a lengthy period of growth and innovation. The Journal published its first full-color figure in 1928. In the ensuing years, the Journal's circulation broke into the tens of thousands, and a sister journal, the *AJVR*, was introduced in part to deal with the enormous number of technical articles being submitted for publication.

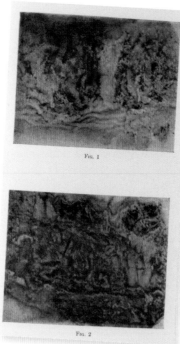

The first full-color images in the *JAVMA* were published in the April 1928 issue.

In 1956, after a two-year study by the AVMA of the benefits of publishing a separate journal devoted to small animal medicine, a decision was made to publish the *JAVMA* semimonthly—on the first and 15th of each month—instead of monthly. The objects were to make each issue of the *JAVMA* less bulky; decrease the lead time between receipt and publication of articles, thereby making the information fresher; and ideally result in the Journal's being read more completely, as subscribers would receive and peruse it twice a month instead of only once.

The *JAVMA* introduced new departments and regular features over the years, and it appeared in new designs and more sophisticated formats. In short, the Journal adapted continually to the needs of its readers, much as its subscribers adapted continually to the demands of the veterinary medical field.

CONTINUED GROWTH

The 1970s saw the *JAVMA* increase the size of its staff and streamline its in-house processes to allow it to better deal with the submissions queue. The number of manuscripts submitted to *JAVMA* and *AJVR* more than doubled between the years of 1970 and 1984. This wealth of submissions, although a great sign for the health of the profession and the Association, also presented some problems. Some were more straightforward, such as the issue of how to simply organize and review each manuscript that came into the Publications Division. Others were more subtle, such as how to present the remarkable and complex range of information the AVMA journals were publishing in a way that was clear and sensible to readers.

It was in response to this latter problem that, in the 1980s, the *JAVMA* staff, led by the editor-in-chief, Dr. Albert J. Koltveit, rearranged the Journal's table of contents into a more practical format that included the sections titled News, Views, Veterinary Medicine Today, and Scientific Reports. They also reorganized the Scientific Reports so that papers would be grouped according to the animal type discussed in each paper. Organizing the Journal along these lines proved quite effective over the years, and the system is still in use today.

THE ELECTRONIC AGE

The 1990s saw the rise of the Internet and a readership that became increasingly comfortable using the World Wide Web to search for and consume information. Under the guidance of the editor-in-chief, Dr. Janis H. Audin, the *JAVMA* and *AJVR* transitioned from print-only journals, adding an online archive of all articles published from January 2000 on.

Another major development during this time was the consolidation within AVMA headquarters of most of the publishing operations. Although the Journals were still printed off-site, the adoption of desktop publishing technology during the 1990s allowed the Journals to transition from traditional typesetting into more modern production processes. Bringing production in-house was key to reducing costs and gave the staff greater control over the final look of the Journals by allowing changes to be made later in the production process.

COVER ART

One of the most striking features of the *JAVMA* is the animal art gracing the cover of each issue. The practice of publishing full-color reproductions of artwork on the cover was quite unusual among scholarly journals in 1973, when the *JAVMA* editor-in-chief, Dr. Arthur Freeman, began the tradition. In the beginning, paintings drawn from the collections of museums and galleries around the world appeared on covers of the first-of-the-month issues, while covers for the midmonth issues merely featured titles of some of the scientific reports in that issue.

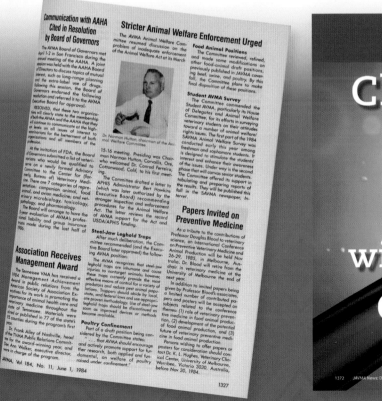
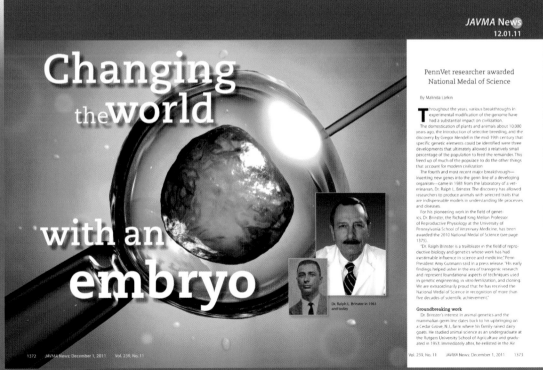

The News section of the *JAVMA* has grown to become more visually appealing.

This changed in 1990, when Dr. Koltveit, now editor-in-chief, suggested that the Journal also publish artwork on the covers of the midmonth issues. In 1990, therefore, the Publications Division announced that it would be accepting original artwork from the veterinary community for potential publication on the midmonth covers. Submissions would be accepted from nonprofessional artists, especially veterinarians, members of their family or staff, veterinary educators, and veterinary students. When the April 15, 1990, issue came out with a reproduction of "Anatone Cowboy" by Dr. David T. Roen of Clarkton, Wash., a new tradition was born.

A driving force in the popularity of the *JAVMA* covers was the decision to assign Dr. Audin, who had an art background, responsibility for selecting each issue's cover art. At that time, Dr. Audin made an effort to choose artwork that highlighted one or more animal species featured in notable news or scientific articles within that issue.

In addition to her work on the *JAVMA* cover, Dr. Audin was later responsible for bringing to the *AJVR* a new cover design that incorporated some of the more striking figures from previously published scientific reports.

In 1995, the *JAVMA* began inviting readers to contact the AVMA about the availability of artwork featured on the cover. From that point on, without exception, the AVMA has fielded calls from interested readers about every single piece of cover artwork, whether it was by a world-famous artist or by a hobbyist artist associated with the veterinary profession.

FEATURES

In addition to the scientific and clinical reports that compose the bulk of the *JAVMA*'s scholarship, the editors over the years have frequently introduced recurring features that strike a different note from the usual content.

Many of these, such as the "Anesthesia Case of the Month" and "Theriogenology Question of the Month" features, were designed to examine a single case or small series of cases through the lens of a specific method or a specific area of veterinary medicine. Others existed simply to inform and entertain, as was the case with the "Reflections" series that Dr. Koltveit ran for years and the "From My Armchair" vignettes from

From My Armchair: W. W. Armistead

Philosophy of Professional Education

Poet Robert Frost is said to have defined a college education as "hanging around until you catch on." That may apply to some college courses, but it is not descriptive of education in the professions—and it certainly does not describe education in veterinary medicine.

Most students—and, unfortunately, some teachers—believe that facts are the only legitimate contents of a science course and that if you hang around until you have memorized most of the facts, you will be educated on the subject. It is a dangerous idea. There is much more to be learned from science education than just science facts. One should learn also to interpret observations, draw inferences, and apply knowledge for problem solving.

Much of the information students memorize to pass college courses becomes obsolete soon after graduation. What we hope will survive, beyond fundamental understanding, are curiosity, habits of continued study, fa... ...ductive reasoning and the ability to translate assorted fa...

There is no room in any of the n... ...dents. And there certainly is no time...

Top: Former AVMA President W.W. Armistead's "From My Armchair" feature
Right: From the December 1954 *JAVMA*, the debut of "What Is Your Diagnosis?"

former AVMA President Dr. W.W. Armistead. Still other features served to augment readers' knowledge of the profession rather than the science of veterinary medicine. This included Harold W. Hannah's popular "Legal Brief" series, which offered valuable commentary on veterinary law, and the "Facts & Figures," which reported results of the AVMA's economic surveys.

Without a doubt, the most iconic *JAVMA* feature remains the "What Is Your Diagnosis?" series. In in-

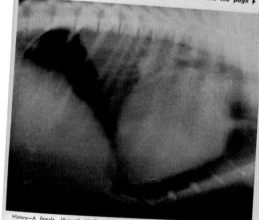

What Is Your Diagnosis ?
Radiograph Offered for Your Study and Diagnosis

Because of the interest in veterinary radiology, the JOURNAL publishes this month, and will continue to do so for the next several issues, a case history and accompanying radiographs depicting a diagnostic problem.

Our readers are invited to submit case histories, radiographs, and diagnoses of interesting cases which are suitable for publication.

Make your diagnosis from the picture below — then turn the page ▶

History—A female, 10-month-old German Shepherd (mixed) had been in excellent health and had developed normally. It had been wormed and vaccinated against distemper. The dog was well until four days before admission when it was believed it developed a cold. At the time of admission, the owner reported finding the dog sitting in a lane a short distance from the house in great respiratory distress suggestive of a diaphragmatic hernia. The owner denied any possibility of the dog having been hit by an automobile or injured in any way. No abrasions or superficial lesions could be found. The dog died three hours after admission.

(Diagnosis and findings are reported on next page)

(465)

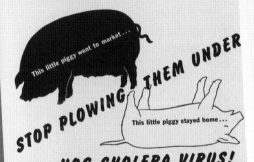
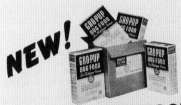

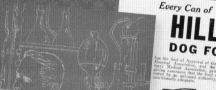

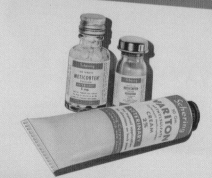
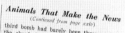
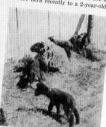
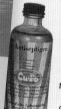
124

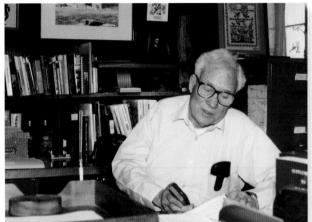

Harold W. Hannah, author of the long-running "Legal Briefs" feature

troducing the feature for the December 1954 issue, the editor-in-chief, Dr. William A. Aitken, wrote, "Because of the interest in veterinary radiology, the JOURNAL publishes this month, and will continue to do so for the next several issues, a case history and accompanying radiographs depicting a diagnostic problem."

The feature invites readers to study the diagnostic images and case history on the first page, make their own diagnosis, and then turn the page to see the outcome of the case as well as a discussion of how the imaging technique was useful in obtaining the diagnosis. Despite Dr. Aitken's initial suggestion that these articles would run for only several issues, the feature remains the JAVMA's most popular even today, almost 60 years after its debut.

AMERICAN JOURNAL OF VETERINARY RESEARCH

In 1940, the editorial staff of the *JAVMA*, realizing that many well-written articles were suffering severe delays in publication or were being rejected outright simply because of a lack of space in the Journal, recommended to the Executive Board and House of Representatives that the AVMA undertake publication of a second journal. The recommendation was approved during the AVMA's annual meeting that year, and accumulated articles that had previously been accepted for publication in the *JAVMA* were published in the first issue of the new journal, which was named the *American Journal of Veterinary Research*.

In an editorial in the first issue of the new journal, Dr. Louis A. Merillat, who, in addition to his role as executive secretary of the AVMA and editor-in-chief of the *JAVMA*, took on the job of editor for the *AJVR*, wrote that the object of the *AJVR* would be "the prompt publication of deserving articles on research and investigation by American veterinarians and their coworkers in the field of veterinary science." In addition, it was expected that publication of the *AJVR* "should gradually transmute the regular JOURNAL into a more useful monthly for members interested in clinical work and yet concurrently provide them with a means of keeping abreast with current advancements in veterinary science."

AJVR covers
through the years

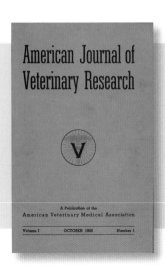

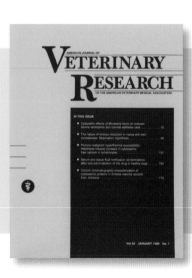

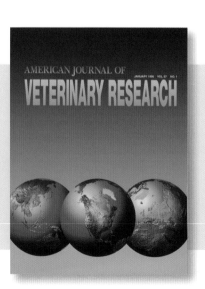

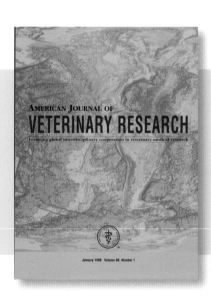

Originally published quarterly, the *AJVR* proved to be so popular among authors that it moved to bimonthly publication in 1959 and to monthly publication in 1968. It continues as a monthly publication today.

At the present time, although the *JAVMA* is a general veterinary journal that publishes manuscripts on any subject germane to the practice of veterinary medicine, for scientific reports, preference is given to manuscripts that have immediate clinical or practical value. In contrast, the *AJVR* currently focuses on the publication of novel research findings that bridge the gulf between basic research and clinical practice or that help to translate laboratory research and preclinical studies to the development of clinical trials and clinical practice. This focus, along with the *AJVR*'s association with the *JAVMA*, means that the *AJVR* has a unique niche among veterinary medical journals.

In addition to serving as a bridge between basic and clinical research, the *AJVR* acts as a type of bridge between nations, seeking to foster global interdisciplinary cooperation in veterinary medical research. According to Dr. Merillat's editorial in the debut issue, "Portraying the worthiness of veterinary medicine throughout the world is another objective" of the *AJVR*, and the *AJVR* has routinely met this goal over the years, publishing research from authors around the world and attracting subscribers from all over the globe.

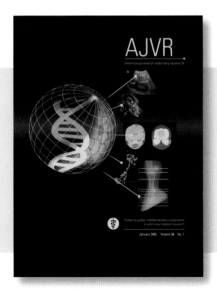
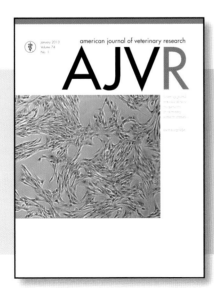

Publication of the *AJVR*

" should gradually transmute the regular

JOURNAL into a more useful monthly for

members interested in clinical work and

yet concurrently provide them

with a means of keeping abreast

with current advancements in

veterinary science. "

– Dr. Louis A. Merillat, 1939–1950 AVMA editor-in-chief

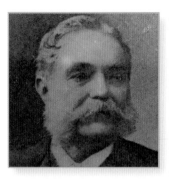

ALEXANDRE F. LIAUTARD

1877–1915

Dr. A.F. Liautard, affectionately nicknamed "Frenchy" by his American colleagues, is considered one of the titans of veterinary medicine in the United States. He was born in Paris in 1835 and graduated from the National Veterinary School of Alfort in 1856. Dr. Liautard was the only one of the AVMA founding fathers to hold an elective office for more than 20 years in succession.

Although Dr. Liautard did some outstanding work as an educator and was a two-time president of the Association, it is for his work on the *American Veterinary Review* that he is best known. He held the senior editorship of the Review from 1877–1915. He returned to France in 1900 and, despite his title, from that point on played no role in the daily operations of the Journal. But he did remain active in veterinary literature, continuing to publish reports and editorials in the Review and elsewhere. Even after the AVMA purchased the Review in 1915, changed the name to the *Journal of the American Veterinary Medical Association*, and appointed a new editor, Dr. Liautard still contributed a monthly feature to the publication until his death in 1918. Veterinary professionals all over the world mourned his passing.

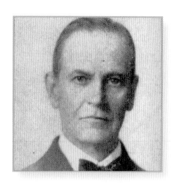

PIERRE AUGUSTINE FISH

1915–1918

In 1915, Dr. P.A. Fish of the New York State College of Veterinary Medicine was named the first editor of the newly renamed *JAVMA*. Previously the editor of Cornell Veterinarian, Dr. Fish brought impeccable credentials and a formidable intelligence to the position, and the expectation was that the new official organ of the Association would flourish under his direction. Instead, just three years later, Dr. Fish relinquished his post to join the military. After the war and through the rest of his life, Dr. Fish remained a frequent and valued contributor to the *JAVMA*.

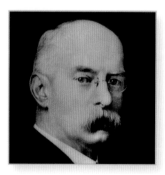

WILLIAM HADDOCK DALRYMPLE

1918–1919

Perhaps the most notable aspect of Dr. W.H. Dalrymple's tenure as editor of the *JAVMA* was its brief duration. The Scotsman had been one of the major players in the early years of the veterinary profession in the United States and was elected president of the Association in 1907. Unfortunately, after being named Dr. Fish's successor in 1918, Dr. Dalrymple had to relinquish the post to Dr. John R. Mohler the very next year because of ongoing health issues.

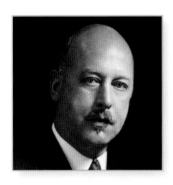

JOHN ROBBINS MOHLER

1919-1923

Dr. J.R. Mohler was another of the greats, a Philadelphia man distinguished by his career with the Bureau of Animal Industry and his election as AVMA president at a young age. He also did excellent work on the AVMA's journals for many years as an associate editor, but, as was the theme during these years, his tour as editor of the *JAVMA* was over shortly after it began, and it doesn't appear that many developments of note occurred on his watch.

Dr. Mohler took up the editorship in 1919, when Dr. Dalrymple stepped down. But, just four years later, in 1923, the offices of editor and secretary were combined, and Dr. H. Preston Hoskins took up the job in Dr. Mohler's place. Dr. Mohler subsequently became an associate editor and continued to work with the Association journals for many years, in addition to serving in myriad other positions that won him many accolades in the veterinary community.

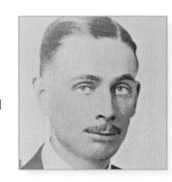

HORACE PRESTON HOSKINS

1923-1939

In a 100th anniversary retrospective of the AVMA, Dr. J.F. Smithcors wrote of Dr. William Horace Hoskins, AVMA president from 1893-1896, that "one of his greatest legacies to the veterinary profession was his son, Horace Preston Hoskins, long-time secretary and editor of the JOURNAL." The prosperity of the journal during the younger Hoskins' lengthy reign as editor (1923-1939) confirms this statement. Dr. H.P. Hoskins, a 1910 graduate of the University of Pennsylvania, was the first editor to fill the role in a full-time capacity and oversaw such innovations as the use of full-color illustrations and the addition to the *JAVMA* of a section of abstracts.

The circulation of the Journal began to grow in earnest while Dr. Hoskins was editor, and his steady leadership was a calming influence on a publication that in recent years had seemed to be casting about somewhat. In addition to the valuable books and reports that Dr. Hoskins authored and his years heading the *JAVMA*, he would later go on to contribute further to the veterinary literature by editing The North American Veterinarian.

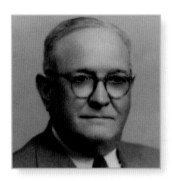

LOUIS A. MERILLAT

1939-1950

In 1939, one of the most honored figures in American veterinary history stepped into the role of editor-in-chief. Dr. L.A. Merillat, the acclaimed co-author (with Dr. Delwin M. Campbell) of the two-volume classic "Veterinary Military History" as well as many other articles and books on veterinary scientific and professional subjects, would edit the AVMA's publications for the next 11 years, until his 1950 retirement. At that time, he was named editor-in-chief emeritus, a title he retained until his death in 1956.

Perhaps the most notable development under Dr. Merillat's watch was the introduction in 1940 of the *AJVR*. The Association introduced the *JAVMA*'s sister journal ostensibly to expedite the publication of an overgrown backlog of technical articles, but under Dr. Merillat's guidance, the *AJVR* quickly began to garner a significant reputation of its own. More and more submissions began appearing for the *AJVR* from authors who previously had sought publication elsewhere, and before long, bimonthly publication was under consideration.

The year 1940 also saw the separation of the editorship and the executive secretary position when Dr. Merillat stepped down from his role of executive secretary to focus on his work with the publications. And that work bore fruit, as circulation for both Journals continued to grow under his leadership. By 1941, *JAVMA* subscriptions exceeded 7,000, while the subscription base for the *AJVR* was already approaching 2,000.

Meanwhile, Dr. Merillat wielded his pen as masterfully as ever, frequently publishing provocative but rigorously composed editorials, and his leadership style inspired in the staff of the Journals the deep loyalty so many others had felt for him during his earlier years in veterinary education, in the military, and in his role as AVMA president. The same meticulous craft that went into the composition of Dr. Merillat's editorials also shaped each issue of the Journals during his tenure. That sure hand would be missed over the next couple of years, as the AVMA Journals once again entered a time of uncertainty at the top.

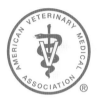

RAYMOND C. KLUSSENDORF

1950–1951

In August 1950, after Dr. Merillat's retirement, the AVMA promoted associate editor and assistant executive secretary Dr. Raymond C. Klussendorf to the editor-in-chief position. Dr. Klussendorf's work as an associate editor had prepared him well for the role, but early the next year, he announced that he would be leaving the AVMA to pursue other opportunities.

Although Dr. Klussendorf's time as editor-in-chief was short, he had worked for six years on the AVMA's publications and was highly regarded for his energy, enthusiasm, and appreciation of the problems facing veterinarians. *JAVMA* articles of the era stress that he was a man of vision who understood the professional and scientific developments of the time and used that knowledge effectively with his many contacts in the field. No doubt the *JAVMA* and *AJVR* would have benefited further from these traits, had Dr. Klussendorf chosen to stay on as editor-in-chief for a lengthier term.

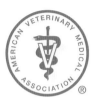

C.R. DONHAM

1951–1952

In the wake of Dr. Klussendorf's exit, the AVMA named Dr. C.R. Donham editor-in-chief on an interim basis in April 1951. The assignment was to last only as long as it took to complete the search for a new editor-in-chief. The AVMA was fortunate that Dr. Donham had just retired from his career as a professor in Purdue University's Department of Veterinary Science, in that he was now free to edit the *JAVMA* and *AJVR* until a suitable replacement came aboard. Dr. Donham did so ably, holding the line during a tough transitional period for the Journals.

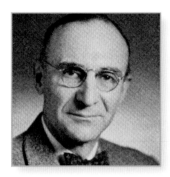

WILLIAM A. AITKEN

1952-1959

In February 1952, Dr. William A. Aitken, of Merrill, Iowa, accepted the Association's offer to become editor-in-chief of the Journals. He was an accomplished speaker, a prolific author of well-received scientific reports, an experienced teacher and private practitioner, and a well-known figure in national veterinary circles. In short, he was perfect for the job. Accepting the position was not an easy decision for Dr. Aitken—numerous friends reportedly had to talk him into it. Some observers may have taken this reluctance as a bad sign for the Journals, which, with three new editors in as many years, had already undergone their share of upheaval since Dr. Merillat's retirement. Dr. Aitken even stated when accepting the position that he would serve for "not more than five years."

Instead, Dr. Aitken spent more than seven years as an outstanding editor-in-chief of the Association journals. His main motivation in assuming the editorship was his desire to help the veterinary profession better understand and control such diseases as shipping fever, erysipelas, and hog cholera. Over the course of his editorship, Dr. Aitken did just that. Through a steady campaign of editorials, editor's notes, shrewd manuscript selection, preparation of abstracts, and interactions with authors, he either directly or indirectly stimulated much of the subsequent work on these diseases.

At the same time, Dr. Aitken took up the editing of the Journals with such zeal and single-mindedness that it became practically a way of life for him. His term as editor-in-chief saw the *JAVMA* grow from 12 issues per year to 24, while the *AJVR*, which had been publishing just four issues per year when Dr. Aitken came on board, grew to six issues per year. And Dr. Aitken's uncompromising editorial style—he was known to challenge practically every sentence of submitted material—paid dividends by producing journals that measured up to the highest standards, setting an example for other scientific journals around the world.

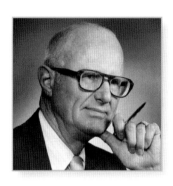

DONALD A. PRICE

1959-1971

Prior to his time with the AVMA, Dr. Donald A. Price had already gained recognition in the veterinary literature for co-authoring an influential 1952 report that described the bluetongue virus in Texas sheep. So Dr. Price's reputation preceded him when he joined the AVMA staff in 1958 as an associate editor. He was then appointed editor-in-chief in 1959 on Dr. Aitken's retirement.

The pairing of Dr. Price with the AVMA's publications was described as a "perfect fit" by Dr. Price's friend Dr. Walter F. Juliff. "He had that curious scientific mind," Dr. Juliff said, "and also that knowledge and obsession with the English language." These qualities served the *JAVMA* and *AJVR* in good stead, as they maintained their pattern of growth and their position as two of the most prestigious veterinary medical journals in the world during Dr. Price's 13 years as editor-in-chief. In addition to the special reports and editorials Dr. Price published in *JAVMA*, he was the author or co-author of numerous scientific reports published in other professional journals. These valuable contributions to the literature of veterinary medicine resulted in his being the first veterinarian elected a fellow of the American Medical Writers Association.

On Jan. 1, 1972, Dr. Price moved on to become AVMA executive vice president. He left the publications in robust health.

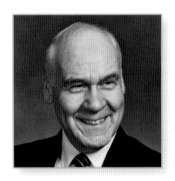

ARTHUR FREEMAN

1972-1984

Dr. Arthur Freeman first joined the AVMA staff in 1959 as an assistant editor responsible for helping produce the *JAVMA*. At that time, Drs. Price and Freeman were the only two scientific editors on the Journals' staff. During his early years as an assistant editor, Dr. Freeman reviewed the scientific articles himself, but as authors began increasingly to submit articles involving commercial products and technical subjects, Dr. Freeman found that he often needed to turn to outside reviewers for help. This led to his and Dr. Price's instituting a system whereby all submitted manuscripts were submitted to reviewers outside the AVMA office.

Dr. Freeman was promoted to editor-in-chief in 1972, when Dr. Price became executive vice president. Over the next 13 years, Dr. Freeman introduced numerous important innovations to the Journals, such as popular features that, in some cases, still run in the *JAVMA* today. Under Dr. Freeman's direction, the *JAVMA* also started regularly publishing artwork on its cover and adopted a larger (8- by 11-inch) format. This larger format led to a doubling of advertising income within two years.

Circulation continued to increase as well. Between 1972 and 1985, when Dr. Freeman moved on to become the next AVMA executive vice president, *JAVMA* circulation increased by more than 60 percent, from 27,000 to 44,000. Over the same time, the Publications Division budget tripled, advertising income quadrupled, subscription income unrelated to dues increased 75 percent, and the Publications Division grew to be the AVMA's largest, with 21 people. By any measure, Dr. Freeman took an already thriving operation and propelled it to an even higher level of performance.

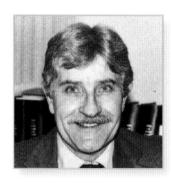

ALBERT J. KOLTVEIT

1985-1995

Dr. Albert J. Koltveit came to the *JAVMA* as an assistant editor in 1969. Prior to joining the AVMA, he had worked as a private practitioner in mixed animal practice, as a scientific writer for a private company, and as an extension veterinarian at the University of Illinois. This combination of experience prepared him well for the long, distinguished career he would have in the AVMA Publications Division.

Dr. Koltveit became editor-in-chief and director of the Publications Division on Jan. 1, 1985, when Dr. Freeman assumed the executive vice presidency. Dr. Koltveit innovated in a number of ways over the years, including reorganizing the table of contents and introducing several well-liked features such as "Reflections" and the still-popular "Animal Behavior Case of the Month." In these moves, one can see why Dr. Koltveit was known as an editor who was especially sensitive to the needs of his readers, someone who was willing to change the presentation and offerings of the Journals to provide clarity and the type of information his readers sought.

In retrospect, however, it seems that one of Dr. Koltveit's greatest accomplishments may have been simply having the vision to foresee the electronic future of publishing and to prepare the AVMA publications accordingly. Although he didn't have the budget at the time to embrace the newest technologies as fully as he would have liked, he was a vocal advocate for the possibilities of electronic communications in his final years as editor-in-chief, and this approach paved the way for the *JAVMA*'s transition into the 21st century. He was especially proud of hiring his successor, Dr. Janis H. Audin, who went on to leverage these technologies and oversee the eventual conversion to desktop publishing. "It was the crowning achievement of my career," he would later say.

Dr. Koltveit retired from the AVMA in April 1995.

who discussed the island's animal health infrastructure after a devastating earthquake early in the year.

The 2011 convention in St. Louis featured a celebration of World Veterinary Year—the 250th anniversary of the founding of the first veterinary school, in Lyon, France. The Poultry Science Association met in conjunction with the convention. The AVMA, AAHA, and other organizations announced they had formed the Partnership for Preventive Pet Healthcare to address a decline in pets' veterinary visits.

At the 2012 convention in San Diego, the partnership launched a program to help practitioners promote preventive care for pets. The AVMA re-emphasized programming for veterinary technicians at the convention and provided sessions for veterinarians to meet the new training requirements for maintaining accreditation with the Department of Agriculture.

Plans were proceeding for the 2013 convention in Chicago, with the intent of making the convention an integral part of the celebration of the 150th anniversary of the AVMA.

MORE THAN A MEETING

The annual meetings of the AVMA have come a long way since the 1860s, when the Committee on Intelligence and Education deemed no papers from the meetings worthy of publication. The convention now offers educational sessions on dozens of tracks to appeal to attendees in all aspects of veterinary medicine.

Wherever it travels from year to year, the AVMA convention remains a gathering place for thousands of members of the veterinary community—to share in the festivities, the camaraderie, and the memories.

AVMAconvention
2009 seattle

AVMAconvetion
2011 st. louis

AVMAconvention
2010 atlanta

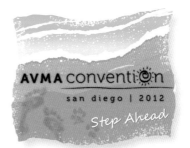

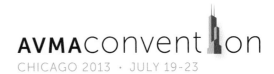
CHICAGO 2013 · JULY 19-23

Rooted in knowledge

David Banasiak

Over the past 10 to 15 years, many changes have occurred in the field of veterinary education. Several American universities are exploring plans to establish new veterinary schools, even as state and federal governments cut funding for education. Schools in the U.S. and Canada are raising enrollment rates to accommodate a growing demand among potential students. Interest in acquiring accreditation from the American Veterinary Medical Association's Council on Education is on the rise as veterinary schools around the world look to the COE's Standards of Accreditation as the gold standard and actively seek recognition under those requirements.

But this was not always the case. While the first veterinary school opened in France in 1761 and was followed by other schools in Great Britain, Germany, and across Europe, America throughout much of the 18th and 19th centuries remained largely indifferent to veterinary education. Thirty-six veterinary schools would be established in Europe before the first American school opened. Early American colleges focused their educational mission on preparing graduates to be ministers or priests. The publication "120 Years of American Education: A Statistical Portrait" estimated that prior to the Civil War, a quarter of all college graduates became ministers. Until the 1800s, America had no veterinary schools, and the few schools founded in the early 19th century were plagued by ignorance, apathy, and greed.

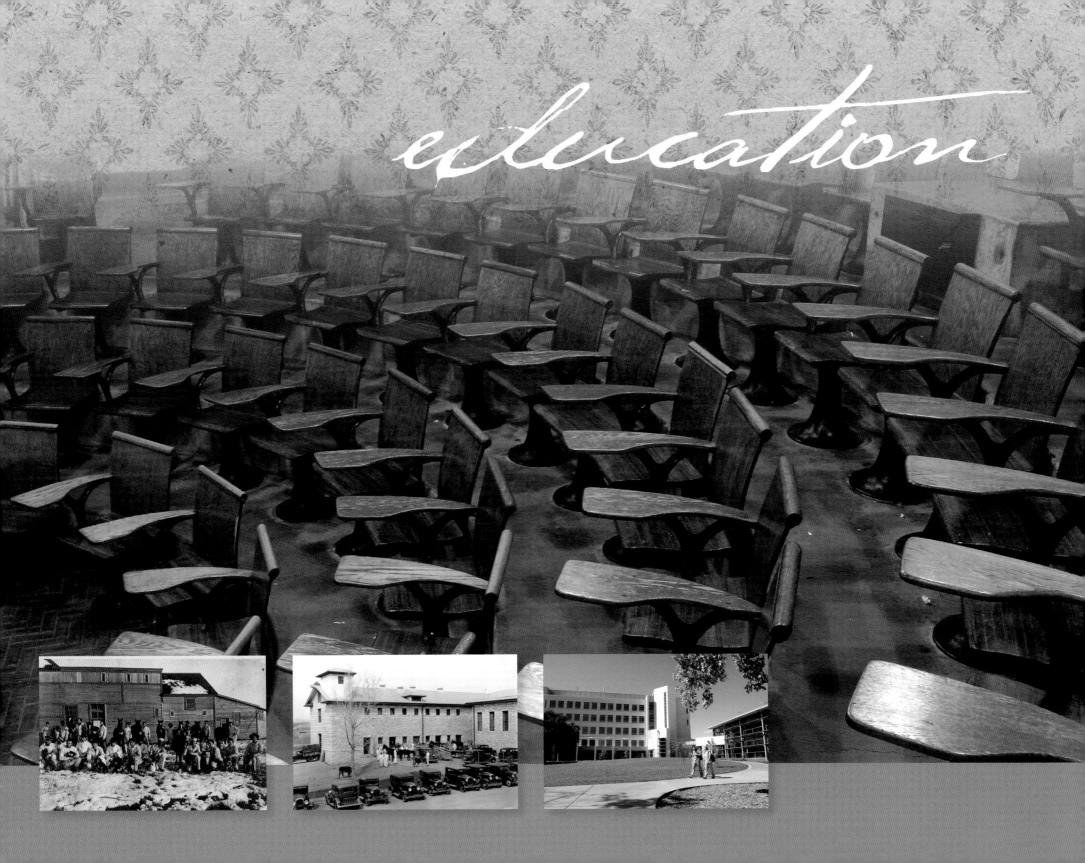

education

"Nobody was laughed at more than the horse doctor. Horse doctors were suppose to be a coarse, ignorant group who had made a failure of blacksmithing or farming and had turned to 'doctoring.' That they actually knew anything about medicine was an absurd notion."

– Dr. R.J. Dinsmore in his book "'Hoss' Doctor"

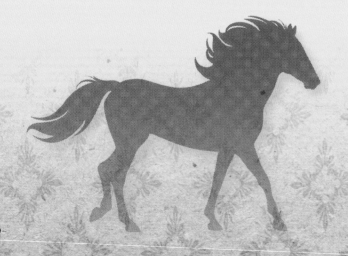

VETERINARIANS GET NO RESPECT

When Dr. Joseph Bushman, a veterinarian practicing in Washington, D.C., during the Civil War, declined President Lincoln's request to serve as a veterinary sergeant in a cavalry regiment in the U.S. Army, his decision was about respect. In Dr. Bushman's native England, veterinarians were commissioned officers in the British army, an advanced rank justified by the high regard afforded veterinarians as trained professionals. Dr. Bushman, a graduate of the Royal Veterinary College in London who had also studied veterinary medicine in France, was a member of a select group of individuals in America: veterinarians who had graduated from a reputable veterinary school.

Dr. Bushman's refusal to serve at a lower rank was justified, and eventually he received a commission to serve in the Quartermaster Corps, where he was assigned to work in the Giesboro horse and mule depot of the Army of the Potomac. He would later be a lecturer at the Kansas State Agricultural College.

But the Army had good cause to disrespect Dr. Bushman's profession. During America's early years, veterinary education, when available, was of dubious quality. The young nation's growing population of livestock and horses was cared for by blacksmiths, farriers, physicians, and a few European-educated veterinarians. Those interested in practicing veterinary medicine trained themselves as best they could from the scant literature available. If they were lucky, they might apprentice themselves to a European-educated veterinarian. Dr. Charles Wood, third president of the United States Veterinary Medical Association, for instance, began his career as a blacksmith but switched to veterinary practice as a self-taught veterinarian.

When it came to receiving professional health care, companion animals fared even worse than horses and livestock during this period. As Katherine Grier writes in "Pets in America," veterinarians considered them useless animals and not worth the effort to treat. Pet owners didn't share this view of their pets and sought health care for them, which, when they could find it, was often provided by pet shop owners. Grier mentions that in 1884, George Walton, a Boston dog dealer, also advertised himself as a dog doctor.

THE FIRST TWO

The two veterinary schools operating in the U.S. before the Civil War—the Boston Veterinary Institute, which opened in 1854, and the New York College of Veterinary Surgeons, which opened in 1857—did little to dissuade the Army or the public of their skepticism toward the veterinary profession. These schools were privately owned and profit-driven, and their brief existence was troubled by squabbling, inadequately trained faculty; a lack of committed students; poor admission standards; and unethical behavior.

It is no wonder, then, that the term "horse doctor" took on a derogatory meaning, being a term that, with one meaning, marginalized the work performed by veterinarians by referencing only a single species treated and, with a second, ridiculed the inadequate and shoddy education received in veterinary schools of the time. Dr. R.J. Dinsmore in his book "'Hoss' Doctor" had this to say on the subject: "Nobody was laughed at more than the horse doctor. Horse doctors were supposed to be a coarse, ignorant group who had made a failure of blacksmithing or farming and had turned to 'doctoring.' That they actually knew anything about medicine was an absurd notion."

Faculty at the Boston Veterinary Institute frequently pressured the administration to admit uneducated students. The institute's president opposed these demands, and eventually, the struggle over admission standards became irrelevant when the school closed after four sessions, having graduated only six students.

Of the two early veterinary schools in the U.S., the New York College of Veterinary Surgeons is often considered America's first practical veterinary school. According to a Feb. 23, 1858, column in The New York Times, the NYCVS was "organized under appointment by its trustees of Capt. Ralston, as Veterinary Principal and Professor of Theory and Practice; Thos. D. Andres, M.D., as Professor of Anatomy and Physiology; and John Busteed, M.D., as Professor of Surgical Anatomy and Surgery." The article goes on to say that Ralston was an officer of cavalry in the British army and a graduate of the Royal Veterinary College.

The NYCVS' time span of operation, 1857-1899, was beset with internal divisiveness, resulting in faculty members and students breaking with the college to found rival schools. The severity of the discordance caused the college to suspend operations from 1873-1877. During this period, in 1875, Dr. Alexandre Liautard left after a quarrel,

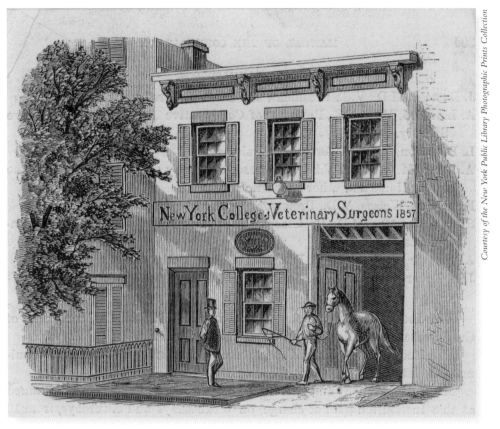

Courtesy of the New York Public Library Photographic Prints Collection

The New York College of Veterinary Surgeons

taking with him most of the students, to open the American Veterinary College in New York.

In 1877, another discontented group left to establish the Columbia Veterinary College. At the college's official opening in September 1878, The New York Times reported: "The college has been organized by Professors and students who seceded from the New York Veterinary College owing to a disagreement with the Board of Trustees."

Despite these struggles, the New York College of Veterinary Surgeons continued operations, becoming, as The New York Times reported in 1897, the first veterinary college to offer a special class for women interested in becoming veterinarians. Unfortunately, a Dec. 30, 1899, fire resulting in an estimated $20,000 loss and the death of 24 horses forced the college's closure. During its time span, the NYCVS graduated 291 students.

Another school that struggled to establish itself during this time was the Veterinary College of Philadelphia. Two attempts to open the college, in 1853 and 1857, both failed because of faculty disputes. The college was reorganized as the Pennsylvania College of Veterinary Surgeons, and in 1866, made its third attempt to open, but it folded by 1870 with a depleted treasury, having failed to attract a sufficient number of students. Dr. Robert Jennings, part of the group who worked to open the Philadelphia college, said it failed because "young men of education and respectability would not engage in a profession of so low a standing."

The Pennsylvania College of Veterinary Surgeons was acquired by Dr. Robert McClure, who opened it as the Merchants' Veterinary College. Under Dr. McClure's leadership, the new college experienced its first commercial success. The college offered diplomas granting the degree of Doctor of Veterinary Medicine and Surgery for a fee of $100, or approximately $2,200 in today's dollars. But that was not all students received. Dr. McClure threw in several books he had written, including "Diseases of the American Horse, Cattle and Sheep." To add a touch of respect and authenticity, diplomas were issued under the name of the defunct Pennsylvania College of Veterinary Surgeons and included the forged signatures of creditable medical men.

Dr. McClure's success, however, was short-lived. The forged signatures drew the attention of the authorities, and in 1877, he was convicted of forgery and sentenced to nine months in jail and a $2,000 fine.

Dr. McClure's imprisonment was not the end of the college, though, as it continued to grant diplomas, offering instruction under a preceptorship system whereby students were apprenticed to practicing veterinarians.

VISIONARIES CALL FOR CHANGE

Before the carnage of the Civil War emphasized the need for trained veterinarians, visionaries observed that disease in animals could have an impact on human health. These forward-thinking men advocated for the study of veterinary medicine as a science and for the establishment of veterinary schools. The Philadelphia Society for Promoting Agriculture, with such famous members as George Washington, Benjamin Franklin, and Noah Webster, was at the forefront in the call for veterinary education. In 1805, Richard Peters, president of the Philadelphia Society, offered a gold medal for the best essay promoting veterinary knowledge and instruction.

Others added their voices to the call. In 1807, physician Benjamin Rush, delegate to the Continental Congress and signer of the Declaration of Independence, called on the Medical School of the University of Pennsylvania to create a veterinary department. He gave nine reasons why physicians should study the diseases of animals, the first being: "By studying the disease of our domestic animals we rescue them from the hands of quacks." Unfortunately, he went unheeded until 1884, when the university opened the Department of Veterinary Medicine.

> "By studying the disease of our domestic animals we rescue them from the hands of quacks."
>
> – Physician Benjamin Rush, 1807

While Rush's calls for a veterinary department would take years to germinate, hope for the improvement of veterinary education would come from another quarter. On June 9-10, 1863, a group of about 40 dedicated men met in New York City, guided by a petition advocating for the formation of a national veterinary association and condemning the inferior state of veterinary education. The petition, strongly promoted by the American Veterinary Association (of Philadelphia), also urged the advancement and diffusion of veterinary knowledge.

It stated: "Whereas, Veterinary Science in this country has been kept in comparative obscurity in consequence of its having been confined mainly to the hands of men uneducated in the anatomical and pathological relations of the various diseases to which our domestic animals are subject, as well also as to the therapeutic action of the remedies used in combating disease. This deplorable condition of the veterinary profession has been the means of excluding the qualified practitioner from the army in the United States. The losses to the national government in consequence from the purchase of large numbers of horses unfit for duties required of them, having amounted to millions of dollars. …"

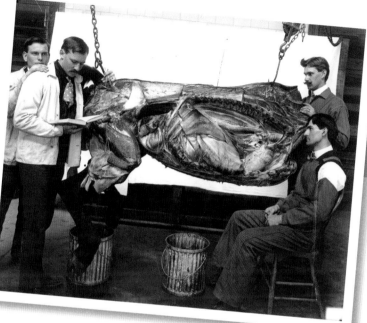

Equine anatomy dissection class at The Ohio State University, circa 1895

Conceived with a commitment to advance and promote veterinary education, the United States Veterinary Medical Association moved to achieve these aims by forming the Committee on Intelligence and Education in 1863 as one of its first standing committees. The CIE would become the grandfather of the current Council on Education, and it is one of the few committees of the AVMA to trace an unbroken lineage to the founding of the Association.

Documented activities of the Association's early years are meager and scarce, but it is known that in 1871, the USVMA passed a resolution calling for the New York College of Veterinary Surgeons to administer an entrance examination to "further the object of a higher grade of education." No record has been found of NYCVS's response to this request.

This resolution appears to be the Association's first attempt to persuade schools to improve the quality of veterinary education, but it had no effect. The fledgling Association had no muscle, no leverage to induce schools to adopt reforms. Many years would pass before their efforts would pay off, and during that time, the Association

would require help from government agencies and the economics of the veterinary marketplace. The Association also would have to overcome the opinions and practices of its own members.

DO AS I SAY, NOT AS I DO

At least one prominent Association member was hypocritical in his calls for reform. Dr. Alexandre Liautard, the eighth and 14th president of the USVMA and the founder of the American Veterinary College (which served for many years as an unofficial headquarters of the Association), advocated higher standards for veterinary schools, including a three-year curriculum; however, he refused to adopt these standards himself and continued to maintain a two-year course of study at his college. His college also declined to participate when, in 1877–1878, the Association called for a congress of veterinary schools and veterinary departments at agricultural schools to discuss improve-

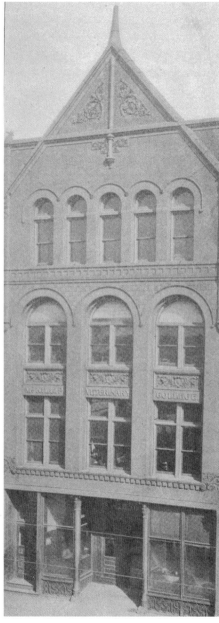

Early photograph of the McKillip
Veterinary College of Chicago

ments in veterinary science standards and the veterinary curriculum.

As the editor of the *American Veterinary Review*, which later became the *Journal of the American Veterinary Medical Association*, Dr. Liautard used the Journal to criticize competing veterinary schools. After hearing that the new McKillip Veterinary College had opened in Chicago with a two-year program, he wrote in the September 1895 issue of the Review: "The McKillip Veterinary College will open as a two-year school. What a pity."

Dr. Louis Merillat notes another instance of Dr. Liautard's flip-flopping in the book "Veterinary Military History" when he relates Dr. Liautard's response to the 1897 decision of the Board of Regents of New York State to set a standard of a high school education as the matriculation requirement to attend a veterinary school. Dr. Liautard was quoted as saying: "The recent action of the Board of Regents of the State of New York at the instigation of our own State Society is a strike at the very foundation of the profession of veterinary medicine." Shortly after this incident, Dr. Liautard retired and returned to his native France.

Why the actions of the New York board of regents angered Dr. Liautard is a mystery, considering that five years earlier, in 1892, the USVMA unanimously adopted an amendment requiring that any future applicant for membership "shall be a graduate of a regularly

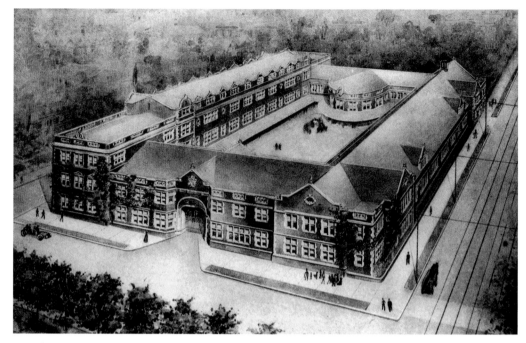

Aerial view of the University of Pennsylvania, 1910

organized and recognized veterinary school, which shall have a curriculum of at least three years, of six months each, specially devoted to the study of veterinary science, and whose corps of instructors shall contain at least four veterinarians."

THE MORE THE MERRIER

From the end of the Civil War in 1865 until 1900, 32 additional veterinary schools opened in the United States. During that same period, 19 of those schools closed, some lasting only a couple years. No standardization of education existed between schools, and quality remained haphazard and irregular. The public was largely apathetic concerning the need for properly educated veterinarians, and even some members of the profession were unwilling to change or indifferent to reform.

American Veterinary Review in 1877 consisted of a collection of papers from the 1876 annual meeting. The Review, now the *Journal of the American Veterinary Medical Association*, went on to publish a wide variety of reports with findings on animal health.

At the time of the Association's 50th anniversary in 1913, the constitution and by-laws stated that one object of the AVMA was "to cultivate medical science and literature." Dr. John R. Mohler, then president, reflected on five decades of progress in the knowledge of animal diseases. He said, "As chemistry and physics have advanced from alchemy, and astronomy from astrology, so has veterinary medicine progressed from empiricism and become scientific."

In 1940, the Association created the *American Journal of Veterinary Research* to publish the overflow of manuscripts from the *JAVMA*. The *AJVR* grew from a quarterly publication in 1940 to a bimonthly publication in 1959 to a monthly publication in 1968. The *AJVR* focuses on reports that bridge basic and clinical research, while the *JAVMA* focuses on manuscripts with immediate clinical or practical value.

In 1941, the AVMA established the Council on Research. A primary initial project of the council was raising and awarding funds for research fellowships. In 1963, the fellowship program became the basis for formation of the AVMA Foundation, now the American Veterinary Medical Foundation.

The Foundation later discontinued the fellowship program because of competition from federal agencies, but it began to provide scholarships for veterinary students and funds for research projects. A more recent additional focus has been funding for disaster preparedness and response activities. Entering the 21st century, the research council continued to promote veterinary research. On recommendations from the council, the Executive Board gave approval for the AVMA to provide funds toward two major National Academies studies: "National Need and Priorities for Veterinarians in Biomedical Research," which came out in 2004, and "Critical Needs for Research in Veterinary Science," which was released in 2005.

In 2007, the research council proposed the concept of the Institute for Companion Animal and Equine Research. The AVMF recently has been collaborating with other organizations to develop the Animal Health Network as an effort to embody this institute to fund research on feline, canine, and equine health.

The AVMA added a goal to the 2012-2015 strategic plan to "advance scientific research and discovery." The accompanying goal statement is for the Association to support "promotion and appropriate funding of veterinary scientific research and discovery to ensure the advancement of veterinary medical knowledge." Among the subsidiary objectives is advocating for research to support evidence-based veterinary medicine.

PANEL ON EUTHANASIA

Many have said that the AVMA Guidelines on Euthanasia are the gold standard for acceptable procedures and agents for euthanizing a spectrum of animal species. Each of the eight editions to date has summarized contemporary scientific knowledge to provide workable guidelines for veterinarians on methods for inducing death in animals as painlessly and quickly as possible when euthanasia is necessary.

The euthanasia guidelines date back to the 1960s. The Council on Research appointed five veterinarians in 1961 to serve as a Panel on Euthanasia, directing them to study methods of euthanasia for unwanted or fatally diseased small animals. Panel members approached the task by drawing on their own training, reviewing the literature, and visiting animal shelters. The 1963 document, then known as the Report of the AVMA Panel on Euthanasia, was nine pages long and comprised sections on more than a dozen euthanasia methods, with each section describing the method of euthanasia and most sections listing advantages and disadvantages as well as recommendations. The panel concluded that the best method of euthanasia for individual animals was intravenous administration of barbiturates.

In 1969, at the request of the research council, the Executive Board appointed a seven-veterinarian Euthanasia Review Panel to update the work of the first panel. Panel members considered euthanasia not only of cats and dogs but also of "birds, rodents, and other small species" and large animals. The 1972 panel report follows almost the same format as the first report, with the addition of a discussion of behavioral considerations and a table on the efficacy of four inhalation anesthetics for euthanasia.

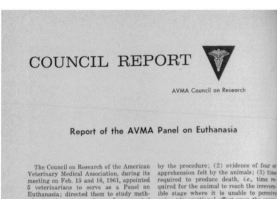

The Executive Board appointed a euthanasia review panel in 1977 consisting of six veterinarians and one public representative. For the 1978 report, the panel added a table on mode of action of euthanasia agents and expanded the table on efficacy of inhalation anesthetics for euthanasia. The report also offered examples of recordings of physiologic activity of dogs undergoing euthanasia by various methods.

The fourth euthanasia panel, again with six veterinarians and a public representative, convened in 1984. In the 1986 report, the panel expanded the information on euthanasia of laboratory animals and food animals. The report retained the table on mode of action of euthanasia agents and provided an extensive table on characteristics of agents and methods of euthanasia. According to the postface, the panel report "calls attention to the lack of scientific reports assessing pain and discomfort in animals undergoing euthanasia."

The fifth euthanasia panel convened in 1992 with seven veterinarians. The 1993 report had tables summarizing agents and methods of euthanasia by species, acceptable agents and methods of euthanasia, conditionally acceptable agents and methods, and some unacceptable agents and methods. One section covered special considerations for horses, food animals, "nonconventional" species such as zoo animals and wildlife, and animals

in fur production. In an acknowledgement, the panel stated that 130 individuals and organizations provided input for the report.

The sixth euthanasia panel convened in 1999 with 15 veterinarians and two nonveterinarians representing a variety of groups. The 2000 panel report, appearing in the *JAVMA* in 2001, provided more information about euthanasia of free-ranging wildlife and information about adjunctive methods of euthanasia. The report had grown longer with each edition, and the sixth edition reached 28 pages.

At a meeting in 2006, the Executive Board approved a recommendation that the AVMA convene a panel at least once per decade to produce the AVMA Guidelines on Euthanasia. In interim years, the Animal Welfare Committee would handle requests for inclusion of new euthanasia procedures or agents. At the same meeting, the board, on recommendation of the committee, approved the first interim revision—addition of maceration as a method of euthanasia for chicks, poults, and pipped eggs. The AVMA posted the euthanasia guidelines, with the revision, on its website in 2007.

In 2009, the AVMA formed 11 working groups to begin a broad-based update of the euthanasia guidelines. The groups consisted of more than 70 representatives from fields such as veterinary medicine, animal science, animal control, and animal agriculture. The panel solicited input from AVMA members on draft guidelines, eliciting several hundred comments. The new AVMA Guidelines on Euthanasia are about three times the length of the 2007 guidelines. They cover vertebrate and invertebrate species. The report does not cover slaughter and depopulation, which are to become the subjects of separate guidance documents.

AVMA VETERINARY MEDICAL ASSISTANCE TEAMS

When Hurricane Andrew hit Florida in August 1992, it became painfully apparent that people are not the only victims when disaster strikes. The category 5 hurricane devastated the state's veterinary infrastructure and left thousands of animals either dead or homeless. It was then that the AVMA began the work of organizing volunteer veterinary professionals into regional teams that could deploy to disaster areas to help animal victims.

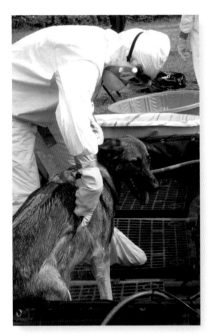 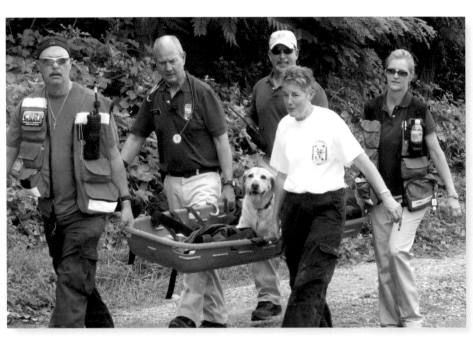 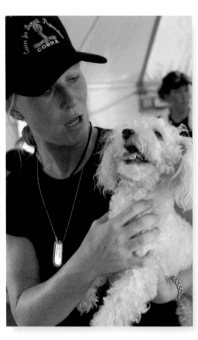

AVMA Veterinary Medical Assistance Teams

The AVMA Veterinary Medical Assistance Teams were officially established in May 1993 by a memorandum of understanding between the AVMA and Office of Emergency Preparedness of the U.S. Public Health Service. The agreement incorporated veterinary services into the federal government's national disaster response plan. The VMATs were a private-public partnership fashioned after the medical teams deployed to disaster sites in support of human casualties of catastrophic disasters that overwhelm state and local resources. In August 1994, the AVMA and the Department of Agriculture's Animal and Plant Health Inspection Service signed an agreement authorizing the VMATs to assist the USDA during animal disease outbreaks. Then in January 1998, the AVMA and American Veterinary Medical Foundation signed a statement of understanding with the American Red Cross in which that organization recognized the AVMA and AVMF as the only national organizations representing the entire U.S. profession of licensed veterinarians.

Ultimately, four VMAT teams were developed, based in Minnesota, Massachusetts, Maryland, and North Carolina. Each team consisted of approximately 22 members from public and private veterinary practice with a broad range of skills—including wildlife, exotic, and aquatic medicine expertise as well as expertise in toxicology, pathology, surgery, and emergency and critical care. Veterinary technicians, academicians, and epidemiologists were part of each VMAT. Team members were trained in hazardous materials handling, animal triage, restraint, and transport as well as disease diagnostics and humane euthanasia. VMATs deployed during federally declared disasters at the request of local and state officials, once it was determined that veterinary assistance was needed. The job of the teams was to assist the local veterinary community with caring for animals and providing veterinary oversight and advice. A member of the AVMA Scientific Activities Division continues to coordinate the Association's emergency preparedness and response activities, including the VMAT program.

The mission of the VMATs has evolved over the years. The program is now a private endeavor of the AVMA and AVMF focusing on providing early assessments of animal-related needs during disasters, offering basic treatment of affected animals, and training state and local responders to provide animal-related disaster relief when called on. But in their early years, the VMATs deployed often. On 9/11, 51 individuals, including members of all four VMATs, deployed to the World Trade Center in New York City, the site of the terrorist attack that killed nearly 3,000 people. There, they supported the efforts of local veterinary responders to provide medical care for the search-and-rescue dogs that were used to scour the rubble for survivors. From Sept. 11 until Oct. 31, the VMATs provided more than 900 treatments to some 300 SAR dogs at the disaster site.

Four years later, when Hurricane Katrina devastated the Gulf Coast region, the federal government for the first time deployed all four VMATs, with two teams deploying to Louisiana and the other two to Mississippi. The teams provided medical care for injured animals, including SAR dogs; coordinated animal relief efforts on-site; assessed the local veterinary infrastructure; and addressed public health issues. Additionally, the AVMA pledged $500,000 to match donations to a new fund created by the AVMF to provide relief for animals and veterinarians affected by the hurricane. The Foundation continues to offer disaster-related grants, with funding available to cover the costs of training, reimbursement for supplies, and repairs for veterinary practices damaged during a disaster.

Hurricane Katrina made it clear that many animal owners would not be willing to evacuate from a disaster area without their pets, prompting Congress to pass the Pets Evacuation and Transportation Standards Act of 2006. The AVMA supported the leg-

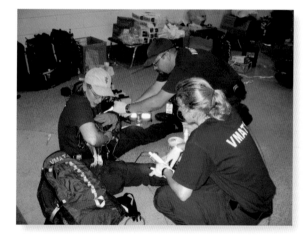 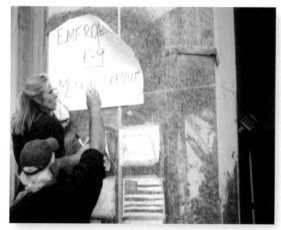

The AVMA Veterinary Medical Assistance Teams assisted with veterinary care during the response to Hurricane Katrina (left) and 9/11 (right).

islation, which granted the Federal Emergency Management Agency authority to help state and local governments develop emergency and evacuation plans that take pets and service animals into account. The AVMA's commitment to ensuring the safety of every family member is evident by the Association's many initiatives in this area. For example, the Executive Board established the Committee on Disaster and Emergency Issues in 2001 to, among other things, advise the AVMA on the veterinary profession's role in emergency and disaster issues. The AVMA has created brochures and a Web page with instructions on ways of incorporating animals into emergency response plans.

PUBLIC HEALTH

Whether it's testing for dangerous concentrations of *Escherichia coli* and *Salmonella* at a processing plant, vaccinating pets against rabies, or monitoring wild birds for the deadly avian influenza virus, veterinary medicine has always been a public health profession. Leaders of the nascent USVMA had a clear understanding about the relationship of veterinary medicine to human health and encouraged the inclusion of veterinarians on municipal sanitation boards. Butchers and policemen were more likely than veterinarians to be meat inspectors, which provoked Dr. Alexandre F. Liautard in 1879 to write in the *American Veterinary Review*: "Especially needed are veterinarians as meat inspectors, for no other can be so well fitted to detect the presence of disease in an animal intended for slaughter, or evidence of its previous existence in the meat that is offered for sale."

A handful of boards of health, notably in New York City's borough of Brooklyn and the state of New Jersey, recognized early on the connection between human and veterinary medicine, and, since the early 1880s, counted veterinarians as members. Henry

Butchers and policemen were more likely than veterinarians

to be meat inspectors.

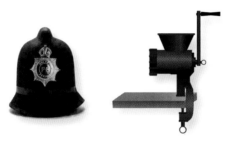

Bergh, founder of the American Society for the Prevention of Cruelty to Animals, called on government to take advantage of the skills and knowledge of veterinarians to combat animal diseases—particularly rabies, glanders, trichinosis, and tuberculosis—to the benefit of the public. "Not only is the skill of the veterinary practitioner applicable to diseases and accidents of domestic animals, but his learning and experience should be employed by the state in a sanitary point of view." By the close of 1885, the number of state veterinarians had grown to 15.

Today, Bergh's vision has been realized, as the number of state veterinarians has grown to 50. Moreover, with thousands of veterinarians working for the USDA, CDC, and Department of Defense, among others, the federal government is one of the largest employers of veterinarians. The veterinarian's role as a protector of public health has often gone unnoticed, however. Dr. W.H. Lowe, speaking before the AVMA in 1900, said, "People recognize and appreciate much quicker and in a fuller sense what veterinary medicine does for their pet animals and for themselves, in a commercial sense, in

protecting the animal wealth than they do for what the science does for the health and lives of the people themselves."

Despite this lack of recognition, the AVMA's commitment to promoting human health and well-being through the profession has never flagged. Helping direct the Association's efforts in this important area is the Council on Public Health and Regulatory Veterinary Medicine. Working with the Food Safety Advisory Committee, this council recommends AVMA support for programs designed to prevent, control, and eradicate animal diseases, and it studies problems associated with zoonoses and ensuring a safe and adequate food supply of animal origin. Each May, the AVMA hosts National Dog Bite Prevention Week to help reduce the nearly 5 million dog bites that happen every year. Additionally, the AVMA advocates for legislation expanding the number of veterinarians working in public health–related areas of practice and sufficient funding for food safety and biomedical research programs.

Through many policies, scientific backgrounders, and online resources, including podcasts and KeepOurFoodSafe.org, the AVMA offers the public and policymakers timely information about various animal-related threats to human health, such as bovine spongiform encephalopathy, zoonotic pathogens potentially used as biological weapons, plague, and West Nile virus. The AVMA also promotes human health and well-being by championing the special relationship between people and pets known as the human-animal bond. Veterinarians strive to maximize the potential benefits of the bond to both the animal and owner. Grief over a pet's death can be as profound as the loss of a friend or family member. To help these pet owners, the Association has promulgated guidelines for providing support to people coping with the loss of a companion animal.

ONE HEALTH

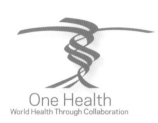

One Health
World Health Through Collaboration

Closely associated with veterinary medicine's public health role is the concept that human, animal, and ecosystem wellness are interconnected and dependent on one other. Luminaries within the medical community have understood this relationship for centuries. Hippocrates, the father of Western medicine, instructed physicians to consider how seasons, weather, and environment might impact a patient's health. Calls for a holistic approach to medicine have been voiced by the likes of Giovanni Lancisi, Louis-Rene Villerme, Rudolf Virchow, William Osler, Louis Pasteur, Robert Koch, Rachel Carson, and James Steele. In his book "Veterinary Medicine and Human Health," Dr. Calvin Schwabe called it "one medicine," which has grown into the present-day one-health movement.

The recent increased interest in one health began in earnest in 2006 when AVMA President Roger K. Mahr called for the creation of a national commission uniting veterinary and human medicine for the purpose of improving and protecting animal and public health worldwide. In his address before the AVMA House of Delegates, Dr. Mahr said, "Animal health is truly at a crossroads. Its convergence with human and ecosystem health dictates that the 'one world, one health, one medicine' concept must be embraced. We need our colleagues in human medicine, public health, and the environmental health sciences. Together, we can accomplish more in improving global health than we can alone, and we have the responsibility to do so." With their training in population health and comparative and preventive medicines, veterinarians are uniquely qualified to lead the one-health charge.

Dr. Mahr's proposal ultimately led to formation of the nonprofit One Health Commission in June 2009. In addition to the AVMA, member organizations include the American Medical Association, American Public Health Association, Association of American Veterinary Medical Colleges, and Association of American Medical Colleges. The mission of the One Health Commission is "the establishment of closer professional interactions, collaborations, and educational and research opportunities across the health sciences professions, together with their related disciplines, to improve the health of people, domestic animals, wildlife, plants, and our environment."

One of the commission's first efforts was to hold the One Health Summit in Washington, D.C., to raise awareness of the importance of transcending institutional and disciplinary boundaries to improve health for all species. Currently hosted at Iowa State University, the One Health Commission is overseen by a board of directors comprising veterinarians and physicians, with Dr. Mahr serving as the chief executive officer.

The one-health concept has gained widespread acceptance in academia and government in the United States and around the world. Adoption of the one-health approach is partly a response to the fact that most emerging and re-emerging diseases are zoonotic. In 2009, the CDC established a One Health Office, now within the National Center for Emerging and Zoonotic Infectious Diseases.

AVMA AWARDS

At a meeting of the USVMA in 1875, members agreed that two prizes be given each year for the best papers on any veterinary subject. The number of accolades the Association awards has expanded along with the size of the veterinary profession and the noteworthiness of veterinarians' contributions to human and animal health. Today, with financial assistance from the AVMF, its donors, and partners, the AVMA gives out more than a dozen awards each year. The winners are esteemed members of the veterinary community and others who have dedicated themselves and their careers to veterinary medicine.

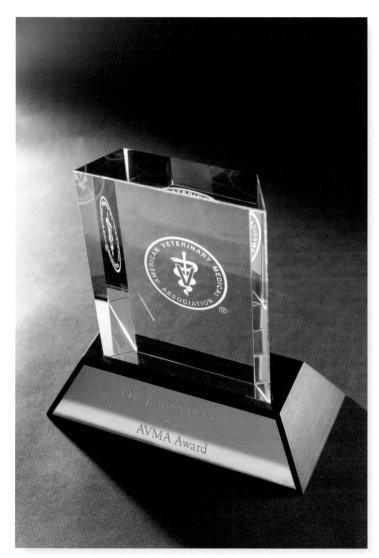

Established in 1931, The AVMA Award honors an Association member who has advanced veterinary medicine in its organizational aspects.

a diverse range of disciplines, from agriculture, public health, humane education, animal welfare, clinical practice, and research to government activities and professional education.

The list of AVMA awards is as follows: The AVMA Award, Bustad Companion Animal Veterinarian of the Year Award, AVMA Meritorious Service Award, AVMA Advocacy Award, AVMA Animal Welfare Award, AVMA Humane Award, AVMA Lifetime Excellence in Research Award, AVMA Practitioner Research Award, AVMA President's Award, AVMA Public Service Award, AVMA XIIth International Veterinary Congress Prize, AVMF/American Kennel Club Career Achievement Award in Canine Research, and AVMF/Winn Excellence in Feline Research Award.

The AVMA Award is considered the highest honor the Association can bestow on a member. Established in 1931, The AVMA Award recognizes distinguished Association members who have contributed to the advancement of veterinary medicine in its organizational aspects. Veterinarians who have exerted outstanding leadership in building stronger local, state, or regional associations, or who have contributed to the improvement of the national organization, are eligible for the award.

Also notable is the award named for the late Dr. Leo K. Bustad, a former dean of the Washington State University College of Veterinary Medicine and a past president of the Pet Partners (formerly Delta Society). The Bustad Companion Animal Veterinarian of the Year Award honors the outstanding work of veterinarians in preserving and protecting human-animal relationships. This award is co-sponsored by the AVMA, Pet Partners, and Hill's Pet Nutrition Inc. The Bustad Award includes a $5,000 grant to the winner with a $5,000 grant to the veterinary college or not-for-profit service program of the veterinarian's choice to further work in improving human–companion animal interactions.

Lasting alliances

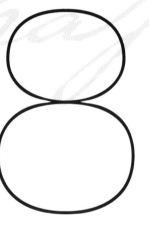

Susan C. Kahler

Partnerships, strategic alliances, and coalitions have enabled the American Veterinary Medical Association to enhance its offerings, strengthen its voice, fund valuable initiatives, and promote common goals. These liaisons have helped advance the profession's mission in areas ranging from legislative advocacy to pet wellness to veterinary continuing education. Collaborating entities have run the gamut from nonprofits to government agencies to corporations.

A few relationships have stirred controversy. In the mid-1990s, the profession became polarized over whether to continue teaming up on a common goal by endorsing the Doris Day Animal League's Spay Day USA, torn by concerns that the sponsor also advocated an end to the use of animals in production agriculture and research. Con-

troversy also arose in 2005 over the propriety of joining forces financially with Heifer International to provide recovery aid to impoverished families in South and Central Asia after a tsunami hit the region, although few would dispute the good AVMA did in raising $1 million.

Most AVMA partnerships have been straightforward and fruitful. The four entities most closely linked to the AVMA in long-lived partnerships are the Auxiliary to the AVMA, American Veterinary Medical Foundation, AVMA Group Health & Life Insurance Trust, and AVMA PLIT. Their collaboration with the AVMA collectively spans 250 years.

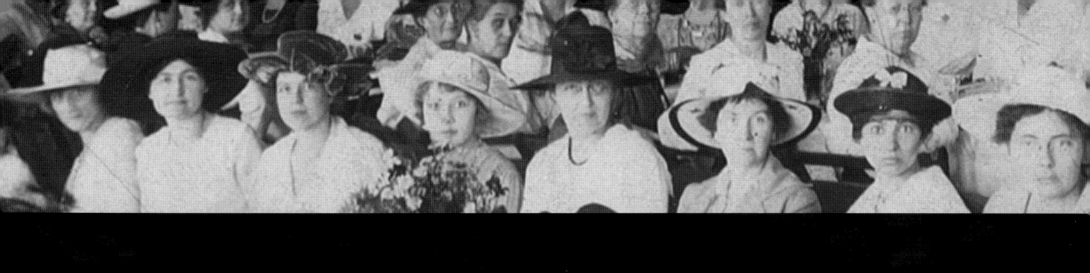

partners

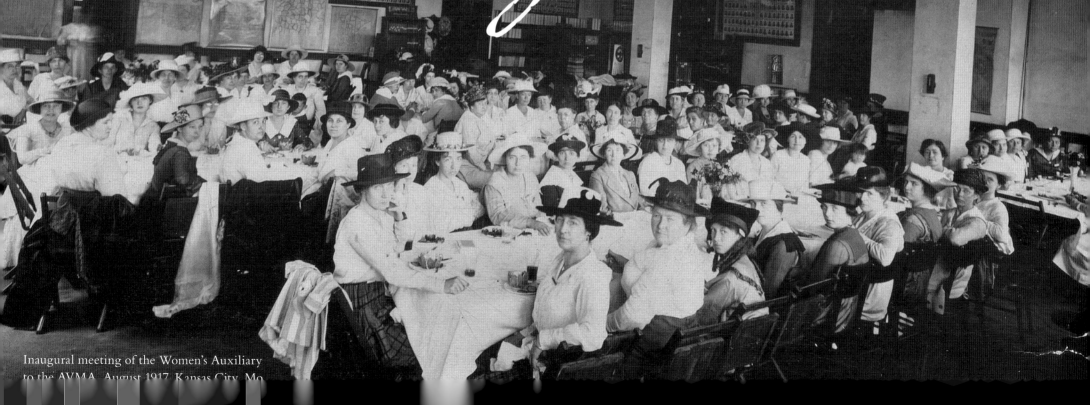

Inaugural meeting of the Women's Auxiliary to the AVMA, August 1917, Kansas City, Mo.

AUXILIARY TO THE AVMA

The oldest of these four AVMA partners is the Auxiliary to the AVMA. In fact, the Auxiliary holds the distinction of being the first auxiliary to the healing arts established in the United States.

It was during World War I, before women had a vote, that the Women's Auxiliary to the American Veterinary Medical Association was formed at the Kansas City Veterinary College in Missouri. The date was Aug. 22, 1917.

Membership was open to wives, daughters, mothers, sisters, and widows of veterinarians. The 55 original members set annual dues at 50 cents and elected Mrs. W. Horace Hoskins of Philadelphia as their first president; 12 years later, she would be honored as the Auxiliary's "mother." Each state was to select a secretary to report to the national auxiliary.

For women who just wanted to support their husbands' profession and have fun in the process, the Auxiliary met with some stiff opposition, as told in the Auxiliary's 75th anniversary history, from which many of these highlights through 1992 are excerpted.

Even before the organization was created, some veterinarians had taken their wives to AVMA meetings. The women got together for food, fun, and "the swapping of ideas on how to be a good wife to a veterinarian." But some men thought the presence of women hampered their social freedom, and it was a generally held opinion that women had no place in their husband's business.

At the 1918 AVMA Annual Convention in Philadelphia, opposition leaders stationed themselves at the Auxiliary's meeting-room door to block entry, but supporters prevailed. In 1923 in Montreal, challengers again tried to dissolve the Auxiliary but were foiled, and Canadian women were admitted for the first time.

AN EVOLVING MISSION

Having prevailed, the Auxiliary launched into its work of supporting the veterinary profession, adapting its objectives over the years to meet the changing needs.

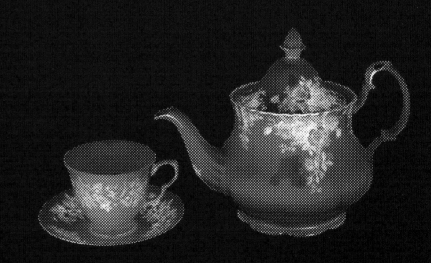

The women got together for food, fun, and "the swapping of ideas on how to be a good wife to a veterinarian." But some men thought the presence of women hampered their social freedom, and it was a generally held opinion that women had no place in their husband's business.

In 1918, the Auxiliary adopted a constitution and bylaws with the objective "... to give necessary financial assistance to the family of any veterinarian engaged in war work if his life has been forfeited in pursuance of such work, or if he has been temporarily or permanently disabled."

With the need for war relief over by the 1919 convention in New Orleans, the Auxiliary sought new ways to serve and amended its constitution to state that its object was "to give necessary financial assistance to the family of a veterinarian if he has been temporarily or permanently disabled."

The only such request ever made and filled was $50 to a family for fuel in 1921.

In 1920, the Auxiliary appointed a committee to study the suggestion of providing financial aid, in the form of loans, to veterinary students. The loan committee consulted with college deans and AVMA members. The following year, after hearing the committee's report, the Auxiliary authorized a student loan fund and amended its objective to state: "The object of the Auxiliary shall include a loan fund to be used for the assistance of needy veterinary students." That year, a student at The Ohio State University received the first loan, of $175.

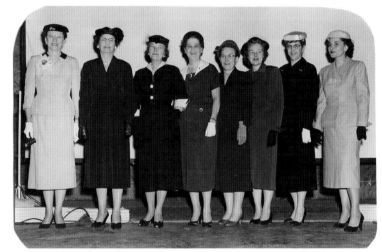

Auxiliary officers, 1956-1957

Within four years, requests for student loans had increased beyond the Auxiliary's resources, so the AVMA placed $2,000 from the Salmon Memorial Fund at the disposal of the Auxiliary, which, in turn, paid the AVMA 4 percent interest on the amount used.

$175 first student loan, given to a student at The Ohio State University, 1920

Demand for loans reflected the events of the day. The Stock Market Crash of 1929 drove up demand, as did the Great Depression. In 1947, demand dropped, with many returning World War II veterans receiving educational grants under the GI Bill of Rights. By 1954, the AVMA had accredited 19 colleges, driving demand back up.

To generate resources for loans, the Auxiliary at various times borrowed from the AVMA, limited the number of loans it made to students, conducted a membership drive, and established a Memorial Fund for donors to honor friends and relatives.

In 1951, AVMA President Clarence P. Zepp Sr. appealed for the Auxiliary's help with fundraising for the AVMA Research Trust, which had been created five years earlier. During 1951, the Auxiliary made only one student loan, so it was looking for other ways to serve veterinarians. As a result, the Auxiliary became more active in public relations and research fundraising.

Within 10 years, the Auxiliary achieved its goal of conducting a campaign to raise $75,000 for fellowships through the research fund.

Up to then, the Auxiliary had been involved in various public relations efforts. In 1945, it produced the booklet "What the Veterinary Profession Means to the Public." At the AVMA's request, in 1955 the Auxiliary set up a radio committee to sponsor a public relations program. AVMA members carried out radio, and, later, TV programs, arranged and coordinated by Auxiliary members. The new Auxiliary committee assisted constituent auxiliaries with these public relations activities. In 1975, the Auxiliary introduced its public relations guide "Is There a Veterinarian in the House?"

In 1973, the Auxiliary appointed a panel to compile a list of books that would enhance the profession, and two years later, the organization distributed its first "approved booklist" to librarians across the country.

The Auxiliary's popular Marketplace of States, an AVMA convention event featuring items offered by constituent auxiliaries, often netted thousands of dollars for the student loan fund and other educational projects. In 1976, the Auxiliary donated $10,702 for the veterinary exhibit at the Museum of Science and Industry in Chicago, and in 1991 it contributed $10,000 for partial funding of an AVMA Congressional Science Fellowship. The Auxiliary even compiled and sold cookbooks and raised money to purchase an automatic flagpole for the first headquarters building the AVMA owned in Schaumburg, Ill., in 1975.

SOCIAL CONVENTIONS

The Auxiliary has always teamed work with pleasure. Even in 1917, some patriotic veterinarians' wives served a luncheon before the organizational meeting, observing the wartime "wheatless Wednesdays" by serving a suitable Boston brown bread, a veal salad, and ice cream in cantaloupe halves. At the 1918 AVMA meeting in Philadelphia, a group of veterinarians took their wives on a side trip to Atlantic City to "jump the breakers." The women were dressed in ruffled caps, black stockings, and daring knee-length bathing suits.

Whether a moonlight cruise on the St. Lawrence or a glass-bottom boat ride along Catalina Island, an excursion to Mount Rainier or a clambake in New England, Auxiliary members found fun amid their work and encountered history along the way. In 1933, they visited the Chicago World's Fair, and in 1959, the Truman Library in Independence, Mo., where former President Harry S. Truman addressed them. Aviatrix Amelia Earhart spoke at an Auxiliary luncheon held for the wives of foreign visitors at the 1934 New York meeting.

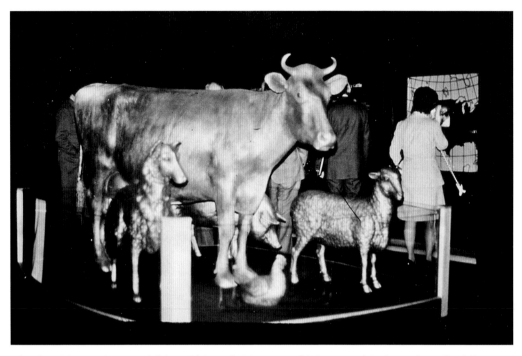

The AVMA veterinary exhibit at Chicago's Museum of Science and Industry benefited from Auxiliary support.

In 1978, the Auxiliary adopted the following pledge: "As members of the Auxiliary to the AVMA, we pledge ourselves to these goals: To assist in informing the public of the value of veterinary services. To assist selected veterinary students with loans and awards. To strengthen the bonds of friendship among those connected with the veterinary profession." The Auxiliary introduced a media kit two years later to help with public service announcements.

Besides public relations, the Auxiliary undertook many educational and fundraising projects. It began selling jewelry bearing the Auxiliary crest and released the handbook "Today's Topics for Veterinarians' Wives" in 1969. Incentive awards were presented to a graduating student and a fourth-year student's spouse at each veterinary college, and to state science fair winners. The Auxiliary sponsored various student auxiliary activities and created an honor roll for constituent auxiliaries that achieved certain benchmarks.

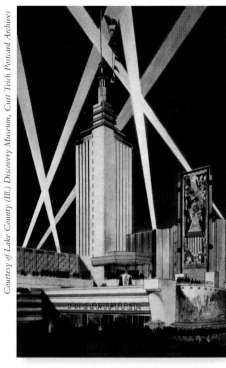

The Women's Auxiliary celebrated its golden anniversary in 1967 in Dallas' Baker Hotel. Auxiliary board members costumed in clothes fashionable in 1917 served as hostesses. Entertainment was a look at "Hats and history" from 1896-1967. Decorating the tables were dolls dressed by constituent auxiliaries in fashions of the preceding 50 years. Charter members Lillie Grossman and Margaret Lockhart cut the anniversary cake.

DOWN TO BUSINESS

The Auxiliary amended its constitution and bylaws in 1924 to provide for its Executive Board, and in 1930, a movement was begun to encourage formation of state auxiliaries, laying the foundation for the Auxiliary's House of Representatives, later called House of Delegates. By the 1947 meeting, there were 25 well-organized state auxiliaries. In 1939, the Women's Auxiliary to the American Veterinary Medical Association was incorporated in Illinois, where the AVMA office in Chicago was handling the student loan fund. The articles of incorporation were amended in 1977 to change the name to the Auxiliary to the American Veterinary Medical Association.

The Hall of Science at the 1933-1934 World's Fair in Chicago included an AVMA exhibit. The Auxiliary visited the fair.

The 1946 meeting was the first where membership cards and dues receipts were issued, marking the first time that membership was considered independently from attendance at the national convention.

Each Junior AVMA organization at a veterinary school had an auxiliary by 1948, and five of these student auxiliaries had affiliated with the AVMA Auxiliary. 1949 was a year of sweeping changes, according to the Auxiliary's 75th anniversary history, as the organization set aside its old structure and adopted a new constitution. In 1950, a Foreign Relations Committee was created to be the liaison with the Women's International Veterinary Auxiliary.

Courtesy of Lake County (Ill.) Discovery Museum, Curt Teich Postcard Archives

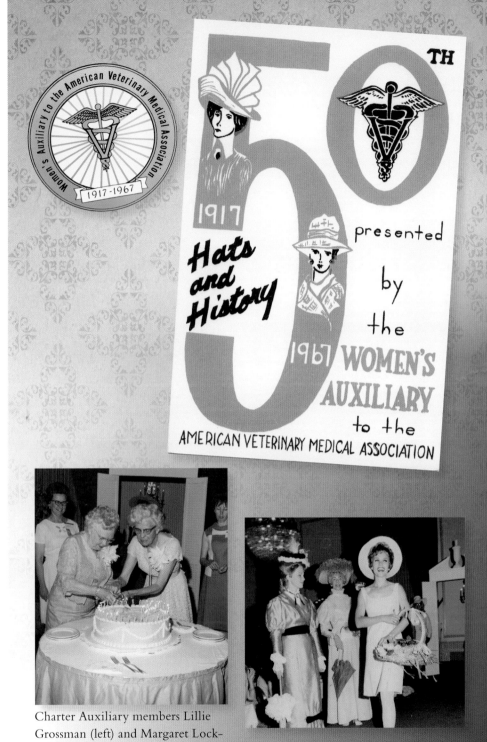

Charter Auxiliary members Lillie Grossman (left) and Margaret Lockhart cut the golden anniversary cake.

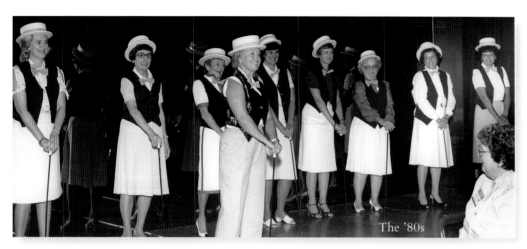

The '80s

CHALLENGING TIMES

The gender shift that eventually led to employed female veterinarians outnumbering males in 2009 was associated with a corresponding decline in Auxiliary members. In its first 40 years, the Auxiliary saw its membership increase from the original 55 charter members to 6,000. Membership peaked at more than 10,000 in 1971. But by 1990, the number had fallen to 6,460, and by 2000, it was 2,765. As of July 2012, the Auxiliary had 303 dues-paying members and 644 life members.

Ginger Morton, 2011-2012 Auxiliary president, takes a sanguine view. "There has been a strong trend of ladies joining the veterinary field, and this, too, opens doors for a new face for the Auxiliary through male spouses."

Ironically, a bright spot was the August 2012 installation of the first male president in Auxiliary history. Greg Mooney of Mount Gilead, Ohio, husband of Dr. Marty Mooney, a 1978 graduate of The Ohio State University, has been active in the AVMA and Ohio VMA auxiliaries for 34 years. He retired as a lieutenant colonel in 1997 after 20 years of active duty with the U.S. Air Force and with the Ohio Air National Guard.

At its 1959 meeting, the Auxiliary adopted a new constitution that closely paralleled the AVMA's. Each state or provincial auxiliary was allowed a delegation of one to seven members. That fall, the Auxiliary set up its office in the AVMA headquarters in Chicago, which led to a closer relationship and exchange of ideas. The Auxiliary HOD began conducting all the organization's business in 1964. Representation was based on one delegate for every 50 members in good standing.

The Auxiliary had an office supervisor until 1968, when the title became executive secretary. AVMA staff member Lavina Davenport served in that position from 1959-1974, when the Auxiliary office was moved to Manhattan, Kan., and Maxine Caley became executive secretary. In 1992, the Auxiliary moved into rent-free space at AVMA headquarters in Schaumburg, Ill., and Chris Kanalas served as executive secretary until 1999. Temporary directors were engaged until Jan Knewtson became secretary-treasurer and took over administrative duties out of Iola, Kan., from 2004-2010.

The name of each Auxiliary president is listed on a plaque displayed at AVMA headquarters since it was presented to Executive Vice President Ron DeHaven at the 2011 AVMA convention in St. Louis.

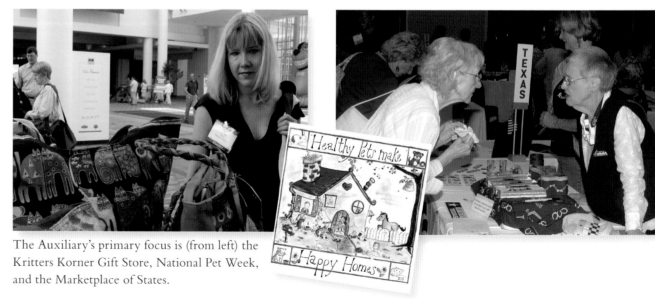

The Auxiliary's primary focus is (from left) the Kritters Korner Gift Store, National Pet Week, and the Marketplace of States.

C O N T E N T S

INTRODUCTION

YOUR EDITOR'S COUNSELOR in such matters insists that we must have an introduction that will bring what we have to say up to this point, but not beyond into what more properly belongs in subsequent volumes.

For in those we hope to reveal the ultimate human resources that will make possible lifting the world out of its still seemingly ever-deepening crisis.

In the present volume we deal quite fully with the importance of human capital, once recognized but subsequently deliberately buried to allow our deregulated banks to continue their irresponsible escapade that threatens the survival of our civilization.

And as though to make that important point, *The Globe and Mail* (12/08/09), "Virgin Atlantic unveils first commercial spaceship" by Urene Klotz, Mojave CA) meets our need to an extent that we had not dared dream of.

"Virgin Atlantic Airways yesterday unveiled the first passenger spaceship, a sleek black-and-white vessel that represents a gamble with a sky-high price tag to create a commercial space and tourism industry.

"The company hopes the winged, minivan-sized Space-ShipTwo will rocket tourists into zero gravity beginning in two or three years.

"'This will be the start of commercial space travel,' Virgin Atlantic Airways founder and billionaire Richard Branson said at the launch in California's Mojave Desert. 'You become an astronaut.'

"The project with a $450 million (US) budget, would see the construction of six commercial spaceships that would take passengers high enough to achieve weightlessness and see the curvature of Earth set against the backdrop of space.

"A twin-hulled aircraft would carry SpaceShipTwo to an altitude of about 18 kilometers before releasing it. The spaceship would then fire its onboard rocket engines, climbing to about 104 kilometers above Earth.

"The trip would take about two and a half hours, and passengers would experience about five minutes of weightlessness.

"Some 300 aspiring astronauts have put down deposits for the $200,000 ride, which includes three days of training.

"Eventually, Virgin Galactic, the offshoot of Virgin Atlantic that is marketing space travel, hopes to cut the ticket price to be competitive with that of air travel between the US and Australia.

"The unit is considering also providing suborbital travel between destinations that would cut the length of a flight between the US and Australia to about 90 minutes from about 15 hours or more.

"A 10-month atmospheric test-flight program is expected to begin on Tuesday and would be followed by extensive flights into space before passenger travel is scheduled to begin in 2011 or 2012."

The major lesson of that is that education changes the very nature of the human race. The realities brushed upon by the Greek and Renaissance philosophers that redefined what man saw and measured and, hence, what man was and could be, has recreated him in command of the outer spaces.

At the very time that more earthbound specimens are finding it tougher keeping even an automobile firm non-bankrupt and adequately fueled, others are learning to re-assess such problems in outer space with a lavish saving in time and fuel.

William Krehm
January 2010

Correction and Apology

Your editor, having entered his latter nineties, experiences some difficulties in remembering names even of those whom he has the greatest reason for not forgetting. Thus, it happened that in the third volume of *Meltdown* I garbled the name of Ursula Hicks, my encounter with whom was the most positive thing that I experienced at the conference at Cambridge University that I attended some three years ago.

Professor Hicks is with the University of London, and in the special sessions that she organized at that Cambridge conference those adhering to the present Cambridge's current pre-Keynesian orthodoxies received a haven. When I recounted the abandonment of the ceiling on interest rates by the US Treasury behind the back of President Truman – at the very beginning of the Korean War! – she joined me in speaking the date of that treachery in unison

Paul Martin's Unique Opportunity for Atonement

IN THIS AGE when the history of economic thought is being buried ever more deeply, it is encouraging that students are learning to treat the computer as a friend rather than foe. Thanks to a freshman York University student, Chris Wiseman, son of one of COMER's leaders, we have before us the document "Implementation of Full Accrual Accountancy" from a website of the Federal Government, www.fin.gc.ca/toce/2001/fullacc_e.html.

There couldn't be better timing for this document coming to light. Without a clear distinction between current and capital spending, no industrial corporation could ever have produced a balance sheet that didn't declare it bankrupt. However, until very recently our federal government has avoided capital budgeting (a.k.a. "accrual accountancy") like the plague. Whenever Ottawa built a bridge or a building, it wrote off the expenditure in the first year. This enormously exaggerated current spending, and in subsequent years the government books carried non-financial investment at a single dollar. Obviously that showed our government eternally on the verge of bankruptcy, unless it was doing away with enough essential public services. That bogus "debt," displayed without the balancing investment that much of it had paid for, was used as a multi-pronged argument: (1) for the Bank of Canada pushing up interest rates "to fight inflation due to the growing deficit and debt"; (2) for raising taxes unnecessarily to balance such hopeless bookkeeping *and* paying these excessive interest rates; (3) for slashing social programs essential for the proper functioning of society; (4) to spread the legend that government is always inefficient and irresponsible, in contrast to the private sector, which is always thrifty, efficient, and honest. To top this performance, over the past forty years our governments disregarded the recommendations of at least three royal commissions to bring capital budgeting into their accounts.

That is the very stuff of major scandal. It can match any of the mega-ripoffs on Wall St. And over those forty-odd years, the economy developed in a way that required ever more expensive infrastructures, both physical and human. From the semi-rural country that was Canada before WWII, it became urbanized. Its high-tech economy had need of a far more educated population. Women, whose full-time attention was indispensable for the extended and indeed even for the nuclear family, became an essential part of the commercial labour force. That left the family dependent on government help for internal services that a mother holding an outside job could no longer provide. Even though education and health are stored in private minds and bodies, investment to improve them enriches the government's tax base and hence is an assured government investment. More-over, both health and education, far from depreciating, go on appreciating as they are handed down to later generations.

The Very Stuff of Scandal

In the 1960s, investment in human capital was fleetingly recognized by economists as the most productive of all investments. But despite that, the persistent edging-up of the price index since the 1960s due to the deepening layer of taxation in price to pay for such services was confused with "inflation." That should have been identified as a very distinct "structural price rise" rather than attributed to an excess of total demand over available supply. To make matters still worse, the tools to rein in this ill-defined "inflation" were narrowed down to a single one: raising interest rates high enough "to do the job." Interest, however, happens to be the revenue of a social group that needs no encouragement to become parasitic.

While Washington goes on searching for Bin Laden and Iraqi Major Tools of Destruction, they have overlooked the role of Wall St's sanctification of high interest during the 1970s in provoking the wave of fanatical Muslim terrorists to destabilize the world. And yet the Koran does condemn to hell-fire those who persist not only in usury, but even in collecting plain interest. Thus the absence of serious accountancy in the government bookkeeping of the West has been a key factor in the bloody chasm that has come to separate an alarming portion of the Muslim world from the West.

The crowning of interest as the one stabilizer of price and the economy, led to a massive transfer to money-lenders not only of a large cut of the national product, but of power. And that not only made possible the massive bail-out of our banks in the early 1990s, but the further deregulation of the financial sector. That allowed the bank holding companies to acquire stockbrokers, financial underwriters, merchant bankers, insurance companies and derivative boutiques. In this way the exponential growth of the financial sector came to gorge on every other part of the economy and on weaker countries to which much real production was shifted. But these new involvements are incompatible with banking proper. Once banks took over stock markets, they themselves became vulnerable to high interest rates, since high rates are poison to anything connected with the stock market.

The founding fathers of economics considered interest a portion of the profit paid by the producer for a loan of the money needed to run his business. If it even approached the total average profit, the economy was headed for a break-down. Since the 1970s, however, it has been seen not as a component of gross profit, but as subject to no ceiling. It fiddles the tune to which the rest of society must dance That has upended the world economy.

This was a major factor in the belated recognition of accrual accountancy that governments had resisted over many decades.

But how to bring it in, after having surrendered the real economy for decades to the banks? Perforce it had to be slipped in by stealth. At the beginning of 1996, the Clinton administration in the US smuggled in accrual accountancy treatment of *physical* investments of government.[1] It was presented as an increase in government savings, which it was not. What was brought into the asset side of the government books was not held as cash but had already been invested. What Clinton needed and got was just a more favourable statistic that would give him an improved rating for government bonds and bring down interest rates, but that would *not* stir up the sleeping dogs of the right. Carried back several years, it enhanced the government balance sheet by some $1.3 trillion. That was a major factor in the lower interest rates that brought on the greatest stock market boom on record.

It took Canada another three and a half years – and the refusal of the Auditor General to approve its accounts unconditionally – to follow in the footsteps of the US. The compromise between the then Minister of Finance, Paul Martin, and the Auditor General at the time took many turbulent weeks in the making. And when it came in, it included a self-demeaning statement by the Auditor General. A deal had been struck as though the recognition of a fundamental law of accountancy was subject to back-stage arm-twisting. The Auditor General declared that since no new money had been brought into the treasury by the change in accountancy, it warranted no increase in government spending.

This was an obvious distortion of the facts. The bailout of the banks in 1991 from their heavy speculative losses had been achieved by doing away with the statutory reserves requiring them to deposit with the central bank a modest part of the short-term deposits they received from the public. Those reserves earned them no interest and put at the disposal of the Canadian government over $120 billion dollars of interest-free money. Now that amount was returned to the banks, which directly or indirectly lent it to the federal government. In the following years the federal government slashed its grants to the provinces by a like magnitude. And the provinces cut their financial support to municipalities. Now that the interest-burden to the federal government has been somewhat reduced by the recognition of its non-financial capital assets, it had to be brought in with extreme caution: for it could blow carefully nurtured reputations for "fiscal responsibility" sky-high. So the Auditor General was forced to declare that it put no new money in the hands of Ottawa for necessary programs.

Capitalism would not be capitalism, were it not possible to borrow against properly valued, income-producing capital assets to finance further investments. Instead, Finance Minister Paul Martin bargained the Auditor General into publicly denying that basic principle of accountancy. Constraining auditors in a not dissimilar manner has earned Wall St. operators fines and even jail sentences. Why should ministers of the Crown get away with doing exactly that? Instead of coming clean with the public, Paul Martin hived off the money saved through the introduction of accrual accountancy as reserves to bolster his boast as champion budget balancer.

Only a single paper published word of the introduction of accrual accountancy when the bill was passed in mid-1999 – Conrad Black's *National Post,* that was desperate for new readers. No debate on the bill took place in Parliament. When the translation of the measure into actual budgetary terms was reported in mid-2003, a new Finance Minister, John Manley, mentioned the contribution of accrual accountancy to his budgetary surplus, but the Liberal caucus that had voted in the bill bringing in accrual accountancy in 1999 didn't seem to know what he was talking about. Within a couple of days the usual senseless number-crunching took over. An epoch-making measure in the history of the land was reduced to a matter of surplus versus deficit.

A Freshman Student Digs Up What Paul Martin has Buried

But now an alert freshman student has fished out of the Internet the actual text of the "Implementation of Full Accrual Accounting in the Federal Government's Financial Statements." That helps us close in on some key hushed-up facts.

To begin with, we must correct the title of the document "Implementation of Full Accrual Accounting in the Federal Government's Financial Statements." In the case of private firms financial and physical assets give a true picture of the asset side of their balance sheet. That is not so in the case of governments. Their revenue is primarily taxation, and thus their main capital asset is their investment in human capital. Economists in the 1960s, pondering the rapidity with which Germany and Japan had reconstructed their economies from the wreckage of the war, concluded that investment in human capital was more productive than the physical capital, which had been so widely destroyed.[2]

Quoting from the government website document unearthed by Chris Wiseman: "What does full accrual accounting mean?

"1. Capital assets will be recognized on the Government's financial assets. This will have no effect on the net public debt (gross liabilities less financial assets), but it will have an impact on the accumulated *deficit* (net public debt less non-financial assets)....

"3. In moving to accrual accounting, the Government will change its accounting policy with respect to Aboriginal and environmental liabilities. Environmental liabilities are currently not recognized in the financial statements and Aboriginal liabilities are not fully recognized."

This represents two instances of "internalizing" capital destruction that had been put out of mind by conventional economists as "externalities." There is nothing external to the economy in unemployment, broken-up families, epidemics, undernourishment. This modest beginning of bringing two major instances of capital destruction into the balance sheet must be expanded to take in *all* supposed "externalities." But the Auditor General of the time, Dennis Desautel – God bless him – had stood up to Paul Martin's arm-twisting at least on this important point.

However, in the first declaration of our new government's fiscal policy, it breaks its agreement that was the price of the

Auditor General giving unconditional acceptance of Ottawa's balance sheets of two years. Why are the "environmental and liabilities" mentioned in item three disregarded in the new Finance Minister's statement? To say nothing about all the other deficits in maintaining our physical and human infrastructures? That serves a timely warning of what the Martin regime will bring Canadians, unless we reclaim our democratic right to be properly informed with meaningful accountancy.

An adequate treatment of these "externalities" calls for bringing systems theory into our economic reckonings. This sets up all areas of the economy that are essential for the system as a whole to survive. It becomes important accordingly to monitor *all* subsystems to prevent one subsystem from cannibalizing another. They do have distinct food chains, but these overlap. For example, all non-market systems depend mostly on government funding. And they have need of an economic theory that derogates no subsystem as an "externality." If, for example, the government claims to balance its budget by cutting vital items in the educational budget, that must be entered as a deficit. For its results will certainly show up in deficient educational standards of the population in years ahead.

The "Backgrounder on the Implementation of Accrual Accountancy" ends on this rather inconclusive note:

"It is premature to provide estimates on the impact of these changes. Departments and agencies are in the process of quantifying their assets and liabilities. *These will have to be reviewed by the Auditor General* [our italics – this is obviously a condition of the bargain between the previous Auditor General and the government]. As a result, the impacts will not be fully known until the audited financial statements for 2001-02 are finalized."

And there is a table of the expected direction of these changes.

For example, both the environmental liabilities are expected to show increases in the net debt and accumulated debt. As are "Aboriginal Liabilities." There is no mention of the conditions of health, social welfare, and education, which are under provincial jurisdiction but depend heavily on federal grants for their funding.

Our New PM Owes the Nation an Explanation

This leaves our new head of government, Paul Martin, owing the electorate an explanation. When the Liberals took over the government, Mr. Martin as incoming Minister of Finance organized a huge conference at the luxurious Metropolitan hotel in Toronto to which friendly journalists were invited, supposedly to consult, but actually to speak each his or her three minutes of assent to his budget-balancing intentions. Those who had proposals that dissented from the Liberal party line were left cooling their heels outside the conference room. That included notably three members of COMER, the late John Hotson, Jack Biddell, who had headed Trudeau's price control agency for Ontario, and myself. Among our proposals a notable feature was accrual accountancy.

The previous Conservative government of Brian Mulroney had bailed out our banks from their massive gas and oil and real estate speculations. This had been done by shifting massive

amounts of federal government debt from the Bank of Canada from where the interest paid on it returned to the federal government substantially as dividends. For since 1938 the federal government has been the central bank's sole shareholder. Now the borrowings of the federal government shifted directly and indirectly to the chartered banks whence the interest paid on that debt does *not* come back to it. That was the hidden essence of the bailout, adding as much as $8 billion a year onto the interest on the government's debt. That debt – driven into the sky both by the use of high rates "to lick inflation" and by the growing burden of interest paid by the government to the stricken banks. And this was extracted from an economy depressed by those same interest rates. It was, moreover, no one-shot bailout. It was an *entitlement* returning each year like the summer solstice. Most of Canada's government debt directly and indirectly can be traced to that hidden *coup d'état*.

Had the new Minister of Finance, Paul Martin, lent ear to a succession of Auditors General or to COMER, he could have avoided slashing grants to the provinces supporting vital social services. Even today the government, according to the above-cited "Backgrounder on Accrual Accountancy," will not be in a position to tell the public what the real deficit might be for some years. How then could the new Finance Minister almost a decade ago have been so sure of the extent of the actual deficit as to deprive millions of Canadians of their livelihoods? This was accomplished by welching on his party's promise to do away with the Goods and Service Tax, and to allow the Bank of Canada to continue its deflationary policy. Sooner or later Mr. Martin will have to answer for this sorry record.

Millions of Canadians were deprived in this way of jobs and a proper education. Families were broken. There is no way in which their lives can be made whole again. Obviously, nobody can sue a Prime Minister, properly elected – if you ignore the complete suppression of all key information about the government debt. Canadians tend to be charitable to their new governments. Paul Martin must not fail to take advantage of this honeymoon period. When freshman students, can punch up the truth about hushed-up legislation it would be dangerous for Mr. Martin to stick to his old tricks. If he flubs this opportunity of atoning for his past, he and his government will incur an awful fate. He must remember that other high-flier, master of glib deceptions, Brian Mulroney. And the wreckage he brought to *his* smashingly successful party.

Our media is full of the scandals on Wall St. where the state prosecutor and the Security Exchange Commission are fining financial houses for as much as $1.4 billion requiring them to restate their earnings of previous years. None of the reinstatements of their accounts were of the magnitude of those the Canadian government is currently engaged in. And in almost all cases their firms' auditors were in cahoots with the executives in cooking their books. That was not the case of the Government of Canada. And now it is evident that what passed for "fiscal responsibility" was in fact "fiscal irresponsibility" that directed billions of revenue from the vital infrastructures of the country to financial speculators.

Rather than repeating his infamous consultation scam of a

decade ago, the new PM would be wiser to expiate his sins with frankness. Doing away with the GST, as promised by his party a decade ago, would be an astute first step in that direction.

William Krehm

1. The reader is urged not to take this on faith. The change can be found in the National Savings figure for January 1996 of the Bureau of Economic Analysis of the US Department of Commerce.

2. Krehm, William (1975). *Price in a Mixed Economy – Our Record of Disaster.* Toronto: Thornwood Publications. Chapter 13, "Society's Forgotten Capital Assets."

Consulting Dostoevsky on Our Split-Personality Economy

WE HAVE ENTERED a critical period in which conventional economics has developed a split-personality. One half of its doctrine turns up at every critical juncture to brand the other half a liar. It calls to mind Dostoevsky's short story, *The Double*. A modest government bureaucrat, Yakov Petrovich Golyadkin, is always being mortally embarrassed by the other half of his split personality. No matter what he tries, it always pops up as another person – same name, same address, same appearance, but with just the character traits that he tries hard to suppress in himself. That double invariably compromises him before the very people he wishes to impress, his superiors in the government service, the fancy social acquaintances whose receptions he tries to crash, the expensive restaurant where he intends to spend a limited amount, while his double, unknown to him, goes on ordering ten times as much as he can afford, and embarrasses him when he tries arguing with the waiter when the bill is presented. The amazing thing in the tale is that nobody but the hero seems to recognize that there are two Golyadkins with quite contradictory characters. Instead they blame the noble-minded Golyadkin for the social gaffes and the crude self-promotions of his unwanted twin.

In official economics the Golyadkin of the self-balancing market is supposed to deliver to us the blessings of a "level playing field," a flat price level, higher efficiency, fiscal responsibility, the trickle-down of the blessings it bestows ever more lavishly on those at the top. However, its double, who is in the driver's seat, instead of these promised blessings has given rise to the greatest bonanza of the legal profession in the constant stream of civil and criminal prosecutions against some of the largest US corporations.

Now let us shift to evidence of the damage that the cynical, grasping "other Golyadkin" has heaped on the "noble" Golyadkin of his own dreams. *The Wall Street Journal* (1/12, "Railroad Logjams Threaten Boom in the Farm Belt" by Scott Kilman and Daniel Machalaba) informs us:

"In a harbinger of potential snags across the US, a sudden boom in the farm sector has combined with shortages of railcars and crews to delay freight trains and lead to higher delivery costs for farmers across the country. The Lord knows that US farmers have waited long enough for such bonanza. But now that it seems to have come, it is being allowed to dribble away, because the 'fiscal responsibility' of the other economic Golyadkin – Wall St.'s itch for ever mounting speculative profits – has prevented it from maintaining its transportation infrastructures to meet the growing world hunger. This is crippling our farmers' ability to supply it when the weather has finally given them a break."

Trains a Month Late

"The demand for grain-hauling equipment is hot because the Farm Belt is humming after five years of recession. Grain prices are profitable for farmers in large part because corn and wheat exports have soared 24% since September 1, a reflection of poor harvests this year in Europe and elsewhere. But failure to deliver their goods is cutting into potential profits.

"That is because years of cost-cutting on both personnel and equipment have left railroads short-handed, forcing them to scramble to deal with the unexpected surge in both the agriculture sector and the economy in general.

"Indeed, delivery times for everything from lumber to containers of consumer products have started to climb. And that could eventually lead to higher prices for items ranging from breakfast cereals to cars.

"'We are going to see logjams, bottle-necks and service disruptions as rail freight picks up with the rest of the economy,' says Tom Finkbiner, a former railroad executive who is now chief executive of Quality Distribution Inc. of Tampa, Fla., the nation's biggest bulk trucking firm. He is also chairman of the University of Denver's Intermodal Transportation Institute.

"About 40% of the nation's grain is transported by railroad, with most of the remainder being carried by trucks and barges. The delays are sparking fears that bottlenecks might also arise in other sectors of the US economy as they also get busier.

"Farmers in Reynolds, ND, for instance are still waiting for a train scheduled to arrive November 1. As a result, the economy of the tiny farm town is slowing. Reynolds United grain elevator has stopped buying wheat from growers because it can't move the 270,000 bushels it already has bought. The cooperative is dependent on Burlington Northern Santa Fe Corp., the second-biggest railroad to move its wheat to market.

"This year the train shortage is far more severe than usual during harvest season, resulting in higher expenses for everybody from Washington state potato growers and Arkansas chicken farmers to owners of cattle feedlots in Texas. To keep their plants supplied with Midwest grain, some feed mills are turning to trucks, a more expensive mode of transportation than rail.

"The conditions of the nation's rail fleet has deteriorated in recent years, particularly so its grain-hauling equipment. According to Steven McClure, president of the rail-leasing unit of CIT Group, 68% of railroad-owned grain cars are more than 20 years old.

"Burlington Northern, for instance, was caught off-guard by the record corn harvest and a bumper wheat crop. It had allowed its fleet of grain-hopper cars to shrink 24% over the past five years to 26,500 cars. In addition to equipment, the railroad industry is short of skilled workers. For example, Union Pacific Corp., the nation's largest railroad, didn't move quickly enough to replace retiring locomotive crews.

"The farm sector's demand for trains this autumn is particularly strong thanks in part to the need to move soya beans to ports to export to China, which is buying US soya beans at a record pace. The domestic appetite for grain is strong, too. A rebound in the consumer demand for beef is lifting cattle price to record highs.

"Grain industry officials say the logjams are the worst since 1997, when railway mergers left the Farm Belt in knots. The added expenses threaten the recovering agricultural sector."

The mergers, which notably included most prominently the privatized Canadian National Railways, was designed for maximum stock market effect. And once the bumper profits were taken as capital gains, to maintain those higher stock prices and push them further, management had to cut every possible cost to the bone. That was brilliant stock-market efficiency, but is turning out disastrous railroading.

"Transportation is a big part of the cost of making food, so the train shortage will help keep upward pressure on food prices already being pushed higher by rising cattle and crop prices.

"For the food industry the rails are getting more expensive in all sorts of ways. For instance, the charge for leasing one grain-hopper car for one month has doubled over the past six month to about $300.

"Even the customers getting relatively prompt service are having to pay a lot to make sure that happens. West Central Cooperative in Ralston, Iowa, is a priority for Union Pacific because the farmer-owned grain-elevator network is large enough to fill a 100-car shuttle train, the type of grain train most efficient for the railroad to handle. But the premium the cooperative can pay above the basic rate to guarantee on-time arrival – a price established through a secondary market much like the scalping of a sport ticket – has more than doubled to $250 a car in recent weeks."

Dostoevsky as Consultant for Washington

If we were to try putting the non-functional parts into which the world's food crisis has split up – entirely like Dostoevsky's hero – we, would come up with the following:

1. Governments – especially that of the US – go on subsidizing their farmers to grow grain and other foodstuffs. At the same time international organizations like the IMF and the World Bank pressure emerging and third world countries to remove the tariffs that protected them from competition. They force acceptance of such a course by manipulating the debt of these vulnerable lands. With their dependence on debt renewal, this means the surrender of their sovereignty in determining their national interest. As a result food production in these poorer land languishes, and they become more and more dependent on imports for their food. Now it appears that the developed nations have not even kept their transport systems in shape to deliver the food that they have forced the less developed countries to count on.

2. At the same time, the US government, to bail out their commercial banks from their speculative losses, is doing less and less of its financing through its central bank at effective near-zero interest rates. And having done that, in the hope, we suppose, that they might gamble more successfully next time around, they were deregulated so that they could acquire brokerage houses, underwrite mergers of railways and other large corporations, design and sell derivatives, insurance, and other financial specialties basically incompatible with banking. However, these give them an inside knowledge of other corporations' affairs, and have helped them get into trouble with the law. The US courts are clogged with a record number of cases in which banks – and three of our five big Canadian banks are amongst these – even designed the scams of companies like Enron that are now facing criminal charges. It also added immensely to the power of the large financial conglomerates, and advanced one of their most lucrative lines of business – arranging mergers of already immense corporations and privatizations of publicly owned services This almost invariably enhanced the stock market capitalization of their stock And to maintain that capitalization, costs and staff were slashed right and left. This was a key factor in the shortage of both rolling stock and staff that is crippling American farm exports. The railway mergers including the takeover of Union Pacific by Canadian National Railways added to the need for brutal cost-cutting that has left the continent's greatest railway systems practically *non compos* to help the world in its great hunger.

Efficiency Measured in Speculators' Loot

Efficiency was conceived entirely in terms of speculators' loot rather than improved services. Surely the railways could have been put and kept in tip-top shape for future needs. With growing unemployment because of the loss of overseas markets, what better way of keeping our work-force trained and employed? But financial derivatives took over. These are unregulated gambles in abstract features of a real asset – for example, interest yield, the currency in which that is denominated, its rate of growth These ghost-like numbers in turn can be optioned, or shorted. And they trade in many times the transactions of useful products. Because they are not regulated, nobody knows the identity or solvency of the counterparty – the guy left holding the obligation to pick up the bill for the lost gambles. That is hazardous enough for the financial gambler. But you cannot deliver grain to hungry nations abroad on even successful derivative plays. You need adequate rolling stock prepared well in advance. But the other half of the economy's split personality may have cut costs to the marrow of the bone, to deliver a proper balance sheet that would support the corporation's railway shares on the stock market.

That personality of the reigning economic doctrine, as disunited as Dostoevsky's hero, is making a raging contribution to doing the world in.

William Krehm

The Astounding Conversion of Finnolly Servus

IF THE WEATHER had been rainy, Finnolly Servus would not have gone to the Peace Demonstration. In a moment of rash enthusiasm, caught from two university students, he had agreed to go. When he told his wife her eyes widened and her eyebrows nearly disappeared into her blonde bangs. All she could say was "Oh." That did not mean that she disapproved. She was just struck dumb at something so alien to her image of her husband, the "Financial Adviser." Still, he had been behaving a little strangely of late, going on about the banks creating money as though that was not a good thing, and praising the acumen of two old ladies he had met at a lecture.

"But I told Fay and May and the students I'd go, and Professor Sparks will be there, and" (he almost sighed) "it looks like a sunny day."

"You're going today? What time?"

"We meet at Woodlawn Park at 1:30."

"Oh, well that's all right. I'm having my hair done this morning. I'll be back before noon."

Finnolly stared. "Would you like to come along?" he stammered.

"Well, if you don't mind. We've certainly heard enough about this invasion. Killing people to get oil for SUVs. is not my idea of the way things ought to be."

It was Finnolly's turn to say, "Oh," and pause open-mouthed. "I didn't know you paid any attention to the war news."

She put her hand on her husband's arm. "Finn," she said, "everybody's talking about it, and the government doesn't seem to be listening. Maybe I don't understand how you get an Initial Public Offering or do a Leveraged Buy-Out, but I do know what a dead body on television looks like, and it's wrong."

Finnolly looked at his wife with a new softness in his gaze. This was the spirit he had married nearly twenty-five years ago, when he was barely out of university, but he had thought it long gone.

"Okay!" he said emphatically.

The demonstration was more than interesting. It was exhilarating to be one of a crowd of 12,000 people, of all ages, shapes and sizes, who seemed to be united in thinking that cooperation is better than competition. Finnolly was beginning to agree. He carried a sign he had been handed: "PEOPLE BEFORE PROFITS." Mrs. Servus, in jeans and a broad-brimmed hat, walked beside him.

They had picked up three students, then parked the little BMW and joined a crowd that flowed toward the park. There they had heard speeches. One speaker talked passionately about the folly and destructiveness of war, but what the Servuses particularly noted was his point that war transfers wealth. War transfers wealth from the average citizen/taxpayer to the shareholders of arms-making corporations, and war transfers wealth from the losers to the winners. These, the speaker emphasized,

are the two basic motivations for the current war. All other claims, he maintained, are pretenses or delusions. He got a lot of applause.

The crowd, which filled every square yard of the park was now funnelling out for the two-mile march to the Embassy.

The students had located Fay and May, and Finnolly rather proudly introduced his wife to them. As they walked along in a little group, he expressed concern that the older ladies might find the walk too difficult.

"Oh, no," said May, "we're wearing our Wallabies. Yesterday we were in a walkathon for conservation. We walked fourteen miles along the Bruce Trail."

Sylvia Servus marvelled at their energy. She had yet to learn that it came from a sense of doing something worthwhile, something to affect the course of affairs.

The marchers had been urged to stick to the route and to keep the march peaceful. All along the route they were reminded of that by the presence of police in pairs standing in store doorways and at the corners of every block.

"The police seem to be friendly," observed Sylvia to Fay.

"These ones are," said Fay.

"There are others?"

"There will be," said Fay, ominously. "Prof. Sparks says we have to make a clear distinction between two police functions, and not mix them up. One function is to keep criminals away from decent citizens. The other function is to keep decent citizens away from government."

Whatever is she talking about? thought Sylvia Servus. A policeman is a policeman, isn't he? He rides in a cruiser, and gives speeding tickets, or he directs traffic at an accident, or if somebody is breaking into your house, they come when you call. Of course, there are the plain-clothes detectives. But all of these, it seemed to her, were concerned with protecting decent citizens. She was just about to ask Fay to explain, when her husband took up the point.

"In the dictatorships," he said, "people don't call the police if they are in trouble, because the main business of the police is to protect the government."

"That's right," said Fay, "So when you see police attacking decent citizens, you must be in a dictatorship."

"Are we going to see that today"? asked Mrs. Servus, with sudden insight and some alarm.

The conversation ended when they were overtaken by a vigorous marching "band." The musicians beat upended water jugs and pails and sang a faintly recognizable version of "Onward Christian Soldiers." But the lyrics seemed to be new.

Forward all brave citizens
Marching as to war
If they refuse to listen
We need to raise a roar.
So-o-o (a big-voiced young man led the chant.)
Stop the BS, stop the gore
We want no part of your bloody war.

Finnolly wrote these words down. He added them to a set of rather clever slogans he had been copying from placards carried by the marchers. The slogans, he realized, represented a wide spectrum of interests, but they were all focussed on opposition to war. There were the public housing advocates: "Stop the War. There Are Already Enough Homeless." A man who claimed he was a monetary reformer waved: "Bring the Boys Home; Send the Bankers." When he saw "No FTAA: Fast Track American Aggression," Finnolly felt a little embarrassed at his own previous support for the exploitive treaty. A very elderly lady being pushed in a wheel chair held a sign that said, "Don't Cripple Democracy." Finnolly laughed. A band of marchers behind a Green Party banner carried placards relevant to their environmental concerns: "No War for Oil"; "Renewable Energy," "DU Kills Children." These were illustrated by quite well-executed pictures of sinking oil tankers, graceful windmills, smiling suns, and sad-faced children. Finnolly ran ahead with his camera to get pictures of them as they approached. He found a vantage point on the sidewalk and began snapping.

Suddenly his arms were seized, and two big men drew him back to the wall. One reached for his camera. Finnolly hung on to it.

"We've been watching you," said the man who held him from behind. "No pictures," said the other, as he tore the camera out of Finnolly's hands, opened it, swiftly pulled the film out and then dropped film and camera to the pavement. The man behind released him. Finnolly Servus was not a big man. From workouts at the gym he was fit, however. He had not been a big child, but had learned that he could stop a bully by striking back. As he looked at the broken camera, and the man before him repeating, "No pictures," something snapped. "Who the hell are you?" he said and his fist snapped out with all the force from his back foot to his shoulder. He might as well have attacked a steel post. The big man parried the punch as though brushing off a spider web and with his other hand delivered a body punch that lifted Finnolly off his feet and left him seated on the ground. By the time he had regained his breath, they had disappeared down an alley. But not before Fay had shouted a quite unlady-like epithet after them.

Gordon Coggins

To be concluded.

The Entrenched Redistribution of Society's Revenue

THERE ARE a lot of sobering lessons from the unending docket of corporative scams before the US courts. Having achieved a radical redistribution of the national income, the group in power is determined to preserve that conquest, no matter by what means.

This requires that we go beyond simple money-crunching. Shifts of wealth of such proportions from one to another social group, in earlier history were usually brought in by a successful military operation or a basic revision of the legal code. The recent one was achieved through underhand improvisations that established beforehand a basic redistribution of both income and power. That is a perilous state of affairs, because it leaves everything in place for further power grabs, with yet more suppression of information that would warn of what was underway.

Thus in the US prosecution of miscreant CEOs, the charges are of fraudulent corporative governance. But the mounting frequency of such charges and the imaginative mutations of their models is a sure sign that such flaws of governance extend from corporations to that of our democracy as such. Often in the teeth of legislation still on the books, the reality has taken on patterns that cannot be openly avowed. That was so from the very Treasury-Fed Pact signed behind President Truman's back in 1951. And thus, a perduring clash has arisen between the legal code supposedly in force, and the ongoing income redistribution. The realm in which the dominant power operates is basically an ideological rather than a constitutional one.

Of course, the clash between fact and fiction in *our political governance* reduces the penalties for infringing the old legal system. Individuals may be punished, but for corporations the penalties are rarely beyond what can be absorbed as a "cost of doing business." The real cost is borne by the victims – either the general public or to that part of it that aspires to participate as shareholders in the ongoing redistribution of the national income.

Mr. Spitzer's Historical Precedents

To probe the significance of the billowing corporative governance litigation, we must delve into historical precedents, for example, the trials of the nabobs of the East India Company went on, some ending in convictions, others in acquittals, but the abuse of the real victims, the Indians, perdured. The citizens of Britain's Indian possessions, passed from the private East India company to the British Crown only a century later. when India became formally a possession of the British Crown. If we are not careful, such a complete legitimization of the corporative realities is what we may be heading towards today.

The same may be said of the piracy on the high seas of Drake and others, even when England was not at war with Spain. The precious metals highjacked in this way not only widened monstrously the gap between the wealthy merchant-pirates and their sailors and workers, but between the English and Spanish nobility. Only much later was piracy brought under the law of nations.

Meanwhile, it is revealing to study the structures of the more recent indictments of corporative governance that are clogging the US courts.

The current *plat du jour* is "market timing" – a by-product of the multi-storied structure of the mutual fund industry. Let us go to *The Wall Street Journal* (2/12, "A Fight at Invesco Spotlights the Toll of 'Market Timers'" by Susan Pulliam and Tom Lauricella):

"In 1998, stock prices were surging and mutual-fund companies were thriving. But inside Invesco Funds Group, a clash was looming between fund managers and the company's senior management. Portfolio managers were angry about a new breed of fast-moving traders who were quietly changing the rules of the mutual-fund business. These investors, many of them large hedge funds, were quickly moving tens of millions of dollars in and out of Invesco funds. Their goal was to profit from fleeting discrepancies between the fund's official prices, set each day at 4 p.m., and the shifting prices of the stocks held by the mutual funds.

"The 'market timers,' as they were known, were creating havoc for portfolio managers' carefully plotted strategies – and cutting into returns for long-term investors. All this rapid [in-and-out] trading rang up higher transaction costs, which fund companies spread evenly across all shareholders. Moreover, the trading prevented fund managers from buying all the stocks they wanted, because they needed plenty of cash on hand to settle the [time] traders' sales." The departing market timers sold their stock back not to the market but to the mutual fund.

All the market timers had to do, was calculate the value of the shares the mutual fund owned, and compare it with the aggregate market value of those same shares. If the discrepancy were big enough they needed only short the shares in question using for the purpose the money they got by redeeming their holdings of the mutual fund shares. The strategy was fool-proof only if they were allowed to sell their mutual fund shares after hours, at a price that had been set long before at 4 p.m.

Market Timers Make the Big Time

"Today, market timers are at the center of a massive probe rocking the mutual-fund industry. Many funds face allegations that they banned market-timing for ordinary investors, but permitted it for big players.

"Invesco not only permitted them, but even encouraged them by making special deals with large hedge funds. In a stormy internal debate some Invesco fund managers argued that the timers should be banned because of the toll they took on ordinary shareholders. They believed that their bosses were willing to accommodate the timers to stem the flow of money away from their funds during a down market. The portfolio managers watched helplessly as the timers played a cat-and-mouse game to move their money in and out of Invesco funds."

The very institution of a mutual fund that invests in other mutual funds, which can do the same by putting their money into yet a third group, raises questions. Though perfectly legal in itself, it gives rise to many-storeyed structures. And you can spell that as you wish, "many-storeyed" or "many-storied." For to innocent investors there is always the hope that at each level the brilliance of the local manager will compound that of the manager one level higher or lower. More certain is fact that it does multiply the fees – and the possibility of maneuvers to fleece innocent hopefuls. It is like a wrestler entering the ring with an additional joint in his arms and legs. It would give him extra powers to grab and surprise.

"Invesco gave dozens of big investors permission to rapidly trade its funds. One was Canary Capital Partners LC, which began trading Invesco funds several years ago and was eventually allowed by Invesco to trade roughly $400 million among its funds, according to people close to the mutual fund inves-

tigation by NY Attorney General Eliot Spitzer and the Security and Exchange Commission. The hedge, run by Edward Stern, often traded after the 4 p.m. close, according to documents released by Mr. Spitzer. This permitted Canary to buy funds whose underlying securities had already risen or were likely to rise the next day. When the fund's prices caught up with the prices of the underlying securities, Canary would pocket a profit. Mr. Spitzer likened the scheme to betting on yesterday's horse races.

"For decades, Invesco was a sleepy outpost of the burgeoning fund industry. Launched in 1935 by a traveling salesman, it was still a small player in 1990, with assets at a relatively modest $1.8 billion. In 1997, Invesco merged with AIM funds to form Amvescap. One year after the merger, Mark Williamson, a former mutual-find executive at Nationsbank took over. The new CEO ramped up the marketing of Invesco's growth-oriented funds. Assets jumped 50% in his first year to $31 billion at the end of 1999. The push for growth ushered in the market-timers. Former fund manager Jerry Paul estimates that $200 million of the $1 billion in his high-yield-bond fund came from timers who traded rapidly in and out of his fund. 'It was a pain.'"

Serious Consequences are Inevitable

"The money washing through Mr. Paul's fund typically came from hedge funds, loosely regulated investment pools for wealthy individuals and institutions. For the most part, Mr. Paul and the fund managers didn't know their identities. Among the market-timers were Canary Capital Partners LLC, a hedge-fund and customers of American Skandia Inc., which set up investment vehicles that permitted such trades, according to documents released by Mr. Spitzer.

"It isn't necessarily illegal for mutual fund investors to engage in market-timing. But regulators and the NY Attorney General say that some fund companies misled investors by contending they were attempting to discourage market-timing. They also may have run afoul of the law by cutting deals from which regular investors were excluded."

A field that awaits urgent analysis is the "trickle down" effects of multi-digit "white collar" crime into the lower "blue collar" level. Since one result of the former is the ravaging of producing companies and their non-executive pension funds, and the outsourcing of industrial operations, it results in massive unemployment, destitution, cynicism, dysfunctional families. The media is abundantly served with crescendoing crime at both social levels.

William Krehm

The Blind Paradoxes of a Degenerate Economic Theory

THE REPLACEMENT NEEDS arising from the Iraqi war and the transformation of China from a frugal Communism to a dream-boat of capitalism have begun pulling the world out of its depression.

However, that is producing more problems than it is likely to solve. For its solutions somehow mix up matters basically irreconcilable: growth with destruction: prosperity with massive joblessness, crushing debt with prosperity. population explosion in areas like China India, with depopulation in Africa and the former Soviet Union.

The confusion of irreconcilables is as apparent in the ideologies as in the policies they beget.

Thus *The Wall Street Journal* (5/12, "Inflation Creeps Back into Euro Zone Outlook" by G. Thomas Sims) highlights a corner of the broader canvas: "Frankfurt – Inflation is creeping back on the radar screen of the European Central Bank. The ECB yesterday kept interest rates on hold, as expected but sharpened its rhetoric about the risk of inflation as the world's No. 2 economy picks up steam. Its comments reinforced expectations that [interest] rates could rise next year and propelled the euro to a new high against the dollar of $1.2155 before falling back.

"Jean-Claude Trichet, president of the ECB, repeated that inflation will hover around 2% in coming months. But he dropped last month's judgment that the longer-term outlook for inflation was 'favorable.' Now Mr. Trichet said he expected only a 'gradual and limited decline' in inflation."

Solving Society's Problems by Interest Rates

"We judge that we have to remain vigilant,' Mr. Trichet told reporters after the bank left its key interest rate at 2%. Despite the slightly tougher tone on inflation, he didn't signal that a rate increase is imminent. During the past $2^{1}/_{2}$ years, the ECB gradually cut its key rate from a peak of 4.75 as Europe succumbed to the global economic slowdown and inflation became less of a concern.

"Some central banks around the globe already are beginning to raise interest rates. This week, Australia's central bank raised borrowing costs for a second time in as many months. The Bank of England left its rate on hold yesterday after its first increase in four years in October. The US Federal Reserve, however, has signaled that rates will remain low for some time. The US, after all, is waging a war, implementing a tax cut for the folks who count, and approaching a presidential election – all at the same time.

"The source of the ECB's disquiet on inflation is a new twice-yearly economic projection compiled by staff and presented at yesterday's meeting of the bank's top policy makers. Six months ago, the projections showed inflation would likely fall on average to 1.3% next year – well below the central bank's target of 'close to but below' 2%.

"Inflation in November was 2.2%, after 2% in October, despite high unemployment and an economy weaker than the US and Japan. The ECB blames higher oil prices, new taxes and rises in food prices after a hot summer."

Here you run into the nonsense deductions at the heart of official theory. The ECB blames higher oil prices and the dearer food supplies due to a scorching summer for the rise of the price index from 2% to 2.2% since October. But how would higher interest rates – the ECB's sole response to higher prices – possibly remedy these identified arch-villains in the price rise? The shortage of oil in large degree is due to the romance of the Americans with SUV's, a romance that has now started spreading to China. Our planet warming is probably due in whole or in part to the pollution of our atmosphere.

How does one inject a bit of logic into this empire of dogmatic greed?

W.K.

Exercising for Systems Theory

IT WAS APPROXIMATELY thirty years since economists had shown any interest in systems theory. There was a passing flicker of attention to it in the early seventies when Jay Forrester had been commissioned by the Club of Rome to forecast the adequacy of oil supplies at the going rate of consumption increase. Working with data that could only be supplied by the petroleum corporations, his predictions of a relatively short-term oil crisis turned out to be on the pessimistic side. That had its part in the disappearance of economists' preoccupation with systems theory. A bum prediction based on the only statistics of available supply was misrepresented as a convincing proof that the "pure and perfect market" would continue to provide the world's oil needs.

There was a far deeper factor at play: systems theory is the polar opposite of economists' ploy in declaring non-market factors "externalities." That simply shoved non-market subsystems of the economy – the ecology, households, the public sector, health, education, and so forth – out the back door. Obviously this negates the very essence of systems theory – that the ability of a system to go on functioning depends on all its subsystems being in working order. No subsystem must be allowed to devour the resources essential for the operation of another. Hence no subsystem can be seen as an externality; no market – including notably our financial market – must be allowed to embark on a course of exponential increase. For that would imply pillaging everything in sight, including all non-market subsystems.

So remote is this constraint from the established concerns of economists, that it is going to take some exercising to get used to. However, it may be helpful to note that good investigative journalists do examine such abuses, and expose false claims by identifying an important public interest being violated. That is the very building block of systems theory. Expand it to take in all non-market subsystems and check to see whether the market – or any other subsystem – is not encroaching on essential resources of another, and you will have a fair notion of systems theory.

Let us try this out on some current examples. Right on the front page of *The Wall Street Journal* (12/11) there are three stories that fill the bill.

"An Unusual Pitch from French Giant: Nukes are Green" by John Carreyrou: "Paris – Blackouts this year in the US, Scandinavia and Italy were a stark reminder that the world has yet to figure out how to meet its energy needs.

"Areva SA, a large but little-known company owned by the French government, thinks it has the answer: nuclear power.

"The world's biggest builder of nuclear reactors and re-cycler of nuclear waste, Areva, aims to go public next year. It is pitching itself to potential investors on the controversial premise that nuclear power is making a comeback – and that the industry that spawned Chernobyl is actually good for the environment."

Applying High Fashion to Nuclear Power

"To make its case, Areva is embarked on a global market-ing campaign that takes as much from the fashion industry as it does from the grubbier world of electricity production. Areva CEO Anne Lauvergeon hired a former top executive from fashion house Hermes to gussie up nuclear power's image. She sponsored a yacht in the America's Cup race. She's run television ads with the slogan: 'We've got nothing to hide. Come see.'

"To prove that point Ms. Lauvergeon had cameras installed at a nuclear-waste recycling plant in Normandy, the largest repository of radioactive material on Earth. They piped live shots of the plant's interior to a Web site for public viewing. The French government ordered the cameras turned off for security reasons after the Sept. 11, 2001, attacks."

In short, the immense dangers of human error and terror-ist theft of nuclear materials had simply been declared exter-nalities. The French government stepped in to stop some of the more scandalous aspects of this misrepresentation. Systems theory seeks to catch the sources of social catastrophes by estab-lishing routine defences of the public interest.

In the same issue of *WSJ* one column to the left of the article on French nuclear enterprise, is another item that can serve as a useful exercise in limbering up our minds: "Costs of Trucking Seen Rising under New Safety Rules" by Daniel Machalaba).

"The first major changes in truck-driver work hours since 1939 are expected to reduce highway fatalities, but also contrib-ute to the biggest increase in trucking rates in two decades.

"The changes, mandated under new federal safety rules that take effect in January, are designed to reduce fatigue among truck drivers, a major cause of accidents. The new rules increase the time truck drivers must set aside to rest in each 24-hour period to 10 hours from eight. The total time a driver can be on duty will fall to 14 hours from 15. Drivers also will be required to include as work hours time spend waiting at loading docks and fueling their rigs.

"Wal-Mart Stores Inc., which unsuccessfully opposed the new rules, believes the more stringent 14-hour rule will reduce the drivers' daily work time by 6% on the average and cause it to add 275 new drivers and 300 new trucks to handle the same amount of cargo. 'The rule will impose serious costs on society,

not only on motor carriers but on shippers and receivers as well,' the company said in a regulatory filing."

Proclaiming Highway Deaths an Externality

That should be an easy misrepresentation to see through. Road accidents, fatal and otherwise, have simply been pro-claimed by Wal-Mart as an externality. Internalize it into soci-ety's costs, and Wal-Mart's argument is exposed as self-seeking nonsense.

On the far left column in the same issue *WSJ* is yet another article that makes a similar point, "Universal Care Has a Big Price: Patients Wait" by Elena Cherney. "Toronto – In Canada's public-health system, which promises free equal-access care to all citizens, medical resources are explicitly rationed. For the country as a whole, that works – Canada spends far less on healthcare, yet health outcomes of its citizens are generally as good as those in the US.

"But the trade-offs are steep: Canadian hospitals are slower to adopt the latest technology, meaning patients have more limited access to cutting-edge medical equipment. Health of-ficials may use expensive drugs more selectively. There are fewer specialists for patients to see.

"The riskiest trade-off of all is troublingly long waits. Once patients see a family doctor and get a referral for specialist care, it can take weeks or even months to get an appointment. In some parts of the country patients waiting for admission to a hospital sometimes find themselves waiting for hours and even days on gurneys in the corridor, and receiving treatment there.

"A study this year by the Organization for Economic Coop-eration and Development found waiting times for elective sur-gery are a 'significant health-policy concern' in about one half the group's 30 members, including the UK, Australia, Sweden, Denmark and Spain. Waiting times weren't a problem in the US, the group said.

"In Canada, the long waits stirred a public outcry and a government inquiry when a 63-year-old heart patient at St. Michael's Hospital in Toronto died in 1989 after his surgery had been canceled 11 times.

"To tackle this crucial problem, Canada is turning to 'cardi-ac-care coordinators.' Their job: to make sure waiting doesn't kill patients.

"In Canada, one way hospitals restrain costs is by trying to always run at capacity. It's more efficient to run a hospital that way, just as it's more efficient to fly an airplane with every seat full. But running at capacity means lines always form. Waits for certain surgeries in Canada can be up to two years. Health care spending accounts for 10% of Canada's Gross Domestic Product, while in the US, it consumes about 14%. Canadian patients can choose their own doctors, and they never have a bill for their care. Canadian physicians, who are paid by the gov-ernment, generally earn much less than their US counterparts. Despite Canada's lower health-care spending, patient outcomes in a number of areas, including cancers and heart-disease, are similar. Overall, life expectancy in Canada is 79.4 years, com-pared with 76.8 in the US, the OECD says.

"Many factors affect longevity, of course. Nearly one-third of

Americans are obese, for instance, compared with 15% of Canadians. And since millions of Americans are uninsured, many may not get access to the care they need."

"Some US experts say that waiting lists are a sign that the health-care system isn't wasting money on unnecessary procedures, equipment or personnel. 'If you don't wait in a medical system, there's a problem,' says Ted Marmor, a health-policy expert at Yale University. The question,' Prof. Marmor says, 'is whether people are waiting inappropriately.'

"In Ontario, the cardiac-care network works to strike this balance. The network consists of 17 hospitals, and 50 surgeons who share heart-patient cases. There are government guidelines: at St. Michael's, six scheduled surgeries are allowed each day. Cardiac-care coordinators are assigned the task of making sure that waiting doesn't kill patients. They must juggle the elective and urgent cases so that all six operating-room slots are filled every day – and no one is left waiting more than the recommended length of time."

Adding New Subsystems to Health Analysis

"Today, most urgent and semi-urgent heart patients are treated within two weeks. Non-urgent patients wait an average for 49 days for surgery. Some patients say that waiting isn't too bad a price to pay for their free medical treatment." The problem was brought under control by setting up a neglected subsystem – that of urgent heart surgeries with its own rules and goal.

So far so good. But yet another crucial subsystem has been omitted here. In 1991 a bill was slipped through Canada's parliament without press release or debate to bail out Canada's banks from their gambles in gas and oil and real estate. It took the form of doing away with the statutory reserves that banks had to redeposit with the central bank as a modest proportion of the deposits they took in from the public. The story is already retold in the page 1 article.[1]

With great understatement, let us say that total cost to the federal coffers has amounted to another 2% of the GDP. By retracing these deplorable steps – the end of statutory reserves and the deregulation of the banks *even to a modest extent,* one half of the 4% lesser amount of the GDP spent in Canada compared to the 14% figure spent on health-care in the US could provide spare elbow room in our health system to cut down unreasonable waiting periods.

This would make available for dealing with the waiting problem for surgery another subsystem of the economy – our monetary subsystem as redesigned some twelve years ago. That could be used to reduce any *unreasonable* waiting periods in our otherwise excellent health system. The eternal question – Where is the money coming from? – needs only an honest ear to the answers that are embedded in our history.

William Krehm

1. To make available detailed information on this key subject, COMER is making available two historic books for a token $10 plus shipping and handling – Bill Krehm's *The Bank of Canada: A Power Unto Itself* (Stoddard, 1993) and Bill Hixson's *It's Your Money* (COMER, 1997).

Letter to the Editor

Dear Charles Michael,

Thank you for your letter of September 6.

Let me begin by saying that the discussion that you have initiated is precisely what the public needs and is not getting.

You perceive a flaw in our argument #1: "*You basically argue for accrual accountancy for the government because properly recording the assets it owns would improve the balance sheet sufficiently to allow more room for fiscal maneuver rather than to be obsessed about deficits.*" That is not our view. We argue for accrual accountancy for government finances and for the economy as a whole. because only with it can we know what is happening in our economy. Of course, liabilities in pensions, loan guarantees and all else essential should appear on the balance sheets, just as they mostly do in the case of private firms. As would the government investment in human education, health, and social welfare, which was proven in WWII by T. Schultz to be the most productive of all possible investments. Of course, this would be governed by the needs of society and the economy. Likewise, necessary maintenance of the environment, physical and human infrastructures. All this must be reported truthfully as well as the off-balance sheet borrowings. If that is to be done, they must appear as an investment (at cost). If they are needed but are not made, they must be shown as a debit that contributes to the government deficit rather than to its balancing.

I would not presume to know whether the government balance sheet would appear in surplus, balance or in deficit, were all this done, but I do know this: We must not let our water system, or our air deteriorate until we come down with epidemics that we thought had been conquered or with new ones that our neglect has helped create. Government deficits were proved in the 1930s and during War II as necessary during a depression or to help us deal with a major crisis. If we don't deal with that crisis, the government accounts may appear to be balanced, but will prove to be disastrously otherwise. What is involved is bum accountancy.

Were we in deficit after having brought in serious accountancy, we must see to it that all available workers who wished to work have the opportunity to do so at some socially useful task – including notably such public investment. This would forestall the unpleasant surprises under which the world is reeling. Where would the money come from? Where did it come from to finance WWII and the postwar reconstruction? By the use of the central bank to create a substantial amount of the money supply rather than assigning that function almost entirely to the private banks. These money-creative powers must not be used for deregulated private speculation that give rise to far more problems as the economy is looted for unbridled private interests.

Perceived flaw #2: "*Instead of its one blunt interest rate instrument, you urge the central bank to also increase (or re-establish) reserve requirements so as to manage the money supply without imposing high rates on those most vulnerable to them. But, if reserve requirements are raised, it will drain liquidity out of the banking system. Will not the resulting liquidity squeeze force mar-*

ket interest rates higher anyway? What's the difference."

There is more than a single difference. First: the raising of interest rates as a stabilizer targets everything that moves or stands still in the economy – for example, mortgages that merely come up for renewal rather than speculative gambles in building and stock market investment for quick profit alone. How much liquidity higher reserve requirements will drain will obviously depend on how high the reserves are raised. But the higher reserve requirements should be accompanied by jaw-boning whereby bank managers will be informed that further investment in overdeveloped areas should not be financed. That was commonly done before it was decided to leave everything to "the market."

Secondly, the goal of a flat price ("zero inflation") is simply not achievable when rapid urbanization and industrialization are underway throughout the world. Who in his right mind moves from a town of 10,000 to New York City and expects his living costs to stay flat? How could humanity expect that when it as a whole is making just such a move? In addition we are in a state of constant technological revolutions, for reasons good and bad. These require a quite different level of education and physical infrastructures. A few historians like Fernand Braudel have seen that clearly. But economists have shut their eyes to these non-market factors by declaring them "externalities."

"That, embedded in the cost of everything is creating [much of] the inflation that central banks are supposedly warring against. How are you going to measure the effect?" To begin with by having an honest economic theory that recognizes the effect: and gives it a separate name rather than "inflation" – we use "structural price rise." And secondly by having governments stop bullying their statistical departments into conforming with established theory. And by having an educated public and an intellectually free university system discuss the merits and the dangers of any economic policy. It was the Auditor General in Canada who after three or four Royal Commissions had recommended serious accountancy over some four decades who finally won the point. But neither in the US nor in Canada were the measures even mentioned let alone explained in the press. The effect is the easiest in the world to calculate: deduct from the GDP the total revenue of all levels of government to eliminate the double reckoning of taxation – once as the mark-up of the price of the private sector via taxation, and secondly through the governments' own expenditures. We need, too, a profession of economists that is not wholly dependent upon academia at the mercy of government or is rewarded many times more richly by serving the stock market.

"My college economics texts said that a cost increase such as quadrupling oil prices in 1974 or your embedded taxes do not create inflation. Indeed, if the money supply remains constant or only increases in line with population or economic growth then such an embedded cost increase is actually deflationary. Other prices decline to offset the rising embedded cost. Thus, to be inflationary, the rising embedded cost must also be accommodated by a rising money supply which puts the problem back in the lap of monetary expansion. Am I wrong in this? Has the theory changed since my college days?"

You are right insofar as that is what the old textbooks said. You are wrong insofar as that theory has created so much trouble throughout the world that even the US Fed and BIS have abandoned it – in stealth of course – and are now arguing that some 2% of "inflation" is useful. But is that inflation or just the cost of the non-market sectors? Why has nobody challenged this abandonment of the Paul Volcker and Bank of International Settlements position that even the slightest price index increase, were it not suppressed with high interest rates, would bring on the sort of hyperinflation that hit Germany in 1923? Did this not imply that were interest rates pushed up high enough, Germany's defeat in WWI would have been erased retroactively, there would have been no reparations, no occupation of the Ruhr industrial heartland by the French army, no general strike to protest it, and virtual civil war in Germany? Why has nobody in the major parties challenged this? After all, most of the present government debt in the US was brought about by the long bout of double digit interest rates to suppress the price rise that we now learn was partly "beneficent."

Incidentally, the US actually introduced capital budgeting in stealth as of January, 1996. You will find its first appearance in the January 1996 Bureau of Economic Analysis figures of the Department of Commerce. In essence it ended the one-year write-off of physical investments by the federal government. Government investment in human capital – education, health, social security – still remain unrecognized. The purpose was to provide a single statistic that President Clinton needed to bring down interest rates, without offending Wall St. Carried back several years this produced an improvement of the government balance sheet of some $1.3 trillion. But it was misrepresented as "national savings," which it was not since it had already been invested and was not held in cash. With a wink and a nudge, it did improve the rating of the agencies of government bonds and hence brought down interest rates. That had the effect of re-electing Clinton and produced the riotous stock-market boom. An important detail of your research is to look up the above-cited issue of the BEA.

Let us deal with a very few matters at a time Send me your next bunch of objections, and pull no punches. And do check those vital BEA statistics.

All best,

Bill Krehm

Mr. Michael wrote from Denver, Colorado.

Guns and Very Salty Butter

With the Iraqi war overlapping far beyond its officially proclaimed end, the "Guns and Butter" theme of Lyndon Johnson has come to the fore once more. And confronted with his reelection problem, President Bush, translates the butter into tax-cuts. That adds a dimension of snake-charming to budget process. No surprise that the portion of the media still unembedded in the White House is increasingly sceptical. *The New York Times* (7/12, "President Both – Bush Can Have Both

Guns and Butter, At Least for Now" by Niall Ferguson) remarks: "In *The Rise and Fall of the Great Powers*, the Yale historian Paul M. Kennedy developed this zero-sum model into a sophisticated theory of how empires work. In essence, you need wealth to fight your rivals, but if you devote too much money to war, your wealth tends to stagnate. That's because (according to the theory) investment in the arms industry is less conducive to long-term economic growth than investment in sectors that ultimately satisfy some kind of consumer demand.

"A simpler version of this idea suggested a trade-off between military spending and personal consumption. 'Guns' are paid for by raising taxes, and this leaves people with less money to spend on 'butter.'

"The Bush administration is currently engaged in an audacious – some would say reckless – experiment to disprove this theory. President Bush's response to the question Guns or butter? is 'Thanks, I'll take both.' Bush's second term depends on his being President Both.

"In the rump to Thanksgiving two measures symbolized the administration's conviction that it can grab those horns and take a ride. The first was the approval of a $401 billion military appropriations package for next year, the biggest ever. The second was Congress's approval of a Medicare overhaul that increases the spiraling costs of the system by adding a drug prescription benefit.

"But these are only two parts of a wider guns and butter policy. Consider the administration's commitment to spend $87 billion on the reconstruction of Iraq and Afghanistan. That comes on top of the initial military costs of 'regime change' in both countries. Plainly, some costs of Iraq's recovery will be borne by other foreign donors and by sales of Iraq's oil. Moreover, these costs are coinciding with increasing American donations to helpful countries. Aid to Jordan, for example, has soared from an annual average of $225 million over the past five years to $1.5 billion this year.

"After decades of decline in relation to gross domestic product, the combined economic and military budget looks set to rise in relative terms under President Bush. Yet this same president has pushed through three big tax cuts. Recall that the US has broken the guns or butter rule before. Under President Reagan, from 1979 to 1986, military spending leaped from 4.8% of GDP to 6.2%, while personal consumption rose from 62% to 65%. The crucial point is that in the short term, at least, fiscal policy is not a zero-sum game: a government can easily increase military spending without reducing consumer demand if it finances the higher spending by borrowing rather than taxation. The downside is that such debt-financed fiscal policies led to inflation in the past. In the late 1960s and in the late 1980s, deficits were partly financed by printing dollars, which ultimately led to higher prices."

The New York Times piece goes on to its punch-line: "To critics of the White House, this is part of what they would call the Enronization of public finance."

Modesty inhibits us from claiming priority in pioneering such revealing if unkind comparisons, but there is scarcely a scam revealed by zealous New York Attorney General Eliot Spitzer in his prosecution of big corporative sinners that has no precedent in government financing. And not alone in the US.

Hitting Reality Square on the Nose

Moreover, the distinguished economist Robert Eisner pointed out that when so-called "inflation" (in real life a very hybrid thing[1]) attains a certain level, it shrinks the real burden of the government debt and stimulates the economy. Eisner used to be a much quoted economist in the eighties and early nineties, but is never cited today, when in fact he is more than ever needed.

Such is the fate of economists who hit reality square on the nose.

When Niall Ferguson, a professor of financial history of the Stern School of Business at New York University, refers to "guns and butter" policy under Reagan and Lyndon Johnson leading to "inflation," he trivializes the issue. For part of the upward price gradient is due to *essential* growth of government investment in physical and human capital. To mix up essential investing with discretionary "spending" is to confuse the problem.

Moreover, much indispensable government investment is not only on physical things like subways, roads, bridges, buildings, but on education, health, and social security.

The surprising rapidity of the recovery of Japan and Germany from WWII, contrary to economists' expectations, resulted in a temporary recognition of public investment in human capital as the most productive of all investment. Without it the marvels of Silicon Valley would have been impossible. That such public investment is largely lodged in private minds and bodies is irrelevant; for it vastly broadens the tax-base. On the other hand, military spending implies the destruction both of physical and human capital, at home and abroad. Given the responsibilities of a lone superpower in a world that it has chosen to globalize, that is no way to balance its budget or win popularity contests. It leaves it no option to investing money to help underdeveloped countries, in a way that would improve the relations between peoples and nations and allow lessening military budgets. A more peaceful program of economic governance would also provide much needed markets for our productive economy in a healthier and more perduring way than by smashing up other folks' lands.

The moral of all this is, that the best of professors have just scratched the surface of the "Guns or Butter" dilemma. To dig further, we must reexamine the basic assumptions of conventional economic theory.

William Krehm

1. That is the sum of honest-to-goodness "inflation" that is really due to an outstripping of supply by aggregate demand, plus what I have identified 35 years ago as "structural price increase" due to a deepening layer of taxation in price that reflects the vast increase in indispensable public investment in both human and physical capital.

The Summers Logic: Economic Growth Versus Social Progress

The Goals of Economic Activity

Economic activity is performed by agents who judge activity goals subjectively, seen in relation to their path-dependent socio-economic background and self-centric value projections. Agents' goals might conflict with each other, but they are also inter-dependent. The value projections formed by the agents on each side of an exchange will only reach their final form during the exchange session itself, then it will be dependent upon what each agent believes the counterparty's projections and market understanding are.

In consideration of this, an important conclusion is that economic theory cannot alone define goals for economic activity. In the case of macro economic goals, they must align the conflicting goals of the individual agents. Because of the agents' subjective value projections, economic analysis used in isolation cannot perform the task. It can only be done by including other social value systems, such as politics, ethics, human rights considerations, etc.

The World Bank Memo

Much debate based on neoclassical economics ignores this principle. An egregious example of this surfaced in a leaked internal World Bank memo, written in 1991 by its then chief economist, Lawrence Summers. Here are the memo's main points:

"The measurements of the costs of health impairing pollution depends on the forgone earnings from increased morbidity and mortality. From this point of view a given amount of health impairing pollution should be done in the country with the lowest cost, which will be the country with the lowest wages.... I've always thought that under-populated countries in Africa are vastly *under*-polluted, their air quality is probably vastly inefficiently low.... Only the lamentable facts that so much pollution is generated by non-tradable industries (transport, electrical generation) and that the unit transport costs of solid waste are so high prevent world welfare enhancing trade in air pollution and waste."

If we accept this logic as valid, it must be so for all economic activity. So, why stop with applying it to the export of toxic waste to the Less Developed countries? Why not extend it to all activity with an economic content? For example, is it then not economically inefficient to let young men and women from rich households expose themselves to the dangerous tasks of being soldiers in Iraq. Volunteers for the armed force ought to be screened for not having too high household incomes before being accepted. Seen in this light, when young Dan Quayle and George Bush ducked from being sent to front duty in Vietnam they, in fact, only performed their national duty at its fullest. Furthermore, it is not only morbidity and mortality that destroy peoples' income earning potential, sending people to jail also does. This makes it very uneconomical to treat everybody as equals for the law. When meting out justice income poten-

tial must be considered, and rich people should receive lighter sentences, ensuring that they do not spend too long time in the income destroying situation of languishing in a jail.

The problem of Summers' extreme market logic is caused by using money to measure the social efficiency of conflicting choices. One of the characteristics of money, listed at the beginning of most economic textbooks, is its use as a unit of account. In line with this, we habitually use money as a measuring tool when we want to compare different kinds of economic output. But if we use it as the *only* measure of the activity taking place in a society, the logic turns around and dictates that only what can be measured in money can count as a socially valued activity.

There are, of course, different ways of measuring human welfare. When statistics index living standards, whether for individuals, social groups or countries, it commonly is done by measuring the money equivalents available for *buying* goods and services. This is a narrow definition that creates problems when seen in larger contexts. It ignores the impact of the self-centric interest conflicts of agents, and therefore becomes misreading when translated into aggregates. Especially important in this respect is that the impact of welfare-decreasing externalities by localized economic activity will not be recognized.

That means that if there is no extra-market system to impose the costs or benefits of externalities upon market prices, there will exist a value differential between the broader social measure of life quality taking such factor into account, and the narrow economic measure of living standards that simply aggregate each individual's output in market terms. This difference can be called the living-standard life-quality differential, or LS-LQ differential for short. It can be used as proxy for the difference between a narrow measure of economic growth and a broader inclusive measure of social progress.

Neoclassical economics has denied that the LS-LQ differential can be a significant factor by proposing the Coarse Theorem. This postulates that if property rights are well defined, information complete and there is no transaction costs (including costs of litigation) all externalities will either be negotiated away or compensated for. Since none of the preconditions of the Coarse Theorem are realistic under real world conditions, the theorem is a typical example of a neoclassical claim that cannot pass a Popperian falsifiability test.

The Employment Problem

Since the externalities cannot be gotten rid of with claims such as the Coarse Theorem, it follows that economic activity in general takes place within socio-economic surroundings where externalities create a LS-LQ differential. It appears, that this could be solved with a system of appropriate taxes and subsidies, which would adjust prices for the LS-LQ differential. But our current economic system, organized around market exchanges would make this problematic for other reasons, one major one being its effect upon employment patterns, which would create a major stumbling block, even if the political will for such adjustment were present.

Under the current economic organization, employment in general is traded in time-framed discrete units, which can only exist in either-or states. In other words, a person is either employed and earns a money income, or is not, earning no money income at all. This is different from other types of factor incomes. Thus, for example, when money is deposited in a bank, the bank does not consider the money as a discrete unit, but intermediates it. In this way, the interest income one gets is not tied to individual loans on the other side of the bank's operations.

Much of the negative externalities are caused by the overproduction of, in a LQ connection, useless goods, or by an inefficient transport system. However, reducing such negative externalities is very likely to reduce a society's output as measured in LS values, which in the short term might cause massive disruptions of employment. Think, for example, what would happen if bicycles and small electric cars were promoted for short-distances. A key economic sector within the current economic system might fall apart as demand for its products dropped. This would threaten to create an uncontrollable economic downturn, instead of accomplishing the desired structural change.

Therefore, only by creating an effective system of work intermediation that can shield individuals from the negative income effects of structural changes, can externalities and the LS-LQ differential be attacked. This is not an easy task, not only because technical difficulties, but because current public sentiments under influence of neo-conservative propaganda disguised as economic theory, would find it hard to accept the underlying principles.

The Summers memo ends with: "The problem with the arguments against all of these proposals for more pollution in LDCs ([the arguments of] intrinsic rights to certain goods, moral reasons, social concerns, lack of adequate markets, etc.) could be turned around and used more or less effectively against every Bank proposal for liberalization." Not only so, Mr. Summers, it is the arguments against all neoclassical reasoning put forward in defense of socially destructive economic policies.

Dix Sanbeck

Keeping Track of Our Prowling Banks

THE SUN is shining on our banking system again. Or it merely the Klieg lights of overdone PR? Under the caption "TD back in black for 2003" (27/11, *The Globe and Mail*, by Sinclair Stewart) we are informed: "Toronto-Dominion Bank, tarred with its first annual loss in corporate history last year, steered its way back to profitability in 2003 with a $989-million profit.

"The results may not rival those of Canada's other banks, but they do mark a significant about-face from 2002, when a lending debacle pushed TD $160 million into the red.... Profit in the fourth quarter ended October 31 was $480 million or 73 cents a fully diluted share, compared with a loss of $219 million or 34

cents in the final three months of 2002. Because of an abrupt improvement in the credit outlook, the bank is now reversing its aggressive loan-loss provision effectively providing a lift to the quarterly numbers.

"During a conference call with analysts, CEO Ed Clark made a point of addressing a report earlier this week by Enron Corp's court-appointed examiner that suggested TD 'aided and abetted' company executives manipulating the company's financial statements.

"Mr. Clark described the collapse of Enron as 'deplorable' but pointed out that TD was not involved in structuring any of the company's complex transactions. He added that TD employees interviewed by the examiner denied any knowledge that Enron was cooking its books to mislead investigators, and said that the bank recognizes it is no longer enough to 'take the word just of the company or its auditors.'"

That is one of the great understatements of the year.

"In the final three months of fiscal 2003, TD actually recorded an $83-million credit for loan-loss provisions. That reduced the bank's 2003 provisions to a paltry $186 million, a far cry from the more than $2.9 billion booked in 2002. The numbers were affected by a tangle of one-time items, which together boosted the bottom line by about 10 cents a share."

"A review of reports prepared by Enron's court-appointed examiner reveals that at least four of the nine financial institutions singled out for 'aiding and abetting' the company's fraud hedged their exposure to Enron with credit derivatives.

"But TD stands out among the group because it used the derivatives far more extensively and earlier than the other banks."

A Surplus of Derivatives

"TD began using derivatives in June, 1999 – 2.5 years before Enron's demise. The derivatives more than offset its exposure to Enron, allowing the bank to book a 'net gain' on its loan during the first quarter of 2002. By contrast, Credit Suisse First Boston, a Tier 1 banker to Enron – [i.e., with a closer formal tie to that company] – did not start buying credit derivatives until three months before the company collapsed. It is owed $417 million by Enron.

"TD spokeswoman Dianne Salt confirmed this week that the bank's credit protection actually exceeded its loans to the company.

"One bank analyst, describing the move as 'extremely unorthodox,' said this is a classic example of a bank using derivatives for risk taking rather than risk minimization. In his fourth and final report on Enron released this week, examiner Neal Batson implicates TD for continuing to provide funding to the company – using derivatives to offset its exposure – even though bank officials knew the financial statements were being manipulated. As a result of the varied roles that TD played for Enron, it had access to substantial information about the company."

That inside information that bankers have of their clients' affairs is one of the many reasons why banks should never have been deregulated to participate in every sort of gamble incompatible with banking. When you add to that the inside information that bank holding companies through their stock brokering, underwriting, derivative boutique and other arms have of their clients' affairs and add it to those that even plain vanilla-flavour bankers always had, and consider on top of that that each of these new functions has its specific temptation to seduce banks from the stony path of virtue, you see that the pious pretences of an "even playing field" are poppy-cock. The playing field in fact is tilted so close to vertical that even bank CEOs that conduct Sunday school classes, find it impossible to show Satan the door.

Once you start improvising a special morality that you consider open to you because of the variety of big hats you wear, just about anything goes.

The TD Bank on its own admission set aside reserves for losses far beyond what proved necessary. That had several questionable effects. By merely releasing much of those excessive reserves the following year, it was able to score an amazing recovery from losses to earnings. This was a cagey way of goosing the price of its stock.

Freddie Mac is one of the two US government-sponsored mortgage agencies that buy up and syndicate mortgages to free up private lending institutions for further loans on houses. Ever since last summer the financial markets have been in turmoil because Freddie Mac restated its income of the past three years to correct a gross understatement of its profits. *The Wall Street Journal* (10/6, "Freddie Mac Ousts Top Officials as Regulators Prepare Enquiries") tells the tale:

"These surprising developments sent investors fleeing from Freddie Mac's debt toward the security of US Treasury Bonds. The market impact was muted, however, in part because Freddie said the restatement would make its profits and capital bigger than previously reported, not smaller. But after a thorough-going investigation, the regulator, the Office of Federal Housing Enterprise Oversight, fined Freddie Mac $125 million for creating the misleading impression that the profits of that institution have been rising at a dependably steady rate."

There lies the Achilles heel of the entire growth compulsion. To have grown excessively means that your growth becomes immediately capitalized, as does your rate of growth and the expansion rates of such growth to infinity.

All these are built into the market price of the company shares. Unless all the factors contributed to that valuation continue into the indefinite future at the present rate, that unsustainable rate of growth, and the price into which it has been embedded must collapse. And obviously, where earnings are built on pillaging the reserves of the nonmarket subsystems of the economy and society, they must continue forever to support such a progression. It becomes a bloody game of musical chairs: Eat or be Eaten. The graph of such a growth rate starts nearly flat and in no time at all stands vertically. That verges on the mathematics of the atom bomb – the exponential function. It cannot be maintained. The understatement of current earnings may be a desperate effort to make it last as long as possible.

Hence, too, the quick, surreptitious exits from the game by those with inside information. Derivatives are a choice way of organizing that exit, since, not being regulated, they do not have to be declared. No outsider knows when the bank peddling a questionable deal to investors, may actually be shorting its position by selling more derivatives than its positive holdings.

Our banks sell derivatives, and to keep that lucrative department thriving, they must devise ever more ingenious games that can be played with their products. Like Bill Gates designing new version of Windows, in part to give away his competitors' products and put them out of business. And like bootleggers given to drink they make abundant use of derivatives themselves. Mr. Clark, quoted in the above-cited article, declared: "You can make a lot of money staying in the loop," went on to say that his firm is "never going to get caught as a counterparty" on a credit derivative. That "getting caught" is definitely a Freudian slip. Smart fellow, that old Vienna Jew!

William Krehm

"Monetary Reform — Making it Happen"

THIS FINE BOOK by James Robertson and John M. Bunzl announces a coming together of society's defences on two distinct fronts – monetary reform represented by James Robertson, and John Bunzl's Simultaneous Approach. Hopefully, it may prove the harbinger of further alliances in other vital areas.

Robertson provides the historical perspective in the efforts of Thomas Attwood, an early 19th-century monetary and political reformer.

"A family banker aged 29, in 1812 he made his mark with the manufacturers and artisans of Birmingham by leading a political campaign against the monopoly enjoyed by the East India Company and other British Government restrictions on overseas trade. That campaign confirmed that business owners and the working people – both of whom who had sprung from the industrial revolution and were unrepresented in parliament – could work together in their common interest that conflicted with those of the rural land-owning classes. The latter still monopolized parliament and government. For ten or fifteen years his energies were directed to monetary reform, but then he was to play a key part in the successful passage of the great parliamentary *Reform Act* of 1832.

"The industrial revolution was straining monetary institutions. In 1797 the effects of the Napoleonic Wars had driven the Bank of England off the gold standard; the exchangeability of its banknotes for gold sovereigns had been suspended. Between 1810 and 1819. Attwood campaigned, unsuccessfully, against the parliamentary 'Bullion Report; which recommended that the number and value of banknotes in circulation should be reduced and their exchangeability for gold be restored.[1]

"Attwood and his colleagues of the 'Paper Money' School were in effect calling for money to be *redefined* to include paper banknotes as well as gold coins and bullion. Today this has been long accepted. Banknotes are recognized, along with coins, to be 'cash.' Like coins they are now issued debt-free by an agency of the state, the Bank of England. Although British banknotes still say 'I promise to pay....' that is a meaningless survival from past history.... Everyone knows they are cash.

"The challenge we face today is similar to Attwood's. But our definition of money should now be extended to include, not just banknotes and coin, but also the electronic bank-created money in our current bank accounts. Although some people say that that is something distinct from money called credit, it is now clearly recognized to be money immediately available for spending. The Bank Charter Act of 1844 eventually resulted in a Bank of England monopoly of the banknote issue in England and Wales. Scottish and Northern Irish banks still issue their own banknotes, but these must be backed by Bank of England notes. However, the number and value of the banknotes issued are simply what is needed for the convenience of the public. They play no part in controlling the total value of the money supply. That is done by regulating interest rates, to control demand for the non-cash, bank-account money created by commercial banks and issued to their customers' accounts as interest-bearing loans. That commercial banks still create this official-currency money for private-sector profit has become a glaring anachronism.

"As pressure grew for parliamentary reform in the 1820s Attwood recognized that monetary reformers would have to work together with campaigners for other radical issues. One of these was the campaign to repeal the Corn Laws, which imposed a tariff on imported grain and imposed dearer food on urban working people. In 1829 Attwood succeeded in bringing these various campaigning groups together under the banner of the Birmingham Political Union for the Protection of Public Rights, a new 'general political union between the lower and middle classes of the people. Its first priority was to campaign for reform of the House of Commons, which had become, in Attwood's words, 'the seat of ignorance, imbecility and indifference.' who specialized in the pursuit of power, influence, and corruption.

"For over two centuries political democracy has been spreading through the world, thanks to Attwood and others like him. But our capacity to control and harness the power of money for the public good has lagged far behind. So much so that failure to bring the workings of money and finance into line with economic justice is damaging confidence in political democracy itself. An international monetary system based on one or two superpower currencies such as the US$ and the euro profits the countries that issue those currencies at the expense of the rest of the world.

"For us in Britain the euro highlights the link between democracy and the money system. In spite of efforts to persuade us that scrapping the pound and replacing it with the euro would be a progressive step, people are increasingly doubtful. Why can't we use the euro as a parallel currency, alongside the pound, rather than a single currency managed by a remote, centralized authority imposing one-size-fits-all interest rates and money supply on millions of diverse people and places? Surely 21st century pressures to become more globalized *and* more localized call for a more pluralistic monetary system. This would allow different currencies and means of payment to evolve at local to global levels, enabling people and organizations to choose whatever currency they find most useful for different purposes. As well as national currencies, continental currencies and a global currency, we should be encouraging currencies issued by local government authorities for local circulation, and non-official payments systems set up by community groups (like LETS)."

This articulates an issue already very much in the air. Thus *The Wall Street Journal* (9/01/04, "State and Local Programs Seek to Aid Uninsured" by Laurie Mcginley) informs us: "Muskegon, Mich. – States and local communities, frustrated by the federal government's failure to stem the growing ranks of the uninsured, have begun experimenting with their own initiatives to expand health coverage, especially for low-income employees of small businesses. Many of the initiatives are small and in nascent stages, started with seed money provided by state and federal governments or nonprofit foundations. They could be snuffed out if the states' beleaguered financial picture doesn't substantially improve." The answer is, of course, alternate currencies at various lower levels, that will limit spending to the availability of unused local human and material resources. In short this is one of the many welcome mats that are already out for the Simultaneous Policy solution.

But nowhere have I encountered improvisations generalized so clearly into essential principle as in the Robertson-Bunzl book. That would give local bodies the choice of providing employment against payment in local as well as national or international currencies. In that way human ingenuity could throw up defences against the monopoly of international conglomerates.

But to make this possible the same recognition and simultaneous policy must be extended to embrace two further areas.

One is the recognition of public sector investment, both in physical and human capital. In the US this was smuggled into the government accountancy under the misleading heading of "savings," which it was not since it was not held as cash.[2] In this way the Clinton administration, beginning with January 1996, was able to show a surplus and through the improved ratings resulting on federal debt bring down interest rates. In Canada, "capital budgeting" (a.k.a. "accrual accountancy") became law in mid-1999 with neither explanation nor debate in parliament or in the media.

Unless the Simultaneous Policy crusade embraces serious accountancy in the public sector, its efforts will be frustrated by the present hysteria for balanced government budgets. Without the distinction between government investment and current spending, you simply have no accountancy. Try introducing such bookkeeping in the market sector and see what would result.

Capital is, after all, what capitalism is supposed to be about. CEOs of private corporations who horse around with company assets even risk ending up in jail.

It is important to note that since the revenue of governments is mostly taxation, it is the tax-base that counts rather than whether an investment in human capital – say education or health – ends up in physical bodies and minds or in the government jurisdiction.

Closely connected with that is the fact that a flat price level ("zero inflation") is simply unobtainable in a highly technological, rapidly urbanizing world. Except, of course, under conditions of severe depression. Nobody in his right senses who moves from the countryside to London, Tokyo, or New York expects his living costs to remain the same. How then can humanity expect to when making a similar move? Price index increases may mean one of two very different things: real market inflation, properly defined as an excess of aggregate demand over supply. Or it may simply designate that the output of the public sector has increased as a proportion of the total national output, and hence the layer of taxation in all price has deepened.

Significantly even the US Federal Reserve and the Bank for International Settlements in recent months have come to distinguish this as "beneficial inflation" and identify it as up to 2% price increase. We identified it under the name of "social lien" almost 40 years ago. It makes no sense to give two different, in fact contrary forces, the same name. You will find no instance of that in any serious science.

To make such nonsense possible, conventional economists have declared all non-market subsystems of our mixed economy "externalities" – i.e., shoved them out of the back door so that they could devote themselves exclusively to the attainment of flat-world economics. But unless you enter the cost of what should be but has not been done to preserve the environment, or public health, you are running up a deficit that will catch up with you with dreadful penalties. Such have already appeared under the labels of AIDS, SARS, Mad Cow Disease, and even Terrorism.

Finally, we must come to grips with the fact that economic theory is misusing mathematics. Much has been made of the "higher mathematics" on which price theory has been based for over a century. But to use the infinitesimal calculus, the "marginal utility" people who assume a "pure and perfect" market that is self-balancing, posit all actors on it to be of such negligible size that nothing they do individually can influence the price level. Obviously this is nonsense in the age of Microsoft and General Electric – a clear case of the customer cut to the cloth.

It is high time that we brought some professional mathematicians into our conferences on heterodox economics to tell economists what mathematics can and what it cannot do. Likewise it is absurd for economists to close ranks and consider that only they, with their tattered record, have a right to be listened to when the economy comes up for discussion.

William Krehm

1. There is a reference to the Attwood brothers in Marx's *Capital*, Vol. 3, p. 547, Moscow 1962: "Let us now listen to a private banker, Twells, an associate of Spooner, Attwood & Co., since 1801. He is alone among the witnesses before the BC (Banking Committee) who provides us with an insight into the country's actual state of affairs and who sees a crisis approaching. In other respects, however, he is a sort of little-shilling man from Birmingham, like his associates, the Attwood brothers who are the founders of the school. He testifies: '4488. How do you think that the Act of 1844 has operated? If I were to answer you as a banker, I should say that it has operated exceedingly well, for it has afforded a rich harvest to bankers and [money]-capitalists of all kinds. But it has operated very badly for the honest industrious tradesman who requires steadiness in the rate

of discount, that he may be able to make his arrangements with confidence. It has made money-lending a most profitable pursuit.'" And there follows a jeremiad of exploitation of the producing economy by the banks and financiers.

2. The US statistic is to be found in the "national saving" figure of the Bureau of Economic Analysis figure of the Department of Commerce, where assets of some $1.3 trillion were discovered – still not counting government investment in human capital such as education, health, and social welfare.

Another Apple Ripe for Falling from Newton's Tree

CHINA is rapidly becoming industrialized and is conquering world markets with labour costs one tenth those of Japan or the US. And she is invading the world agricultural market as well. Her population numbers 1.3 billion, but her problems are hardly of lesser magnitude. Domestic market size has always been a key factor in world trade – if accompanied with enough power. And power readily enlists military conquest towards that end. Small powers with hinterlands to go with their city core like Holland and then England rapidly replaced city states like Venice and Florence, and small countries like Britain and the Netherlands and Portugal acquired colonial empires as cheap, controlled sources of labour and raw materials. Japan's history has been interpreted by historians in this sense. Right-thinking economists, however, have been elaborately trained to pay little heed to history. Today China is well on the road to dwarfing the United States in economic mass.

But size is only one key factor. China, violently aroused from the slumber of centuries by the fading Communist regime, is rapidly adding the advantages of a modern education and technology to it to its ancestral reverence of learning. That formidable resource has been reinforced not only by the highly educated elite of its Diaspora in East Asia, but those, who, fleeing the Communists' regime, learned in the West to wed Confucius with Newton and Einstein. And now she is not only shifting from the bicycle to the automobile, but using that as base for export. And inevitably that is building up a lust for a due share of the world's oil reserves In the long run this is certainly creating as many problems as it seems to be solving. The gap between the rewards of the budding capitalist and the mass of Chinese workers is greater than in the Britain of Charles Dickens.

Meanwhile the United States has been shedding its real productive advantages. It has outsourced to countries like China and India first its simpler industrial processes to deflate its own costs and evade its own tax system, and then surrendered more and more of its technology and even its management and marketing strategies to them. By this means it is resorting to a massive deflation of its real production to leave more room for the hyperinflation of its financial sector.

The absolute power of Wall St. is expressed in the pricing of its financial assets: the rate of growth achieved tends to be extrapolated into the indefinite future and incorporated, into its current price. The result is a striving towards exponential growth in which the rate of growth of the rate of growth and hence all higher derivatives of that growth equal the value attained by the underlying function. That however, is the mathematics of the atomic bomb. Result: the spread between speculative fortunes made on Wall St. and those in the productive economy match those between the economic leaders and the mass of peasantry and workers in nominally Communist China. Both are unsustainable.

A Striving Towards Exponential Growth

It is becoming clear that growth – a single scalar figure with no sense of direction – is entangling us ever more hopelessly in this maze.

For the past decades COMER has made use of systems theory that shows the perils of such an arrangement. A subsystem is a component of a system that by definition pursues a distinct purpose from other subsystems but is essential for the functioning of the system as a whole. An automobile is a good example. To move safely, its mechanical subsystem, its engine, its fuel sub-system, its electrical and electronic sub-systems must each be in working order. Trying to average out their efficiencies can only lead to disaster. If a single one falters it becomes a hazard to the driver and the congested traffic on our roads. Conclusion: no subsystem must be allowed to devour the essential resources of another.

But the world economy, scrambling after exponential growth, has neither time nor space for such a careful coordination of our economic subsystems. Systems theory is the basic solution. But we are ever farther from thinking in terms of serious solutions. We are still at the diagnosis stage. And for that we must go back to the methodology that has enabled scientists to put men on the men and probe the surface and subsoil of Mars. This at a time when governments are riotously undermining the chances of human survival on our home planet.

Over the past 40 years some of us in COMER have tracked the disintegration of official economic theory. As technology led to a mixed economy, and the public and private sectors became every more intertwined, official economists retreated into "number crunching," i.e., manipulating *absolute numbers*, i.e., scalars proclaimed "key statistics" – GDP, growth, whatever. COMER, however, introduced into economics the concept of "vectors" as opposed to "scalars."

To pursue the compelling comparison between the proper use of mathematical thinking in its home territory of physics and its illiterate misuse by conventional economists, I will contrast the use made of a very basic principle by physicists and official economists.

Number-crunching Replaces Analysis

For the purpose I will use as reference a standard text, *Principles of Mathematical Physics*, by William V. Houston, Professor of Physics, California Institute of Technology.[1] In the preface the author explains: "This book has been written as the text for a course which I have given for several years to juniors, seniors and first-year graduate students." And this is what he has to say about Scalars and Vectors (p. 76): "A scalar quantity can be represented by a single number, while a vector quantity requires for its representation a vector. A vector is a line whose length, on a certain scale, represents the magnitude of the quantity, and whose direction is the direction of the quantity represented. Completely to represent the direction, it is necessary to distinguish between the origin and the end of the vector, and a vector is considered unchanged when it is moved parallel to itself. The location of the origin is usually of no consequence, and a vector is considered unchanged when it is moved parallel to itself. Though the position of the origin is usually not important the distinction between the origin and the end is always significant since the interchange between the two gives the vector the opposite direction."

The importance of the vector concept in economics is that it tracks the changed effect when a measure crosses the boundary between subsystems. In doing so it enters another vector field. "If, with every point in space, there is associated a certain vector, that whole set of vectors is said to constitute a 'vector field.'" A vector entering that field from outside interacts with these vectors and its quantity and direction undergo change. High interest rates which may be a boon to financial corporations, may have a disastrous effect in the household in causing families to lose their homes and end up on the streets.

We Need the Vector Concept to Understand a Mixed Economy

There is one property of vectors that has a particular importance for economic thought. Again I quote the Houston book:

"In the study of a physical problem it is usually necessary to establish a system of coordinates in which the various material bodies can be located. The position of the bodies, expressed in terms of these coordinates, are then the variables in the equations that state the laws of physics. Although these equations will contain the explicit reference to the coordinates used, it is difficult to believe that the relationships expressed should depend upon the coordinates in any essential way. The laws of physics should be relationships between physical things, and these relationships should be true regardless of the language used to state them. In fact, it has long been taken as an axiom that the laws of physics must be expressible in a form which is the same for all systems of coordinates."

There are various ways in which this is achieved in physics. For example, depending upon their convenience in the problem studied, the coordinates can be measured on straight lines at right angles to one another, or inclined at other angles. Or they might by a radius vector and the angles between it and the rectangular line coordinates just described. Translated into economics the coordinates, in the above passages, would have to include price, by far the main coordinate in a market, and one of the important ones in a mixed economy. The use of "zero inflation" as the main policy goal, or even the notion of a single world currency, unless the price were adjusted to economic realities, is a grotesque distortion of what economic theory should be about.

The notion of vectors whose values are entirely independent of coordinates in which they are expressed and change their values and directions as they are affected by the new *vector field* they enter on crossing the boundary between two subsystems of the economy is fundamental in this necessary remaking of economic theory suitable to a mixed economy.

But there are also principles of variation in mathematical physics that are "the equivalent to the Newtonian equations of motion and which can be derived from them. Instead of describing the motion of a particle directly in terms of its acceleration, it describes the path followed by a particle in terms of a quantity which has a stationary value compared with other possible paths. For example instead of using velocity and acceleration which depend on coordinates of space which we wish to eliminate, we deal with such things as momentum and energy, which does not depend on space coordinates.[2] When you integrate a function the result contains an arbitrary constant. That is another way of saying that the integral is independent of any set of coordinates since that arbitrary constant can invalidate means that the expression is independent of any spatial coordinates. From the statement that the variation of a certain integral is zero can be derived the differential equations that describe the motion. This principle provides a statement of the Newtonian equations which is independent of the coordinate equations used, and from which the differential equations can be derived with a minimum of effort. The variation principle is of little or no assistance in solving the equations, but it does provide a convenient means of writing them in any desired coordinates.

Another Apple from Newton's Tree

"This so-called Hamilton's principle is not the only principle of variation which can be used for mechanical problems. Others, notably the principle of least action, can be, and often have been used." Maximization of the GDP and Globalization and Deregulation the current militant dogmas of official economics, however, can be summed up as a "principle of *greatest possible action*," the exact opposite of the basic principle of mathematics and physics.

In comparing alternate paths that differ only slightly from the sought minimal path, we use the paths (expressed in coordinates) diverging from the minimal path over a slight passage of time. Expressing them as a function of time, we eliminate the coordinates of space from our equations. That helps us to the desired goal.

Note that is the sort of elimination we did when we applied Gaussian modular congruence to eliminating the variables of public deficit and debt from our policy model.[3] We can take as our target the public treasury, the state of which depends on the balancing of two variables – its income and expenditure. To eliminate revenue we choose a consumer tax that hits the most vulnerable section of the population. To reduce the spending we shift central government debt from the private banks to the central bank. In Canada, as in the UK, since the one shareholder of the central bank is the government, virtually the entire interest paid by the central government on such debt held by the central bank reverts to the government as dividends. But even in the

US, where private banks are the shareholders of the Federal Reserve System, roughly the same proportion of the interest paid on such debt held by the Fed reaches the government because of the ancestral monarch's monopoly of coining precious metals. Instead of dealing with taxes (the income of the treasury) and its expenditures, we deal with the results of these two contrary variables taken in equivalent dosages so that spending and taxation are eliminated from our equation. By balancing this paired reduction of contrary measures for neutral effect, we have in fact eliminated the joint effect on "balancing the budget." Step Two is purely passive. As the benign indirect effects of these two measures – lower interest rates and lower consumer taxes – work their way throughout the economy a bonus of positive effect will appear. Repeat dosages of the same variables, or other desired pairs of measures of contrary but positive effect will be justified.

What I originally formulated through Gaussian Modular Congruence can also be arrived at by Hamilton's variation principle.

Joint sessions of mathematicians and open-minded economists must be a feature of future Conferences of Heterodox Economists, that are enjoying much current popularity.

Another apple is ripe for falling from Isaac Newton's tree. Universities must not miss the occasion.

William Krehm

1. New York: McGraw-Hill Book Company, Inc., 1934.

2. This relationship between "independence from a particular set of coordinates" will be more readily grasped by the inquisitive reader with enough curiosity about economics and a timidity about mathematics, if we start with the differenciating operation that concerns itself with the rate of change of the value of a function f with respect to infinitesimal changes in the value of three rectilinear coordinates of space x, y, z, – df/dx, df/dy, and df/dz. If f has a constant term c, that, of course, won't change with the space variables and the dc/dx is therefore zero. Turn the process around to the contrary operation of integration. Since any constant terms in f would have disappeared in the differentiation process, in the opposite integration you are free to insert *any number of arbitrary free-standing constant terms*. That signifies independence from any given set of coordinates since the value of the integral is indeterminate.

3. Krehm, William (2002). *Towards a Non-Autistic Economy – A Place at the Table for Society* (p. 165). Toronto: COMER Publications.

A View of Globalization from the Cayman Islands

IT IS AN IRONIC FACT that one of the key features of modern globalized capitalism, offshore banking, was invented by some obscure comrades in charge of managing the foreign reserves of the old Soviet Union. During the early Cold War years, they were apprehensive about depositing their accidental dollar holdings in American banks where they risked being frozen if a political confrontation arose. The solution the comrades came up with were to deposit the dollars in London, since the Brits have never been quick to mix the sacred art of banking with the base art of politics. And while they were at it, why not open their own bank in what was still the banking center of the World? In this way, the Russians ended up having a bank in London, mainly dealing in "red" dollar deposits and lending.

For America's big corporations a dollar is always green, no matter where it comes from. They quickly saw the advantage of having access to dollars outside of America, where the banking system at the time was strictly regulated. Nor did it take long for the British banks to realize that the Russian comrades in their midst had hit upon a significant financial innovation. Therefore, they hurriedly followed in their steps and started to open departments specializing in unregulated dollar deposits and lending. Offshore banking as a wider phenomenon was born.

In the early days, tax considerations weren't an important facet of offshore banking. It started out mostly catering to corporate customers, that were interested in the lower rates and quick decisions available to customers with the right corporate credentials. In the early period, this new market for eurodollars (as it came to be called) was mostly used for corporate America's expansion in post-war Europe. But it didn't take long for wealthy individuals to realize that the low level of regulations also was beneficial for what today is euphemistically termed "tax planning."

The Outsourcing of Jobs and Profits

In London, while regulations for foreign accounts were low there was still a demand for a paper trail documenting all transfers. Therefore, when the focus started to shift towards deposits, for which the main objective was tax evasion and even money laundering of criminal income, offshore banking activities started to move to new destinations. The preferred choice became small jurisdictions with no prior international banking activities and thus no laws covering them. Most importantly, many of these small jurisdictions saw the luring of these deposits to their shores as a potential bonanza for moribund and underdeveloped economies, and were thus ready to protect the deposits by refusing to engage in information sharing with authorities in the depositors' home countries.

In recent decades, another prominent feature of the ongoing globalization has been the outsourcing of manufacturing to developing economies where labour costs are much lower. However, the question of labour cost is not as simple as it appears. The direct labour cost going into a product can be as low as one

21

percent of its final sales price, as recent revelations regarding manufacturing conditions for Nike products have shown. It is also worth noting that products, when they are brand names as Nike's are, have higher price inelasticities, which translates into higher abilities to absorb labour costs. Thus, seen only from a price consideration, much of the outsourced production could probably – using normal profit standards – be kept in the US by accessing the growing pool of workers within its borders forced to accept whatever minimum wage work they can get. Clearly, it appears that there are other factors behind the trend of offshore outsourcing of the corporate production activities.

Here the tax havens come back into the picture. Offshore production in a global economy creates new possibilities for reducing tax liabilities, that don't exist if a company both produces and sells within its home country only. To take advantage of this, when moving a production offshore, it is typically accompanied by the establishment of a subsidiary in a tax haven to which ownership of the so-called soft assets, such as patent rights, brand names and company logos, are transferred. The tax haven subsidiary will thereupon invoice the offshore manufacturer for the "right" to use these soft assets.

This transform the soft assets from balance sheet items into costs embedded in the products when they return to the home country. Since the tax haven subsidiary is fully owned and operationally controlled, the cost structure of the whole process can be geared up and down so that profits in the home country disappear no matter what sales prices can be fetched in the home market. Sometimes the process is refined by moving the main company itself – either as an empty shell registration or as a skeleton corporate headquarter – to the tax haven. This leaves a subsidiary with all the rest of normal corporate functions, such as design, marketing, distributing, and the majority of the corporate executive staff, in the original home country.

A key aspect emerging from the whole process is that it is increasingly tailored to focus on the corporate elite's interests, at the expense of ordinary shareholders. For example, the corporate elite can have part of their remuneration hidden as "consulting" fees paid to shell companies and bank accounts the executives themselves have set up in the tax haven, with the money coming from the revenue accruing to the subsidiary that holds the soft assets.

The Culture of Free Riders

Interpolating from a sample of credit card transaction records, the IRS concluded that upwards of two millions Americans access funds held in tax haven bank accounts by credit cards, while tax returns only reported 170,000 accounts. In the Cayman Islands alone, deposits totalled more than $800 billion, which equals one-fifth of all deposits within the US. A conservative estimate is that upwards of $70 billion in taxes are lost every year due to the hiding of income in the tax havens. However, since the Bush Administration cut the IRS' auditing staff drastically, it has essentially been reduced to the role of an onlooker.

The growing problem of tax evasion occurring in tax havens spurred the OECD into action in 1998, with the Clinton Administration signing onto the process. Forty-three identi-fied offshore tax havens were notified that they would have to comply with a certain level of information exchange, otherwise they would be the target of countermeasures. Despite the fact that both the demands and the contemplated countermeasures were very weak, they were too much for the Bush Administration, who in 2001 gave the activities in the tax havens another free pass by declaring that the OECD demands were "not in line with this administration's priorities." Anybody surprised here?

The OECD initiative had brought all the market extremist out on the war path. According to them, tax "planning," as everything else, should be left to free, unregulated market forces. That we are talking of asymmetries of almost incomparable proportions doesn't matter. Forget the fact that a developed country burdened with upholding a sophisticated socio-technical infrastructure has to raise taxes to pay for it, while a tax haven like the Cayman Islands (with barely 40,000 inhabitants, many of them expatriates connected to tax haven activities) has little to take care of.

In this case, the market extremist logic cannot even considered a fig leaf for the culture of free riders that has come to prevail among the current elite. Outsourcing profits and income to the tax havens has become another nail in the coffin for the dying principles of the welfare state. As the rock singer Perry Farrell put it: "Your true nature is how you treat the weak." Using that measure, there is not much doubt about the nature of the crowd that took over the White House during the Texan *coup d'état* of 2000.

Dix Sanbeck

REVIEW OF A BOOK BY JOSEPH STIGLITZ, NEW YORK, 2003

"The Roaring Nineties"

STIGLITZ' FIRST BOOK, *Globalization and It's Discontents*, was an exposé of the operation of the IMF and the World Bank by an insider. His exposure of the disastrous impact of the "Washington Consensus" policies in the developing world led to his departure from the World Bank (he was senior vice-president). Unfortunately, despite the overwhelming evidence, the book was not widely read and had little impact.

This book is a damning indictment of the economic policies of the US federal government for the past 20 years. Even the Clinton administration comes in for some heavy criticism. While Stiglitz credits Clinton with good intentions (he was part of the administration) and even a few good policies, such as the tax increase on the wealthy, on most issues he was unable or unwilling to withstand the ideological attack from the neo cons.

The Clinton "New Democrats" enthusiastically endorsed the Reagan-Bush deregulation/privatization agenda, with disastrous results. Stiglitz documents how telecom deregulation led to "frenzied overinvestment," tremendous overcapacity and a bloated stock market bubble which inevitably burst.

Banking deregulation also contributed to the bubble. The

repeal of Glass-Steagall allowed the banks to participate fully in the tech bubble. Unfortunately for the public, in the pursuit of their profits and fees, the banks utterly failed to exercise "due diligence."

Giving free rein to the market was supposed to protect the public interest but the opposite occurred. Stiglitz is scathing in his denunciation of corporate behaviour. The plethora of stock options for executives – $1 billion from the Sprint – World Com merger alone – he characterizes as "theft." The same CEOs who plundered their own companies used their influence, backed by hefty campaign contributions, to emasculate the regulatory framework. Enron's role in energy deregulation, and its subsequent theft of billions from California ratepayers is a case in point, but there were many more. Accounting firms like Arthur Andersen were caught up in the miasma of corruption and falsified the books to keep the bubble going. When it burst thousands of workers lost their savings and pensions but the CEOs made off like bandits with their loot. Only a token few will ever do jail time.

The same CEOs who were stealing from their own companies were pushing the government to lower taxes on corporations and the rich. The Clinton administration did raise taxes on the rich early on, but was unable to withstand the pressure and implemented a "huge" capital gains tax cut in 1997 which Stiglitz calls a "pure gift to the rich." Bush has continued this policy by abolishing the inheritance tax and the dividend tax while simultaneously running up huge deficits. Stiglitz demonstrates that these kinds of tax cuts do little to stimulate the economy, but they do undermine the government's fiscal position and render welfare programs untenable.

On globalization, Stiglitz is clearer than in his first book The US today "must get its way" and "rejects the rule of law." The IMF and World Bank act as agents of the Treasury Department to maintain US economic hegemony. He condemns the US for hypocrisy in imposing free market policies abroad while doing the exact opposite at home. For example, US production costs for cotton are twice the international price, but the US subsidies, the bulk of which go to wealthy corporations, is greater than the value of the cotton produced! Small cotton farmers in Africa and elsewhere are the losers. In one sense, the policy is consistent. The same widening gulf between rich and poor being pursued at home is being promoted abroad. Financial liberalization, pushed hard by large US banks and the IMF, has caused financial crises and misery for many countries, but has been a bonanza for US and European corporations which bought up the bankrupt companies at fire-sale prices.

There are some problems with this book. Although Stiglitz deplores the cancerous growth of the financial sector and its destructive impact on the political system, he seems unaware of the true nature of banking and the explosive growth of public and private debt. However, he remains an unapologetic Keynesian and rejects the supply side nonsense that has so bedevilled our economic discourse these past 25 years. As an insider, and a patriotic American, he speaks with authority. This book needs to be widely read. But that seems unlikely.

David Gracey

The Astounding Conversion of Finnolly Servus

FAY RUSHED UP to Finnolly Servus, where he sat, stunned, on the sidewalk, catching his breath and staring at his broken camera.

"Are you all right?" she asked.

"I'll recover," he said tersely, getting to his feet, rubbing his midriff.

"Now you've met the other kind of police" she said. "They could have been private cops, though."

"Private cops?" questioned Finnolly.

"Yes, there are now twice as many private police as public police. It used to be the other way round. But you'll soon see the other kind of public police, too. Look up"

On a roof overlooking the street, he saw two figures: one with a camera; one with what looked like a gun.

They rejoined the march. As they got closer to their target location, certain buildings were fronted with a line of masked police carrying large black shields and holding long black truncheons. Were they protecting good citizens from criminals, or protecting government from good citizens? The answer wasn't clear.

When they had almost reached the packed square where the Embassy building stood, the marchers ahead of them stopped and then began reeling back on them. "Tear gas," somebody shouted.

Finnolly looked around for Sylvia. She had almost caught up with him. He took Fay by the arm and struggled back through the milling, undecided crowd, working his way toward his wife. His eyes were beginning to sting. Some of the marchers were leaving the street by a lane. May and Sylvia joined them. Finnolly changed direction. Then he saw his wife turn back. He waved her on, and, with Fay, struggled toward the entrance to the lane. They hadn't quite reached it when a helicopter, flying low over the street, drove the crowd to press against the buildings on either side. Finnolly held Kay firmly by the arm and became part of the funnel flow of bodies into the lane.

"Now I know why I didn't want to be at the head of the parade," joked Kay, and then more soberly "Those kids up front must be really getting it. Maybe the wind will change."

They did not catch up with Sylvia and May until the lane debouched into another street, where they gathered on the sidewalk behind a newspaper box.

"I'm sorry, Finnolly," said May, "I didn't intend to get you and Mrs. Servus into anything like this. I'm really sorry.

"Call me Sylvia," said Mrs. Servus, still dabbing her eyes with a handkerchief. "I wouldn't have believed it if I hadn't been here."

Finnolly was concerned. "Are you all right, Syl?"

"Of course I'm all right."

She had not seen his altercation with the private cops. The time did not seem right to report it.

"Here's a restaurant. Shall we go in for a coffee?" he said.

The restaurant was already crowded, but people shifted over to accommodate them. Almost all eyes, including the waitresses,' were constantly directed to the TV screen over the bar. The camera looked down on the crowd before the Embassy, probably from a window on the other side of the square. In front of the Embassy the police in riot gear stood three deep. On the boulevard in front, a crew was setting up a speaker system. Three people standing on a folding table held microphones.

"See the people on the lower right," said a rather youthful bald head next to Sylvia, pointing at the TV. "They're going to try to broadcast. They couldn't get permission, but they're going to try anyway."

As they watched, a phalanx of policemen separated from the main squad and formed a flying wedge in the direction of the would-be broadcasters. As they closed the distance, many of the crowd, instead of moving aside, sat down. The police squad eventually slowed to a stop. More sitters crowded in. The police group raised their truncheons.

The camera gyrated wildly and swung off the scene. The screen switched to a commentator at a news desk. "And those pictures from Patrick Mulligan at the Peace March we received a few minutes ago. It looked as though the demonstrators were trying to set up a loudspeaker system, for which we know they do not have a permit. We have lost contact with Patrick temporarily, but we will continue to follow this story."

"It looks bad," said May. "If that's how it started, and then they used the tear gas, we have had some people hurt."

"But what's so terrible about a PA system that they had to attack those people just sitting there? It could have been us!" said Sylvia.

"The truth," answered Finnolly, sagely, and then added, "I wonder what they did to Mulligan."

"Probably the same thing they did to you," said Fay, "but he'll be OK. Don't expect to see that scene again on the six o'clock news, though."

Fay was right, the evening news, in all the media, showed only shouting demonstrators, waving placards or raising fists.

For some time after the march Finnolly thought about wealth transfer. He devised what he later came to call the Servus Law of Money: "Money goes where money is." That is, the rich get richer and the poor get poorer. It was the law of the free market economy. (He had seen quite enough as an insider to know that the idea, popular in the business press, that unregulated markets eventually make everybody rich was a complete and utter crock.) What he wanted to get clear was a better alternative. That came to him when he was discussing it with Sylvia.

"Wouldn't it be best," she asked, "if everybody had enough money and nobody had too much?"

"Sure, but how do you decide how much is 'enough' and how much is 'too much'?" Finnolly resisted.

"You told me a while back that the chief executives of companies now make 400 times as much as the common workers in their companies. That's too much, isn't it?"

"OK, I guess it is. Suppose we cut it to 100 times. But how much is 'enough'?"

"Well, what do people actually really need?" said Sylvia with remarkable clarity. "They need healthy food and to have a warm home in winter. They need clothes."

"They need to be able to afford health insurance, and to get their children educated," said Finnolly, somewhat surprising himself.

"Do they need a car?"

"Hmmnnn." Finnolly thought about that. He finally said, "I don't think a car is a NEED. It's certainly something everybody wants."

"So couldn't you just figure out how much money would meet those real needs?"

"Sure. It has been done. The figure is called 'the poverty line.'"

"Well, double that, and I would call it, 'Enough.'"

"You make it sound simple, dear. But how do you do it?"

"You're the financial man. Figure it out."

"But there is the law of money. Money goes where money is just as sure as water runs downhill."

"So put a dam in it."

Finnolly thought about it for a week. What puts a dam in the natural flow of money from the poorest to the richest? He came up with three things: collective bargaining by workers, redistribution by government, and, as an unfortunate last resort, robbery or revolution. All three he realized had been on his hit list. He also saw that executive compensation had so egregiously outpaced the workers' wages because for two decades governments and unions had been in retreat.

It now seemed crystal clear to him that democracy – government of, by and for the people – had also been in retreat. Finnolly Servus, middle-aged capitalist, had recovered a youthful lesson he had learned from his Grade Twelve history teacher: democracy is worth fighting for.

It was an astounding conversion.

Gordon Coggins

BOOK REVIEW

In Memory of a Great Sacrificed Canadian

Origins of the Modern Japanese State – Selected Writings of E.H. Norman. *Edited by John W. Dower. Edited with an introduction on E. H. Norman, "Japan and the Uses of History," by John W. Dower, Pantheon Books, Random House, New York, 1975.*

JUST IN CASE a younger generation may not know the name E.H. Norman, let me quote from Dower's introduction: "Norman's death and the subsequent neglect of his work in the West provide a saddening chapter on the politics of postwar American scholarship in Japan. In his own words, Norman was 'addicted to history,' and the brief tribute to Clio with which this volume begins suggests the intimate link which he perceived between historical consciousness and man's fate. Although he did his doctoral work in Japanese history at Harvard, his prior training was in at Victoria College in Toronto and Trinity College in Cambridge in ancient and medieval European history. His parents were missionaries in Nagano prefecture, and he lived in Japan from birth until his mid-teens. [His work] breathes both an enviable knowledge of the West as well as the East, and a sense of humility before the 'delicate tracery' of historical change."

Norman died by suicide, run over by Washington's great McCarthy machine that churned out sentences of guilt by association. The main charge was that he had attended Marxist study classes at university, and had thus met individuals who years later became Soviet agents. But given Washington's fulsome wartime propaganda build-up for Joe Stalin ("Uncle Joe"), responsibilities for that were far-flung. In that respect Washington made little distinction between the servile dictators it had imposed and sustained in Central America and its great Soviet ally. President Roosevelt himself was quoted saying of President Anastasio Somoza, a gangster type sustained by the US in Nicaragua during an entire era: "He is a son of a bitch, but his *our* son of a bitch." That *bon mot* covers much of Washington's foreign politics to this day.

The McCarthy committee was stone-deaf to much revealing evidence of style. It is not difficult to distinguish a great independent thinker from the stylistic flat-footedness of an ideologue. And no agent – of Washington or of Stalin – could produce the sensitive, profound handling of history by E.H. Norman.

The great turning point in Japanese history was the end of the period when the Emperor was shorn of all actual power and secluded in Kyoto, while shoguns – formally his servers – took over. This was known as the "shogunate" or the "Bakufu" (literally the "tent government" or military headquarters). It was "one of the most conscious attempts [anywhere] to freeze society in a rigid mold. Every social class, and every subdivision within it, had its own regulations covering all the minutiae of clothing, ceremony and behavior. The criminal code, severe even by feudal standards, distinguished between *samurai* – the warriors – and commoner." The late Shogunate held "It is enough to follow the books of old, and there is no need to write new ones." Scholars who pursued their studies in "Dutch learning" (the Dutch were the only foreigners tolerated) were even executed. "Its slogan was 'revere officials and despise the people.' Recent Western scholarship has challenged this view of peasant immiseration by revealing increased productivity beyond what was recognized at the time Norman wrote, and postulating that this contributed to an over-all rise in living standards. What Norman did observe was that misery and disaster were recurrent: that economic growth and changes in the mode of production per se may have altered the nature of the burden on the little man, but that the dispossessed can be crushed beneath the wheels of change."

Sound familiar? It should. There is in fact a tendency among critics of Norman's view that sees in modernization a virtue in itself that solves problems by "trickle-down." But he pointed to the relative lack in Japanese culture of compassion for the weak and unfortunate. In the poisoned atmosphere of the 1940s, he emphasized that this was the legacy of the *cultural mold* rather than any inherent *racial* characteristic.

"Norman's interpretation of Japan's rapid transition from feudal society rests to a large extent upon the *timing* of this development, 'the fortuitous concurrence of two processes: (1) the death agony of feudalism and (2) the pressure exerted on Japan by the Western nations.'

"The Western threat to Japan was primarily economic. Following the treaties of the 1850s, the influx of foreign manufactures heightened the domestic economic crisis by destroying home industries such as cotton, sugar and pulp and causing drastic fluctuations in the money economy. In this way, Western imperialism contributed to the turmoil which culminated in the overthrow of the Shogunate. This economic pressure was perpetuated through the fixed tariffs imposed on Japan under the unequal-treaty system, which served as a reminder to Japan's leaders that their development stood in danger of being stunted like China's. This gave urgency to their objectives of creating a strong state and influenced both the priorities which characterized economic growth, entailing a curtailment of social and political reforms. Japan's comparatively successful transition to a modern state was accomplished in part because *for reasons of their own* the Western powers did not attempt to clamp Japan in the vise of neocolonialism during the period when the country was most vulnerable. The threat, however, nevertheless remained, and the game of international power was played by Western rules. Japan acquired extraterritorial rights in China before she had shaken herself free of similar foreign privileges in her own land."

The Samurai Heritage

In his *Japan's Emergence as a Modern States* (1940), Norman wrote "Japan has been handicapped by her late entry on the stage of world politics and by her economic insufficiency. [However, she recognized that] unity of purpose and action among the great Powers can never be maintained long. The conclusion was drawn that Japan's opportunity would come at the moment of sharpest tension between the powers. Patience, good judgment, and the will to strike fast and hard at a moment's notice have continued as characteristics of Japanese foreign policy. In this way she acquired with a comparatively small output of energy what other nations of greater economic strength have achieved only after long wars, setbacks and even defeats. The Japanese Empire was built in the course of thirty-five years or so. During that time she engaged in three victorious wars, 1894-5 (with China), 1904-5 (with Russia), and 1914-8. None of these exhausted Japan unduly. Nor did her next great advance of 1931-3, by which Manchuria was pried loose from China with only desultory fighting. As a yardstick to measure the success of this policy one might mention the continual reverses suffered by the immense empire of Tsarist Russia during the 19th and early 20th centuries."

Japanese history unrolled in a matrix of such improbable circumstance that no economic model developed in the West, Marxist or other, could possibly provide a neat fit. The *samurai* – the warrior caste – were originally peasants and landowners as well, but the introduction of cannon from the West, caused cities and towns to throw up walls. To keep them in line the samurai were brought to live within the fortifications or leave their families there as hostages. Absentees, they leased their plots to plain peasants, who paid rent in rice, the only existing currency. To lessen their exposure to the instability of rice prices, this was soon transmutted into coin. And to handle the resulting transactions the samurai turned to the lowest and most contemned of social groups – the outcast *etas* alone excepted – money lenders and merchants. By marriage or partnerships these were brought into alliances with samurai families to handle the complex money transactions. For though murderously adept in wielding the two long swords that marked their status, the samurai had no knowledge of the simplest arithmetic. With the restoration of the Meiji monarchy (1867-8), the sale of land plots was introduced to protect the usurious loans for which they served as collateral. From such humble beginnings arose the grand alliances of banks and world industries – the *zaibatsu*. This historic nexus still contributes to the reluctance of the Japanese banks to foreclose on historic customers, as the American model requires.

A Matrix of Improbable Circumstance

The presence of so many landless samurai, the shrinking pensions that replaced the land that once was theirs, weighed heavily on Japanese politics. Some of the now redundant samurai acquired forbidden Western learning and helped bring it into the educational system. Others agitated for foreign wars – against China and Korea and Russia – that would give them an outlet for their rusting martial talents. Sober statesmen, meanwhile, restrained them until a central government and a central policy, and a navy and army had been created to make such wars a likely bet.

These multifaceted powers of analysis shows up as well in its planning its industrial rebirth after the shattering defeat in the Second World War. Little was left to the self-balancing market. Having so little foreign currency, they sought out the lines of export as their ultimate goal to leave a maximum of net export revenue. Certainly the bill was not filled by textiles, one of their main exports before the war, could not fill the bill, since the cotton and yarn had to be imported. They identified heavy machinery and automobiles. But first they had to develop the supporting base for that. Hence they concentrated on steel and iron, electrical and eventually electronics.

Over the years they resisted American pressure to allow their currency to float upward to reflect the triumph of their exports. A contrary course would have meant pushing up further the unaccustomed level of unemployment for Japan – in the 6 and 7% range. Today, their automobile industry is competing successfully with the Americans in the US market. That contributed to their bank problem of the last decade. Like the rest of the first world they are shifting a lot of their manufacturing to China and other Asiatic countries.

To a visitor to Tokyo is impressed with the tip-top shape of its infrastructures after a decade of slight "economic growth." Its subway system, its trains, railways, its educational system frequently make one ashamed of the potholes in all these back home.

In the 1950s and considerably before Senator McCarthy appeared on the scene, Washington was using scholarly research on Japan as an ideological weapon. In that it was pursuing the pattern pioneered by it in Central America and continued in many other parts of the world. In the seventies one of the world's semi-hushed up scandals was revealed when a congressman forced the revelation of the bogus Congress for Cultural Freedom set up by the CIA to commission thousands of articles misinforming the public about rightist coups throughout the world. Fraudulent academic texts were financed that still feed misinformation into the educational system. Newspapermen were rewarded with genuine scoops that could guarantee them lucrative reputations as reward for planting misleading misinformation in their publications. No less an eminence than Arthur Koestler turned out to have been ensnared in that web.

That caught up with H.E. Norman. Far from relying mainly on Marxism, his scholarship on Japan stood in the way of the ideology that Washington was developing to deliberately replace Marxism at its own game. The same Foster Dulles who bestrode US Latin American policy in the 1950s made his power felt in academic views on Japan. Quoting Dower again: "As far as Japan is concerned, the intellectual tasks formulated by the [US] government in the late 1940s and early 1950s had been met by the main line of Japanese studies in America. It penetrated the Japanese intellectual world and attacked progressive scholars, de-emphasized militarism and was gentle with capitalism. It met Dulles's subtle concern with emphasizing the social superiority of the Japanese by concentrating on the successes of the prewar era and the positive features of its traditional social and value structures. It presented Japan as a counter-model for developing countries and deliberately focused upon the more attractive aspects of Japan's emergence as a modern state.

"Norman's views have scant currency within the university establishment. The dark, harsh night of his people under feudalism has been replaced by the roseate dawn of early modernity. [The view was propagated that] the tragedy of modern Japan was largely a dilemma of the interwar period could certainly never be shared by a Chinese or Formosan or Korean nationalist, or by the great majority of Japanese during the earlier period when 'things had gone so well.'

"The thrust of such preoccupations has been extremely significant in shaping many recent interpretations of Japanese external behavior. Japan's dilemma becomes an unfortunate problem of growth, much like acne in adolescence, which might have been avoided if a few salves had been applied before the unsightly condition erupted. What has not been seriously examined is the extent to which the Japanese experience was similar to that of theoretically more advanced capitalist countries.

"Norman's axiom was: it is the effect rather than the motive which should be of primary concern to the historian. In some of his shorter pieces he called attention to the nature of Japanese behavior abroad: atrocities, military occupation, military corruption and disobedience (as opposed to the prevailing image of fanatical discipline), organized prostitution in subject areas, and the crucial role of the narcotic trade in Japanese activities in China, used to both finance aggression and, it was hoped, to debilitate Chinese resistance."

Washington's Cultural Hoax in Japan

None of this fits into the official Washington model of "modernization" or more currently Globalization and Deregulation. Even as it brings the world ever greater disasters, it goes on admitting but a single remedy: more of the same. And it was to that fatal flaw in our power structures that Norman fell victim.

"On August 7, 1951, Professor Karl August Wittfogel testified before the Senate Committee on Internal Security that he knew Norman from his attendance at a Communist study group in 1938. This began the public hounding of Norman that led to his destruction six years later, but the impact of the Senate Inquisition was broader. These were the hearings which wracked and eviscerated Asian studies in the US, and which made taboo even the using of terms like "feudal heritage," and the asking of scholarly *questions*, which could be equated with positions held by communists.

From there the case against Norman patched together in Washington moved on wheels. "Morris introduced a 1940 letter taken from the files of the Institute of Pacific Relations (IPR), indicating that Norman, then assigned to the Canadian Legation in Tokyo, might be persuaded to write for *Pacific Affairs* under a *nom de plume*. The letter also suggested that 'very secret messages' concerning IPR business might be sent care of Norman." Another witness testified that "secret messages" mentioned in the letter referred to the possibility of research manuscripts and involving IPR branches in Tokyo and Shanghai. Such secrecy was considered potentially necessary given the state of war between China and Japan. In fact, no such messages were ever sent through Norman.

"Eugene Dooman of the State Department testifying before the committee on September 14th leveled a further distorted, and ultimately fatal charge against Norman, namely, that together with the John Emmerson of the State Department he had abetted the growth of the postwar Communist Party. The issue involved the release of Communist leaders Shiga Yoshio and Tokuda Kyuchi from prison (where both had been incarcerated since 1928 and were released under a general order from General MacArthur)." Dooman stopped short of pointing the finger at MacArthur as a Communist agent on like grounds, but went on: "John Emmerson of the US State Department and Norman went in a staff car to the prison and brought Shiga and Tokuda back to their homes.

"The initial Wittfogel accusation against Norman drew [an] immediate response from the Department of External Affairs of the Canadian Government: Mr. Norman was subject to the normal security investigation by the proper authorities of the Canadian Government, according to rules which apply to all members of the Department of External Affairs. Subsequently, reports reached the Department which reflected on Mr. Norman's loyalty and alleged previous association with the Communist Party. These reports were very carefully and fully investigated by the security authorities of the Government, and as a result Mr. Nor-

man was given a clean bill of health, and he therefore remains a trusted and valuable official of the Department.

"On August 16 Lester Pearson, Secretary of State for External Affairs, also released a statement reaffirming confidence in Norman, castigating the subcommittee and expressing 'regret and annoyance that his name had been dragged into their hearings on the basis of an unimpressive and unsubstantiated allegation by a former Communist.' Norman at the time was head of the Far Eastern desk in External Affairs, and in a strong gesture of confidence Pearson brought him as his chief adviser to the Japanese peace treaty conference at San Francisco the following month. After affixing his signature to the treaty documents, Pearson handed the gold pen with which he had signed for Canada to Norman, 'I'm giving this to the person who really did the work.'"

Then comes a significant paragraph:

"Although Pearson and his government staunchly defended him, a more complex background to the events of 1951-2 became apparent after Norman's death. It was learned then that as early as 1950 he had been subjected to a gruelling six-month investigation by the Royal Canadian Mounted Police, during which he purportedly acknowledged his earlier, and mistaken, 'campus flirtation with Marxism.' Pearson himself later claimed that Norman himself had requested the investigation (apparently after an accusation had been directed against him by a Canadian ex-party member). The 1950 report remains closed, and the precise sequence of events is confused and opaque, replete with secret informants, alleged mistaken identities, fallacious and amended reports and seemingly inconsistent dates. It was of considerable significance, however, for although the Canadian Government concluded that Norman was not a Communist and his loyalty and integrity were beyond question, the information was in fact made available to the US Government, presumably to the FBI, as a matter of routine exchange of security information. And it appears to have subsequently made its way into the hands of the witch-hunters of the Senate sub-committee."

This is an automatic procedure that was in place before Norman's tragedy and proceeds right to this day, as witness the recent deportation by the US of a naturalized Canadian to Syria, where he was subjected to imprisonment and torture. It reduces Canadian sovereignty over its citizens and officials to mere road-bumps before the whim of the US secret services. Paul Martin's statement, made in April 2003 is hardly reassuring on the point: "Canada has to take a more sophisticated approach to ties with the US…. Multilateralism is a means not an end." That would seem to take care of our sovereignty as well.

But back to Norman. "In 1953 Norman was appointed High Commissioner to New Zealand, a minor post which he repeatedly described as exile. Three years later, however, he was recalled to assume a position of immense important – Ambassador to Egypt. With the Suez crisis of 1957, [came] a period of sheer physical and mental exhaustion – an exceptional personal accomplishment. For Norman is credited with having persuaded Nasser to permit the entry of the UN peace-keeping forces into Egypt in the wake of the British, French and Israeli invasion. Lester Pearson later received the Nobel Peace Prize for his endeavors in the Middle East at this time; much of the real work and accomplishment, it has been suggested privately by a senior Canadian diplomat, was Norman's. At this moment, the Senate subcommittee renewed its accusation, in hearings on 'The Scope of Soviet Activity in the US.' The reopening of the old inquest came at a time when Norman was, by all accounts, exhausted by his endeavours He wrote to Pearson [that] he believed this could only embarrass his government and threaten the fragile Middle East peace. His behavior became erratic. On a doctor's advice he drafted a telegram requesting a temporary holiday leave, to be sent on April 4th. However, on the morning of that day, he [went] to the apartment building where a friend lived, and took an elevator to the ninth floor and walked to the roof, and walking backward, fell to a parking lot below. He died instantaneously, aged forty-seven One of the two letters he left, to a friend, read "I have no option. I must kill myself, for I live without hope."

That message is timely for Canada as a nation, as our new government takes over.

William Krehm

From Knavery to Norm

FROM AN ABERRATION, knavery in high places is well on the way to becoming the norm. From the style of impatient over-achievers, it has become the very substance of our economy.

Along with ever bolder fraud in our globalized world, there is the whine of governments in the richest lands about their inability to meet society's most elementary needs: "there is no money." The environment is in clear rebellion against its mistreatment. War and terrorism, new and old diseases are taking an ever greater toll. No reserves are set aside for geological disasters.

The Wall Street Journal (29/12) carries several stories that report this alleged lack of resources that seemingly makes it necessary to pilfer the allotment to one indispensable program, before we can address another ("Brain Drain – Initiative to Leave No Child Behind Leaves out Gifted-Educators to Divert Resources From Classes for Smartest to Focus on Basic Literacy" by Daniel Golden). "Springfield, Ill. – To make sure even the most disadvantaged students learn the three R's, Congress two years ago passed a law known as No Child Left Behind. National test scores suggest it is indeed helping the weakest students.

"There's just one problem: it may be leaving behind some of the strongest.

"The 2001 law, championed by the Bush administration, calls for all public-school students to be proficient in reading and math by 2014. Schools must make steady progress toward these goals. They face penalties if they don't continually raise their proportion of proficient students, both overall and within various racial and other categories. Schools that miss milestones can be required to pay for outside tutors and let parents transfer children elsewhere. But a school faces no penalty if top students tail off as long as they remain proficient."

Surely a world engaged in investigating life on Mars can grasp the idiocy of robbing all Peters to pay all Pauls. Especially when either group, if neglected, is sure to become a cankerous problem.

"To abide by the law, schools are shifting resources away from programs that help their most gifted students. Because 'all the incentives in No Child Left Behind are to focus on the bottom or the middle,' says Stanford University education professor Michael Kirst, 'reallocating resources there makes sense if you want to stay out of trouble.'"

The underlying assumption of that judgment is that the world is not already in deep trouble. From the President and our central bankers down, each one concentrates on the pie cut dearest to his heart, rather than on the pie as a whole. Scant wonder that the entire pie should be hitting the world square in the face.

"Illinois eliminating its $19 million in state funding for gifted-student programs this year, is spurring California to reduce funding for such initiatives by $10 million or 18%, a deeper cut than the cash-strapped state imposed on other education programs." And the *WSJ* goes on to list the entrenchments of programs for gifted students across the world's richest nation.

"This shift in the delicate balance between the pursuits of excellence and of equality may create a more knowledgeable US citizenry overall. But reducing programs for the best students also could make it harder to replenish – and diversify – the country's ranks of top intellectuals and scientists.

"The effects may be felt most by gifted low-income minority pupils whose parents haven't the option of shifting them to private schools or of providing outside enrichment to compensate for cutbacks. Seven-year-old Devlon Ross lives in a ramshackle house opposite a pawnshop in Springfield. He and an older brother recently slept several nights on bare mattresses in a front room because a raccoon gnawed through their bedroom ceiling.

"In kindergarten, Devlon scored in the 99th percentile of an intelligence test making him the only African-American at his elementary school to qualify for services for gifted children. In first grade, during weekly sessions with a specialist, he arranged cubes in intricate patterns and solved logic puzzles designed for older students.

"But this fall, Springfield dropped that program after state funding for it vanished. Devlon now daydreams in the back of his second-grade class, rarely raising his hand. His report card brims with 'unsatisfactory' grades, and he has been suspended four times. His mother says he is bored and needs 'that one-to-one attention.'

"'I believe we could do away with affirmative action [in college admissions] if the needs of these young, bright minority children are met at an early age,' says Susan Rhodes, gifted-education coordinator in Springfield. 'But No Child Left Behind leaves them behind, because it doesn't let us spend money on children already meeting the standards.'

"Before the program of Plymouth, Mass. for the gifted was

discontinued, eighth-grader Marina Ramsay says she studied everything from robotics to the stock market. She won first prize in the state science fair for a project on the effects of magnetic fields on plants. Now, in science this year, Marina says, she was assigned to 'memorize the order of the planets in the solar system. I learned that in kindergarten.' The parents are considering teaching her at home next year.

"The Jefferson Middle School in Springfield landed on a watch list for showing insufficient progress under the law. It responded by targeting 60 low-scoring students for improvement and putting them in classes of just 20. The move increased high achievers' class sizes to 30 or more. English teacher Barbara Boosinger, a former Jefferson 'teacher of the year,' says that though she prefers teaching high achievers, she switched to the lower track because of the smaller classes."

That indicates the complexity with which factors recognized and unrecognized interrelate for unexpected results. That is especially the case when the vital question of funding solutions remains unrecognized as *essential investments for society's future*.

W.K.

A Letter to the Long-Overdue Canadian Enquiry on Abuses in the Margin Accounts of Our Banks' Brokerages

SINCE the US investigation of mutual funds, brokerage and underwriting analysts have shown a scandalous victimization of their most vulnerable clients, it would be logical for Canada's supervisory authorities, whoever and wherever they might be, to examine the practices of stock brokers – to see how they treat their most vulnerable clients – those with marginal accounts. We must remember that these have already suffered disproportionately from the revealed abuses of the stock analysts – mostly in the employ directly or indirectly of the same banks and at the hands of the underwriting arms of the same conglomerates.

In marginal accounts, the client puts up money for usually 50% in the case of stocks over $3, and the bank finances the balance against the collateral in the account. Fair enough. But the banks, in addition to the interest they charge, also rent out the clients' shares that serve them as collateral to people wishing to short the stock. This rental stays with them as a second income from these margin loans. They thus use the client's collateral to help knock down the price of his shares. That already is not playing nice. Brokers in the US have been sent to jail for less than that – *when they prey on customers with greater clout*.

I have a friend who had for years accumulated a producing mining stock, because of his experience with the competence and honesty of its management. It was priced well below $3 and hence could not serve as security. However, for convenience

he left these shares in the margin account to avoid the expense and trouble of registering them in his own name. There were plenty of dividend-paying shares in the account that did serve as collateral for the banks' loans to the account. My friend is a conservative soul who was a client of the TD's brokerage firm for 15 years before TD took it over. Never before did he have trouble keeping his account in good standing. After September 11/01 when stock markets caved in, he sold stock for the purpose. In addition, two of the companies whose shares were in the account had already notified their shareholders that deals had been approved for them to be taken over by substantial companies listed on the Toronto Stock Exchange. The proceeds of those take-overs coming in within two weeks or so were enough to put the account in good standing. Since the collateral stock was in the brokers' name, notice of the deals had been sent him by TD Green Line. Twice my friend alerted the customers' representative of TD Green Line and asked him to bring the attention of his back-office to the impending take-overs. He assumed that this was done. Then to his dismay, he found out that some 19,000 shares of his mining stock had been sold out, at its rock bottom price for several years because of the Twin Towers. Since then the stock has since steadily mounted to 8 times the sell-out price in a period of little more than two years. That stock, sold out at $2.30, was within six months at 5.50. Currently, it is well over $18.

My friend wrote to the predecessor of Mr. Clark as TD CEO, Mr. Baillie.[1] He sent a copy of his file on the sell-out of his carefully accumulated mining stock over the years, and asked why he was not told that the sale of the marginable shares in his portfolio that would be taken over in a couple of weeks could not be taken into consideration. (That was standard practice in most brokerages before banks took them over.) Had that been done, he could have sold shares of *his* choice that were actually serving as collateral, or put up further cash, which he was in a position to do. In reply they asked him whether he could produce a tape to document such a request. Brokerages, of course, do have expensive installations to preserve their conversations with clients. To expect a modest margin client to have similar installations was disingenuous. When my friend tried contacting the Ontario Securities Commission on the matter he was confronted with a recording – "if the matter is a disagreement with your broker, retain a lawyer." That, too, was disingenuous since suing a bank would run up far great legal fees than the loss imposed on the client. As a settlement my friend proposed that TD cover his loss on the stock and commissions from the sell-out to when he was able to buy back his position at a well onto double the sell-out price.

Will Canada Follow the US on Broker Investigations?

When he got nowhere in his correspondence with the bank, my friend carefully filed the interchange of documents against the day when the OSC – given the involvement of Canadian banks in the investigations south of the border – will be obliged to introduce similar enquiries into our banks' behaviour on our stock markets in Canada. From recent press releases it seems that a national stock market supervisor to replace the present provincial ones seems imminent. That is why my friend informs me that he is brushing off the dust of his file on the incident.

But isn't anybody with a margin account asking for trouble? In financing the purchase of stocks over $3, the ratio of margin financing is usually 50%. Our banks in acquiring their miscellaneous brokerages, derivative boutiques, underwriting, merchant banks as a group show in an increase in their leverage of assets to cash on hand of 11 to one in 1946 to a present 380 to one. And what is more, the $1 of their own money in that denominator was originally government money.

In 1991 to bail out the banks from their speculative losses in real estate and gas and oil financing were assigned over 95% of the money creation, much of the base for which had been loans of the central bank to the government. Since the federal government is the sole shareholder of the Bank of Canada, the interest on the federal debt the central bank held returned to the government in the form of dividends. The bail-out did away with the statutory reserves – 10% of the chequing account and other short-term deposits the bank s took in from the public had to be redeposited with the central bank on an interest-free basis. That made it possible for the government to borrow from the central bank in that amount within the constraints in force. Now such borrowing by the government has been shifted directly and indirectly to the commercial banks and the interest paid on such loans stays with them. And this was no one-shot bailout, but an annual entitlement recurring every year. More amazing still, in the following years the banks were deregulated and empowered to acquire all these other financial institutions that are incompatible with banking – because they are high-risk gambling of frightening leverage. It was after the restructuring of our banking system to bail out the banks and then deregulate them took the money out of Ottawa's coffers that made necessary the slashing of its grants to the provinces – and was passed on to the municipalities that has created the crisis in our health, system,

In these circumstances, the very talk of "level playing fields" is a cruel joke. That is the hidden dead rat under the floorboards of our public life that has given rise to the public cynicism about banks, politics and politicians.

William Krehm

1. In an earlier issue we dealt with the spread in the current practice of doing away with employee pensions at the very time that more pensions of high executives of large corporations are having their pensions increased in a number of imaginative ways. In the case of Mr. Baillee the five consecutive years on which an agreement was signed with him his retirement pension bonus was based were would be at his choice in the last ten years of his service. This works out exactly to avoid the year of disastrous losses to which the Enron excess reserves contributed. That liberality could possibly be connected with the success of the TD bank's maneuver of shorting more Enron stock than was needed to hedge the financing of the Enron stock holdings by the partnerships in which Enron was involved.

Mr. Martin's Pinocchio Nose

AS OUR NEW Prime Minister installed himself in the chair of his long desires, an unseemly load of plots within plots began appearing. The term "plots" in this context can be taken in either of two meanings.

Paul Martin himself is very much a plot within a plot. Son of a social-minded medical doctor who ran against Trudeau for the leadership of the Liberal Party, he emerged as a business tycoon, head of Canadian Steamship Lines. On October 2002, Alliance MP James Rajotte directed a question to the government about the value of the orders CSL had received from Ottawa. On February 14, 2003, came the official reply: the Martin companies had chalked up a grand total of $137,000 government business. Since Mr. Martin was already slated as the up-and-coming PM, it is unlikely that the answer did not undergo scrutiny before being released. The companies have been handed over to Mr. Martin's sons, and are based in an offshore tax shelter, but still are close enough to enjoy orders from the Canadian government. Undaunted by the skimpiness of the official reply, the Alliance researchers continued digging. On they moved to Lansdowne Technologies Inc., a subsidiary of Canada Shipbuilding and Engineering, and came up with a figure of $161 million for all companies in the CSL group.

That raised more than eyebrows, but after a few days of public astonishment, still further plots within plots on the capital scene had taken over.

Enter the Auditor General

On February 11th, Auditor General Sheila Fraser minced no words in delivering her report on an "outrageous" and possibly criminal abuse of hundreds of millions of government dollars funnelled to friends of the federal Liberals. Public Works Minister Stephen Owen told the *Toronto Star* (11/02) that 13 separate cases involving payments to advertising agencies through the government sponsorship program have been referred to the RCMP for criminal investigation in light of Fraser's findings and more could be on the way. Fraser, whose auditors spent 18 months examining the more than $1 billion in advertising and sponsorship programs as well as other government operations, expressed shock over the way government officials handed out contracts to Liberal-friendly firms without regard to the rules. Millions of dollars were shifted around in questionable transactions. The report put a question mark over $100 million of the $250 million spent on the sponsorship program following the 1995 Quebec referendum. "A single thread of many strands is woven into the scandals that now shroud the federal government." If you are a federal Liberal office-holder ask not for whom the bell tolls. "[That thread] spins from the corruption of the Quebec contracting horrors around the suspicious purchase of Challenger jets and flows through Shawinigan, former prime minister Jean Chrétien's home town. Follow it and reach the inescapable conclusion that in this capital the line that must separate public policy from partisan politics has not just been crossed, it has been obliterated. Here cabinet ministers, mandarins, appointed officials and crown corporations collude to mislead Parliament and to fritter away taxpayers' money on foolish projects with no visible connection to national interest." That scathing indictment is boldly written in Auditor General Sheila Fraser's startling review of irresponsible Chrétien government schemes (*Toronto Star*, 11/02, James Travers).

The response of the Martin crew was strangely bumbling. "First the PM blamed his testy relationship with Mr. Chrétien and those around him for his ignorance of the Quebec sponsorship scandal. Mr. Chrétien's tactic [at such junctures] was to repeat over and over the same line and frustrate his opponents. The Martin strategy left many Liberals scratching their heads in disbelief. 'Talk about Mismanagement 101,' said one veteran Liberal. 'Call an enquiry? Dumb move. First Paul knew nothing, then it was a 'sophisticated group,' referring to Mr. Martin's explanation earlier this week that a small group of civil servants was to blame. Today it is 'I only knew in 2002.'

"A poll conducted immediately after the release of the Auditor General's report, showed the new government dropped nine percentage points this month, down to 39% of decided voters from 48% in January.

"'Outside of an election period, I've never seen numbers move like this,' said Darrell Bricker, president of the polling firm Ipsos-Reid. The Conservative support jumped from 24% from 19%, while the NDP nudged upward 2% to 18%."

It is all very well for Mr. Martin to blame his predecessor for the Auditor General's report, but here, too, there is an important plot within a plot, ignored because it has been surreptitiously declared *verboten*. There is a long history of conflict between Auditors General and governments of Canada, since at least three Royal Commissions and a series of Auditors General recommended over almost 40 years the introduction of capital budgeting (a.k.a. accrual accountancy) to no effect. Such resistance of governments in Canada to serious bookkeeping, cannot fail to arouse auditors, unless they consent to their profession being reduced to just another scam.

Mr. Martin's Previous Encounter with an Auditor General

When a corporation or an individual buys a building, or makes any physical investment, it depreciates the capital asset over its term of usefulness, and enters the depreciated cost as an asset on its balance sheet to set off the debt incurred for the investment. Not so our government. It writes off the entire investment as current expenditure. That, of course, contributes to a current deficit, and subsequently the building appears on the balance at zero or a token dollar. The end result is a "misleading" net debt, which is used as an argument to cut or not make vital social or environmental investments on the false grounds that "the money is not there." That passes for "fiscal responsibility" – a particular specialty of Mr. Martin during his term as Finance Minister.

This scenario came to a climax in 1999 when the previous Auditor General, Denis Desautels, (under whom Ms. Fraser served as deputy) refused to give unconditional approval to the government balance sheets for two years unless capital budgeting were brought in. However, Finance Minister resisted doggedly over many weeks and exacted from the AG a humiliating statement that since no new money had been brought into the treasury the more realistic balance sheet in no way justified an increase in spending. The recognition of the crucial investment by government to provide the ever costlier infrastructures of a modern, high-tech, and rapidly urbanized world was essential for an understanding of our mixed economy. Deny it, and you guarantee growing unemployment, crime instead of education, deteriorating health and environment. There is no way of looking after these needs unless you treat such infrastructures as investments. Otherwise you open the door to pillaging government assets by privatizing them for a song. To "reduce the debt" you provide fat, fast profits for speculators.

But here, too, there was a "plot within a plot": the tough bargaining between the AG and Finance Minister Martin was kept from Parliament and from the media. The only mention of it in the print media was in Conrad Black's *National Post*, which was desperate for readers.

In our January issue ("Paul Martin's Unique Opportunity for Atonement") *ER* quoted a document fished from the internet by a freshman student at York University, but kept from more accessible media. We quote from our comment, "Capitalism would not be capitalism, were it not possible to borrow against properly valued income-producing capital assets to finance further investments. Instead, Finance Minister Paul Martin bargained the Auditor General into publicly denying that basic principle of accountancy. Auditing auditors has earned Wall St. operators fines and even jail sentences. Why should ministers of the Crown get away with exactly that? Finance Minister Paul Martin hived off the "improvement" in the balance sheet as reserves to bolster his boast as champion budget balancer."

Fished from Internet

And the government document, "Backgrounder on the Implementation of Accrual Accountancy," states: "In moving to accrual accounting, the Government will change its accounting policy with respect to aboriginal and environmental liabilities. Environmental liabilities are currently not recognized in the financial statements and aboriginal liabilities are not fully recognized.

"This represents two instances of 'internalizing' capital destruction that had been put out of mind by conventional economists as 'externalities.' There is nothing external to society in unemployment, broken families, epidemics, undernourishment, This modest beginning of bringing two major instances of capital destruction onto the balance sheet must be expanded to take in *all* supposed 'externalities.'" These are capital investments, if made, capital liabilities if not attended to.

Once again, what was learned in the past about dealing with the major problem has been suppressed.

And here again Mr. Martin has much to answer for. One of the first things that Mr. Martin did when he took over the Finance Ministry was call a grand conference of economists for "consultation" at the most expensive hotel in Toronto. The participants, however, were carefully chosen to tell Mr. Martin exactly what he wished to hear. Four members of the COMER board were denied admission. The February 1994 issue of *Economic Reform* reported, "A crucial stretch of our history has been suppressed as is evident from the survival of provisions still in the *Bank of Canada Act* that are rarely mentioned, let alone applied.

"Our banks are well on the way to becoming government pensioners. According to Bank of Canada figures bonds issued or guaranteed by the federal government and held by the BoC have dropped by 37% between 1987 and the same month of 1993. But over the same period similar securities in the portfolios of our chartered banks have risen by 768%. The fly in this balm is that when the economy starts recovering and prices point up, the BoC will raise interest rates 'to lick inflation.' That will collapse the value of the banks' fully leveraged bond holdings and much of their capital will go up the chimney."

To bail the banks out from their speculative adventures throughout the world, the Bank for International Settlements had declared the debt of OECD (i.e., most developed) countries debt free requiring no additional capital to acquire. The previous Mulroney Government Canada had abolished the statutory reserves that required the chartered banks to redeposit 10% of their chequing count deposits with the central bank. Those deposits had earned them no interest. That allowed the central bank to restrain any perceived "inflation" without raising interest rates. Such a tool was highly important, since it lessened the dependence on high interest rates to fend off perceived inflation. Higher interest rates hits everything in the economy that moves. It is also the revenue of a group that needs no encouragement to become parasitic.

That is one of the things that the COMER spokesmen wished to warn the new Finance Minister about. Instead he chose to uphold what the Mulroney government had done and in fact was to lead to the break-up of the Conservative party.

It was to hide some of the paper trail – that real balance sheet of our government books – that Finance Minister Martin in 1999 bargained so long and fiercely with Auditor General Desautels.

The details of the pressures on the Auditor that led to the compromise of the 1999 agreement should be reviewed by a special enquiry. The suppression of vital economic information makes a mockery of democratic process. The further deregulation of our chartered banks from their speculative losses in areas incompatible with banking was followed in Mr. Martin's watch as Finance Minister with his granting them still more scope for gambling. It made it possible for them to become involved in unsavoury stock market scandals of the US – three of our five really large banks have been massively fined by US supervisory authorities. They have blackened the name of Canada abroad.

Mr. Martin's aides have pointed his being kept apart from the politics and practices Quebec wing of the Liberal Party, that were directly under the control of the former Prime Minister. The same might have been said of Mackenzie King who looked after the broader agenda of the Liberal party during his long leadership while Erneste Lapointe headed the hard-knuckled party machine in Quebec. But because King's social policies in nationalizing the Bank of Canada were progressive, the overall result of his leadership were decidedly positive. In Martin's case the orientation of his Finance Ministry was to confirm the dismemberment of that progressive role of the Bank of Canada under the Conservative government of Brian Mulroney. It is not excluded that this policy, if persisted in, may yet result in the Liberal Party sharing the fate of its great historic rival.

William Krehm

A Further Thought on the Robertson-Bunzl Proposals

THE WALL STREET JOURNAL (15/1/04) carries a front-page spread, "J.P. Morgan Chase to Buy Bank One" by John Sapford, Joseph T. Hallinan, Laurie P. Cohen and Monica Langley. It informs us that "J.P. Morgan will take over Bank One Corp. for roughly $58 billion in stock, forming the second largest bank in the US. The newly created colossus will have loans and assets of $1.1 trillion, trailing only Citigroup. Under the terms of the deal, Bank One shareholders will receive 1.32 shares of J.P. Morgan for each share held. Those shares value Bank One at $51.77 a share, representing a 14.5% premium of its 4 p.m. trading price of $45.22 on the New York stock exchange yesterday."

Point number one to be made: This constitutes a further concentration and additional "money creation" not by the central bank or the government but on the stock markets. It will make a definite contribution to further unemployment, and to the next stock market bubble-and-bust that will leave governments still more bereft of "money" to look after society's most urgent needs – the environment, health, education, and addressing the social roots of terrorism.

Back to the *WSJ* piece: "The merger is the latest indication of a strongly held belief among the nation's top bankers: size matters. Bolstering that conviction is the success of Citigroup, which has $1.2 trillion in assets. Being huge offers two advantages. One, banks can swiftly concentrate on areas of the financial market that are hot. Two, large clients like being able to have all their financial work – loans, underwriting, and mergers and acquisitions – handled in one place, since it gives them leverage to reduce their costs." "Reducing their costs" is a code word for firing more staff.

However, two equally important "advantages" are passed over in silence: (1) The fewer the banks left, the smaller the internal reserves required for the chequing and other short-term deposits created. That is because of the greater likelihood that cheques written by any client of any arm of the financial conglomerate will prove an in-house transaction that obviates many cheques issued by one client of the bank being cleared in favour of a client of another bank and thus drawing down the first bank's cash reserves. (2) It increases the inside information of corporation clients at the disposition of the merged banks. That information is a valuable asset for stock market manipulation, and leaves the "level playing field" that we hear so much about ever more up-ended.

Fleshing out and advancing the proposed Robertson-Bunzl combination of monetary and other necessary reform ideas reviewed in our last issue, appears an essential riposte to this new bank merger offensive. For it clearly must bring on further hyperinflation of the financial sector. To meet this new aggression, we must formulate carefully elaborated proposals for money creation at every level of government and non-government communal effort, and invite knowledgeable criticism.

Only the central bank is in a position to undertake the financing of such long-term projects as a new subway system.

The Bank of Canada charter, for example, provides for direct loans to the federal government and the provinces or to any other corporation – which would include municipalities – if the loan to them is guaranteed by either the federal or a provincial government. However, these provisions, still in the Bank of Canada's charter, have not been used for decades except in loans to the federal government on a very reduced scale. A loan from the central bank to the federal government implies the near total return of the interest paid on it to the federal government as dividends, for since 1938 it has been the sole shareholder of the BoC. (But even in the US where the local Federal Reserve banks are privately owned, roughly the same proportion of interest paid on federal loans goes back to the government as a right of seigniorage – an extension of the ancestral monarch's monopoly in coining precious metals.)

This opens the way for loans to the provinces, and even to the municipalities under guarantee by one or the other or both higher levels of government, with a negotiated agreement of Ottawa to transfer a portion of the interest payments going to the federal government from such guaranteed debt returning to the borrowing government to reduce the effective interest rates to the borrower. The central bank's interest rate in its entirety would, of course, already be far below the market. Such lower effective rates for the financing of socially necessary programs would already tend to lower market rates, because federal loans from the central bank broaden the *monetary base* – even by the old banking rules. Government borrowing from private banks heightens their leverage for creating interest-bearing debt that they are in a position to use for all sorts of gambles that deregulation has opened to them – stock market activities on their own account as well as to finance their clients, underwriting, highly leveraged derivative funds that may short currencies throughout the world.

But at the municipal and communal levels (LETs for example) there would be no need to have the entire loan arranged in a single currency of the various sort proposed. Even in municipalities where a variety of industries exist, the purchases required for a project would usually necessitate not only products and services originating in other parts of the country and even abroad. And for that local currencies would be useless. With proper preliminary analysis of how much of what currency components would be needed in a given project, the financing could be negotiated in federal legal tender to cover purchases from other parts of the country and abroad, provincial or state currency to cover items of such origin, and local municipal and local non-government currency (as in LETS) to cover part of the local labour employed.

Local currency could be almost entirely used not only for services such as care for the elderly, making existing homes more heat-conserving to help with the power shortage. Planned economy? – that baleful charge. We plan our economy, well or poorly, every time we go shopping, take our temperature, prepare a meal, go to the banks. Why should we allow demagogy from on high to proscribe planning in the infinitely more complex field of public finance? Especially when the use of central banks to finance capital investments by public bodies has been severely curtailed over recent decades.

William Krehm

Reply to a Request from Australia

JOHN HERMANN, of COMER of Australia, has suggested that we draw up as "a reasonably detailed statement of COMER's philosophical position." The most up-dated version in print is probably my *Towards a Non-Autistic Economy – A Place at the Table for Society* (COMER Publications, 2002).

We guide ourselves by what we conceive to be the problems of the economy, and relate those to the needs of society for its survival. We hold that the degenerate discipline of official economics has replaced the methodology of the founders of economic theory – Benjamin Franklin, Adam Smith, David Ricardo, with a caricature of the differential calculus. This it has achieved by increasingly suppressing intellectual freedom in our universities, in parliament, and our media. Its practitioners may object when we seek out what is relevant in the core of mathematical analysis, that we are talking over the heads of the public.

We are not running for election to any public post, and by the nature of any serious discipline we must address ourselves in part to qualified economists, professional or otherwise. Simultaneously, of course, we must attempt to explain to a broader audience what we are attempting to do and why we are devoting so much of our lives to it.

An example: one of the great breakthroughs in 20th century physics was the development of quantum theory, the full mathematical apparatus of which is beyond the understanding of the citizen lacking some minimal command of mathematics and physics. But one of its conclusions is that by his very investiga-

tive intervention the physicist disturbs the object of his investigations. This has a tremendous relevance in economic theory and its current crisis. The late French economist, François Perroux, produced what is probably the best economic counterpart of quantum theory in his concept of the Dominant Revenue. This holds that in every period the revenue of a given economic group (which can be a subset of Marx's "classes") is taken, in its mass and rate of return, as an index of the welfare of society as a whole. That is true, said Perroux, in terms of the prevailing power distribution. As that changes, so does the Dominant Revenue. Thus the British landowners and their Corn Laws were – by the Reform Bill – replaced with the industrialists preaching free trade, so long as Britain retained a virtual monopoly of industrial development.

Maths Can be Stunningly Simple

After the resounding failure in the 1930s of the first attempt of the financial community to take over, this was replaced with an alliance of government investment and a sector of industrial capitalists, with the trade unions as junior partners, while the banks were bailed out and relegated to the doghouse. With the US Fed-Treasury-Accord negotiated behind the back of President Truman in 1951, power began to be retrieved surreptitiously by the financial community. Deregulated and globalized, it is in utter control today. In exercising that control it is running up a new record of disaster.

To such an extent that we must dip further into the great heritage of mathematics to find tools to break this usurpation. Surely dimension theory is highly relevant. Initiated by Galileo, this teaches that bigger is not always better and can even mean increased vulnerability. The principle of Least Action which runs like a red thread through both mathematics and physics from ancient times, also has something pertinent to tell us. Systems theory requires that no subsystem can be allowed to devour the resources of another, if the system as a whole is to function. As does Gaussian modular congruence analysis that simplifies many problems by eliminating multiples of a given modulus to deal only with remainders. We do that with modulus 7 when we refer to the eighth day with the name of the first, Sunday, instead of dropping the week concept and giving every successive day since Adam bit the apple a new name.

Mathematics is not always bewilderingly complex. It can be stunningly simple. For example, probably its most important application to our mixed economy, is what we learned in our first-year high-school algebra classes: to solve linear equations with n independent variables, we need n different equations. In economics this is known as "the Tinbergen counting rule" that has been violated unconscionably. When central banks in the 1970s proclaimed interest rates "the one blunt tool" for managing an economy that was being deregulated and globalized – i.e., the number of independent variables were being multiplied beyond counting. Qualified mathematicians and physical scientists must be enlisted in this campaign to reconquer intellectual freedom for economic studies in our universities, government and the media.

John Hermann suggested a statement of our attitude towards

the sundry efforts of other reformers – positive or negative. The following is a summary response to that excellent idea.

Post-Keynesianism. We agree fully with their concept of money being *endogenous* rather than *exogenous* in origin, that is, created by the very investment process, rather than brought in from the outside. Just as a worker is paid by the week or month for work *already done*, so the financing of other investment costs is arranged by a bank opening a line of credit which is drawn on as the investment proceeds. The notion that savings must have been made in advance before money is created is misleading. The base for money creation today is the credit of the central government resting on the productive potential of the country that is already there.

However, most post-Keynesian groups have yet to distinguish between *market inflation* and *structural price rise*. The latter component of secular price increase is the result not of an aggregate excess of demand over supply, but of the growth of public investment in physical and human capital within the total output of the economy, i.e., roughly the sum of the output of the public and private sectors. Most investments in human capital – health education, social welfare, physical security, can only be financed by government. And since the basic revenue of government is taxation, that implies a deeper layer of taxation in price, since the private sector is the tax-base of the government. The original development of that idea based on a 60-some page article of *Revue Économique* of Paris of May 1970, was expanded into W. Krehm's *Price in a Mixed Economy – Our Record of Disaster*, 1975.

Georgism. Henry George put his finger dead on the capital appreciation of real estate values in thriving cities as source of many great fortunes, past and present. We have elaborated this position drawing substantially on the work of historians like Fernand Braudel, who emphasize the civilizing role of the cities as centres of science, the arts, education. Price levels have always been higher in large urban centres than in the countryside, reflecting the cost of the huge public investment in these centers to pay for the services they alone can provide. Modern society has become infinitely more complex than when George proposed his "single tax." We need a great variety of taxes, but we should be careful of what social groups they favour and which they may victimize. The spread between the wages of the most unskilled labourers and the large corporate CEOs is a good index for the extent of society's ailments.

In my work, *Babel's Tower – The Dynamics of Economic Breakdown* (1977), I developed a neglected application of the Georgian idea that could reclaim for society part of the vast capital gains that go to fuel speculation today. The various levels of government help plan public transport facilities in large cities such as subways, and hence have considerable advance knowledge of any significant changes in their pattern. That "inside information" should, with the help of low-interest loans guaranteed by the senior levels of government, be used by the various levels of government to acquire options on key plots of land the value of which will sky-rocket once, say, a projected subway route is made public. Some of that capital gain can be appropriated by the government for the financing of the future

facility and kept out of the costs of the future service to consumers in a simple way.

Seizing Some Truths by the Tail

The government will rent the land under long-term lease to developers at the proper time so that much of the capital gain will be kept out of the rents of privileged structures at hubs. Instead of having to buy and hold the land, for years, the developer will have only to finance the buildings erected on such sites, without the costs of land acquisition. The governments can use their capital gains to help pay for their maintenance of the transport service. This would obviate the heavy grants from senior government levels to maintain the transport services of our large cities. This is a very obvious application of Georgian thinking, but it has been not applied, because it runs counter to the ideology in the saddle.

Something similar must be said of Social Credit. Major Douglas had a great neglected truth by the tail, when he emphasized that our inventions, and even our social practices would be unthinkable without the great "social heritage" of philosophers, martyrs, anonymous inventors and scientists, slaves. (He was an engineer by training, but coined the poetical great question, "Must we build machine guns in order to buy a cabbage?") This "social heritage" must not be appropriated entirely by those who patent an invention or a gene and employ it as though it were not based to a significant extent on this vast social heritage. Hence he developed the idea of a social dividend, which would be a modest payment to all members of society. Not enough for them to live on completely, but that would help them survive the rat race, or even to pursue alternate life styles. That is not a complete alternative to the market or our mixed economy, but an important element in humanizing it somewhat, gearing down the drive towards exponential expansion that by its very definition is unsustainable. In that respect social credit resembles Georgian economics – not the total solution but a vital ingredient of it.

Ecological Economics. This is one of the several vital subsystems that must be respected in order that the system as a whole may function. Conventional economics merely labels all such subsystems – other than the "pure and perfect market" – as "externalities." That shoves them out the back door.

Sraffian Economics. Basically this returns attention to the labour value theory of the founding fathers of economic theory, Benjamin Franklin, Adam Smith, Ricardo, that in various guises served as the nexus between theory and reality. It was a strand in the great revolt against marginal utility theory, which in essence replaces real value with the derivatives (rates of growth to infinity). There is in fact a relationship that COMER has emphasized between the derivative value theory in force (the rate of increase) and the speculative instruments known as "derivatives" based on speculative forecasts of a detached aspect of securities.

Complexity Theory. Before we invest too heavily in complexity theory, we must bring into our field of vision such obvious relationships as the contribution of taxation to price rise having nothing to do with an imbalance of aggregate supply and demand. In actual fact that taxation factor in price is counted not once but twice in our GDP – once as the value (at cost) of the public sector and again as the layer of taxation in the output of the private sector. Only when we have exhausted the resources of correctly applied elementary arithmetic, should we trouble our heads about chaos theory. The chaos that exists is largely the result of an overdose of ideology in our thinking.

I trust this may be of help. In any case, let us continue the discussion in manageable doses.

All best,
William Krehm

The Balanced Budget Fetish

THE FEDERAL NDP Election Planning Committee appears committed to a policy of annual balanced budgets as a key plank in our election platform. The rationale is that about 90% of the party members who attended the strategy/planning seminars supported such an inclusion. Similarly, a large majority of the members of recent focus groups, consisting of people who "liked" the NDP but had not voted for us, also supported its inclusion.

At first glance, these numbers are shocking. How is it possible that so many of our members and its supporters have forgotten our party's origins and the basic tenets of Keynesian economics? These numbers are eloquent testimony to the power of the right wing press, business spokespeople, "think" tanks like the Fraser Institute and the C.D. Howe Institute, and countless Liberal, Tory and Alliance politicians – all reciting the mantra of balanced budgets. In the 90s we were subjected to an unprecedented scare campaign about debt and deficits which, though mostly false, clearly had a great impact on the population. Here in Ontario, we have endured eight years of Tory obeisance to the balanced budget (more in rhetoric than reality, it now appears) and the victorious Liberals found it necessary to worship at the same altar (at least until they got elected!).

No doubt a balanced budget is desirable most of the time, but that does not mean a fiscal deficit is a bad thing. After a decade of tax cutting, budget balancing governments in Toronto and Ottawa, we face serious real deficits – in our municipal infrastructure, in public housing, in health care and education. These deficits are seriously injurious to the public welfare, much more so than a financial deficit. As the new Liberal government in Ontario has discovered, a deficit is not the greatest evil of our times.

Why is the right so enamoured of balanced budgets? Well actually they are not! If you look closely, their allegiance is mostly rhetorical. George W. Bush is running a deficit this year of $521 billion – compared to a surplus of $250 billion in Clinton's last year. The Reagan administration ran huge deficits. Here in Canada, the Trudeau Liberals and the Mulroney Tories had massive deficits year after year. In Saskatchewan, the profligate Tories under Grant Devine ran the biggest per capita deficits in history, pushing the province to the brink of bankruptcy.

The right-wing rhetoric about balancing the budget is really about reducing social spending. They love tax cuts (which reduce revenue) and certain types of expenditure, like the military and subsidies to corporations, but they hate social spending of any kind. The balanced budget cudgel is their weapon of choice. If you cut taxes and balance the budget, you cannot possibly increase, or even maintain, social programs. If the pressure is sufficient, you may have to sell off government assets to balance the books – the method of choice for our late lamented Tories in Ontario.

Balanced budgets are a key component of the "Washington Consensus" and are invariably imposed by the IMF on countries being subjected to "structural adjustment." The result is always a shrinkage of the economy, a goal sought by the IMF but inimical to the welfare of the population. It is but one of many IMF tools designed to impoverish the population and improve the climate for bankers, investors and multinational corporations. (See Joseph Stiglitz's *Globalization and Its Discontents*.)

There is a more fundamental issue. In any economic downturn a government deficit is an absolute necessity. The Ontario Rae government was correct in running large deficits during the terrible recession of the early nineties. Unfortunately they were unable to withstand the attacks of their opponents, who cared little about the deficit but wanted to force the government to reduce social spending. By failing to defend their stimulative fiscal policy, they paved the way for the destructive tax and spending cuts of the Harris Tories.

Have we forgotten the important lesson of the Great Depression? In the early 1930s, almost all governments responded to the downturn in the economy by reducing expenditures in an effort to balance the books. Of course this reduced aggregate demand even more and made matters worse. At this juncture, J.M. Keynes, in his masterful and seminal work, *A General Theory of Employment Interest and Money*, demonstrated that the problem was a lack of demand (i.e., spending), and that the only solution was for the government to borrow massively, spend massively and run massive deficits. Roosevelt's New Deal in the US was a partial implementation of this policy. Countries like Sweden and New Zealand went further and ended the Depression in their countries within a few years. When WWII broke out, Canada (like Britain and the US) printed money, borrowed massively, and spent huge sums on the war. Within 18 months we had full employment. The deficits were huge: by 1946 the national debt was 127% of GNP, but the economic stimulus carried the economy through the post-war expansion. Very little of the debt was actually paid off but economic growth reduced the relative size of the debt to 25% of GNP by 1960. Keynes had been proven right and the lesson is still valid today, if largely forgotten. Do we really intend to sacrifice countless workers on the altar of balanced budgets as R.B. Bennett did in the thirties?

More fundamentally, this simplistic nonsense distracts us from a much more important discussion – monetary policy. Many people who worry about *deficits* are really worried about *debt*, and with good reason. In our society debt is escalating at a fearsome rate. Today, household debt averages $66,900 – an increase of 18% in four years. As public (government) debt has been reined in over the past decade, private debt (businesses and individuals) has ascended into the stratosphere and it is far more damaging than public debt. Why, for example, do politicians congratulate themselves on taming deficits when thousands of university graduates have been forced to incur debts well in excess of $25,000 because those same politicians reduced grants for higher education? Are we really better off? In reality, the balanced budget/tax cutting mantra has been used to manipulate us, and now it looks like we are going for the bait – hook, line and sinker!

We need to look at the real problem and educate our public about real solutions. Debt is the problem, monetary policy is the solution. Since 1980, we have deregulated the financial system and privatized money creation. In 1991, bank reserves were abolished. Less than 5% of our money supply is legal tender (i.e., created by the government through the Bank of Canada). The other 95% has to be created by borrowing, i.e., by incurring debt. An increasing money supply – about $25 to $30 billion per year – is absolutely essential to maintain economic growth. Thus we are caught. We must increase our debt to maintain economic growth and pay the interest on previous debt. The only way government debt and deficits can be stabilized is for individuals and businesses to borrow more. If we reduce our borrowing, the economy must contract.

Of course, it does not have to be that way. We could re-regulate the financial system. The government could create a greater share of the money supply – say, the 20% it used to create. The Bank of Canada could assume a greater share of the national debt. And the Bank of Canada could make low interest loans to municipalities for infrastructure. By the way, most of these proposals have been adopted as policy at NDP conventions but actually implementing them would entail a tough fight with the banks and other vested interests.

No doubt such a fight would be difficult to win. It is probably a lot easier to tell the public that we have learned our lesson and will behave ourselves in future. It might even win over a few converts – though how we can outdo Paul Martin and the new Conservatives in this area is a mystery to me. The worse outcome, of course, would be to come into power burdened by such an inane policy. Surely we can do better.

David Gracey (Scarborough Southwest NDP)

Canadian Banks on Wall St. Come Home to Roost

FOR YEARS, Canadians received the unending reports about the Global Crossings, Enrons and other Wall St. scandals with the classic Canuck reaction: what can you expect of the Yanks? It couldn't happen here. So ingrained was this sense of national piety that no great heed was given to the detail that three of our five giant banks were actually involved in the largest US scams, Global Crossings, and Enron. So deeply rooted was the conviction of our national purity that when Nortel – Canada's communication superstar – fell from $124.50 to

pennies in a matter of weeks, it didn't even rate an enquiry. Had we not witnessed the crowning of Paul Martin as head of government? It was a period when much of the last bailout of our banks from their speculative rumbles of the 1980s had been put to bed in complete stealth by a long perfected technique of Mr. Martin – simultaneously saying different things from the two sides of his mouth.

Learning about our Banks from the US Courts

So by the circuitous route of US prosecutions we arrived at the screaming headline in *The Toronto Globe and Mail* (7/02, "CIBC mulling US settlement" by Sinclair Stewart and Shawn McCarthy): "Canadian Imperial Bank of Commerce is considering a settlement with US regulators over its alleged role in financing improper mutual fund trades, the bank's chairman said yesterday.

"William Etherington, who along with CEO John Hunkin has been leading a wide-ranging overhaul of CIBC governance, said the bank is determined to improve its reputation and deal promptly with the aftermath of its involvement in a series of well-publicized financial scandals.

"One of its former US employees was arrested this week in conjunction with the mutual fund probe, and charged with five felonies by New York State Attorney General Eliot Spitzer. The crusading Attorney General has warned that more charges are in the works, and indicated that he may pursue civil sanctions against the bank itself.

"All of this comes on the heels of an $80-million (US) settlement CIBC struck with the US Securities and Exchange Commission in December over charges that the bank 'aided and abetted' the accounting fraud at Enron Corp.

"Mr. Etherington said, 'We need to put this behind us as we have put Enron and the SEC behind us. What's absolutely the most crucial thing here is the reputation of the banks and the employee morale.'

"One of the most visible changes occurred on Thursday, when the bank dismissed vice-chair David Kassie, an aggressive deal-maker who ran the CIBC World Markets Inc. investment banking unit.

"Mr. Kassie turned CIBC World Markets into the leading underwriter in the country, and even carved out a place for the bank in New York. But during his tenure, the investment bank's freewheeling style landed it in some embarrassing messes, including Enron, Global Crossing Ltd. and Livent Inc."

Then came a revealing passage that discloses the depth of moral rebirth undergone by CIBC as it steps out of the confessional: "'Clearly it was a sad day when we said it's time that we need new leadership, because we are very mindful of what [Mr. Kassie] has brought to the table. But, *I mean, people in his profession, they understand how the game works.*" [Our italics.] It is in fact, writ globally, the second oldest profession in the world.

"Mr. Hunkin has already begun shifting the bank's business mix more toward retail banking and wealth management and has been steadily reducing risk in the merchant banking portfolio and corporation loan book."

Whenever our banks lose big in the mega-gambles their

deregulation made possible, they retreat to something closer to old-style banking. They will take out these trifling losses from the hides of retail customers. But they do so essentially to retrieve their losses, and move into the big-time with the help of fresher versions of Mr. Kassie. The deeper problem, far deeper than the investigations taking place in the US, is the valuation of securities and of the innumerable derivatives of securities by extrapolating the rate of growth of a security, of an industry, of the economy, already achieved. These are built into its market price and hence must be maintained into the indefinite future. Of course, that is impossible, because the entire context in which the golden security functions so spectacularly has been declared "externalities."

Our Financial Atom Bomb

The alleged "risk management" that is ever on the lips of central and commercial bankers' valuations is based on what can be highly vicious financial instruments applied to a single abstracted feature of a security known as a "derivative." These are derived from the rates of growth of a function in differential calculus. The usefulness of this concept is its complete isolation from every context – very much as is official economic theory as a whole. Because it is so isolated, and so stubbornly deregulated, it does not have to be declared – and banks can get rid in stealth of their involvement with a given stock at the very time that they are peddling it to the public. Since speculators are spared not only the risk but the need to take positions in the total security, they can build up wild leverages. That is how hedge funds managed to earn billions out-muscling the world's central banks on occasion in knocking down entire series of currencies like bowling pins.

In their obsession with "rates of growth," economists and the Finance Ministers they counsel overlook that the ultimate "successful" essay in growth rates took place in Hiroshima when the first atomic bomb was dropped. The mathematics of that bomb was the exponential curve defined in an esthetically perfect way: the rate of its growth always equals the value attained by the function itself. That is the rate of growth that the world economy is driven to maintain – the stock prices already achieved. Of course, it is a deal with the devil. When the project is tiny and obscure, and can fix markets in the dark, replacing "market share" for non-existent earnings, the black magic required is a cinch. But the larger its price, the more unsustainable the valuation. And the first time the stock, the economy or whatever, cannot maintain the valuation already built into its worth, the entire house of marked cards collapses. That is what drives deregulated banks to move into scams to safeguard not only the price of their stock – and hence their credit – but the stock options granted high executives. There is no room left for Sunday school morality.

"To defend his shareholders' interests," as the saying goes, and of course his own options, the CEO will be driven to the most criminal improvisations. That is why as laudable as the Mr. Spitzers are, they must be pushed further into the valuations of our stock market and the projections of our finance ministers.

Banking is an indispensable service to a society. When the world's moneys were on the gold or silver standard, without banking the development of the economy was restricted to the growth of the available stocks of those metals. Banks made it possible to limit reserves to enough cash in the till to meet the net clearance of calls on them. That made it possible for banks to lend out many times the actual cash held in their tills. If they ran short, they could borrow overnight from the central bank once that institution was introduced in Sweden and Holland in the late 1600s. It was a cross between a miracle and a potential scam. That is why the Roman Church severely regulated the priests who administered the miracle of its faith – to lessen the temptation to build up an estate for their family, they were pledged to chastity. And they were certainly not allowed to corner the wine or the wafer markets. Not so our deregulated banks and their holding companies.

After their speculative binges of the 1920s that helped bring on the great Depression, the banks were severely confined to banking. They could engage in nothing having to do with the stock market, or insurance, or any other financial industry that depended on pools of capital.

After the world went off the gold standard – even in theory in 1973 – the credit of the central government became the only legal tender. With enough short-term government debt in reserve, the private banking system could lend out up to ten times its cash reserves. That provided the central banks with an alternative to raising its over-night lending rate to prevent inflation. It could simply raise the proportion of the deposits taken in by the chartered banks that had to be redeposited with the central rate on a non-interest-earning basis. That avoided hitting everything in the economy with higher interest rates whenever the central banks thought they saw inflation on the horizon. They could leave the bank short-term rate alone, and raise the reserve requirement that had to be deposited – interest-free – with the central bank. It also gave the central government more elbow room in borrowing from the central bank on a virtual interest-free basis. For since 1938 the government of Canada has been the only shareholder of the Bank of Canada, and thus the bulk of the interest on the debt held by the BoC returned to the government as dividends. Even where the central bank is not nationalized but owned by commercial banks, as in the US, the take of the government from the central bank is not very different from that of nationalized banks – because of the ancestral monarch's monopoly in coining precious metals. Today that has been largely translated into the powers of credit-money creation.

However, since the chartered banks as a group had lost much of their capital in speculative non-banking activities during the 1980s, their bail-out became urgent. In most countries – including the UK and the US this took the form of reducing the statutory reserves to a token amount and making no further use of them. In Canada and New Zealand, possibly because they both had advanced social legislation that ran counter to the prevailing standards of the banking community, the statutory reserves were done away with entirely. On top of that the Bank for International Settlements, a club of central bankers based in

Basel, not only proclaimed the independence of central banks from their governments, but introduced its guidelines on *Risk-Based Capital Requirements* to enforce the solvency of banks. This constituted a shift from legal tender reserves to the banks' capital which was not necessarily in the form of legal tender, but could be in loans, or physical assets. But that enabled the Canadian banks to quadruple their holdings of federal government debt to some $80 billion dollars. The holdings of such federal debt by the BoC, which amounted to over 22% of such outstanding debt in the mid 1970s fell to under 6%. Due both to this shift of debt from the BoC, where it was held at virtual interest-free rates to the banks and the public, the federal debt almost tripled over the next few years.

Now from all points of the compass the failure of this policy has become evident.

Emerging countries are in full revolt against the globalization and deregulation, as their export staple prices are no longer determined by supply and demand, but by the pressure to obtain the renewal of their foreign loans by meeting the export quotas set for them by the IMF. Meanwhile the flow of capital from Latin America has been reversed – on balance away from rather than to these countries.

Globalization and Deregulation have in fact been wired in favour of large nations according to their economic power. The *Financial Markets Center* of Philomont, VA (17/12/03, "Capital Flows Monitor") sums matters up: "For one thing, the large emerging economies that have expanded most impressively – China and India – have consciously resisted some of the main policy prescriptions associated with financial liberalization. For another, stark inequities continue to pervade the global system. In the aggregate, the nations that most urgently need external investment to finance development have become net exporters of capital. In the wake of the 1998 Asian financial crisis, developing countries began a massive build-up of foreign exchange reserves to protect themselves in the event of future crisis. Led by Africa and developing Asia, these countries enlarged their reserve holdings by 98.4% between 1995 and 2002, thereby increasing their reserve coverage as percentages of imports, external debt and debt service."

A Dangerous Reversal of Capital Flows

"At the same time – and for similar reasons – private investors from developing countries substantially increased their deposits in foreign banks. These actions produced a major shift in the global makeup of capital outflows. By the end of 2002, emerging economies as a group supplied a larger share of net outflows ($125.2 billion) than the Euro area ($120.5 billion). And they contributed 23.7% of the net inflow to the US. Most African, Latin American and Central and Eastern European countries continue to rely on capital flows to finance current account deficits and support growth. Still, these exceptions have not substantially altered flows of financial resources from the poor to the rich. Developing countries now have a direct stake in the global system's most egregious imbalance: America's ballooning current account deficit. Over the past decade, the US has become the global economy's dominant importer of both goods and capital. In 2002, net capital inflows to the US amounted to $528.0 billion and absorbed a staggering 75.5% of total net capital outflows from the rest of the world. By contrast, shares of the other six largest net capital importers ranged from just 2.8% for Australia to a mere 1.4% for Portugal."

In 2002, the net liabilities of the US to the rest of the world rose to $2.6 trillion or 25% of the US GDP. The US has become a borrower of first choice and buyer of last resort whose influence extends far beyond its commanding 21.1% share of world output.

Interest rates elevated to the role of the sole means of keeping the world economy in balance, is particularly provocative to the Muslim world. The Koran condemns not only usury as such, but interest itself. Having oil prices denominated in dollars the exchange value of which has been sinking systematically *vis à vis* the euro and other currencies for strategic reasons of the US, is particularly galling to the Arab countries.

The US debt to the outside world is growing at an alarming rate, and any major shift from the dollar to other currencies as reserve money can create a major economic breakdown.

The persistence of ever new major scams occupying the prosecutors in the US, is telling us that a patchwork response to what is clearly a systemic problem will bring no lasting solution. Attention must be turned to the shift of major money creation from central banks to our deregulated gambling banks. It must be stopped. The suppressed record of how the world got into this perilous mess must be brought into the open. The incredible further deregulation of the world financial system after it had been bailed out by ending the statutory reserves must be reversed. The combination of bailout cum further deregulation can indicate only one thing: a further shift of power to the financial community. This certainly is not without linkage to the high cost of funding electoral campaigns.

William Krehm

Ruminations on Rhetoric

T HE GLOBE AND MAIL reports that John MacNaughton, "head of the Canada Pension Plan Investment Board… called on the financial services industry to help shake many Canadians from the misconception that the federal government's plan will eventually run out of money… 'a myth promulgated during RSP time.'" He pointed to last year's report by the Chief Actuary for Canada that "the CPP in its current form is sound for at least 75 years." No doubt his listeners in the Calgary audience began immediately to correct the misconception, which they originally trumpeted from the housetops and from which they have reaped handsome rewards.

The Actuary's welcome announcement about the security of the CPP should alert us to the need for critical appraisal of all the rhetoric coming from the financial sector's spinsters, and their political allies.

In fact, a concerted effort to challenge and correct the rhetoric is a necessary preliminary to real change. For instance, what would be the effect of the following changes? Wherever "taxpayer" appears, substitute "citizen." For "tax cut," substitute "expenditure cut" or "revenue cut." For "freedom of choice," substitute "sale of public assets," and for "choice" in the energy market, substitute "elimination of the public option." In other words, call them what they are. A "free trade treaty," as currently devised, is fundamentally an "unrestricted investment treaty."

"Globalization" sounds like a mighty and irresistible natural force, rather than a product of human choices. Suppose it were called by a term that more clearly indicates the intentions of its proponents, perhaps, "the destruction of democratic national states." For all the wishful thinking and self-deception of the globalizers, the nation state is not obsolete. To distinguish a world order in opposition to globalization, we need to keep the word "internationalism" in common use.

Corporate and government spinsters know the rhetorical cogency of approaching issues in exclusively economic terms, but civic values, moral values, cultural values and national values do not, therefore, leave the planet. To give them the priority they deserve in a democratic society a little "un-spinning" of the economic rhetoric would go a long way.

As we jog down the path to the federal election, we will no doubt hear again and again another old chestnut: "Tax cuts to create jobs." If the politician is talking consumption tax, like the GST, it has a good deal of validity. But applied to income and capital gains taxes, it is about a century out of date. In second stage capitalism, where the dominant revenue was the revenue of the industrialists, giving them a tax reduction had some chance of ending up in job-creation as they built or enlarged their factories. In today's "third stage" capitalism, where the dominant revenue is the revenue of speculative lenders, the lion's share of any reduction is merely recycled into the financial casino.

Joggin Down the Path to the Federal Election

Another election idiocy is the practice of horse-race voting. Grant Devine, commenting on the new Conservative party leadership election recently, referred to it quite unconsciously. People, he said, don't want to *waste* their vote on some one who cannot win (CBC, 20/2/04, italics mine). Now, wait a minute. If anything is a "waste" of a vote, it is voting for somebody other than the elector's preferred choice. Mr. Devine went on to use another term which we could well expunge from the vocabulary of political commentators – referring to an election as a "race." In a race, the aim is, indeed, to pick (and put your money on) the horse that will win. In an election, on the other hand, the aim is to pick the candidate who best reflects your views and plunk your vote down there. The effect of horse-race voters, aided by that darling of political "science," the opinion poll, is real and incalculable.

The old terms "Left" and "Right" are becoming more or less historical terms. For the current scene a more illuminating division would be between borrowers and lenders, which is both an economic and a social distinction. As the United States moves from its republican phase to its imperial phase, that distinction may modulate further into an increasingly useful one – the

opposition of "democracy" and "oligarchy." Watch for lots of "freedom" and "liberty" thrown in – from both sides!

Actually, I wonder if "democracy" can really be resurrected from the morass of meaninglessness it has fallen into. It does have a specific technical meaning from the Greek: *demokratia*, from *demos*, the common people, and *kratos*, strength, or rule. Though Aristotle defined it (rather pejoratively), it has never been better defined than by Abraham Lincoln's linking of "freedom" with "government of the people, by the people, for the people" in his Gettysburg address. Freedom and democracy, he recognized, are hard to define. If you're a lion, you want freedom to hunt and kill anything that moves. If you're a rabbit, freedom is a fence, with the lion securely on the other side.

Lincoln said on another occasion: "With some, the word liberty may mean for each man to do as he pleases with himself and the product of his labor; while with others the same word may mean for some men to do as they please with *other* men and the product of other men's labor.... The shepherd drives the wolf from the sheep's throat, for which the sheep thanks the shepherd as his liberator, while the wolf denounces him for the same act.... Plainly the sheep and the wolf are not agreed upon a definition of liberty" (April 18, 1864).

It could be explosive if we had that kind of clear thinking engaged as our electors and leaders try to uncover that democratic balance which lies somewhere between the tyranny of the masses and the tyranny of the oligarchs.

The Romans had the Key Question — Cui Prodest?

A useful method of judging policies or pronouncements is to ask the three questions: Why is it done/said? Is it necessary/true? and Who benefits from doing/saying, it? If you can riddle out who benefits – not always open and obvious – then you can ask: Why is that group or individual being privileged?

When the government borrows from private lenders instead of from its own bank, for example, it is pretty easy to see who benefits. So ask, why are the shareholders and executives of banks being privileged?

Who benefits from public healthcare? Everybody who gets sick, but also those who don't get sick but enjoy the peace of mind due to knowing it is there. There are other benefits. Employers, who calculate they lose $50 billion a year because of illness-related absenteeism, would lose a great deal more without public healthcare. Also, without public healthcare, their workers would certainly bring healthcare demands to the bargaining table. By this brief analysis, Canadian public healthcare gets a pretty good rating. Try it on American-style healthcare, and rejoice.

The business press and financial industry ads have run a fascinating campaign to persuade us that market forces are democratic.[1] But clear thinking refuses to buy the notion that the characters featured in the articles and ads which Thomas Frank quotes so tellingly – downsized-workers-turned-day-traders, the ladies of the neighbourhood investment club, or the whiz kids in the corporate computer center – are captains of democracy. The real oligarchs still wear suits.

As the United States continues its hypocritical or self-deluded crusade for a muddle-headed extension of "democracy" (read "unrestricted market capitalism"), clear thinking becomes increasingly necessary. Of course, though we hear a great deal from pundits and politicians about "a rules-based trading system," in practice there seems to be just one rule: the United States wins, or it doesn't play. And what do you do with the kid who says, "It's my ball and bat, and I'm going home?" Perhaps Joe Clark deserves the last word: "The goal of economic progress is the extension of human liberty, not…the open-ended servicing of human greed." What clarity and simplicity! But that was in 1976.

Gordon Coggins

1. See Frank, Thomas (2000). *One Market Under God, Extreme Capitalism, Market Populism, and the End of Economic Democracy.*

Gearing Down the Exponential Growth Model

IN THE JANUARY ISSUE OF *ER*, we dealt with the consequences of the deal struck when our present Prime Minister, then Minister of Finance, bargained for weeks with the then Auditor General of the government, Denis Desautels. Mr. Desautels refused to give unconditional approval of two years' balance sheets of the federal government unless it introduced accrual accountancy (a.k.a. capital budgeting). Previous Auditors General and at least three royal commissions had recommended that to no avail. Nothing complicated about that issue. Almost all of us live in houses that have mortgages on them. If they had not, you would have to come up with the entire purchase price in cash to buy it. Or if you rent, the landlord would have had to do that on acquiring it. Fewer houses would be built because the builder or the investor-buyer would have had to put up the entire price in his own money, unless he could use the house as collateral for borrowing a substantial part of its cost or purchase price.

Are Those who Bed-Down on the Sidewalk in Better Shape than our Banks?

Or if you wrote a mortgage on your house, but forgot to put the value of the house on the asset side of your net worth, you would appear to be an undischarged bankrupt and you could not borrow a dime except at usurious rates. If our banks noted only their debts but not their assets on their balance sheets, they would appear in worse shape than the homeless who sleep on the sidewalks. For their debt is definitely greater. However, they do list their assets on the scoreboard to offset their liabilities. The folks that sleep on the sidewalks, while having no debt, also have no assets.

However, our governments have pretended that they have no physical assets to offset their debt. When they built a building, a bridge, or a road, they entered cost as a current expense. That grossly exaggerated the current year's deficit and left nothing on the asset side in unused value of their balance sheet in subse-

quent years, yet the facility might last 40 years and the ground under it actually appreciate in value.

But none of this was ever explained in parliament or the media. It took a 20-year-old freshman to dig up in the internet a government document "Backgrounder on the Implementation of Accrual Accountancy" that really put the introduction of accrual accountancy in better perspective. That amazing document bore witness to the hard bargaining that had taken place between "Honest Paul," our Finance Minister of the day and now our Prime Minister, and the Auditor General. It all led to a conclusion on the following inconclusive note:

"It is premature to provide estimates on the impact of these changes. Departments and agencies are in the process of quantifying their assets and liabilities. *These will have to be reviewed by the Auditor General.*" [Our italics.] This was obviously a condition laid down by the Auditor General that stuck in Honest Paul's throat. And that is why someone had to go fishing in the internet to bring it to light in the following passage: "In moving to accrual accounting, the Government will change its accounting policy with respect to aboriginal and environmental liabilities. Environmental liabilities are currently not recognized in financial statements and aboriginal liabilities are not fully recognized."

This represents two instances of "internalizing" vast capital assets of our government if the these necessary investments have been made or as liabilities if they have not. But they have instead been put out of mind as "externalities." There is nothing external to the economy in unemployment, broken-up families, epidemics, undernourishment or about the downloading of programs to the provinces, without the funding to pay for these new responsibilities. The provinces did the same to their municipalities. The present modest beginning of bringing such assets onto the balance sheet must be expanded to take in all "externalities." And an end must be put to the objective of "Honest Paul" of paying off the national debt. By balancing a budget that ignores the greater part of the government's physical capital assets, and does not even mention the investment in human capital – education, health, social security, he would: (1) have to collapse the economy; (2) leave the land without legal tender, since federal debt is the only base money in the land today. What then would Honest Paul pay off the debt with – paper dollar bills of a different colour?

Is Non-accounting "Anti-inflationary"?

Also left unclear is whether the readjustment of the necessary government physical and human investment is carried backward and over how many years.

But most important of all: such adjustments must not be considered as involving just a lump sum of money. In the world today, neither gold nor silver is the money-base as was the case a century ago. Instead it is the central government's credit that supports a huge inverted pyramid of money creation. Most of our money creation is done today not by the central bank but by the commercial banks on the stock market, and in a great variety of other gambles. Many of these involve books cooked as badly as our government's, but usually in the opposite direction, exaggerating their net worth to send their share prices into orbit.

The curious detail in all this is that it is hushed up, supposedly because of the fear of it being seen as "inflationary." But the real inflation in our society is not in the provision of health, education, and social services or environmental conservation. The eventual costs of not providing such public investment measures will be far greater than attending to them in a timely way. They will produce more crime, more jails, more anti-terrorist spending, more SARS, more Mad Cow disease, more wars than spending for real values. In the long run there will be immense savings by avoiding even the strictly monetary cost of neglect. Our economy has become a double-tiered affair – with severe deflation produced by Globalization and Deregulation in the real economy that allows the wiping out of real production; and hyperinflation of the financial superstructure.

Virtual non-interest bearing loans to our government from the central bank have been replaced with interest-bearing loans from banks and "the market" to governments. Globalization and Deregulation incorporates into the current value of securities and derivative aspects of those securities by extrapolating the rate of growth – fictional or real – already attained into the remote future.

A further point. The recognition of a tiny portion of the government's essential capital investments as assets, or treating them as liabilities, does more than distort the balance sheet of an individual, a corporation, or a government. We need only delve into history to appreciate that. For centuries the only credit available to workers was the pawn-shop. And lending them money at any usurious rate was deemed a charity. All they could put up as security was the tools of their trade, or their scant personal possessions. That is why throughout the Spanish-speaking world to this day pawnshops are called, ironically enough, Monte de Piedad – Mount of Piety. In the nineteenth and early twentieth century cooperative banks – called "savings and loans," "trust companies" or "Building Societies" arose to make home mortgages available to the working class. For banks would not and even were not allowed to touch home mortgages. These "building societies" raised money – not by taking in deposits – that was no good for financing the purchase of a house because a deposit can be withdrawn and a home must be financed over at least a couple of decades. Instead, they originally raised their money by selling shares, and those who wished to finance acquiring a home would wait their turn if the society's capital was still inadequate.

The important thing is that by opening up the purchase of homes with reasonable financing to millions, the capitalist system itself benefited enormously. And when the Roosevelt administration during the thirties introduced government mortgage insurance, and the banks were authorized to invest in government-insured mortgages (in 1967 in Canada) the capitalist system prospered as never before. And before long the lowly worker who for centuries could only borrow at pawnshops, became as a much sought-after consumer whose borrowing needs were feverishly sought after and even promoted by the capitalist market system. At the present time credit-card

controlled by banks is one of the few things really going in the world. To the extent that it is bound to be a prominent factor in bringing on the next bust.

From Pawnshops to Credit Cards — the Story of Loans to the Lowly

On the other hand, governments whose credit is the only legal tender, are today being denied creditworthiness in a mega-scam that for sheer brass vies with those of corporation heads that are hogging the headlines today. That is why governments, allegedly "to balance the budget," are selling off their railways, public power systems, roads, schools, educational and health institutions for a song. And the promoters who pick up these bargains at once, jack up the price of their services, and let the facilities decay. The British railways, the CNR and Ontario Hydro are outstanding examples of this.

Since the present model of deregulated globalized finance is dangerously unsustainable, the goal must be to gear down the rate of growth of the financial sector, while shifting money creation from the private financial institutions to financing government investment loans on a near-zero basis. The provisions for doing that are still to be found in the *Bank of Canada Act*.

William Krehm

Situational Economics — A New Approach to Value Determinism

A MARKET-CENTERED VERSION of neoclassical economics is the current basis for policy- making in most Western countries, especially in the United States. However, despite its popularity with policy-makers it does not offer consistent explanations about how economic activities develop in modern societies. Empirical data in at least three major areas run contrary to its claim of creating efficiency and general progress. First, income disparities have risen dramatically since the late 1970s with the created productivity gains being usurped by the top, leaving the bottom 80 percent with no gains in inflation-adjusted terms. Second, policies dictated by short-term corporate interests have largely left negative externalities unattended, leaving a ticking bomb under society as we know it. Third, infrastructural deficiencies, due to the constant policies of tax reductions, have left the bulk of the citizens with falling life qualities in run-down inner-city neighborhoods or dysfunctional middle class suburbs, while an increasingly wealthy elite retreat to gated communities. Here, they employ a growing number of private servants and security personnel, recreating a life-style that is more and more reminiscent of the feudal elite of pre-industrial Europe.

Many of the economists of the preceding Keynesian period had come to believe that the market-centered theories of neoclassical economics were inadequate, both in response to economic crises – Keynes' own work dealt mainly with this problem. In a broader way it found expression in Galbraith's famous book, *The New Industrial State*. Galbraith contends that for the capitalist system to work properly, there must exist what he calls "countervailing forces"; various types of social forces that act as a counterweight to the concentration of economic power, and, by extension, general social and political power. In an unregulated market system these will be concentrated in the large corporations.

By the 1970s, Keynesian economics were pushed to the background by supply-side economics, advocated by a group of conservative economists who wanted to return to a pure version of neoclassical economics, where only markets mattered and governments played a minimalist role. The problem faced by Keynesian economics was that even though it had shown the practical defects of neoclassical economics, it had not been able to conclusively break away from its theoretical basis. Therefore, it had no strong riposte to face the supply-side onslaught.

The Need for Countervailing Forces

Galbraith had realized that market activities in industrial societies, large-scale manufacturing and distribution units dominate economic activity and translate into a concentration of power. Hence the need to establish countervailing forces outside the narrow system of economics capable of counteracting these tendencies. However, he left the question there and didn't attack the problem of the value determination of the neoclassical system.

A major step forward in this respect came when George Soros formulated the concept of reflexivity. With reflexivity, Soros describes a phenomenon where the valuation of a current trade is dependent upon an expectation of a future value (for the sake of simplicity we assume a single value in the future; in reality, it is often a complex number). However, when one arrives at that point, it is discovered that the observed value has partially risen due to the previous trade. This interdependence undermines the notion that economic value can be represented by simple, rational numbers.

Soros' concept of reflexivity does not cover the dichotomy between the supply and demand sides that arises during economic exchanges. Neoclassical theory assumes that the principle of marginality will always establish a value at which an exchange ought to be executed. Agents who do not exchange at this value will be driven out of the market. However, for this to work, markets have to be perfect, information equally available to all, and the time-spatial continuum cannot have any influence upon economic activity. These are unrealistic conditions that undermine the neoclassical principle for value determinism.

To replace this, a new approach of situational economics is proposed. Among other things, this is based upon the notion that there exist different causalities for microeconomic and macroeconomic phenomena: A situational-probabilistic causality for microeconomic activity, and an indeterminate dualism for macroeconomic relations.

Under normal conditions, buyers and sellers will only consider their own interests during the exchange, i.e., they confront each other with agent-centric interests. Sometimes, a seller will sell an identical item to many buyers. In such cases, the buyers will desire the items to different degrees. According to the standard economic approach, they express this in the price they are willing to pay. On the other hand, buyers can often buy an identical item from more than one seller. Once again, the price at which the sellers are willing to sell expresses different degrees of willingness to part with their goods.

However, the value projections emerging during such encounters are not mechanically arrived at. The sellers and buyers, the self-centric agents, will not only form their value projections in a subjective way dependent upon their personal understanding of economic and social relations, but also upon their estimate of the opposing agent's understanding. This means that the value projection an agent forms regarding an object of exchange is arrived at "situationally." It will change with time and location, but will also depend on who the opposing agent is. Since this happens on both sides of an exchange, all value projections connected to exchanges are "situationally" interdependent, i.e., they form partly in response to one another.

Because of this, the value projections connected to microeconomic exchange events will, unavoidably, contain irrational elements and can never be arrived at by the application of deterministic principles alone. This means that, while the ability to foresee the outcome of economic events is partially based upon an understanding of certain economic principles (for example, that higher prices reduces demand), to be effective, an economic agent or forecaster must also judge the weight of factors forming the value projections. This includes influence from established economic and social power systems, as well as the agents' abilities to shape events towards their specific agent-centric interests. For example, an advertising campaign by a seller can enhance the product's inelasticity and thus reduce its price-demand responsivity. Under such circumstances, a deterministic approach breaks down and must be replaced by a situational-probabilistic approach. According to this, the ability to assess probabilities and one's skill in pattern recognition and judgments become crucial elements when engaging in economic activity or making forecasts.

That also implies that aggregations will not represent an average of outcomes according to a set of economic principles.

When we move to the macro level of economics we face a different situation. In principle, macroeconomic phenomena do not describe events but relations between aggregations of micro events. Therefore, while all microeconomic phenomena are discrete, macroeconomic phenomena are not.

The Breakdown of Determinist Price Formation

The interest in macro relations is based on the assumption that knowledge of them tells us something about the direction of economic trends. For example, if a homeowner reads in the newspapers that interest rates are falling, it makes sense to postpone the refinancing of a mortgage.

On the public level, knowledge about macro relations makes it possible to implement policies that either optimize the revealed economic tendencies, or influence them towards more desirable goals. To achieve that, we must know how to read the available microeconomic data, but understand what drives the tendencies.

Because of the nature of their microeconomic basis, there will always emerge a cluster of possible interpretations of the macro relations. Employing a traditional methodology, all of these appear to be equally valid. With no adequate internal analytical method available to choose one interpretation over another, the question moves out of the realm of economics into other social value systems.

It is worth noting that existing path-dependent misalignments have a tendency towards self-reinforcement. Growth begets more growth as expressed in money terms. To escape this trap, the different interpretations of the macro relations must proceed by comparing the economic options with general humanistic values, advocated by Western philosophers such as Bertrand Russell and paralleled in the concept of *ren,* central to the Chinese social philosophy of Confucianism.

Dix Sandbeck

Storm Clouds Again over the East

WITH THE US elections around the corner, a new wave of synthetic optimism is overwhelming the world. For local optimism these days, courtesy of Globalization and Deregulation, must embrace the entire world or be ruled out in your hometown. More than that, the cheerful prospects are more easily improvised in far-off places about which we know little. That is why a new bust is in the making before we have quite come out of the previous one.

The East Asian crisis of 1998 moved on with disastrous effects to Latin America, Russia and indeed the entire world. Since then tons of further deregulation and globalization have been prescribed to the world in an ultimate triumph of homeopathy, in which the cure of the disease resembles the symptoms.

Not surprising, then, that the major storm clouds of the day should be gathering over the scenes of the late Asiatic credit bubble. *The Wall Street Journal* (20/01, "After Credit Binge in South Korea, Big Bill Comes Due" by Hae Won Choi and Gordon Fairlough) recounts: "Seoul, South Korea – A household crisis rocking South Korea provides a chilling warning to developing nations throughout the world: doling out credit cards to boost consumer spending can juice growth in the short run, but the ultimate consequences can be dire.

Credit-card Defaults Win the High-jump Race

"South Korea once boasted one of the world's highest saving rates. But in a sharp about-face over the past few years, consumers – with government prodding – have gone on a credit-fueled buying binge. Now, the bill is coming due, as credit-card defaults traumatize families and rock the nation's financial system. Between 1999 and 2003, South Korea's total outstanding credit-card debt grew more than five-fold. By the third quarter of last year, Korean consumers had run up a collective credit-card balance of $57.47 billion, compared with $10.95 billion at the end of 1999.

"South Korean regulators say the nationwide credit-card delinquency rate, the percentage of loans more than 30 days overdue, jumped to 13.5% in November, compared with 2.6% at the end of 2001. Some industry executives, however, say the actual proportion of bad loans may be as high as 30%, given aggressive efforts of lenders to mask the problem. In the US, by contrast, bankers are wringing their hands over data that show Americans hit a record-high credit-card delinquency rate of 4.09% in the third quarter of 2003.

"Debt-related murder-suicides and other crimes have become a regular staple of South Korean newspapers and TV news broadcasts. Last summer, a 34-year-old woman pushed her two daughters, ages 3 and 7, out the window of the family's 15-floor apartment. Then holding tight to her 6-year son's hand, she jumped, too. Police say the woman was distraught over $25,000 in credit-card debt that she and her husband, a construction worker, couldn't pay.

"Because Korea's social structure makes family members feel accountable for each other's debts, one person's credit problems often ripple through entire families and social networks, curbing the spending of large groups of people and prolonging a slump in consumer spending.

"Bad loans are putting a serious strain on South Korea's financial institutions, which are still recovering from the Asian financial crisis of the late 1990s. Earlier this month, banks had to rescue the country's largest card insurer with a $3.19 billion bailout package.

"As countries in the region tried to get their economies rolling again, many nudged banks to make consumer borrowing easier to strengthen domestic consumption and reduce the countries' reliance on exports. South Korea even offered consumers tax breaks for credit card use.

"Some government are now trying to rein in consumer credit. Thailand has raised income requirements for cardholders and Taiwan has strengthened controls on card issuers. Singapore is clamping down on aggressive card-marketing.

"Much of the pain from Asia's bad loans could be offset as the countries' export industries pick up steam. Even so, analysts worry that credit problems could make Asia's economies extremely susceptible to external shocks and further constrain growth.

"Kim Sang Mi got in on South Korea's credit boom at the beginning. One of the first things she did when she moved to Seoul in 2000 was to go online and apply for two credit cards. She used them to buy furniture and appliances for her new apartment. Then she branched out into hip clothes and fancy cosmetics, things she couldn't get in the small town where she grew up. She started going out with friends to restaurants and bars, charging nearly everything. She says she wanted to take advantage of the tax breaks offered by the government. 'I wanted to blend in like the people of Seoul,' says Ms Kim, now 27 years old and an accountant in an online game company."

Capitalizing an Unknown Future

Note the ingredients of this powerful broth – a migrant to the big city, online, credit-card, an account in an online game company, and above all tax-breaks! All devices for shoving planning into the future. Meanwhile the piper goes on piping and nobody, least of all the government, worries about paying him. All that is left "to the market," which gets manipulated by the government and an economic system that capitalizes the unknown future.

"About a year into her shopping spree, Ms. Kim was struggling to pay her bills. She started taking cash advances on some of her five cards to make payments on the others."

This was pyramiding bogus money creation with no nexus between the debt-money created and the consumer's ability to pay, or with society's needs.

"Ms. Kim borrowed thousands of dollars from her friends and family, wiping out much of the savings of her brother and parents. Then early, last year, after she had run up a tab of more than $42,000, her juggling act failed. Her card companies pressed her to restructure her debt. To do that her brother and parents had to sign as guarantors. Under her new deal with the card companies, Ms. Kim must devote nearly her entire salary of about $1,100 a month to card payments for the next three years. She seldom goes out and volunteers to work late so that she can get free meals from her company. Her brother pays most of her rent and living expenses, and for the past two months about half his salary has gone towards paying her card debt."

"Unsustainable household debt has led to serious declines in consumer spending. In the first nine months of 2003, private domestic consumption fell 1.1% compared with a 6.8% year-on-year increase in 2002.

"LG Card lenders have had to bail it out for the second time in three months in early January, essentially agreeing to acquire the card issuer by swapping $1.69 billion in outstanding debt for equity. LG Card's creditors, including some of the largest banks, also promised to lend a fresh $1.39 million to keep the company afloat. Finance ministry officials pointed to a report by LG Card's auditors which estimated the potential cost to creditors at $22.51 billion. They also feared a contagion effect. If LG Card went out of business, it could lead to a cascade of delinquencies at other card issuers, since many Koreans use cash advances on one credit card to make their payments on others."

That is the reverse side of the counterfeit coin of deregulation and mergers. It is all champagne and waltzes on the way up, and rat poison once the bills come in.

"The current mess has its roots in a South Korean government campaign – starting in 1999 – to strengthen domestic consumption. The government established rules allowing consumers to deduct some credit-card purchases from their taxes and pushed for low interest rates to stimulate spending. It also lifted a ceiling on cash advances. Previously, individuals had been allowed to take out only about $600 in cash through their credit cards. The government further slashed taxes on luxury goods and cars to encourage spending. *The government push came as the country's banks were casting about for a new way to make money after the big corporate bankruptcies of the late 1990s.*

Household lending and credit cards in particular were seen as a potential source of new profits." [Our emphasis.]

From Frying Pan to the Fire

It was a straight case of jumping from the frying-pan into the fire. "For decades South Korea's banks had focused on funnelling money from depositors to the nation's massive family-controlled conglomerates, such as Samsung Group and LG Group. The banks had little experience in consumer spending. Korea had no independent organization that tracked individuals' credit-worthiness. Companies set up street-corner booths, getting signatures and issuing cards on the spot without in-depth credit analysis for credit lines of thousands of dollars. Between 1997 and 2003, the total number of credit cards more than tripled, hitting 72.8 million, or about two cards for every person over the age of 17. It escaped the monetary sages that all this was money-creation.

"New loans were extended with scant proof they could be repaid. The goal, some bankers say, was to hide the real number of nonperforming loans. In some cases, delinquent borrowers were given new loans with a six-month or one-year moratorium on repayments." In essence the banks were granting these reprieves to themselves.

"Woori Finance Holdings Co., the country's second-largest financial institution, 87% owned by the South Korean government, first disclosed this practice at the end of September, when it had to meet stricter US accounting standards to trade on the New York Stock Exchange." That means that South Korean "risk management" has been leaking into the governance of the New York Stock Exchange when it was still faced with meeting its then CEO's take-home pay.

"Youm Eun Ha, a 27-year-old bookkeeper, says that when she fell behind in payments to LG Card in September, the company restructured her loan, despite her objections, and gave her a six-month moratorium on payments. Ms. Youm said LG told her that if she didn't restructure, it would garnishee 50% of her salary every month."

W.K.

The Perils of Ignoring the Great Legends

THE DEFINING QUALITY of the great Greek legends is that human kind seems fated to act out their plots again and again on an ascending scale. Thus, Oedipus killed a wayfarer at a crossroads because he failed to recognize him as his father, king of Thebes. As a result all his triumphs were doomed to dust. He did solve the riddle of the sphinx and was rewarded with the crown of Thebes, unwittingly marrying his mother whom he had in fact widowed. When what he had done in his blindness was disclosed, he tore out his eyes. His mother-wife, Jocasta, hanged herself.

With such grim warnings, we are driven in reading our Wall

Street Journal to give heed to another great legend: the cleaning of the Augean stables. The king, Augeus, kept 3,000 oxen in his stables without cleaning them in 30 years. Hercules, put to the test, tidied them up in a single day – by turning the river Alpheus to flow through the stables.

Our applause goes to NY Attorney General Eliot Spitzer and others for their tireless broom-work on Wall St.'s stenchy stalls. But will the Augean stables ever be tidied up without a diversion of the Potomac River?

Take the *WSJ* issue of 27/01, page C1, "Money & Investing" section, carries the beginning of six articles, and every one of them has to do with major accounting, statistical, and other scams: no matter how fast Mr. Spitzer sweeps and shovels, a peg ever on his nose, there is no visible drop in the new scandals that surface.

"US Investigates Cattle Trades" by John R. Wilke begins: "Federal Regulators are investigating whether some commodity traders last month had advance knowledge that an animal in Washington state tested positive for mad cow disease. Investigators with the Commodity Futures Trading Commission (CFTC) are interviewing possible witnesses, reviewing documents and phone records, and examining trading patterns on the Chicago Mercantile Exchange, the commission's enforcement chief said yesterday. At issue are investors who took short positions in live-cattle futures, betting on a price decline, in the days just before the Dec. 23 announcement by US Department of Agriculture Secretary Ann Veneman.

"The investigation was triggered by concerns that the market-sensitive news leaked, either by the government or elsewhere, before the USDA's announcement. The CFTC's definition of insider trading is narrower than that of the Security and Exchange Commission, and the range of civil charges it could bring against investors with any advance knowledge of the USDA announcement would depend on where, when and from whom they got the information. It isn't clear, for example, whether an employee of a slaughter-house could be charged. But any employee of the USDA or the Iowa testing lab could potentially face charges if found to have traded on early knowledge." In short it will all depend on the crossroads where the miscreant encountered the father he didn't recognize, and on his relationship with his unknown dam. In short the Oedipus legend is still going strong, and "investors" – the very term used for eyeless speculators is eloquent of the mess we're in – will prosper grandly from even a disaster like Mad Cow.

∾ ∾ ∾

Without leaving the *WSJ* front page let's move to the extreme left column "Ahead of the Tape by Jesse Eisinger." "Cheesed Off Wall St.'s baloney has a first name R-E-S-T-R-U-C-T-U-R-I-N-G. No answer to any business problem has a more magical ring for investors and analysts. So when Kraft reports its fourth-quarter earnings today and holds an analysts' meeting, the solution to its current revenue shortfall and management shake-ups is clear, at least to the Street: Cut costs and offload assets.

"Deutsche Bank's Eric Katzman forecast that it will announce plans to fire about 10% of its staff, around 6,500 people,

saving roughly $75,000 a head.

"But Kraft is already wildly profitable, especially by standards of the food industry. Its operating margin was almost 21.7% in 2002. It fell last year to a still-high 20.1%, estimates Prudential's John McMillin. The average in the food industry is around 17%.

"Kraft's problems don't appear born of bloated infrastructure. And Kraft continues to dominate its major food categories."

Mathematics of Atom Bomb Takes Over

What does this point to? As COMER has long emphasized, our stock market valuations increasingly capitalize not the return on capital, but *the rate of growth* of that return, and *the rate of growth of that rate of growth of return*, and so forth to infinity. All that is summed up by graphs that strive to stand vertical. Such graphs embody exponential growth, which is the mathematics of the atom bomb. Of course, the first thing they destroy is sustainability. Kraft may believe that it alone is preserving its rate-of growth valuation, while other firms are concentrating on their direct returns and cherishing their staff to instill loyalty and thus conserve Kraft's market for it. But the fact is that all CEOs are "restructuring" for quick exits with the spoils.

∾ ∾ ∾

In the extreme right column of the same page se have the story "Sun Life Unit Reaches Pact in Fund Probe:" by John Hechinger and Tom Lauricella:

"Massachusetts Financial Services Co. has reached a tentative agreement to pay $225 million in penalties and cut its management fees by $125 million to settle charges that it improperly allowed fast-moving traders to skim profits from long-term investors in its mutual funds, say people familiar with the matter.

"If made final, the settlement with New York Attorney General Eliot Spitzer and the Securities Exchange Commission would result in the second-largest penalty exacted so far in the four-month-old mutual-fund scandal.

"Under the terms of the tentative agreement, MFS, a Boston-based unit of Sun Life Financial Inc. would pay $175 million in disgorgement and $50 million in fines. The fee reductions, which would be part of MFSs agreement with Mr. Spitzer's office but not the SEC, would amount to $25 million annually for five years.

"MFS is also expected to agree to a number of changes in the way the firm oversees its funds and to provide greater information about the fees it charges investors. Eighty-year-old MFS, the nation's 11th largest fund firm – and by its reading of history, the oldest – has about $140 billion under management, including $76 billion in mutual fund assets.

"Mr. Spitzer's focus on fees, rather than fines, has been shunned by the SEC, partly because some regulators and other critics fear he has used his prosecuting powers to set prices. But Mr. Spitzer has called fund fees the '800-pound gorilla' of the industry, and maintained they should be cut when companies violate the trust of shareholders.

"While the fines and fee cuts MFS is said to have agreed to are substantial they are smaller than those imposed on Alliance Capital Management Holding Inc. Alliance, another big mutual-find firm, agreed to pay a $250 million fine and to make management-fee reductions of 20% for the next five years estimated to total about $350 million. The company neither admitted nor denied wrongdoing. (Did Oedipus really have no inkling that the wayfarer he met at the crossroads was his royal father, or that Queen Jocasta was his mother? The gods are still out on that one.)

"The differing sizes of the settlements reflects the different actions taken by MFS and Alliance. The amount of the market timing at MFS appears to have been larger than at Alliance. But top executives at MFS don't seem to have negotiated the type of deals with market timers that Alliance officials made.

"In these arrangements, market timers made sizable investments in Alliance-run hedge funds and mutual funds in exchange for the right to market time certain other mutual funds. Through these arrangements Alliance was able to earn greater fees off both the market-timing assets and the long-term investments in these other products."

The Delights of Market Timing

"Market timing" allows favoured clients to buy mutual funds at their closing quote established at 4 p.m. each day in the interval in between two such even though the prices of the stocks held by them may have risen. This cuts into the fund earnings that can be distributed to mutual fund holders not so favored. It is betting on horses long after the race has been run.

On the same page is another article "Marketing Charges in Mutual Funds Gain More Attention" by Christopher Oster that enters further into yet other suspect practices in the mutual fund business.

"A little understood category of marketing charges costing investors an estimate $10 billion a year is gaining increased attention from critics who say it should be amended or eliminated completely. The charges in question, approved in 1980 under Rule 12b-1 of the 1940 *Investment Company Act*, will get more scrutiny today at a Senate subcommittee hearing called to examine the 'hidden costs within mutual funds.'

"Fund analysts say the problem with the rule is that few investors understand how 12b-1 dollars are spent. Said Jeff Keil, a vice president at fund-researcher Lipper Inc. and co-author of a recent 100-page report on 12b-1 fees, says that part of the problem is that the 12b-1 fees are intended to give fund companies flexibility in how to use them, but that has contributed to the fees also being shrouded in mystery.

"In adopting 12b-1 fees, the SEC reversed its long-held position that a fund's assets shouldn't be used to help sell more fund shares and made it legal to use money to pay for marketing and distribution expenses. That cleared the way for no-load groups – such as Vanguard Group, an early proponent of using investment assets for marketing – to better compete with broker-sold funds, Mr. Keil says.

"Before 12b-1 fees, funds sold through brokers carried front-end commissions known as 'loads.' But with the new rule in place, fund companies gained flexibility to structure loads in a variety of ways that were more popular with investors because they charged less money in upfront fees. For example, because fund companies could collect annual charges of as much as 1% in the form of 12b-1 fees, fund companies were able to introduce several share classes, some of which carried back-end sales charges that declined over time and others that charged so-called level loads spread over several years. As a result 12b-1 fees have essentially replaced commissions in many cases In 2000, the Investment Company Institute, the main fund trade group, released a report that said that 63% of 12b-1 fees were paid as commissions to brokers. A separate 32% of the fees went to administrative services such as payments to outside companies that do record-keeping and others services to current shareholders.

"One of the concerns about the rule's use is that load funds can be presented to an unsophisticated investor as the equivalent of a no-load fund."

∾ ∾ ∾

We were planning to go on to the other three tales of horror all on the front page of a single issue of the *WSJ*, when scandal struck at the very heart of the royal house of Thebes, pardon me, the Liberal regime in Canada. And that made it necessary to preempt the space for our lead article. For Canada, deemed so pure, that is still has to have a single commission of enquiry, now, may or should, end up with a half dozen.

William Krehm

When Half-empty
Is Not Half-full

"HALF-EMPTY" is the equivalent of "half-full" only when you are talking about glasses of water. It does not apply to a society where scams and corruption are making daily headlines, and information is severely rationed. The case of government heads and corporate CEOs coming clean on half the evidence must be seen as a failed 100% cover-up.

To illustrate this important principle, we are offering a cluster of seemingly unrelated items. However, in this era of stock-market-driven Globalization and Deregulation (G&D) few things that matter are unrelated.

It all began with a blast of certainty. Respectable academics assured the public that "There was no alternative" – TINA. The assumption was that they had really analyzed the alternatives to G&D including those that had given us our best years. And now it is increasingly apparent that they had taken it all on not wholly disinterested faith. Today, the more conscientious of these teachers, having learned their painful lesson, hang their heads in shame.

The Globe and Mail (21/02, "NAFTA takes it on the road" by Doug Saunders) is still a believer: "With job losses rampant, this year's US economy may end up turning on the issue of free trade. Before they map out their positions, politicians would be wise to follow [us] down the route of the controversial 1-69 superhighway being built from Canada to Mexico.

"When the construction of the final stretch – Indianapolis to Nuevo Laredo, Mexico – begins as early as this year, it will meet fierce resistance in the Midwest. But it will be heralded in other communities for its promise of trade-driven growth, or at very least a flood of low-pay jobs in places where there were no jobs at all.

"The upcoming presidential vote is very likely to become the NAFTA election. In Bloomington, Indiana, in the rust belt, Democratic candidate John Edwards has won strong support for promising to cancel the deal outright. "He wouldn't need ads,' Democratic strategist Greg Hass said of Mr. Edwards, 'just the word NAFTA is a red cape in the face of a bull. John Kerry, the front-runner, has promised to renegotiate the deal if he becomes president (though he voted for it as senator). And even George W. Bush has started making protectionist noises.

"Back in 1994, when NAFTA came into effect, most US residents paid it little attention. Years earlier, it already had been the subject of a great debate in a hard-fought Canadian election, and the object of passionate hopes and fears in Mexico. But a poll at the time showed that 49 percent had never even heard of it.

"Ten years later, the world has changed dramatically. At the north end of the NAFTA highway, Canadians have largely made peace with NAFTA. It has brought an era of export-driven prosperity. benefiting many regions and sectors, albeit with an even mix of very good information-economy jobs and so-so service-sector jobs.

"At the south end, Mexicans aren't as pleased. The deal has quadrupled exports and raised wages in manufacturing, badly hurt many parts of the agricultural sector by flooding markets with government-subsidized US crops, and left Mexicans, on average, only slightly better off than before."

The trouble with such appraisals is that "average Canadian," "average American" and "average Mexican" are statistical fictions that have never drawn breath. And the welfare of living folks can't be gauged by their jobs alone. The gap between the earnings of stockbrokers, bankers, CEOs and the factory workers and farmers has widened vastly. The insecurity of most people has increased, as government assets are privatized, and their livelihoods have become mere chips in the games of the mighty. To maintain those average earnings constant, you can decrease the money earnings of the lower 80% of the population provided that the income of the upper 20% pushes up much, much faster. If that happens, the "average" will stay the same. But that does not mean the result is neutral. Or even sustainable. Add to that the heightened pollution of the environment that the multiplication of highway, air, and city traffic brings; the breakdown of public health quickens at the very time that new diseases develop and old ones believed controlled reappear.

The truth is that throughout the world society is becoming increasingly a double-deck affair. At the lower level many workers are losing their newly found unskilled manufacturing jobs to still more miserable countries in Asia and Latin America. At the top, deregulated, the transnational financial industries have flourished by means fair and foul. Corporation books have been cooked by the very auditors in collusion with the audited. A variety of dodges couched in irrelevant similes or misapplied mathematics are used to hide reality. Much of the super-prosperity on high is based on wiping out the historic defences of the underprivileged. The pricing system of securities is in fact based on the capitalization of achieved rates of growth of the disparity between the winnings of financial corporations and the increasing misery of the actual producers.

The Fiction of a Flat Price Level

Another fiction is the notion of a flat price level as a valid goal in a society that is becoming increasingly urbanized and high tech. Without the institutions that large cities alone can provide, a modern society would be unthinkable. And attempting to enforce a flat price level with the "one blunt tool" of interest rates vests power with those who control money creation. For today there is no money but credit – neither gold nor silver is legal tender any more. Those who rule over credit hold the world at ransom.

But back to the NAFTA Highway. "In the US, it often seems as if half the population has woken screaming from a ten-year nap. Here in the middle of America, NAFTA has become the hottest word in the political vocabulary. This year's election will be won or lost in the deeply undecided states in America's industrial middle.

"Yet once you've driven a few more miles down this road, it becomes clear that the politics of trade are as complex and layered as a highway interchange. The road is not as straight as it seems.

"If you want to know why NAFTA has suddenly leaped into the political menu here, it's worth following the highway's path into the industrial west end of Bloomington. For decades, this city of 60,000 has been known for the stark town-and-gown division between the comfortable lawns of its state university campus in the east and the trailer homes and the tiny bungalows of its sprawling industrial district to the west. The past five years, however, have nearly wiped out the blue-collar side.

"Jackie Yenna has worked at the General Electric refrigerator factory in Bloomington for 34 of his 51 years. It employed 3,000 people, including his mother, at decent union wages. Not far away, the RCA TV plant had 8,000 employees, and a dozen other manufacturing plants made this a boom town.

"The closings began about five years ago. The GE plant was among the first hit, cutting 1,400 jobs as it moved its operations to other countries, mostly Mexico. Then the RCA factory moved to Mexico, eliminating its last 1,100 jobs in 1998. Mr. Yenna was one of the lucky few to keep their jobs. He and his fellow survivors spend their days nervously awaiting the next bad news, counting the years to retirement and settling for mediocre pay raises.

"Across the central US, the story has been the same, with an estimated three million jobs lost since 1999. And now they're building a six-lane highway to Mexico through the center of the town. The town has risen against it – city councillors have won multiple terms on anti-highway platforms. The jobs of many went down south, and now they have to line up to get jobs helping build a road that'll make it easier to move things to Mexico.

"The angry and hollowed-out American Midwest is packed with unemployed voters venting their disappointment with the Republicans.

"Yet Bloomington has not turned into a squalid ghost town of soup lines. Mr. Yenna says most of the guys laid off in his factory have taken advantage of training to find work in cleaner, better-paying industries, or they have started their own businesses. The unemployment rate in Bloomington is under 3.5%, and the main question is whether you have a good full-time job or a bad one.

"The NAFTA superhighway's route passes through Memphis, and then enters the cotton fields of Northern Mississippi's Delta, one of the very poorest places in the US. Nobody here worries about the NAFTA Highway taking jobs away. Jobs are scarce enough already. The prospect of a burger-grilling job at a roadside fast-food is a real opportunity. The low wages, the lack of business taxes and Mississippi's anti-union laws could make the Delta a competitor for companies that want to be cheap and flexible, but aren't quite up to moving south of the border, perhaps because of the increasing political stigma of such a move. All they need is a decent highway. This is the implication: 'We want what the guys in Nuevo Laredo have got. We want to be the end of the road.'"

Hope Dies at the Road's End

"But Mexico isn't quite what you'd expect either. The stretch of ramshackle cities that hug the Texas border are famously known as *maquiladoras,* low-wage manufacturing centers created in the 1980s as a tax-free, regulation-proof stateless netherworld that has attracted thousands of poor Mexicans seeking any steady work, even for $2 an hour with no benefits.

"The NAFTA Highway ends in Nuevo Laredo, a muddy enclave of high-security industry parks and cinder-block housing across the border from the Texas town of Laredo. Here you will find a Sony DVD factory, a Caterpillar engine-parts plant, and dozens of other small and medium-sized factories. It is one of the more successful towns in one of the three northern Mexican provinces that have experienced wage growth and increased employment from NAFTA. The rest of the country has seen little benefit. A million new jobs have been created in this region since 1994, at average wages 37% higher than in Mexican domestic industries.

"But the past few years haven't been good. Many Mexicans are now finding themselves in much the same position as Bloomington's layoff-plagued workers. NAFTA has put them up against the rest of Mexico and G&D has put them in competition with the rest of the world. Since 2001, more than 240,000 jobs have been lost to Mexican towns deep in the heartland where people will work even cheaper, or to China or southeast Asia. In Nuevo Laredo, a third of the jobs have disappeared, turning it into Mexico's rust belt.

"'Mexico is becoming less competitive in the world,' Jeffrey Davidow, the former US ambassador to Mexico, said in a recent panel discussion. 'Mexico's advantage in the world has gone to China. He was referring to India's recent growth, driven by a highly educated work force and high-tech industries a step beyond mere assembly. But it's not about to happen in these northern towns. *Universities, training programs and incentives to move workers above the bottom rung don't exist.* [Our italics.] And the commitment of Mexican authorities to keep taxes low guarantees they'll never be created. At the end of the long road, the Mexican border is proving to be not so much a source of fear as a subject of pity."

At this point, however, the writer, Doug Saunders, gets carried away with his highway-ladder analogy, mistaking it for a runway which will allow the economy to become airborne:

"The question that Mexico is now beginning to ask itself – how to move beyond the prison of assembly-line labour – has already been answered, it turns out, by the people of Bloomington. The Indiana residents may not know it yet, but they have followed the path of their Canadian neighbours, out of industrial labour into a service economy.

"A decade ago, Bloomington's largest employers were General

Electric and RCA. Today, they are the state university, followed by a major hospital and then a large number of new high-tech industries, most of them in biomedical and computer-related fields that have made Bloomington's east side a boom town.

"While a few of the industrial workers may be upset about the danger of more jobs disappearing to Mexico, most of the opponents say the biggest threat is the prospect of more heavy industry. They see that economy as a thing of the past. Bloomington offers a cultural, educated, natural environment that attracts companies in the knowledge-based economy. Put an interstate through here, and you're just going to homogenize it.

"Bloomington is, in truth, a place much like the areas of Ontario perched at the top of the road. In much of Canada, the growth is in the service industries – an equal mix of really good jobs, requiring education and skill and offering better pay than the old blue-collar work; and bad but plentiful jobs, requiring little skill and providing rudimentary salaries and little security."

"The new economy, with or without NAFTA, has taken us down a strange and winding road, where Mississippi wants to be Mexico, Mexico is turning into Indiana and Indiana is trying to be more like Canada. Meanwhile, Canada is struggling to stay aloft at the top of the highway."

However, it is an illusion that Canada is anywhere near the top of that highway. The head offices of many of its great corporations have long since gone south. As have entire industries. So let us note what is afoot in those countries in a position to creep up on the current economic mega-powers. They may end up with glasses that are really full for only their dominant social groups. Or perish in the attempt to do so.

On the Use and Misuse of Mathematics by Economists

But first a word on the misuse of mathematics by economists, and how we can know whether our glasses are half-full or whether there in fact there is any water in them at all.

It all has to do with how banks and others in the financial sector have come to incorporate into the market price of their shares their supposed knowledge of the future. This they manage by dealing less and less in existing goods and services essential to human life, than in the *rates of growth* of the market values of securities, real or manipulated, on claims to such items. The "rate of growth" of the market value of a security to some chosen variable is known as its "first derivative"; and the rate of growth of that rate of growth, as the "second derivative." The term "derivative" is borrowed from differential calculus: it means "rate of growth" of one variable with respect to another. Thus a derivative to the 10th power, is the rate of growth of the rate of growth of one variable with respect to another – the same process being repeated nine times.

Market operators can manipulate the stock market these days by buying from their friendly bank just the future of the rate of growth in the value of any stock or bond, or of the yield on a given bond in a foreign currency. In doing so and investing in a bet on the future increase in the value of such an abstracted aspect of a bond or a share rather than in the security itself, they can achieve spectacular results:

1. It can give them far greater leverage for their plays. They can place their bets indirectly on an aspect of a far larger number of shares or bonds than if they had to buy the actual security, In this way small groups of very wealthy gamblers have managed to outgun central banks and bring down a whole series of currencies like the British pound and the Italian lira. Hedge funds, open only to those prepared to put up many millions of dollars, have been a feature of the financial world for at least two decades.

2. Once their view of the future growth rates (derivatives) is incorporated into the market price of a corporation share, the slightest shortfall from that forecast market value of the share will bring down the whole house of cards.

There is a very simple but extremely elegant mathematical function that incorporates future increases of growth rates into higher powers to infinity. Its principle is simple: the rate of growth moves up in tandem with the value already attained by the underlying function, as does the growth rate to the second order, and thus on and on to infinity. It is in fact the mathematics of the atom bomb: in the bomb the rate of growth was of unstable isotopes of uranium released which triggered further increases in the growth rates of such releases until the whole blew up over Hiroshima.[1]

The deregulation of our banks that allows them to engage in just about every aspect of the stock market – including notably brokerages and underwriting and merchant banking – has had tremendous implications on the "Is the glass half full or half empty" problem.

To begin with in a price-model that strives towards exponential growth, it is impossible to define what a glass "half-full" might be. It is of the nature of an infinite series in general and of the exponential function in particular, that you can cut it in two and each half will have the identical value as the whole, since by definition there is no greater or lesser infinity.[2] Thus the very concept of "half" ceases to exist. And secondly, whatever the approach to market valuations of shares or GDP or whatever that incorporate endlessly future growth into present prices, the exercise becomes increasingly unstable for the same reason as the bomb dropped on Hiroshima in 1945.

The Wall Street Journal (26/02, "China's Price for Market Entry: Give Us Your Technology, Too" by Kathryn Khanhold) lifts a corner of the curtain on the negotiations setting the patterns of world trade – and much else.

"Beijing – In his two decades pursuing contracts in China for General Electric Co. Delbert Williamson's strategy was always simple: Sell the most power equipment at the best price.

"But by the time Mr. Williamson sat down at a banquet at the historic Dioyutai State Guesthouse in Beijing last March, to celebrate the award of a $900 million contract for high-tech electricity turbines, the formula for GE's success in China had changed drastically.

"In addition to offering a competitive price, Mr. Williamson had to agree to share sophisticated GE technology with two Chinese companies that wanted to eventually make the equipment themselves.

"To be considered in the bidding for equipment contracts totaling several billion dollars, GE and its competitors were required to form joint ventures with the state-owned Chinese power companies. GE was also required to transfer to their new partners technology and advanced manufacturing guidelines for its '9F' turbine, which GE had spent more than a half billion dollars to develop.

"'It was a difficult negotiation,' said Mr. Williamson, 65 years old, who retired this month after 45 years with GE. 'They're interested in having total access to technology and we're interested in protecting our investment in that technology.'"

China's Immense Gravitational Pull

"Chinese call it [exchanging] 'technology for market.' China's leverage is that with its 1.3 billion population, it is – along with India – the greatest potential market and producer in the world." And those two things – the gravitational pull of its potential market, and the equally great menace as a potential supplier competing to fill the high-technological needs of the rest of the world may determine the survival of the human race. The immense populations of a few countries like China, India, and Brazil with what are becoming open-ended societies provide the platforms for challenging the United States.

"Such demands of sharing advanced technology as a condition for present purchases fall into a gray area of international trade law. China officially agreed to phase out many tariffs and technology-transfer requirements as part of its entry in December 2001 to the World Trade Organization. But she didn't sign a key piece of the WTO agreement that would have prohibited such demands. Its government negotiators have continued to ask foreign negotiators to transfer technology and set up research centers to train local engineers.

"That's the trade-off they have to deal with – short-term sales for long-term competition.

"In an effort to gain easier access to markets in China, Motorola Inc. has poured more than $300 million into 19 technology-research centers. A Microsoft Corp. center in Beijing now employs more than 200 researchers. Siemens AG has spent more than $200 million since 1998 working with a Chinese academic institute to develop a mobile phone technology compatible only with the phone systems in China."

In this, China is to an extent following the example set by Japan in the 1960s and 1970s. The difference is in the overwhelming population mass represented by China today. and the cheapness of its labour. Occasionally the US government bans the licensing of technology on defense grounds.

This is playing a key role in China's efforts to step up its power generation, at a time when the market within the US itself for power generation equipment is unusually weak.

"In simple terms, a turbine is any motor in which air, wind or steam spins blades on a shaft to create energy or perform a task – from windmills to pump water to hydroelectric generators that use the force of water behind a dam to make electricity. Modern turbines are highly complex – 40-ton devices capable of generating enormous amounts of electricity using superheated natural gas to spin the shafts. The precise shape of three rows of blades inside a turbine, temperatures reached by the fuel powering them, and the strength and composition of the materials used to make them dramatically affect the level of power each design produces.

"The small gas turbines produced by a partnership between GE and a Chinese government-owned company in the 1980s were capable of generating enough to power 40,000 homes. By contrast the GE gas turbines sold to China today, while cheaper to install and cleaner for the environment, generate enough power to serve about 300,000 homes.

"GE has formed a separate joint venture with Shenyang Liming Aero-Engine Group Corp., under which GE is permitting the Shenyang venture to manufacture the second and third rows of blades inside the turbine, technology that GE initially did not want to give up, according to people familiar with the negotiations. Included in the transfer are technical drawings of a key cooling system and the highly advanced technology of the blades.

"But the Chinese negotiators eventually accepted that they wouldn't get the most secret system for the first row of blades and the technology behind a thermal protective coating for those blades. US export rules prohibited GE from sharing that, because it is used both in the power turbine and aircraft engines. Instead, GE will manufacture the first stage blades in South Carolina and then ship them to the Harbin factory for final assembly.

"Mr. Immelt says that China won't be able to fully exploit what it learns from foreign bidders until its engineers are able to replicate or build upon the advanced technology they do obtain. 'That's going to take some time,' he says. *By the time the Chinese companies accomplish that, GE will have developed significantly more complex new designs.*" [Our italics.]

How then are we to classify this trading of short-term market for longer-term strategic security, both commercial and military? Is it a case of a half-empty and half-full glass? Or is it an example of an economic system ensnared in a compulsion towards exponential growth that must expand ever anew to avoid collapse. And transplanting that model to countries with the vast populations of China or India on those terms can lead to disastrous consequences that we don't even dare spell out. And yet we must, because a model launched on greed-powered gambles can lead the world to a catastrophe that we simply are not facing. It could leave our half-empty glasses not half-full, but shattered, with much blood rather than water spilled over the landscape.

Does Paul Martin pass the half-empty equals half-full glass test?

Our new Canadian Prime Minister provides us with a striking example of the Half-Empty-Half Full-Glass Theorem. For years he looked forward to that post, which his distinguished father had just missed occupying. An immensely successful business man, he rose to control Canada's major shipping line, and spent an impatient decade as Finance Minister under his predecessor. Meanwhile, he burnished a reputation for "fiscal responsibility," to win the approval of the financial community.

Mr. Martin and his Liberal colleagues took office shortly after the Conservative government under Brian Mulroney had shown themselves particularly servile in bailing out Canada's six giant banks from heavy losses in financing speculative real estate, gas and oil, and other high jinx. At the same time banks throughout much of the world had experienced similar misadventures, and the formula for their bailout was set by the Bank for International Settlements. a private club of central bankers based in Basel. Under its *Risk-Based Capital Requirements* commercial bank liquidity was no longer judged by their reserves of legal tender but by their *risk-based capital.* Debt of the most developed (OECD countries) was declared "risk-free" requiring no additional capital for banks to acquire. In this way, instead of the banks putting up cash with their central bank as collateral for the deposits they accepted in chequing accounts, they henceforth needed only concern themselves with having enough till cash to meet their customers' needs. Money (credit) for longer-term loans and deposits they could create with no extra cash. The statutory reserve they used to leave with the central bank as modest collateral for the deposits they received in chequing accounts) had earned them no interest. Those reserves also provided a costless use of credit by the government, that as sole shareholder of the Bank of Canada got back substantially all the interest it paid on the its debt held by it as dividends. These two provisions for the bank bailout made it possible for the chartered banks to quadruple their holdings of federal debt without putting up further cash or even investments.

However, in rushing to the rescue of the illiquid banks, the BIS had overlooked an important detail. It had declared zero inflation the only acceptable goal of central bankers, and central banks' higher interest rates had been declared "the one blunt tool" to enforce a flat price level. But whenever interest rates were pushed higher, the banks' hoard of existing bonds with lower coupons fell in market value.[3]

The result was the utter collapse of the official monetary policy. But since it was essentially a matter of a power grab, that led not to reassessment, but to more cover-up. The control of what could be taught, or even mentioned in the media was tightened. The free discussion of the sort that had existed in the 1930s became impossible. Yet without that freedom, the world could never have worked it way out of the Depression.

And Finance Minister Paul Martin helped pioneer the new trend. Not only were the banks bailed out without discussion in Parliament, but not even a press release on the bill that was to change the very nature of Canada's economy was issued. It took COMER a couple of years to track down the legislation – Subsection 4 of Section 457 of Chapter 46 of the Statutes of Canada 1991. And when we did, the response of bank spokesmen was that the statutory reserves had been "an unjust tax." The powers of money creation historically vested in the monarch, had been transformed into a privilege of the banks.

Without putting up any substantial money of their own the banks were able to take on another $60 billion of federal debt. And depending on how high the central bank was pleased to push up interest rates to "lick inflation" that amounted not to a one-shot bailout, but to an annual entitlement of anywhere from $5 to $8 billion a year. Moreover, it would grow with the economy.

The fact that further extensive deregulation of the Canadian banks took place right after so generous a bailout allows only a single interpretation. Power had shifted from the loose alliance of a sector of the industrialists with the government as investor to the financial sector. The fire-walls that had been set up in the 1930s for good reason between the banks, the stock market, and other pools of capital, such as insurance companies, were razed. It was tantamount to a *coup d'état,* and as such had to be carried out in secrecy, and under cover of a diversion – the campaign against "fiscal irresponsibility." You could have ended up under the impression that the banks had just bailed out the government rather than vice versa.

The transfer of such a massive amount of federal debt to the banks and the market, from a near-interest free loan from the Bank of Canada, tore a gaping hole in government finances. At once, federal non-financial expenses were cut, including the grants to the provinces which helped finance vital programs like health, education and social services. The provinces in turn downloaded social programs onto the municipalities, without adequate financing to support them. The banks had pushed out the most vulnerable portions of the population from the relief lines.

Smuggling in Accountancy

This set the stage for a well-planned campaign for privatizing government assets at all levels, which were treated by the government as current spending. The interests of society were ravaged from all directions – the Goods and Service Tax (GST) that hit the most vulnerable population disproportionately, the rapid increase of university fees and the introduction of user payments for services had been entirely paid for by the state.

The shock of all this was so great, that the governing Conservative Party was practically destroyed in the 1993 elections. When Paul Martin, the new Liberal Prime Minister today, was brought in as new Minister of Finance he had the choice of carrying out his party's promise to repeal the GST, and fill the gap by rolling back the privileges bestowed on the banks.

In the September 1998 issue of *ER,* I described once again how the Clinton administration had addressed the problem of a budgetary deficit by recognizing government investment in material capital as an asset rather than as a current expense.

"Before January, 1996, when the US federal government purchased capital assets such as buildings or computer systems, the Bureau of Economic Analysis (BEA) treated the transactions as current spending and wrote off the investment in a single year. The value of the acquisition thereafter appeared on the government's balance sheet at a token $1. In contrast business firms write off such capital goods over their useful life, and their depreciated value appears on the books to offset the debt incurred to acquire them.

"At the beginning of 1996, BEA quietly corrected this gross exaggeration of the real net deficit. This increased the national savings statistic by $135.2 billion for 1994, $151.1 billion for 1993, and comparable amounts for previous years. 1995 data are available only on the new basis. Carried forward to 1995 and backwards to 1959, the change exceeded 1.25 trillion dollars. The above figures can be found in the *Survey of Current Business* for January–February, p. 13, Indicators, p. 354, and the Federal Reserve Bulletin table A-40.

"Robert Rubin, Secretary of the Treasury, has applied to US foreign policy the arbitrage skills that earned him the chairmanship of Goldman, Sachs on Wall St. Instead of raising the issue of capital budgeting (a.k.a accrual accountancy) as a theoretical issue and applying it across the board, he quietly concentrated on a single statistic. That gave him the improved deficit figure he needed that bond rating agencies go by in setting bond yields. He avoided stirring up the sleeping ideological dogs of the right.

"Our Finance Minister should come out of his lethargy to do the same as the first step in rescuing the looney. The ground has been thoroughly prepared for him. On page 33 of the *Bank of Canada Review* (Summer, 1997) he can read a quotation from the *Public Accounts of Canada 1995-6:* 'Full-cost recovery for many federal assets, including bridges, ports, and telecommunications systems, was never considered feasible (because the asset was a public good) or desirable (for public-policy reasons). The federal government finances the cost of acquiring and maintaining such assets through budgetary appropriations, recording their book value at a nominal $1. Consequently, if these assets are privatized, all of the sale proceeds can be applied against the deficit. The federal government is gradually moving towards full-accrual accountancy, whereby the cost of acquiring physical assets is spread over the asset's useful life."

Finance Minister Martin could have followed the Clinton administration in adopting serious accountancy to reduce the false deficit and find the means to honour his party's promise to repeal the GST. He chose instead to direct available resources to financing further gambles of our major banks on the world markets. The result: three of our five largest banks have been charged with participating in some of the largest and malodorous stock market scams, and have settled with the American regulating authorities for hundreds of millions of dollars. Elsewhere in this issue you can find material from Eric Reguly of *The Globe and Mail* on the record of our banks' in their US adventures financed at such cost to the most vulnerable Canadian taxpayers.

Though Mr. Martin professes a great admiration for the present Auditor General Ms. Sheila Fraser, in 1999 he was locked in a bitter debate with her predecessor Denis Desautels. whose deputy she was at the time. Though their stand-off was ignored by the media, *Economic Reform* in March 1999 reported: "Spread across the front page of *The Bottom Line,* a trade publication of accountants (101/99) you can read: 'Nearly forty years after the federal bureaucracy was told it would have to reform its financial management, the government still has not fully modified its accounting practices, according to Auditor General Denis Desautels. We are still years away from having a financial system that would meet acceptable standards in the private sector. Reform of the financial management system has been on the agenda since the Glassco Commission recommended an ac-

counting process that would provide better information on the cost of government-run activities,' Desautels reports.

"And it's been ten years since Treasury Board approved the Financial Information Strategy (FIS) which is intended to replace the current cash-based system, of charging capital expenses to the accounts at the time of acquisition with a full-accrual process which would amortize the costs over the life of the assets. Desautels also offers a dark warning of what can go wrong when governments 'cook their books.'"

Towards the end of 2003, Mr. Martin finally achieved his heart's desire and became Prime Minister. But it was as though the sharpness of his elbows in pursuit of the post had made the gods jealous. No sooner was he installed, than all the wrong things started happening. First there was the question from an opposition member about the total amount of the orders that his shipping line had from the government during his decade as Finance Minister. The answer came through as $137,000. But a few months later, the same member had researched the record to include subsidiaries of the holding company registered in an offshore shelter received an answer from official sources as a revised figure of $161 million.

Our PM Loves His Auditors General but Pays Them No Heed

And before the dust settled on that one, the Auditor General issued a report that blasted the manner in which $100 million dollars had been paid in commissions on $250 million dollars of contracts had awarded for advertising to Liberal-friendly companies without competitive bids. The Auditor General minced no words in describing her shock, and called for an enquiry.

Mr. Martin, while proclaiming his ignorance of the shenanigans in letting out millions of dollars of contracts without competitive bidding, fell back to expressing his admiration for the Auditor General and her labours. Overnight the polls showed that the Liberals had fallen drastically.

And this is where we come to the final test of whether a half-empty glass always means that it is necessarily half-full. Though Mr. Martin now expresses his admiration for this Auditor General and Auditors General as a group, his record hardly supports that. His least charitable critics in the media seem unaware of his weeks of close bargaining with the then Auditor General Denis Desautels in 1997 on adopting capital budgeting (accrual accountancy) as a series of Royal Commissions and Auditors General had recommended over some decades. But most scandalous of all was that after weeks of acrid bargaining Mr. Martin insisted on a statement from the A.G. that since no new cash had come into the treasury by the shift to accrual accountancy, no new spending is justified. But, of course, that is not so. When capital assets were written off in a single year, the strictly cash deficit that resulted was used as a pretext for slashing important public services. Surely, then, the correction of this non-accountancy should have had the contrary effect. Surely that is good enough reason for questioning Mr. Martin's half-full glass. Symmetry is the very essence of the half-full-half empty glass concept.

Twisting the arm of their auditors has brought major legal trouble into the lives of US corporation heads. There is no reason why Canadian government leaders should be immune to such hazards.

William Krehm

1. The expression is not hard to understand:

    Differentiating (i.e., taking the first rate of growth): the first term 1 as a constant doesn't grow hence it becomes 0, the second simply x grows as x grows and becomes 1 to replace the original first term that has vanished, likewise all succeeding terms move to the left if we take their growth rates, as will the second power growth rates, and since it is an infinite series, there is an endless number of terms on the right to replace those that disappear on the left as we move by single steps to higher derivatives. of the power of x. [The way of differentiating powers of x to x itself is taught in high schools these days.]

    As time marches on, the growth derivatives embodied in the present price are put to the proof. If the market price in any year does not live up to the prediction already embodied in its price, the price collapses, and you have a major sell-off of the stock market and the economy. That is particularly so since most securities in one way or another already serve as collateral for further deals and are incorporated in the price of other stocks valuated in the same way. Derivatives have long been recognized as the instruments of explosive power, but banks and governments have resisted all recommendations that they be regulated. Since they are not regulated, one of the most common scams in which Canadian banks were involved in the Enron scandal in the US was seemingly retaining their interest in common shares while in effect selling unregistered derivatives that allowed them a secret exit with their loot from the deal. Derivatives are in fact. amongst much else, the secret revolving doors in high finance. The resulting hazard is increased for banks loaded up with government bonds bought entirely on the cuff.

2. To handle the problems of infinity George Cantor during the years 1871-84 created a completely new mathematical discipline, the theory of sets, in which was founded for the first time in a thousand years of arguments, back and forth, a theory of infinity with all the incisiveness of modern mathematics. When we equate two sets of things, we mean nothing more than this, that between the members of the first set and those of the second a one-to-one correspondence exists. First Cantor discovered denumerably infinite sets (Hahn, Hans (1956). Infinity. In James R. Newman (Ed.), *The World of Mathematics* (Vol. 3, p. 1,594). New York: Simon & Schuster). In the case of this type of infinity there are as many numbers in the set of all cardinal numbers as in that of all even cardinal numbers. You equate 1 in the first set to 2 in the second set, 2 in the first to 4 in the second, 3 in the first to six in the second and so on to infinity. You have established the correspondence and since the second set will not run out of even numbers since we are talking of two infinite series, the equivalence is perfect.

    But then he discovered other types of infinity and had to distinguish them. So he called his first type Aleph Null.

    This other type of infinity lurks in the spaces between cardinal integers. The space between any two cardinals by infinite decimal factors proves that it is not denumerably infinite, i.e., has a one-to-one correspondence with the cardinal numbers. This infinity is called the *continuum* and designated by *c. C* infinity is greater than

Aleph-Null infinity. In this article we are talking about Aleph-Null infinity, and we should always at least try to know what we are talking about.

3. The story is recounted in Krehm, William (Ed.) (1999), *Meltdown, Money Debt and the Wealth of Nations,* COMER Publications, reproduced from *Economic Reform,* May, 1993 ("The Next Trip to the Vomitorium" by William Krehm) the essentials of the tale: "To replace the [statutory] reserves banks must now increase their capital [not their cash holdings with the central bank] in proportion to their new loans. These proportions are set on a risk basis. Government bonds [of OECD countries that have not devalued their currencies for at least five years], judged risk-free require no additional capital.... But no matter how sound government credit might be, the moment our central bank embarks on its holy war 'to lick inflation,' all existing government bonds will plummet below their cost. Far from being 'risk-free,' in the world of 'zero inflation' any fixed-rate security [considering the leverage with which the banks can now acquire it] is a long shot."

Ruminations on "The Corporation"

THE FILM, *The Passion of the Christ,* appeared on screens in late February amid a brouhaha of pro and con. Jewish spokesfolk warned of anti-semitism. Psychologists feared for the minds of impressionable young children, and Christian Churches chartered busses and bought blocks of tickets. The Christian response was not unanimous, however. Five men at a non-denominational Bible study divided just about evenly the day before the opening: two were keen to go (though one said he would not take his children); one was undecided; and two were going to pass. One of the latter put it rather strongly, saying, he "did not want to suicide-bomb his mind with two hours of gratuitous cinematic gore." All of which merely goes to say that advance publicity does have some effects.

Two weeks earlier another film opened in commercial cinemas across the country. Fresh from winning awards, the documentary, *The Corporation,* made by Mark Achbar, Jennifer Abbott and author, Joel Bakan, essayed the common marketplace. Its advance billing, illustrated by a silhouetted male in suit-and-briefcase costume, with a halo over his head and a pointed tail behind his behind, promised that it starred "7 CEOs, 3VPs, 2 whistleblowers, 1 broker, 1 spy, and a really big mess, with Michael Moore, Noam Chomsky, Naomi Klein, and Milton Friedman as themselves," and "the FBI's top consultant on psychopaths."

X-ray of the Corporation

The film deserves its kudos. It is not a railing litany of corporate abuses, though those are present in abundance. It is an analysis of the modern corporation – its origins, its history, its behaviour, its legal status as a "person" and the character of that "person," derived from "psychiatric" observation. The twenty-odd talking heads are heard mostly in short snippets and sometimes in eloquent juxtapositions, and the cinematic effects are not gratuitous but tellingly deployed. Ray Anderson, CEO of Interface, the world's largest maker of commercial carpet, defines externalities as "making other people pay the bills." As he describes the corporation as "an externalizing machine, just as a shark is a killing machine," the visual presents an elegantly beautiful shark – pursuing a human swimmer. There is a whole series of such comparisons, some explicit, some implied: a corporation is like a sports team, "a group of people working together for their common good," (images of football scrimmage and tug-of-war), a noble, far-seeing eagle (beautiful photography), a hive (with the CEO as queen bee). These are corporate self-concepts. The public concept is represented by Godzilla crushing underfoot a fleeing victim, Moby Dick as seen by Gregory Peck's Ahab, and Dr. Frankenstein being bear-hugged to death by the monster he has created.

One of the most subtle cinematic effects is the use of black-and-white movies and newsreels from earlier in the 20th century, which subtly make the point that the corporation is not an eternal and elemental cosmic fact, but that it does have a history – a birth, youth, and maturity. Corporations we are reminded were originally chartered to serve the public good, and their charter was a gift from the people. The critical point in their history, however, was the declaration by the US Supreme Court in the late nineteenth century that a corporation is in itself "a person." Thus was the modern corporation given its power, until it is now "the dominant institution" of our day. The 14th Amendment of the US constitution, that "no person shall be deprived of life, liberty or property," was passed to protect black people. Of 307 cases brought to court under the 14th amendment between 1890 and 1910, nineteen were brought by black people, 288 were brought by corporations. The judgments in these cases firmly established for the corporations that, "We are a person." Critics note that these "immortal persons…have no soul to save, and no body to incarcerate," but are designed by law to be responsible only to their shareholders. The point of this historical recitation is that corporate persons are the product of human judicial decisions – which can be reversed.

Perhaps the funniest, and saddest, cinematic juxtaposition is the offsetting of Michael Walker of the Fraser Institute with images of child labourers in Third World sweatshops. Walker smilingly explains how the Chinese and Bangladeshis "are starving to death" and saying "come over here and hire us. We will work for 10 cents an hour. Come and rescue us," and, when they will no longer work for 10 cents an hour, he explains, the industry moves on leaving them "all plump, healthy, and wealthy." (Like himself, no doubt.) An investigator reveals from the Nike corporation's own records that, for making a shirt, the workers in Central American shops are paid $3/_{10}$ of 1% of the retail price. It is a priceless juxtaposition of ideology and ugly reality.

Yes, this film has bite. But it keeps its sights firmly on the target. It does not scream liar at the genial Sir Mark Moody-Stuart, ex-CEO of Shell, who convinces the band of protesters picketing his home, that he cares as much as they do about ecology, and poverty and equality; nor at Sam Gibara of Goodyear, who explains that the CEO is not free to do what he would like to. Noam Chomsky puts it very clearly when he compares the corporation as institution, to the institution of slavery: both institutions are monsters with nice people shackled in them.

The film's goal is to promote the shackling of the monster. It gives some lively footage of a California citizens' legal group demanding that the Attorney General revoke the charter of Unocal, the California-based energy company. The official declined to do so, but admitted that the state did have the power to revoke a corporation's charter. This was taken as a small victory, and perhaps a sign of the future.

One-legged Reform

Replacing corporate control with human control, however, is reform with one leg. It won't walk very far. The other leg is to subject the monetary system to the same dynamic: to replace corporate control with human control; more specifically, to return control of the money supply from the chartered banks to democratic governments. As Michael Rowbotham so categorically puts it, "reform of this debt-based money supply system… is more important than the war against poverty and starvation, more important than the movement to protect the environment, the struggle against pollution, the fight against drugs and racism, and the battle for social justice and welfare…for the simple reason that the current financial system is responsible, both directly and indirectly for causing, or at least exacerbating them."[1]

When 97% of the nation's money supply is created, not by the government (as most people have been (mis)led to believe), but by the chartered banks, the whole society is held hostage for the debt payments. The legal imperative laid upon corporate executives to increase profits, regardless of the collateral damage, is certainly socially destructive. But not more so than the economic imperative for "growth" at all costs. The impossibility of ever paying the interest on a debt money supply for which no debt-free money is created to pay the interest, fuels the drive for growth which subverts equity, sustainability, and perhaps human survival itself.

Until democracy can re-assert itself in two government policies – re-instituting the reserve requirements for the chartered banks; and using the Bank of Canada once again to finance government debt at all levels – de-personing corporations will be a half-sided reform.

Perhaps the new Christians to be created by Mel Gibson's spectacular film, will direct some of their new-found charity into the citizens' democratic movement to reform both the Cycloptic corporation and the Charybdian monetary system.[2] It would be a worthy enterprise.

Gordon Coggins

1. Rowbotham, Michael (1998). *The Grip of Death: A study of modern money, debt slavery and destructive economics* (p. 325).
2. Homer's Cyclops looked with a single eye; his Charybdis was a giant sucking sea vortex.

Hats Off to the Speaker
of the Unspeakable

ERIC REGULY, the financial columnist of *The Globe and Mail,* is noted for the insight and forthrightness of his sallies into the realm of the unspeakable – the record of Canada's great banks. His achievement in the field calls to mind that of Maureen Dowd in *The New York Times* on President Bush and his pals. In the issue of 24/02 he did himself proud once more.

"The banks' annual meeting season has started and the bank bosses, in their plywood speeches and stilted answers to shareholders' questions, will drone on about value creation, the necessity of expanding in the US, the attraction of mergers and the like. The bosses, with the possible exception of CBIC's John Hunkin, a familiar face among US regulators, will be treated like gods because banks shares have performed well. No one, sadly, will call them hypocrites. If they were serious about pleasing shareholders, they would forget about the US, forget mergers and lobby to scrap the ownerships that effectively make them immune to takeovers.

"Imagine a bank CEO saying this: Canada has been hugely successful for us. It's a great place to do business and will continue to be a money spinner of sinful proportions. Let my rivals blow their brains out on mergers and overpriced crap in the US. We're staying put.

"It'll never happen. Getting monstrously big is the CEO's mantra and shareholders have been ruthlessly conditioned to expect it, even demand it.

"The Big Six banks, in spite of their (hit and miss) push into the US and overseas markets, continue to make the bulk of their profits in Canada. We're talking many, many billions here. In 2003, the Royal Bank had a profit of slightly more than $3 billion, up 72% from 1999, the last boom year. It is one of the few banks on the planet to have ramped up profits every year in the past three years, when the news was all about recession, bear markets, corporate collapses, and failing loans. The combined market value of the Big Six is more than $160 billion. They trade at an average of 2.3 times their $ 68 billion or so of book value. Based on 2004 earnings estimates, the sextet is expected to earn about $12.8 billion. That would give them a return on equity of about 19%.

"The 19% return, of course, includes all their operations, domestic and foreign. It's difficult to separate the banks' domestic Return On Equity (ROE) from the foreign ROE, largely because the banks tend to report on business lines (such as capital markets or insurance) not geographically. But there's no doubt that US returns are lower than the Canadian returns. This means the Canadian ROE is a fair amount higher than 19%; some analysts thinks it's as high as 25%.

"In short words, the banks' domestic operations, notably its branch and retail operations are licences to print money. And they're becoming even more profitable because of branch consolidation, the widespread use of phone and internet banking, and the ever-rising fees. Forget about becoming an entrepreneur. Become a banker instead.

"[One] big problem about mergers is the potential hit on ROE. Suppose the acquiring bank offers a buyout premium of 30%. This means the purchase price would be equivalent to a lofty three times book value or so, giving the acquiring bank a much lower ROE on its purchase. This would reduce the merged bank's overall ROE. Anyway you cut it, the best way to preserve ROE is neither to merge nor expand in the US."

What even Reguly doesn't dare utter, is the compulsive drive to maintain and even increase the "rate of growth" which has already been extrapolated into the future and embedded into bank share prices. That is what the options to the top executives are based on.

And the stellar performance on the domestic market of the Big Six merely reflects another thing that COMER has insisted on: the bailout of 1991, doing away with the statutory reserves put up as collateral against their chequing account deposits with the BoC, was not a one-time affair. It is an entitlement paid them again and again each year. It gives the banks the interest on their federal debt holdings that the Bank for International Settlements' (BIS) *Risk-Based Capital Requirements* had declared risk-free requiring no additional capital for the banks to acquire. Not surprising that they should have increased their federal debt holdings by 300%. The Bank of Canada reduced its federal debt investment correspondingly. Of course, when the BoC holds federal debt, the bulk of the interest on it goes back to its single shareholder as dividends, and that single shareholder happens to be – ever since 1938 – the government of Canada. In short the shift of so much federal debt from the central bank to our chartered banks added to the federal government's interest payments needlessly, and the resulting deficit served as justification for slashing essential social and other capital programs. That and the deregulation that followed closely on the bailout, gave the banks not only a licence to go out and gamble with public money, but almost obliged them to.

The Canadian Finance Minister became a doting uncle sending his nephew to Las Vegas to live it up and just write him when he ran out of funds. Or better yet, the Canadian bankers mutated into something like a national hockey team who were expected to win glory for our flag abroad. Translating the role of our banks from providing essential services to the Canadian economy into such fervent patriotism, most Canadian columnists overlook how completely the public had been brainwashed. Our banks are not hockey teams, and if we are foolish enough to believe they are, we become the puck in their game.

William Krehm

Belated Opening of the US Oil File

THE WALL STREET JOURNAL (4/02, "In Quest for Energy Security, US makes New Bets on Democracy" by Andrew Higgins) has scored a woefully belated coup. Under the *Freedom of Information Act* it obtained a document that, had it come to light a year ago, could have saved hundreds of American lives. It is a confidential 34-page cable sent in April 1975, by the US ambassador to Saudi Arabia, James Akins. In this he "denounced as 'criminally insane' an idea then floated in the media: America should seize the Saudi oil fields to break an Arab oil cartel and ensure cheap energy for the US. Scoffing at America's 'New Hawks,' he warned that any attempt to take Arab oil by force would lead to a world-wide fury and a protracted guerrilla war. This did not go down well with Washington. Discussion of a military strike never got beyond the planning stage, but the idea terrified the Saudis, who laid plans to booby-trap oil wells.

"A few months later Mr. Akins was out of a job. He believes that his memo 'was basically the cause of [his] being fired.'"

Policy-making in an Ideological Cloud

The article resumes other documents released from the American and British secret archives. They add up to an amazing record of misfire, and describe the ideological cloud in which the leaders of these countries did their thinking. Underlying it all was the ever more powerful thirst of the US for oil that guaranteed a head-on clash with other cultures.

"The episode highlights America's struggle with a quandary that has tormented it for decades: how to deal with countries America doesn't trust and that don't trust America, but that can dictate the fate of America through their control of oil. For a half century the US has veered between confrontation and cajolery to secure a steady flow of fuel at a stable price from the Persian Gulf. The US has jumped from country to country in search of reliable friends.

"Often it has stumbled: the shah of Iran was overthrown. Saddam Hussein mutated from prickly partner to foe. The House of Saud still stands, but wobbles, both at home – where a divided ruling family staggers between reform and reaction – and in Washington, where people ask how an ally could spawn 15 of the 19 Sept. 11 highjackers.

"While many Arabs believe last year's invasion of Iraq was an oil grab, there's no evidence that the US plans to hold on to the Iraqi oil fields or put them up for sale. Still, with the US occupation, the quest for a solid ally in a region holding two-third of the world's known oil reserves has begun afresh. Indeed, occupation officials have recommended a strong, state-controlled Iraqi oil sector, even if that means limited investment opportunities for the US oil companies. Washington's goal in Iraq was reducing terrorism by seeding a democratic government in place of a dangerous tyrant."

"Washington now seeks change by prying open closed political systems. No Gulf producer is a democracy. Of the world's oil reserves, only 9% are in countries rated 'free' by the US research group Freedom House.

"Since 1970, America has scoured the world for other supplies to reduce its dependence on Gulf states. It has poured money into fuel cells and other technologies.

"Much oil has been found and the US has become more efficient in its energy use. But none of this disturbs a hard truth: America's economy depends on some of the world's most anti-American nations. By 2020, the federal Energy Information Agency expects the Persian Gulf will account for 54% to 67% of world oil exports, up from around 30% now.

"The White House believes giving Iraq democratic rule can help a dependence for oil 'on countries that don't particularly like us.' Whether America's initiative works in Iraq, whose oil reserves are second only to Saudi Arabia's, could also have an impact on the Saudis. A big unknown is whether the 'democratic revolution' Mr. Bush promises spreads to the doggedly undemocratic kingdom.

"When invading Saudi Arabia was considered in the 1970s, the US decided it wouldn't even apply strong political pressure on the despotic Gulf states behind the embargo. Secretary of State Henry Kissinger said at the time that pressure could cause instability and 'open up political trends that could defeat economic objectives.'

"[But], in a speech last fall citing the absence of freedom in the area, Mr. Bush said 'it would be reckless to accept the status quo.'

"Also out to overthrow the status quo, however, are America's enemies in the region. Democracy, if it really takes hold there, could amplify the voice of America's foes. Anger at Western use of Arab oil has been a theme for decades of populist rhetoric, both secular and Islamist. Just last month, Osama bin Laden, in a tape played on al Jazeera TV, denounced the US occupation of Iraq, spoke of the oil market as 'the biggest theft in history.' In 1998 the Saudi-born el Qaeda leader said oil ought to cost $144 a barrel, quadruple the present price."

Fighting Wars with Other Countries' Oil

"In the early 1940s, Interior Secretary Harold Ickes wrote a gloomy article warning, 'If there would be a World War III, it would have to be fought with somebody else's oil.' And geologist Everette Lee DeGolyer, returning from Saudi Arabia, reported that 'the center of gravity of world oil production is shifting to the Middle East.'

"Franklin D. Roosevelt, though seriously ill, made a stop on his journey home from the 1945 Yalta Conference to meet the Saudi king. Their encounter on a battleship in the Suez Canal established bonds that, for more than a half a century would tie the two countries: oil and security. It also raised an issue that would divide them – establishment of a Jewish state. The king suggested the Jews get land in Germany.

"America's wish to keep Persian Gulf oil secure took a violent turn in Iran. In 1952, the CIA carried out a British plot to topple an Iranian leader who had nationalized the Anglo-Persian Oil Co. At first the US had no enthusiasm for an idea it saw as the last gasp of Britain's empire. Christopher Woodhouse, an official the UK sent to Washington to lobby for the plan, wrote later how he helped win over the US: 'I emphasized the Communist threat to Iran.'

"The resulting coup against Mohammed Mossadegh brought back the exiled Iranian shah, Mohammed Reza Pahlavi, who promptly invited US companies to join a consortium to run Iran's oil industry. Washington poured in arms, turning Iran into a Cold War bulwark against the Soviet Union.

"On prices, however, Iran's and American interests diverged. The shah became a truculent hawk in the Organization of Petroleum Exporting Countries. Said James Schlesinger, secretary of defence in the mid-1970s, 'It was a great disappointment to Kissinger and Nixon, who thought the shah was a pal of theirs.'

"Saudi Arabia also disappointed. On October 17, 1973, Mr. Kissinger met with other top US officials to discuss the Yom Kippur Arab-Israeli war and the possibility of oil-supply disruptions He reported on a meeting held earlier in the day with the Arab envoys, and describing the Saudi foreign minister as a 'good little boy,' he predicted confidently: 'We don't expect an oil cutoff in the next few days.' Minutes later, an aide rushed in with a bulletin: Saudi and other oil producers had announced an immediate cut in output. Prices leapt 70% overnight and later quadrupled. The US sank into a recession." As usual, Mr. Kissinger considerably oversold his diplomatic magic.

"Mr. Nixon launched a plan to end all imports by 1980. It flopped: imports rose 40% by the target date. Mr. Kissinger turned to the Soviet Union for help, offering wheat in return for oil. The 'bushels for barrels' plan fizzled."

Lobbying for a War Against the Saudis

"Behind the scenes, officials mulled a more robust response to Arab cuts. Ambassador Akins says he knew something was afoot after a barrage of articles appeared championing war against Saudi Arabia. Particularly belligerent was one in *Harper's* under the pen-name Miles Ignotus. Titled 'Seizing Arab Oil,' it argued that 'the only countervailing power to OPEC's control of oil is power itself – military power.'

"Its author was Edward Luttwak, a hawkish defence expert then an adviser to the Pentagon. Mr. Luttwak says he wrote the piece after consulting with several like-minded consultants and officials in the Pentagon, including Andrew Marshall, who remains head of the Defense Department's in-house think-tank.

"Mr. Luttwak says they wanted to demonstrate the merits of 'maneuver warfare,' the use of fast, light forces to penetrate the enemy's vital centers. 'Last year's invasion of Iraq,' he says, 'was the accomplishment of that revolution.'"

Mr. Schlesinger says that the Pentagon concluded that "the only difficulty would be sabotage." Remarkable then, that the same Pentagon should have shut its mind to that perceptive conclusion when it came to last year's Iraq adventure.

One of several recently released British intelligence reports dealt with the same theme. "One outlined a 'dark scenario' under which US policy-makers would use force 'despite their Vietnam experience. This would, of course, be a highly dangerous policy with only slim chances of success.' Military action, the UK intelligence committee warned, would provoke Arab sabotage and leave American European allies 'badly torn.'"

Tony Blair, obviously, pays as little heed to his intelligence, as the Rumsfeld group does to theirs. And we are reminded of George Bernard Shaw's remark that Britain and the US are separated by a common language.

"While weighing ways to punish Arab oil producers, Washington played down the Iranian shah's price aggressiveness. Iran's anti-Soviet stance trumped its unhelpfulness on energy. The US Defense Intelligence Agency gave an upbeat assessment of the shah's prospects in September 1987, saying 'he was expected to remain actively in power over the next 10 years.' Three months later he fled a country in chaos, with Americans held hostage, and with Ayatollah Khomeini in power. World oil prices tripled.

"With Iran ruled by stridently anti-American militants, Washington tilted toward Iraq, which also had a new leader, Saddam Hussein. The Baath Party to which he belonged had first grabbed power after a coup backed by the US against the government of Abdul Karim Qasim, whom the US saw as dangerously leftist. Among his sins he had hosted a meeting that set up OPEC.

"When Mr. Hussein invaded Iran in 1980, Washington, after a period of aloofness, provided Iraq with satellite pictures and other help when it faced defeat.

"A 1988 national security directive enshrined the wooing of Iraq as policy. 'Normal relations with the Hussein regime,' it said, 'would serve our long-term interest and promote stability in both the Gulf and the Middle East.' But Iraq invaded Kuwait in 1990, and began moving troops toward Saudi Arabia. Once again, a partner had become an enemy."

All the while, however, there is another great enemy richly installed within the gates, undermining the world of stable prices and steady growing supply that Washington aspires to. *The Wall Street Journal* (5/02, "OPEC Appears Unwilling to Increase Its Output" by Chip Cummins) writes: "Hedge funds and other speculative investors have been buying oil and other commodities amid signs of global economic growth. Their purchases appear to have exacerbated the recent run-up in crude prices. OPEC officials have worried that if demand eases at the same time as these investors reverse their buy orders, prices could tumble."

Another example of unbridled zeal is the cooking of their books by some of the largest oil companies exaggerating oil reserves still in the ground. That has begun receiving attention from US prosecutors – with traumatic effect on the stock market quotations of the conglomerates involved. But this is merely an extension of the drive for exponential growth that a financial system on steroids imposes on public companies.

Obviously there was a deeply traumatic relationship between the US and UK governments and their inability to see what is in front of their noses. That calls to mind the device of official economists to declare entire areas of reality "externalities." Could that logical distemper have spread from economic theory to military and foreign policy?

William Krehm

Money Illusions

VERY FEW PEOPLE today draw a distinction between money and wealth. To most, the terms are synonymous.

But money is not wealth and the distinction is important. Money is a representation of wealth, and a claim on goods and services, but wealth is derived only from the production of goods and services in the real economy. The quantity of money has a real impact on that production on that and on other factors such as inflation, but it should not be confused with the production itself.

Why does it matter? Because focusing on money distorts our understanding of the economy. Look, for example, at the last budget trimming exercise undergone by the Toronto City Council which resulted in large cuts in many areas, as well as a failure to meet clear needs in other areas such as transit. This was done in order to limit the property tax increase to 5%. Councillors were told quite rightly, that "there is no money" for their expenditures. The debt is $2 billion, with interest charges rising every year. Who could argue?

Suppose instead City Council had asked themselves the question, *"Do we have in Toronto the resources – the labour, the expertise, the machinery, etc., to meet these needs?"* If the answer was no – these resources are not available – then all could see the necessity for cuts. But if, as seems the more likely answer was at least a partial "yes," citizens might question why the lack of money was such a stumbling block.

History provides the answer. In 1861, when Abraham Lincoln and his cabinet were confronted with a demand from the New York bankers for 17% interest on a war loan, they refused. But the war didn't stop. They still needed the men, the guns, the transport, etc. to prosecute the war. These goods were available, or could be produced, in the real economy. The solution was obvious. Lincoln persuaded Congress to authorize the printing of money – greenbacks – which the US government then spent into circulation to purchase the needed materials. They did the job just as well as the money the bankers would have created, and there was no interest attached, and no debt.

The same thing happened when Canada entered World War II. The need was urgent, the resources were clearly available, so the Bank of Canada created millions to purchase the materials.

It is true, of course, that the City of Toronto cannot create legal tender, but the Bank of Canada is authorized to do so on their behalf if the loan is guaranteed by either the province or the federal government.

We live in a wealthy society with plentiful resources, but money is always scarce. (To be accurate, there is abundant money, but a huge chunk of it is tied up in the financial sector – in stocks, bonds, derivatives, options, etc., and does little but chase after itself). We have the resources to maintain good schools, good hospitals, good transit, so why should lack of money be a problem?

Because all money in our society, except the tiny portion (6%) still created by government, comes into existence only if someone is willing to borrow it and pay the interest and the principal on the loan. Such borrowers must be "credit worthy."

Financial speculators of all stripes generally meet the test, so a lot of this debt money disappears into the financial vortex. For the real economy individuals, or companies, or governments must do the borrowing. But as debt loads mount and interest payments rise, bankruptcies increase and lending standards are tightened. The recent lowering of interest rates has helped to keep borrowers afloat but at some point borrowing must stop. When that happens it will be apparent, as it was during the Great Depression, that abundant physical resources do not translate into money.

There is a better way, and Abraham Lincoln found it 140 years ago.

David Gracey

China Bubble — Next Bust?

DOUBLE, DOUBLE, TOIL AND TROUBLE; Fire burn, and cauldron bubble.
– Shakespeare, *Macbeth*

Never, ever has there been an economic cauldron of quite the size of the new Capitalistico-Communist China, in which all manner of fantasy and make-believe are crumbled into the pot. The resulting broth, can easily run up an unprecedented productivity in nightmares.

Let's listen to *The New York Times* (18/01, "Is China the Next Bubble? "by Keith Bradsher): "Dongguan, China – The prospectus for China Green Holdings Ltd. looks like a seed catalogue. Color photographs show the corn, cabbage, pickled plums and other vegetables that the company exports, mostly to Japan. There is even a helpful list of the growing times for broccoli, cauliflower and sweet peas tucked in between tables showing that the company earned $14.1 million on sales of $31.2 million in its last fiscal year. Though China Green's business literally involves small potatoes – cubed and shipped in plastic bags – its initial public offering in Hong Kong was anything but. Retail investors put in bids to buy more than 1,600 times as many shares as were available, making it the most oversubscribed IPO ever in Hong Kong. The stock jumped 58% last Tuesday, its first trading day.

"Japan had its bubble in the late 1980s, when the Imperial Palace grounds in Tokyo became worth more than all the land in California. Thailand and Indonesia had their bubbles in the mid-1980s, when speculators and multinationals poured money into what seemed a Southeast Asian miracle. The US had its Internet and telecom bubble in the late 1990s, when stock prices looked as if they could rise indefinitely and unemployment kept hitting new lows.

"Each of these bubbles ended badly, with millions of families losing their savings and many losing their jobs.

"Recent excesses – from a frenzy of factory construction to speculative inflows of cash to soaring growth in bank loans – suggest China may be in a bubble now. Bubbles can last years, but they seldom deflate painlessly when they do pop. Nobody knows how harmful a sharp economic slowdown would be in China, a country undergoing huge social changes like the migration of peasants to the cities. The Communist Party rests its legitimacy on delivering consistent annual increases in prosperity.

"The Chinese government is showing concern. In the last few weeks, the central bank has tried to dissuade banks from reckless lending while the government has bailed out two of the largest ones, to prepare them for possible hard times as well as planned stock sales. The State Council, China's cabinet, has warned that it will discourage construction of new factories in industries like aluminum and steel, whose capacity has grown swiftly in the last three years.

"Huge billboards in Guandong Province commemorate Deng Xiao-ping's decision, a quarter-century ago to allow capitalism to gain a foothold in a few cities in southeastern China. Practically ever since, China's astounding economic growth has provoked warnings that the boom may not be sustainable. Year after year, China has proved the worriers wrong, although there have been missteps notably when inflation surged and foreign exchange reserves withered in the early 1990s.

"But even by Chinese standards, things have been moving at a blistering pace of late. Official statistics, which the government tends to smooth so as not to indicate big booms or busts, show that the economy expanded 8.5 percent last year, despite the fact that growth came to a virtual halt during the second quarter because of an outbreak of SARS. According to independent economists, however, the Chinese economy actually expanded at an annual pace of 11 to 13% through the second half of last year.

"Strains are already showing. Blackouts have become a problem in a majority of China's provinces, as families with new air-conditioners and refrigerators compete with new factories for electricity. Auto sales soared 75% last year, as prices in a market protected from imports until 2001 drifted down toward global levels. Still, automakers are planning huge factory expansions in the hope that such growth will continue.

"Most economists specializing in China now predict that sometime this year growth will have to slow, at least for the investment side of the economy – the building of new factories, for example. That could prove painful. The US economy suffered severe weakness on the investment side in 2001 and 2002, when the market for telecommunications equipment became glutted. Tens of thousands of lost jobs in that industry, resulted, not to mention steep drops in the stock portfolios of millions of Americans.

"If there were a prospectus for Chinese economy, it would need to warn of a high dependence on sales to America. China exported $125 billion worth of goods to the US in the first 10 months of last year and imported just $22 billion. The resulting trade surplus equaled an extraordinary 9% of China's entire economic output during this period. That has turned Chinese exports into obvious targets during an American election year.

"American trade officials have begun to take the legal steps needed to impose steep tariffs on Chinese products as varied as color televisions, furniture and bras. To avoid a trade war, China has followed Japan's example in sending official buying missions to the US. Shopping for everything from soybeans to communications equipment, they have agreed in the last two months to buy $11 billion worth of goods, by Beijing's calculations. Some of these deals may have happened anyway like the one to import General Motors auto parts for assembly into finished cars here."

W.K.

Financing Municipal Infrastructure through the Bank of Canada

PRIME MINISTER MARTIN'S decision to rebate the GST to cities is nice (about $1 million for Kingston), but it is small potatoes compared to what municipalities could save if the government would use our public bank, the Bank of Canada, to finance public debt. For example, Kingston needs about $250 million for repairs and new construction of the city's roads, bridges and sewers. At 6% amortized for 20 years, this would cost over $21 million per year – more than twice the City's capital budget – so a lot of essential infrastructure does not get built.

However, if the federal government borrowed $250 million from the Bank of Canada it would, effectively, pay only enough interest to cover the cost of administering the loan, which has been as low as 0.37%. Not only that, it would not have to pay it back in 20 years, nor should it. A capital investment should be repaid at the rate of depreciation of the capital asset. For sewers and bridges which have a life of at least 50 years, the payments could be spread over 50 years so that annual payments on $250 million would amount to $5 million per year plus about half a million for administration costs. Financing in this way would mean that Kingston would be able to build all of its essential infrastructure.

If this is so good, why isn't the government doing this, you ask. Good question, because the government did use the Bank of Canada in this way for 35 years – from 1939 to 1974 – when it reduced the use of its own bank in favour of using the private sector almost entirely. As a result, when interest rates went sky high in 1980 and again in 1989 so did public debt – up to about $590 billion for the federal government, 94% of which was due to interest, not the cost of programs and services. Obviously, private banks and other wealthy private sector investors lobbied the government very effectively to get the government to make such a dumb decision. If you owned a bank, would you go to someone else's bank to get a loan?

For municipalities, the best aspect of getting financing through the Bank of Canada would be the independence that would give them. Imagine not having to beg the federal and provincial governments for cash every time a major capital project had to be undertaken. They would only have to convince a banker (the Bank of Canada) that they had the ability to handle the loan they were requesting.

The effect of the 1974 decision has been a huge transfer of taxes to private banks and investors. In 1970, for example, our three levels of government spent $3.3 billion on interest. In 1975, payments on interest had doubled to $6.6 billion. By 1985, it had jumped to $40.6 billion and nearly doubled again by 1995 to $77.5 billion. Since then, due mainly to lower interest rates and some pay-down on the federal debt, interest payments for the three levels of government have been reduced to about $66 billion (2002). Nevertheless, from 1995 (the year that Finance Minister Paul Martin declared war on the deficit) to 2002, Canadians spent $594 billion in unnecessary interest on public debt, the federal government alone spending $344 billion.

A Disparity of Digits

These figures are so large they are almost meaningless unless they are seen in perspective. Example – $2 to $3 billion would provide good low cost housing from coast to coast to coast. We can't find money for housing, but we spend more than 20 times that amount every year on unnecessary interest. Example – health care could use another $3 billion on top of the $2 billion promised by Mr. Martin. We can't seem to find that extra $3 billion for health care, but we spend 20 times that amount on unnecessary interest every year.

On April 3, 2001, Kingston Council passed a resolution asking the Federation of Canadian Municipalities to urge the federal government to: (a) instruct the Bank of Canada to buy securities issued by municipalities and guaranteed by the federal government to pay for capital projects and/or to pay off current debt; and (b) refund to municipalities any interest paid by municipalities to the Bank of Canada.

The authority for doing this rests in Section 18(c) of the *Bank of Canada Act* which states that "the Bank may buy and sell securities issued or guaranteed by Canada or any province," meaning that the mechanism is there for municipalities to get long term financing for capital projects through the Bank of Canada *if* their securities were guaranteed by Canada or a province.

At the meeting of the national board of the Federation of Canadian Municipalities, held on September 8, 2001, two resolutions were passed concerning financing for municipalities through the Bank of Canada; one came from the City of Kingston and the other from Squamish, BC. The Federation forwarded these resolutions to the federal government, but nothing has come of this. Those who oppose this usually say that it will cause inflation, but this is not supported by the facts. The facts are that when the government borrowed to finance the war, then the post war reconstruction of roads, water lines and treatment plants, sewers, housing, medicare, education, research and more, the Bank of Canada held a significant portion of its debt (20 to 30%) paying for it by expanding the money supply. According to some we should have experienced record inflation during this period, but we did not. For example, in 1952 the inflation rate was 2.4%, and while it rose and fell over the years it was never very high, being only 3.2% in 1971 (just before the sudden increase in oil prices).

While municipalities are starved for money to pay for infrastructure our public bank, the Bank of Canada, which could provide the financing, is not used. It doesn't have to be this way. We used it before to finance public capital projects and we can do it again. It is a matter of political will, and this is a good time, politically, to act on this. Politicians are more inclined to listen to proposals from their constituents when faced with an election. In addition to the Federation and the Association of Municipalities of Ontario, it is a made-to-order issue for the new group of small city mayors, Municipalities United for a New Deal, and the group of Big City mayors. It is also an issue for the Canadian Labour Congress because using the Bank of Canada to finance public infrastructure would provide employment for thousands of Canadians and bring down our chronic 7% to 8% unemployment level. Canadians should be pressing these organizations and their political representatives at all levels to act on this. *Write or call, but do it!*

Richard Priestman

References

Bank of Canada Act.

Statistics Canada (2002). *Canadian Economic Observer, Historical Statistical Supplement* (pp. 13-19).

Chorney, Harold (1989). *The Deficit and Debt Management: An Alternative to Monetarism.* Montreal: Concordia University.

Committee on Monetary and Economic Reform (www.comer.org).

Findlay, Don. www.monetaryreform.com.

Krehm, William. *The Bank of Canada: A Power Unto Itself.*

Statistics Canada – the Mimoto analysis of federal spending issued by Statistics Canada in June, 1991, showed that neither inflation nor program spending caused debt to rise. High-interest-rate monetary policy did. High interest rates, it summed up, "bloated government spending on debt charges in the 1980s."

Seeing Ourselves in China's Mirror

IT IS EASIER to see the mote in another's eye than a beam in one's own. To understand our home society better we may note how in China a melange of left-overs from Marx, Mao tze Dung, Hobbes, Darwin and Bush II, have been stirred into a witches' brew to justify the rapid enrichment of those in power.

The New York Times (29/2, "China's Wealthy Live by a Creed: Hobbes and Darwin, Meet Marx" by Yilu Zhao) tells a ghoulish tale that echoes throughout much of the West.

"This is the dark side to China's new wealth. Envy, insecurity and social dislocation have come with the huge disparity between how the wealthy and poor live. Clear signs of class divisions have emerged under a government that long claimed to have eliminated classes.

"China still calls itself socialist, and in an odd sense it is. While the income structure has changed, much that was intended to underpin social order has not.

"The criminal justice system, for example, has remained draconian. When caught, burglars invariably receive lengthy sentences. But there is no shortage of burglars, and the reasons is clear: 18% of Chinese live on less than $1 a day, according to the United Nations. The poor are visible on the edges of any metropolis, where slums of plywood apartments sometimes abut the Western-looking mansions.

"The most recent measure by which social scientists judge the inequality of a country's income distribution indicates that China is more unequal, for example than the United States, Japan, South Korea and India. In fact, inequality levels approach China's own level in the late 1940s when the Communists, with the help of the poor, toppled the Nationalist government.

"In 1980, when the turn toward a market economy started, China had one of the world's most even distributions of wealth. Certainly, China before 1980 was a land of material shortage. As a child in the 1970s and 1980s, I can recall, every family collected ration coupons to get their flour, rice, sugar, meat, eggs, cloth, cookies and cigarettes. Without coupons, money was largely useless.

"Today huge supermarkets offer French wines and New Zealand cheeses. China's business elite have come to believe that the world is a huge jungle of Darwinian competition, where connections and smarts mean everything, and quaint notions of fairness count for little.

"I notice recently that on my most recent trip to China from the US, where I moved nine years ago. So I asked a relative who lived rather comfortably to explain. Is it fair that household maids make 65 cents an hour while the well-connected real estate developers become millionaires or billionaires in just a few years?

"He was caught off guard. After a few seconds of silence, he settled on an answer he had read in a popular magazine.

"'Look at England, look at America,' he said. 'The Industrial Revolution was very cruel. When the English capitalists needed land, sheep ate people.' (Chinese history books use that phrase to describe what happened in the 19th century, when tenant farmers in Britain were thrown off their land so that sheep could produce wool for new mills.)

"'Since England and America went through that pain, shouldn't we try to avoid the same pain, now that we have history as our guide?,' I asked.

"'If we want to proceed to a full market economy, some people have to make sacrifices,' my relative said solemnly. 'To get where we have want to get, we must go through the "sheep eating people" stage too.'

"In other words, while most Chinese have privately dumped the economic prescriptions of Marx, two pillars of the way in which he saw the world have remained. First is the inexorable procession of history to a goal. The goal used to be the Communist utopia; now it is the market economy of material abundance. Second, just as before, the welfare of some had to be sacrificed so the community could march toward its destiny. Marx is used in the end to justify ignoring the pain of the poor.

"What the well-off have failed to read from history, however,

is that extreme inequality tends to breed revolution. Many of China's dynasties fell to peasant uprisings, and extreme inequality fed the Communist revolution.

"While the domestic product has grown at least 7% a year for the last decade, the income of the rich has grown much faster than that of the poor. Political and business elites are merging, as state factories are sold at cheap prices to managers who often have government ties.

"A December article on the People Daily Website, the Communist Party newspaper, gave examples of politician-businessmen buying multimillion-dollar properties for cash in and around New York City and Los Angeles.

"Meanwhile as the Communist Party recruits successful businessmen as new members, blue-collar workers have lost their moral and social standing. Millions have lost their jobs, and older laid-off workers have been described in many publications as 'historical baggage.'

"Often they are of the generation born just after the Communists took power in 1949.

"Sun Liping, a sociology professor of Tsinghua University in Beijing, is one of the few scholars who openly talk about them. 'They are not "historical baggage,"' he said of the unemployed. 'The wealth of the Communist country, the assets of the state factories, were created by them.' He said the reason that the unemployed are not yet despondent is that they 'have put their hopes on their children.'

"There are other ways in which the oddly mixed and cynical legacy of Chinese Marxism presents difficulties for anyone who would try to redistribute wealth. The reform era began with concepts like 'truth,' 'kindness,' and 'beauty' already devalued. In the Maoist period people learned to scoff at such notions. For a few decades, Communist ideals like saving humanity from capitalist oppressions had displaced Confucian teachings like respecting the elderly. That left a moral vacuum when Communism's grip loosened, and nothing has emerged to fill it. We have a very cynical population."

And over the devastation that was left, the West has poured the lava of consumerism, exponential growth, overnight enrichment. The vices of two opposing systems powered by high-technology have interacted to produce a stricken field.

William Krehm

Why Oil Trusts Rule the Roost

UNDER LICENSE of the prevailing self-balancing market theory, corporations claim a knowledge of the most remote future, and lose no time in incorporating these powers into the current price of their shares. Once that is done and prices based on such continued rates of growth have been established, they must be maintained. For failing that, the price of their stock crashes and with it the enterprises for which it is serving as collateral. The slightest shortfall from the rate of growth serving as a girder supporting the corporation's stock price, would thus lead to a string of disasters. There is certainly no possibility of old-fashioned morality intruding in so cozy an arrangement, except in the form of prosecution for cooked books. The anticipated continued increase of future growth rates has been so connected with survival, that honest correctives of the corporative books is becoming synonymous with ruin. For two or three years now, in a crescendoing way, the American and European press have been full of major scandals of depraved books, auditors and banks not only suborned but actually designing the scams. The prevalence and the magnitude of this ever more bulging docket suggests something systemic rather than individual crimes.

It is in fact the end result of the dogma of an all-wise self-balancing market, that in recognition of its absolute wisdom and virtue, simply must be completely deregulated. With flail and fasting, the saints of yore in their wisdom imposed virtue on their weak flesh. In contrast our financial makers and shakers have sought to perpetuate virtue by the multiplication of earthly rewards. This has not only drawn the masses of faithful to these new altars, but made it essential for them to stop at nothing to keep those altars standing.

The latest proof of this predicament is the most convincing yet. The pillars of the temple are still rocking with the Parmalat epic of cooked books and non-existent bank accounts that were supposed to hold fictitious billions of dollars. But now it is a major oil company, Shell Oil, that is hogging the headlines on unflattering grounds. But wasn't this predictable even though none of us predicted it? The main capital reserves of oil conglomerates are in the ground or under oceans, where verification is unavoidably shrouded with much guesswork, hope, and technology. Enron for all its motivation and talent dealt in generated electricity, and the plausibility of its market price could be checked from the number of blackouts, the alleged generators and the power lines. All these were above ground, and the reality of the power delivered could have been confirmed or disproved in no time. The rest was routine auditing and even auditors leave paper trails that are subject to verification once official investigations begin.

But how could world conglomerates like Shell come under such suspicion? Well, for one thing, oil companies have to compete for investors to buy their shares with the banks and the Enrons that the banks may be financing. Hence under the existing deregulated system their high executives may be driven – to maintain, as the saying goes, "a level trading field" – to improve their reserves which are so conveniently stashed beyond auditors' expertise. Accordingly, it came as a shock to read the following heading in *The Wall Street Journal* (12/1/04, "Shell Cuts Reserve Estimate 20% as SEC Scrutinizes Oil Industry" by Chip Cummins, Susan Warren and Michael Schoeder):

"Royal Dutch/Shell Group's disclosures that it overstated its proven reserves by 20% rattled energy investors and is raising questions about whether the oil industry has inflated a lifeblood measure of its future prospects.

"Shell, one of the world's largest publicly traded oil concerns, said Friday that it had erroneously overbooked its proven oil and natural gas reserves by the equivalent of 3.9 billion barrels of oil. The oil portion alone, about two-thirds of the revi-

sion, represents some $67.5 billion in potential future revenue, assuming moderate oil prices of $25 a barrel.

"Reserves are at the heart of an oil and gas company because they represent what can be taken from the ground in the future. Since companies must replace the oil and gas they produce each year just to stay even, reserve growth is a crucial indicator of how well a company is doing. If the reserve size falls, the company is less valuable to investors and its stock price will tumble."

The end result: the stock price of oil giants not only is based on incorporating what the stock is likely to do in the future into the present price of the company's shares, but a foreknowledge of what luck the company will have under sea and land, but of the stability and friendliness to oil companies of the political regimes throughout the world into the remote future. Such powers of prophecy would fall just short of the powers of God Himself. And the Good Book did warn us that He is a jealous god.

William Krehm

Invest

A FUNNY THING HAPPENED on the way to the Conan O'Brien show in Toronto. We all got a lesson in one of the first principles of applied economics: if you want to make money (or save money), you've got to spend money (or borrow money).

Even if a few million dollars that the city of Toronto doesn't really have is invested into something as laughable as bringing in a zany comic – what, invest in something that's not made of concrete, pavement or steel; now that's not funny, that's silly – to spruce up the city's stodgy "brand," and thereby indirectly bring in thousands of cool tourists who will spend their cool millions here, which will create tax dollars that cover the cost of the initial investment many times over – are you putting me on? Is this the way economics really works?

Yes, Virginia, economics is not just about masquerading Calvinism, the wellspring of the popular Canadian view that there's no gain without pain, and no way to show virtue without the essential preparatory work of suffering. Because this legacy of pre-Enlightenment religion is so powerful in Canada – not all the things that make Canada different from the US are positive – we adopt advertising slogans like "the city that works," probably because we think people will want to pay big money to come on a holiday here because it's another opportunity to work, which is the only sure way to scrub away our sinfulness.

This belief should make us laugh louder than anything Conan O'Brien says to make fun of us, but even Conan couldn't get a snicker out of exposing that foible to us.

But I digress. I'm trying to find a way to explain, if only to myself, why Canadians, who mostly don't buy into the neo-conservative mantra that it's bad for governments to spend money on anything other than police and war – who generally believe that governments should spend money on health, education, environment and culture – still cling to the ultimate neo-conservative view that government investment in health, education, environment and culture is evil. Because investment means spending money you don't have, that you haven't earned, that you have to borrow, that you haven't suffered for.

Nobody accepts an idea that stupid, not George Bush, not the Wall Street Journal, not my mom who went through the depression and knows the value of a penny; nobody except the great mass of Canadians treat this idea as unchallengeable truth.

No family budget chief thinks it means the same thing to borrow $5000 for a house, or to borrow $5000 for a major repair on a leaky roof, or to borrow $5000 to fly to Las Vegas to give money to slot machines. The value of the house will go up faster than the interest rate on the mortgage and we get to live in it at the same time, the budget chef will say, and the savings from not having a leaking roof will more than cover the costs of the repair, but the $5000 loan to go to Las Vegas still has to be paid off, even though we have nothing to show for it.

This is budgeting that knows the difference between investment, avoided cost and expenditure.

A neo-conservative trance has made it impossible for us to apply this everyday knowledge to government.

And that's the reason why Toronto, Ontario and Canada are in a budgetary pickle. Because government treasurers who treat a dollar spent on investment, avoided cost and expenditure as if they're all the same will make some costly mistakes.

Any way you slice it, the dollar is still spent, and you had to borrow it, the hairshirt budget chief will say, and someday you'll have to pay it back with interest. This is the error that logicians call "the fallacy of misplaced concreteness." It plays well up here, perhaps because we appreciate the fact that we get another opportunity to suffer.

The Institute for Competitiveness and Prosperity, chaired by U. of T. business professor Roger Martin, has tried challenging this dogma with a report showing that lack of government investment in areas that increase productivity costs Canadian governments $75 billion – please note the b – in tax revenue. We trail the US economy in productivity because we under-invest in things that add productivity and overspend on things that don't, Martin said when he released the report – to virtually no media coverage – in late January at the Davos World Economic Forum.

If governments understood this, they'd know that money grows on trees, and that a 30 million dollar investment in urban tree planting would provide employment (thereby avoiding millions in unemployment insurance), clean the air and reduce ultra-expensive hospital costs related to emergency admissions for lung disorders (thereby avoiding hundreds of millions in healthcare costs), absorb rainwater that otherwise becomes ultra-expensive stormwater (avoiding the billions to expand sewage pipes) when it floods the sewers.

To think about things this way is a bit of a mind-bender for some. It means that we wouldn't ask the stupid question: can we afford to spend money to end hunger suffered by a tenth of the population – mostly kids – in this city, province, and country. We would ask the smart question: when food is so cheap, can we afford to not solve the problem and to spend many times more money on hospital bills and lost educational opportunities. The cost of an investment in healthy food wouldn't even amount to a rounding error in the operational budget of the health and educational system.

To understand this, all you need to know is that smart investment can reduce operating costs, and that it's smart to borrow if your savings are higher than the interest paid to borrow money. There's not a business that wouldn't go broke if it didn't apply this concept every day.

The good folks at the Committee on Monetary and Economic Reform have an explanation that's scarier than mine for why government budget chiefs can't see the difference between a hole in the budget and a hole somewhere else. They blame live bankers, not dead theologies.

Their research shows that it took until 1996 in the US and 1999 in Canada before federal budgets had to acknowledge two things: that certain expenditures (on schools, for instance) created assets that should not be listed in the books as debt, and certain failures to spend (on the environment, for instance) created liabilities that should not be listed as savings.

If we can ever get over economic Calvinism and start to get the budgetary significance of this, we'll be just like Conan O'Brien – laughing all the way to the bank.

And in case you're laughing too hard to remember, the reason we're paying hard cash to bring Conan up here and make fun of us so we'll look good to the world is that we had a big problem with SARS that costs us hundreds of millions in lost tourism revenues – all because a provincial government wanted to save nickels and dimes on public health staffing that could have prevented or limited the outbreak. That's the punchline: there is an expensive difference between investment and operating costs.

Wayne Roberts

The Virus in Our Economic Policy-Making

IMAGINE someone devising a virus that would invade the world's computers to eliminate the words "not" or "no" where they occur in our laws and insert them where they don't. The Ten Commandments would suddenly become a licence to kill, to steal, and rape. The angels would be overworked exchanging the road-signs "Hell" and "Heaven." What a Hollywood thriller that would make! Its producer might even get elected governor of New York state or to the presidency of the US!

More than a smidgen of this has already occurred in our economic policy. We can see signs of it in the budget our own new government handed down in late March. Let's start with a *Globe and Mail* report (22/03, "Budget puts Martin's reputation on the line" by Heather Scoffield).

"With his party languishing in minority territory in polls mainly because of the scandal over the sponsorship funds, PM Martin and [Finance Minister] Goodale want a budget to reinforce Martin's reputation as a good money manager."

Let's pause right there. A good nurse or teacher is a clear enough concept: the goal entrusted to him/her is the health of a patient or the education of a child. But *managing money* is a confusing concept. Money is a medium of transaction, rather than itself an intended beneficiary. In every trade there is a minimum of two parties, and to judge its success you must ask "for whom?" Whenever someone is shortchanged, the other is overpaid. That is why leaving the question of how good Mr. Martin is as "a money manager" must be complemented with another question "for whom?" In fact he is far too good at what he is doing: suppressing information vital for this nation.

"'The whole thing is about proving that the Liberals can handle their money,' said one government source."

The beauty of language is that at times what is not actually expressed is more important than what is uttered. "Handling their money" is even structured like "handling their drink," but in fact it is not the Liberals' money but the nation's. It should not even be alluded to in such terms.

"'The calculation is – and I think it's the right one – that people want to see us managing their money carefully. That's the hallmark of Mr. Martin,' one of his officials said.

"And so the emphasis tomorrow will be on debt repayment, on prudent fiscal management, on staying out of deficit on the $500 billion federal debt. Mr. Goodale has promised to pay off a solid chunk in the 2003-04 fiscal year ending March 31, and every year after."

This raises another problem, hardly less serious than the software virus mentioned at the beginning of this piece.

To make sure of our facts let me call as witness a couple of Canadian currency bills – the $50 and the $20 come to hand.

Over the Queen's right shoulder in the $20 note are the English words "This note is Legal Tender" and in the $50 one over William Lyon King's right shoulder in French, you can read *ce billet a cours légal* which is the same thing. And just to make sure – as is our habit in most things – let's consult our American cousins. On their $1 bill to the right of Washington's ear is an even more explicit statement to the same effect: "This note is legal tender for all debts, public and private." That means that not only can you pay your taxes with that piece of paper, but any creditor who refused to receive it would find his debt no longer valid.

Why stop there? On the £50 note of the Bank of England to the left of Her Majesty's coiffure we read "I promise to pay the bearer on demand the sum of," leaving the problem in what to the bearer. The British, after all, are the world masters of archaic ceremony. Finally the ¤5 bill has not one word on the matter at all, expressing that there is nothing behind the note than the smart paper and the general credit of the European Union. That, however, does not prevent the EU central bank from pursuing a deflationary course as though that there might be anything more behind their bills than that. And that unknown "something" is in short supply and needs higher interest rates and more unemployed to bring it in better balance and keep prices flat.

Our question then is: what would Finance Minister Goodale pay to discharge the promised "solid chunk of the $500 billion federal debt not only in 2003, but every year thereafter." Paper bills of a different colour? Hardly foreign currency – which would be another government's paper, since gold hasn't been recognized as money internationally since the early 1970s. Rejoice Canadians, at least your gold fillings are safe before the Martin-Goodale onslaught! Our government's boast is not prudent fiscal management but a scam that makes the sponsorship scandal seem peanuts. The goal of a flat price level and "paying off the debt" when our aged population is multiplying, and higher technologies and urbanization call for higher public investment, is a pipedream. Outstanding historians like the late Ferdinand Braudel have long recognized that, but conventional economists have for the past thirty years received their thinking orders to elevate it as the ultimate goal of their profession. It has served as the means of shifting a good chunk of the world's income from the productive population to gambling high finance.

A Forgotten Lesson

For if you shrink our money supply, the economy sinks into ever deeper depression as the real value of private debt explodes. That was the lesson of the Great Depression that brought on World War II.

How can a government be so arrogant to make such statements and issue such a budget? The answer: a financial *coup d'état* carried out in secret by the worlds' central banks.

Here is what you must ask our new PM as the election campaign gets under way.

Let him explain why Subsection (4) of Section 457 of Chapter 46 of the Statutes of Canada 1991 was passed without debate in Parliament or press release. This bill snuffed out the statutory reserves that chartered banks had to hold with the Bank of Canada. These involved the redeposit with the Bank of Canada (BoC) of a modest part of the deposits they received from the public in chequing accounts. These reserves helped ensure that the banks would be in a position to honour cheques drawn against their clients' deposits with them. Since no interest was paid by the BoC on such reserves, they amounted to a near-interest-free loan to the Government. The profits of the BoC come back to it, less a modest overhead charge, as dividends; for since 1938 the federal government has been the sole shareholder of the BoC.

These reserves also offered the government an alternative to raising interest rates for controlling inflation, real or perceived. By increasing the statutory reserves, say from 8% to 10%, the BoC could reduce the chartered banks' leverage in making interest-bearing loans. For its own needs, the government could borrow from the BoC, on a virtual interest-free basis within the prevailing restrictions. As the late John Hotson used to say: "find me a banker that does his borrowing at another bank!" Our government alone since 1991 has worn that fool's hat.

The Secret Bunker in Basel

This coup of the bankers was largely designed at the Bank for International Settlements (BIS), a non-government institution in Basel, Switzerland. BIS was founded in 1929 as a clearing house for the conversion and syndication of German reparations collected in German currency into strong currencies. BIS stock can be bought on the Paris stock exchange, but it has had more effect on Canadians' lives than all their elected representatives. Yet BIS's board includes US private banks. And no representative of a government other than the heads of central banks is allowed to attend its sessions. At Bretton Woods in 1943, Resolution Five called for the liquidation of the BIS at the earliest date, because of charges of its complicity with the Nazis.[1]

An unusual feature of BIS is that the voting rights are reserved to the original shareholders, even though they may since have sold their shares. This would include the three large US private banks that took up the subscription of shares reserved for the Federal Reserve, that declined to acquire them because of Washington's isolationism at the time. Anything remotely smacking of democracy is loathed at BIS. That has made it an ideal bunker for plotting the take-over of the world by our high-flying bankers.

To meet the needs of banks throughout the world that had lost much of their capital, BIS designed its *Risk-Based Capital Requirements*. Key to the document was its shifting the measure of bank solvency from the *cash* held to its *capital*. The capital of banks is originally raised in cash, but is not allowed to remain in that form. For cash breeds no interest and is frowned upon as "lazy money." So it gets "invested" in highly leveraged gambles made possible by the deregulation of banks since 1951. This enables them to acquire brokerage houses, underwriting, mortgage and insurance institutions, derivative boutiques, merchant banks that temporarily hold and deal in every type of firm. Moreover, such assets are kept on their books at their "historic" value, i.e., their original purchase price rather than their current value. BIS's *Risk-Based Capital Requirements* declared "risk free" the debt of OECD countries – the most highly industrialized lands. It thus requires no capital for banks to acquire.

This indeed was a core gimmick in the world-wide bank bailout of the early 1990s. You will find it not only the prominent means of bailout out of our banks in 1991. It was also a key feature in the corrupt bailout of Mexico's banks in 1994 that almost brought down the entire world financial system crashing. Only a $51 billion fund put together by world institutions including the US and Canada saved the situation. It catapulted the banks, so recently bailed out, into a position of world power. In combination with the end of the statutory reserves, it enabled Canada's banks to quadruple their holdings of federal government bonds by taking on another $60 billion dollars worth without putting up a penny of cash. Depending on how high the BoC screwed up interest rates, the combination of ending statutory reserves and the BIS new Risk Capital Requirements made possible an annual entitlement of anywhere from $5 to $8 billion dollars a year. And to perfect this scenario BoC Governor John Crow had been imported from the IMF where he had run up a record of bullying Latin American banana republics. In the same spirit he convinced PM Brian Mulroney to put zero inflation into our constitution. However, the representatives of all three parties on the Commons Finance Committee voted against the move, and, as a result the necessary powers for keeping this country free of oppressive debt are still in the *Bank of Canada Act*. However, subsequent governments have acted as though they had been removed. Most of our national debt that our brand-new PM Paul Martin is determined to pay off in a secret medium, dates from that pillage of the Canadian economy for and by the banks.

The victims were the most needy sectors of our population. For to pay that piper the most crucial public investments such as the environment, health, education, all our infrastructures, physical and human have been slashed. A favorite method towards this end was downloading vital social functions from the federal government to the provinces and from the provinces to the municipalities, without adequate funds to finance them.

Rather than do away with the Goods and Services Tax (GST) and bring back statutory reserves to cut the debt service burden, the budget "reinstates Mr. Martin's practice as Finance Minister of putting aside $4 billion in rainy-day funds. Most of that nest egg will go toward reducing the debt at the end of the year unless needed for emergencies." The $4 billion cushion will let Mr. Goodale and Mr. Martin demonstrate that they have no intention of running a deficit, despite the ever greater need for restoring the drastic cuts to social programs in recent years.

Digging up a Key Episode of Paul Martin's Past

To appreciate the enormity of this position, we must disinter a key episode in this country's history. In 1997 after the Auditor General of the day, Denis Desautels, refused unconditional approval of two years' balance sheets of the government, until Finance Minister Paul Martin agreed to introduce a basic principle of accountancy into the government's books – the distinction between capital investment and current spending ("accrual accountancy"). Up to then, despite recommendations by three royal commissions and a series of Auditors General, Mr. Martin – like his predecessors – had disregarded the advice of the Auditor General on how its books should be kept. When the government built a bridge or a road or other capital asset that would serve for years or decades it entered its cost into its books just as it did its outlay for floor-wax or paper clips: it wrote it off wholly in the year when it was built and thereafter carried at a token dollar. In short, it recognized the debt incurred for the investment, but ignored the continuing asset for which the debt was incurred. If you applied such non-accountancy in the private sector, few corporations would be solvent. Nevertheless, Finance Minister Paul Martin at the time resisted bringing in accrual accountancy, and provoked the Auditor General to accuse him of "cooking the books."

Finally a compromise was reached – it was agreed to apply such serious accountancy initially only in two areas – the treaty obligations with the First Nations, and the environment. The non-performance of the government in making good these two non-financial deficits would be translated into financial terms as "liabilities" so long as they were not repaired. Only a single newspaper, *The Financial Post*, desperate for readers, reported this agreement. The compromise left unaddressed initially not only the deterioration of many other areas, health, municipal services, education, social services. These were simply been declared "externalities" as is standard in official economic doctrine. These gaping and growing "non-financial" deficits were wholly ignored in Mr. Martin's budgeting.

A New Demension of Understanding with the Provinces

But if the statutory reserves returned, and if the BoC were once again used for financing loans to all levels of government, all services really vital for the country could be addressed. The only real restraint would be the presence of real resources in the land for the task – material, labour and technology. It is important to note, however, that the net interest received by the BoC on such loans would revert only to the federal government, not to the provinces and not to the municipalities. However, in return for junior levels of government observing federal standards, an agreement could be negotiated for Ottawa passing on all or part of such interest paid to the debtor government. This would open a new dimension of understanding between our governments. It would end the downloading of vital programs to the provinces without the resources to take care of them, so that Mr. Martin could win kudos as a deficit-killer.

If you depreciate capital investments of government in a single year, you not only exaggerate the deficit in that year but you can sell such investments to private investors at 5% of their real value and book the entire sales price as profit that goes to reduce the national debt. Mr. Martin's deal with the Auditor

General provided accrual accountancy in two isolated instances – damage done to the environment and our obligations to the aboriginal peoples still not met be booked as liabilities.[2]

It is important in this connection to note the different ways in which the Clinton Government and Finance Minister Martin smuggled elements of accrual accountancy into their bookkeeping. The Americans, directed by the Treasury Secretary, Robert Rubin, applied the smarts of his Wall St. background without prodding by the government's auditor. He used accrual accountancy across the board for the government's physical investments to head off the next bank disaster that arose from the *Risk-Based Capital Requirements*. In their haste to save the stricken banks the BIS and the international experts it had consulted had overlooked an important detail. Making it possible for banks to load up with government debt on zero margin wasn't smart for an institution that had proclaimed zero inflation as its goal and high interest rates the means of attaining it. For whenever interest rates go up, existing bonds with a lower coupon shed value. It therefore became essential to bring down interest rates so that the banks' bond hoard could recoup their value. American banks had already begun closing their doors because the bond hoards that had been the means of their previous bailout were shrinking due to rising interest rates.

Treasury Secretary Rubin finagled his way out of that oversight of the BIS by introducing accrual accountancy for nonfinancial capital assets, and carrying it back several years. In this way, Rubin improved the balance sheet by a trillion dollars. But to avoid arousing the sleeping dogs of the right, this trillion-odd dollars of ignored assets was called "savings." Savings, however, are held in cash, which was most definitely not the case with the government's belatedly recognized non-financial assets. However, Rubin's change gave the Government the single statistic needed to induce the bond-rating agencies to bring down interest rates. That turned the economy around and assured President Clinton a second term.[3]

In contrast Mr. Martin a year or two later was still resisting pressure from the Auditor General to bring in accrual accountancy. When he was finally prevailed upon to introduce it in a marginal, surreptitious way, it left a huge differential between interest rates in Canada and the US.

That was anything but helpful for keeping Canada in one prosperous piece.

Mr. Goodale hailed his budget as giving Canada "the utmost in accountability" (the *G&M*, 24/03). But there is no accountability without serious accounting. But that is exactly what is getting in ever shorter supply.

William Krehm

1. To fully grasp the issues of the coming federal election, we are making available a limited number at half price a detailed documented account of the Bank for International Settlements – Krehm, William (1993), *The Bank of Canada: A Power Unto Itself*, Toronto: Stoddard. Price is $5 including postage.

2. The particulars can be downloaded from a federal government website www.fin.gc.ca/toce/2001/fullacc_e.html, "Backgrounder on the Implementation of Accrual Accountancy." While Finance Minister Goodale talks so confidently of the reduction of the debt, this key

but hidden document informs us that "It is premature to provide estimates on the impact of these [accountancy] changes. Departments and agencies are in the process of quantifying their assets and liabilities. These will have to be reviewed by the Auditor General. As a result, the impacts will not be fully known until the audited financial statements for 2001-02 are finalized." The implications of this document merited front page spreads across every newspaper in the country but failed to receive a mention in them. It was discussed more fully in Economic Reform of 1/04.

3. The story is told in greater detail in *Towards a Non-Autistic Economy – A Place at the Table for Society* by William Krehm, COMER Publications, Toronto, 2002, p. 125.

Auditing our Auditors

IN OUR LAST ISSUE we carried an article by Gordon Coggins reviewing a movie on the birth and career of a bloodless species, the corporation, that since its birthing less than a century ago has taken over the world. Being bloodless, it cannot itself bleed. In an emergency, it is its shareholders and employees that bleed for it. The corporation does have its corps of well-paid professionals to keep it good and honest – the ministers of its faith, if you wish. But now these spiritual monitors are being caught red-handed breaking the laws and charters that brought this bloodless monster into being.

The resulting scandal can be compared with the simony – the selling of passes into heaven by dignitaries of the Roman Church – that helped precipitate the Reformation and countless civil wars throughout 16th and 17th century Europe.

From a recent *Wall Street Journal* article (25/3/04, "Behind Wave of Corporate Fraud: A Change in How Auditors Work" by Jonathan Weil), we get a glimpse of the soul-searching underway amongst auditors today.

"Consider what happened when James Lamphron and his team of Ernst & Young LLP accountants sat down early last year to plan their audit of HealthSouth Corp.'s 2002 financial statements. When they asked executives of the Birmingham, Ala., hospital chain if they were aware of any significant instances of fraud, the executives replied no. In their planning papers, the auditors wrote that HealthSouth's system for generating financial data was reliable, the company's executives were ethical, and that HealthSouth's management had 'designed an environment for success.'

"As a result, the auditors performed far fewer tests of the numbers on the company's books than they would have where they perceived the risk of accounting fraud to be higher. That's standard practice under the 'risk-based audit' approach now used widely throughout the auditing profession. Among the items the Ernst & Young auditors didn't examine at all: additions of less than $5,000 to individual assets on the company's ledger.

"Those numbers are where HealthSouth executives hid a big part of a giant fraud. This blind spot in the firm's auditing procedures is a key reason why former HealthSouth executives, 15 of whom have pleaded guilty to fraud, were able to overstate profits by $3 billion without anyone from Ernest & Young noticing until March 2003, when federal agents began making arrests.

"A look at the risk-based approach helps explain why investors continue to be socked by accounting scandals, from WorldCom Inc. and Tyco International Ltd. to Parmalat SpA, the Italian dairy company that admitted to faking $4.8 billion in cash. Just because an accounting firm says it has audited a company's numbers doesn't mean it actually has checked them.

"In a September 2003 speech, Daniel Goelzer, a member of the auditing profession's new regulator, the Public Accounting Oversight Board, called the risk-based approach one of the key factors 'that seem to have contributed to the erosion of trust in auditing.' Faced with difficulty in raising audit fees, Mr. Goelzer said, the major accounting firms during the 1990s began to stress cost controls. And they began to place greater emphasis on planning the scope of their work based on auditors' judgments about what clients are risky and which areas of a company's financial reports are most prone to error and fraud."

Getting from the Horse's Mouth who will Win the Race

"Auditors still plow through 'high risk' items such as derivative financial instruments or 'related party' business dealings between a company and its executives. But ostensibly 'low risk' items – such as cash on the balance sheet or accounts that fluctuate little from year to year – often get no more than a cursory review for years at a stretch. Instead, auditors rely more heavily on what management tells them and the auditors' assessments of a company's 'internal controls.'

"If controls over a company's sales and customer IOUs are perceived strong, the auditor might mail out at year end only a limited number of confirmation requests to companies that do business with the audit client. Instead, the auditor would rely more on the numbers spat out by the company's computers.

"For inventory, the lower the perceived risk of errors or fraud, the less frequently junior-level accountants might be dispatched on surprise visits to a client's warehouse to oversee the company's procedures for counting unsold goods.

"In theory, the risk-based approach should work fine, if an auditor is good at identifying the areas where misstatements are most likely to occur. Proponents advocate the shift as a cost-efficient improvement.

"'The problem is that there's a lot of evidence that auditors are not good at assessing risk,' says Charles Cullinan, an accounting professor at Bryant College in Smithfield, RI, and co-author of a 2002 study that criticized the re-engineered audit process as ineffective in detecting fraud.

"Auditors can't check all of a company's numbers, since that would make audits too expensive, particularly in an age of sprawling multinationals. And in many ways, the tools at auditors' disposal haven't changed much over the modern industry's 160-year history.

"Auditors are supposed to avoid becoming predictable. Otherwise, a client's management might figure out how to sneak things by them. It's also important to sample-test tiny accounting entries, even as low as a couple of hundred dollars. An old accounting trick is to fudge lots of tiny entries that appear insignificant individually.

"Facing a crush of shareholder law-suits over accounting scandals of the past four years, the Big Four accounting. firms say they are pouring tens of millions of dollars into improving their techniques. KPMG's investigative division has doubled its force of forensic specialists to 280, some hailing from the FBI. PricewaterhouseCoopers LLP auditors attend seminars run by former CIA operatives on how to spot deceitful managers by scrutinizing language and verbal cues.

"But the firms aren't backing away from the concept of risk-based audit itself. 'It would be negligent not to take a risk-based approach,' says Greg Weaver, head of Deloitte & Touche LLP's US audit practice. 'Auditors need to understand the areas that are likely more subject to error,' he says.

"Mr. Lamphron, the Ernst & Young partner, and his firm blame HealthSouth's former executives for deceiving them. Testifying before a congressional subcommittee in November, Mr. Lamphron said I know we planned and conducted a solid audit. We sought out the right documents and asked the right questions. Had we asked for additional documentation here or asked another question there, I think it would have generated another false document and another lie."

"The pioneers of the auditing industry had a more can-do spirit. In Britain during the 1840s, William Deloitte, whose firm continues today as Deloitte & Touche, made a name for himself by helping unravel frauds at the Great Eastern Steamship Co. and Great Northern Railway. A growing breed of professionals such as William Cooper, whose name lives on in Pricewaterhouse-Coopers, began advertising their services as an essential means for rooting out fraud."

Government Reaps What Government Sows

"But in the US, the notion of the auditor as detective never quite took off. The Securities and Exchange Commission in the 1930s made audits mandatory for public companies. The auditing profession faced its first real public test in 1937, when an accounting scandal broke open at McKesson & Robbins: More than 20% of the assets reported by the drug company were fictitious inventory and customer IOU's. The auditors had been fooled by forged documents. However, the American Institute of Certified Public Accountants, that sets auditing standards, repeatedly emphasized the limitations on auditors' ability to detect fraud, fearing liability exposure for its members.

"By the 1970s a new force emerged to erode audit quality: price competition. For decades, the AICPA barred auditors advertising their services, making uninvited solicitations to rival firms' clients, or participating in competitive-bidding contests. The institute was forced to lift these bans, however, when the federal government deemed them anti-competitive and threatened to bring antitrust suits."

The government then has reaped what it sowed with its militant espousal of "the eternal wisdom of the free market."

"Increasingly audits became a commodity product. Flat-fee pricing became common. The big accounting firms spent much

of the 1980s and 1990s building more-lucrative consulting operations. Many audit clients were paying their independent accounting firms far more money for consulting than auditing. The audit became a mere foot in the door for the consultants. Economic pressures also brought a wave of mergers, winnowing down the number of accounting firms just as the number of publicly traded companies and corporative financial statements were becoming more complex.

"In an October 1999 speech, the then SEC's chief accountant, noted that more than 80% of the agency's fraud cases from 1987 to 1997 involved top executives. While the risk-based approach was focusing on information systems and the employees who fed them, auditors really needed to expand their scrutiny to include top executives, who with a few keystrokes could override their companies' systems.

"When WorldCom was a small, start-up telecommunications company, its outside auditor, Arthur Andersen LLP, did things the old-fashioned way. It tested the thousands of details of individual transactions, and reviewed the items in WorldCom's general ledger, where entries were first logged.

"But as WorldCom grew, Andersen shifted towards what it called a risk-based 'business audit process.' By 1998, it was incurring more costs to audit WorldCom than it was billing, making up the difference with fees for consulting and other work, according to an investigative report last year by WorldCom's audit committee. In its 2000 audit proposal to WorldCom, Andersen said it considered itself 'a committed member of [WorldCom's] team and saw the company as a 'flagship client and a crown jewel of the firm.'"

It had crossed the line separating auditor from audited.

"When questions arose, the auditors relied on answers supplied by management, even though their software had rated WorldCom a 'maximum risk' client, according to a January report by WorldCom's bankruptcy examiner, former US Attorney General Richard Thornburgh.

"They did check to see if there were any major swings in the items on the company's consolidated balance sheet. There weren't any, and from this the auditors concluded that follow-up procedures weren't necessary. Indeed, WorldCom executives had manipulated its numbers so that there wouldn't be unusual variances. Had the auditors dug into specific journal entries they would have seen hundreds of suspiciously round numbers that had no supporting documentation.

"Andersen signed its last audit report for WorldCom in March 2002, saying the numbers were clean. Three months later, WorldCom announced that top executives, including its former chief financial officer, had improperly classified billions of dollars of ordinary expenses as assets. The final tally of fraudulent profits hit $10.6 billion. WorldCom filed for Chapter 11 reorganization in June 2002, marking the largest bankruptcy in US history. Now, out of business, Andersen is appealing its June 2002 felony conviction for obstruction of justice in its botched audits of Enron Corp."

One question – the greatest – remains unasked and unanswered. How much serious accountancy can a financial system based on the incorporation into present stock prices of the extrapolation of the rate of growth already achieved into the remote future? Once such an economic model has been adopted, what sort of accountancy can it stand? It is a model that makes a practice of proclaiming liabilities assets – for example environmental pollution, the break-down of our health and educational systems "growth." Indeed, the very sins of many of our large accounting firms underlie the financial model of ever crescendoing growth that have taken over our financial system. In this age of compulsive mergers, the cops have merged with the gangsters as happened in Capone's Chicago years ago.

William Krehm

WITH A DOFF OF OUR HAT TO ECONOMIC REFORM AUSTRALIA (ERA)

Bubbly from its March–April 2004 Issue

John Hotson Redivivus

Most economists don't understand money, interest and debt. Maybe they don't understand money because they're afraid to, because if they did, they'd have to do something about it, and get into trouble with people who do understand it (the leading bankers).

The situation in "monetary theory" is about where sex education would be if the "stork theory" of how babies got here were the "official paradigm." The facts about money (and baby) creation are well understood. Yet economists prefer fairy tales – like that helicopters drop money on people – to straight forward discussion of the fact that all money today is "rented" from the banks. Nor do economists focus on the great problems – inflation, stagflation and depression – that this causes society.

Why is this? Do economists consider that money, like sex to be a "dirty" subject about which the less accurate the information given the young the better?

Most economists really believe that demonstrating that "if the world were very different from what it is, then things would happen very differently than they do" is a useful way for a grown person to spend his/her time. Thus economists love to "show" that if all markets were "purely competitive" and there was "perfect foresight and factor mobility" and no government "interference," then all sorts of wonderful things would happen and this would be the best possible of all worlds. Of course it cannot be proven because to do so would necessitate setting up an experimental "perfect" world and seeing what happens. We can't and so the world continues the way it is, full of "monopoly distortions," "errors of foresight," immobilities, and government actions.

John Hotson (1930-1996), in The COMER Papers, *Vol. 3 (1993) reprinted in* ERA Newsletter, *March–April 2004.*

An Imagined Interchange

At a recent computer expo (COMDEX), Bill Gates reportedly compared the computer industry with the auto industry and stated, "If GM had kept up with technology like the computer industry has, we would all be driving $25 cars that got 1,000 miles to the gallon."

In response, General Motors issued a press release stating: "If GM had kept up with technology like Microsoft, we would all be driving cars with the following characteristics:

1. For no reason whatsoever, your car would crash twice a day.

2. Every time they repainted the lines on the road, you would have to buy a new car.

3. Occasionally your car would die on the freeway for no reason. You would have to pull to the side of the road, close all the windows, shut off the car, restart it, and reopen the windows before you could continue. For some reason you would simply accept this.

4. Occasionally, executing a maneuver such as a left turn would cause your car to shut down and refuse to restart, in which case you would have to reinstall the engine.

5. Macintosh would make a car that was powered by the sun, was reliable, five times as fast and twice as easy to drive – but would run on only five percent of the roads.

6. The oil, water temperature, and alternator warning lights would all be replaced by a single "This Car Has Performed An Illegal Operation" warning light.

7. The air-bag system would ask, "Are You Sure" before deploying.

8. Occasionally, for no reason whatever, your car would lock you out and refuse to let you in until you simultaneously lifted the door handle, turned the key and grabbed hold of the radio antenna.

9. Every time a new car was introduced, car buyers would have to learn how to drive all over again because none of the controls would operate in the same manner as the old car.

10. You'd have to push the "start" button to turn the engine off.

Growing Troubles in the European Union

GLOBALIZATION seems to be working at least in one respect. Economic and social headaches are no longer confined to a single country or continent, but bring on sleepless nights throughout the world. The latest proof of that is the mounting malaise in the European Union. And that has a vicious potential since, with an aging population, Europe is increasingly dependent on Asian and African immigrants to complement a dwindling labour force. In such a setting, nonfunctional economies can ignite hostilities that most people associate with the Third World.

The Wall Street Journal (13/04, "Broken Pledges May Hit Euro Zone" by G. Thomas Sims) informs us: "Frankfurt – The fiscal framework that binds the network of countries using the euro is once again at a breaking point. This is creating fears of slower growth and higher unemployment in the world's second-largest collective economy and raising a debate about how to revise the system."

Sharp Reversal of Intentions

"This year, half of the 12 euro-zone countries will post budget deficits above 3% of gross domestic product, the maximum allowed under European Union guidelines, the European Commission predicted last week. The violators include the three largest countries – France, Germany, and Italy – as well as the Netherlands, Greece and Portugal. The EU's executive arm and watchdog on budgets sees only 'slight improvements' for next year.

"The fiscal course marks a sharp reversal from the intentions of just a few years ago. In the run-up to currency union in 1999, EU nations pledged to aim for budget surpluses and agreed to apply fines if budget deficits exceeded 3%. But over the past few years, as the economy slowed, tax revenue dried up and countries failed to trim spending, Portugal, Germany and France broke the 3% limit but escaped penalties with promises of getting their budgets in order.

"In November, the commissioner recommended initiating the sanction process against Germany and France, but finance ministers who must endorse any recommendation blocked the move, dealing a blow to the 3% rule enshrined in the Stability and Growth Pact. As a result, the commission is suing EU finance ministers before the European Court of Justice in hearings beginning in about two weeks.

"Many economists believe the growing list of countries struggling to limit deficits further waters down a pact that is drowning. To be sure, many of the world's largest countries are accumulating budget deficits. The US is projected to post a deficit of 4.5% of GDP this year; but it had budget surpluses as recently as the late 1990s. Many European countries have only a short history of fiscal austerity, so the credibility of the five-year-old-currency is at stake."

To this add the detail that the American budgetary surpluses in the latter 1990s were due to the initial recognition in 1996 of Washington's physical capital investments as such rather than as current spending.[1] That, however, was not advertised, for ideological reasons – governments are not supposed to be able to make "investments" though the health of the opining economist's mother and children may be at stake. Accordingly, a trillion dollars of the federal government's assets were for the first time booked as "savings," in the January, 1966 figures of the Bureau of Economic Analysis of the Department of Commerce. However, by no stretch of the imagination were they "savings", since they existed not as cash, but as roads, buildings, bridges, penitentiaries. That coup that revolutionized the fiscal statistics of the US cannot, however, be repeated. The value of the depreciated physical assets of the federal government has already been incorporated into the budget balance. Unless of course you go on to recognise government human investment in such areas as education, health, social welfare.

For economists – in the remote 1960s when they were allowed to think about the problems of the economy instead of wishing them away in a "pure and perfect world" that never existed – that was considered meaningful economics. But recognizing public investment in human capital would leave the whole corpus of equilibrium economics in a shambles. For it recognizes the market itself as the only force capable of dealing with the problems of the world – by pushing out of sight and mind everything that doesn't provide more chips for the world's financial gambling. That has brought us a growing harvest of war, terrorism, unemployment, starvation, and disease. Now it threatens to pull apart the EU – a daring experiment in its day.

"The European Central Bank – which steers the euro-zone economy and manages the euro – has become increasingly vocal in the pact's defense. In a report last week, the ECB argued that the indebted countries would cause consumers and businesses to factor higher taxes and possible default into their decisions, hampering growth and employment. Also, spending countries will have to pay higher interest rates on their debt, eating into funds that could otherwise be used for investment and growth, the ECB said."

Nothing Irresponsible about Going Back to What Worked

Of course, the ECB, like Washington, Westminster and Ottawa, utters nary a word about the proposal that governments borrow directly from their central banks, say as much of their needs as they used to until the 1970s. In that way they would get back almost all the interest they paid. This happened either as dividends, in the case of central banks owned entirely by the government as in Canada and Britain, or by right of the government as heir to the ancestral monarch who had the monopoly for coining precious metals. That, of course, would leave the banks without a yearly entitlement to finance their gambles. Once the electorate was convinced that this solved the deficit problem – and countless others for which such financing could be used – the percentage of the national debt financed in this way could be stepped up cautiously beyond the 1975 figure. During WWII Canada's proportion of its debt financed through its central bank had not exceeded 16%. Surely there is nothing more responsible than going back to what worked, and then carefully proceeding along that path in careful further steps.

But wouldn't that bring back runaway inflation? That is another myth that must be disposed of. The real surge of prices began when interest rates came to be used as the sole blunt tool to flatten out price. The tremendous urbanization and technological revolutions that took over in the post-war period inevitably required more public services. Nobody moving from the countryside to New York City expects his living costs to remain the same. How then can economists expect just that when humanity as a whole makes such a move? More public services mean higher taxes which become a deepening layer in price. This is not due to an excess of demand over supply, but to an increase in the share of public services in the total economic output. It is 34 years since my first writings on this ignored factor were published[2] but it has been an ideological pillbox for the deregulated financial sector to deny this obvious relationship. This past year, however, even the US Federal Reserve and the

Bank for International Settlements have begun talking of some 2% of "inflation" as "good" inflation. That is like describing medicine as "good poison" rather than as medicine.

"With the European pact fraying, an overhaul is growing more likely. Some economists have suggested that a new pact focus less on deficits and more on overall debt, arguing that debt levels have greater implications for the long term well-being of a country."

Let us take up that important point. In the 1960s Theodore Schultz was awarded a Nobel Prize for Economics for recognizing public investment in human capital as the most productive that could be made. He arrived at that conclusion through his experience as one of the hundreds of economists that Washington had sent to Japan and Germany after WWII to predict how long it would take those formidable economies to rebuild. In retrospect, Schultz concluded, they were dreadfully wide of the mark in their predictions. He decided that was because he and his colleagues had concentrated on the physical destruction of plant and equipment, housing and physical things, and overlooked that the highly educated, motivated populations were still basically intact.

Once you include human skills and training as an investment, you cannot exclude health and social welfare, for they look after the vessels in which skills and education are kept and protected. Moreover the rate of depreciation of human investment is far slower than that of any physical plant. Educated, healthy parents produce and nurture more productive children, who pass on that investment to their own young. Amongst physical investments, the longer-term ones are the most uncertain. It is a tenet of banking that the terms of their assets must match that of their liabilities. Trouble sooner or later lurks in any disparity between the two. Transfer that rule to human investment by government and you will at once appreciate that financing it through the central bank is an arrangement smiled on by the gods. You educate your population to its talents, and protect that investment by looking after its health and social needs, and much of that investment will help real productivity for generations. Financed by the central bank, it will not only be virtually interest free, but can be amortized over generations. No need to shorten the write-off period as is done to encourage physical private investments.

But we have dealt with only the ground floor of the leaning edifice of economics. A vast educational and training structure was reared in the early postwar decades to educate the skilled workers in developed countries. As we outsource more and more of our skilled workers, importing them from Third World countries, and send more and more of our skilled jobs abroad, is it not inevitable that we should have less and less use for these educational facilities? So even though the investment was only marginally recognized in our public accountancy, are we not, instinctively deeming it less and less useful, and writing it off? That is something that should be pondered.

The European Union is increasingly dependent for its manual labour on immigrants from Africa and Asia. Leave them and their children undereducated, treated as a lesser breed, and you are guaranteeing endless trouble ahead. Recognize

human investment for what it is, and make more of it where it is needed, financed by the central bank over a realistic term of depreciation, and the reward will come not only from earth but from heaven.

William Krehm

1. Krehm, William (2002). *Toward a Non-Autistic Economy – A Place at the Table for Society* (p. 125). COMER Publications.
2. Krehm, William (1975). *Price in a Mixed Economy: Our Record of Disaster.* Chapter 13, "Society's Forgotten Capital Assets." Toronto.

REVIEW OF A BOOK BY FRANCIS HUTCHINSON AND BRIAN BURKITT, ROUTLEDGE, LONDON, 1977

"The Political Economy of Social Credit and Guild Socialism"

THIS REMARKABLE BOOK on the history of social credit was given to me by Michael Rowbotham some years ago. I must have read it carefully at the time for my margin pencillings are much in evidence. But clearly it required the disturbing developments in the intervening years for me to make a greater effort to appreciate fully some of the conclusions that Major C.H. Douglas had arrived at. The problem was that he was using an approach that varied from that of less unconventional reformers – to the point that they did not even grasp what it was that he was seeking and to an extent actually found. Reflecting that, his solutions and even his language seemed clumsily at odds with the accepted vocabulary and grammar of economic thinking, right or left. Even his A and B Theorem which seemed to us an unschooled blunder of an engineer lost in the labyrinth of accountancy and economic thought.

But the misadventures of the world are forcing us to penetrate the obscurities of his language that barred access to many potential allies.

But a bit of background. "The writings of Major Douglas gave rise to the social credit movement, popular throughout the inter-war years. Douglas's earliest books, *Economic Democracy* and *Credit – Power and Democracy*, first appeared in serial form in the socialist journal the *New Age* in the period immediately following World War I. Close examination of the early Douglas/ *New Age* texts alongside the literature of guild socialism reveals that the editor of the *New Age*, A.R. Orage, provided Douglas with a great deal more than editorial support in the formulation of the original texts. Without Orage's guild socialist contribution [the Douglas doctrine] would have provided unpromising material for a popular debate which was to be sustained over two decades throughout the English-speaking world.

"Guild socialism and Douglas had this in common: In their different ways they both questioned the deep faith that Marxist and most brands of socialism shared with the prophets of capitalism – that economic growth was in itself beneficent and necessary, and ultimately liberating. The guild socialists questioned this on esthetic, philosophic and social grounds under the influence of William Morris, John Ruskin, and even of Robert Owen.

The guild socialists saw in excessive industrialization an undermining of the elements of pluralism and local autonomies in earlier societies. Current Globalization and Deregulation with its destructive effects on the environment, the family, the multiplicity of life styles, is only an explosive manifestation of this trend. As important as the effort to safeguard the jobs of workers may be, it is an uphill struggle, given the concentration of power in the financial sector. The incorporation into current price of the rate of growth already achieved brings with it the need to continue that growth, and its rate of its growth into the distant future. The slightest shortfall of this commitment triggers the collapse of the price structure. And since share values serve as collateral for further financing, it becomes unsustainable. The mathematics of the model in fact are those of the atom bomb.

An Unequalled Thoroughness

Douglas-Orage review the nature of money from the ground up with a thoroughness that has few if any equals. "Douglas stressed that production does not create money. It is possible to imagine a producer in a system of single-stage production [i.e., without the purchase of intermediate goods and hence not incurring costs that have need of money]. Having access to land (which has not been bought) and a discarded spade, and having saved seed potato and horse manure (discarded A), it is possible for a producer to plant, tend and harvest a potato crop at no financial cost. The crop can be put in a discarded sack and sold to a neighbour for £5. Has the producer created £5? Or any money at all? That is the sort of maddeningly basic question Douglas was given to asking.

"Nevertheless, at the point of exchange no value is created. However sophisticated the system, production of all commodities follows the same pattern as the potato example. All production requires inputs from the natural world which the economy cannot create. All production requires human inputs. First, an inherited body of knowledge, as in the ability to save seed, cope with pests and drought and so on. Second, a 'producer' who may be employed or self-employed, but who comes to the task physically developed from infancy to maturity and still requires social care. Neither form of 'human input' is produced through exchange on the market. Wealth creation can take place outside the exchange economy.

"Money is a commodity itself. In a single-stage production a large proportion of subsistence requirements can be seen to be produced outside the formal economy. Hence in newly monetized economies 'cheap' labour occurs because subsistence requirements continue to be provided from outside the cash economy.

"Money has no intrinsic properties, only those which people choose to give it. Hence a comment such as 'There is no money in the country with which to do such and so' is meaningless, unless it is an indication that the goods and services required to perform the task in question do not exist and cannot be produced. In that event it would be useless to create the money equivalent of the non-existent resources. On the other hand, it is misleading to argue that the country 'has no money' for

social betterment or for any other purpose, when it possesses the skills, the labour and the material and plant to create that betterment. The financial system in the form of the banks or the Treasury can, if they so wish, create the necessary money in five minutes. Indeed, they are creating money for 'necessary' tasks every day, and have done so for centuries.

"Money can be described as a 'ticket system' whereby money 'tickets' or grants the right to participate in the economy. The ticket office [of a railway] is not the place where the measurement of productive capacity should take place. To orthodox economists steeped in general competitive equilibrium theory the dynamic relationship between money creation and policy formation in production and distribution was incomprehensible.

"'In popular belief, banking is understood to be no more than a private pawnbroking transaction between borrower and lender: lenders place their savings in a bank, and borrowers take that same money to invest in new machinery, labour and materials. In reality the banker is in a unique position of lending something without parting with anything, and making a profit on the transaction' (Douglas, 1923). 'The bank lends new money; bank loans create money and the uses to which it can be put are dependent upon these transactions' (Douglas, 1922c). 'Every credit transaction affects the interests of every person in the credit area concerned, either through its effect on prices or through the diversion of the energies available for production purposes' (Douglas, 1922c). 'An overdraft, arranged perhaps on the basis of the title deeds of a factory, facilitates production. However, the overdraft is new money exactly as if the banker had coined goods for sale' (Douglas, 1920). Hence the granting of credit by a financial institution is more realistically viewed as the creation of a mortgage on future production than as the allocation of the past savings of industry. The term 'deposits' is highly misleading, implying something deposited for safe keeping, like jewels in a safe deposit. Bank deposits are not like that. The deposits of commercial banks are to them liabilities, although they are assets to their holders."

Our Censored Textbooks

"As later explained by *Encyclopedia Britannica*, 1979) – a bank that received, say, $100 in gold might add $25 to its reserves and lend out $75. But the recipient of that $75 would himself spend it. Some of those who received gold in this way would hold it as gold but others would deposit it in this bank or in other banks. If, for example, two-third were deposited, some banks would find $50 added to deposits and to reserves and would repeat the process. When this multiple expansion process worked itself out fully, total deposits would have increased by $200 bank reserves by $50 and $50 of the initial $100 would have been retained as 'currency outside banks.'"

You will find that process explained in even greater detail in just about any textbook on economics published in Canada prior to 1991 when the bill was passed abolishing statutory reserves that banks had to redeposit as security against the deposits received in chequing accounts. By that the key mechanism of banking had been suppressed. That, of course, and the speculative banking orgies that have taken over since banks were deregulated to empower them to acquire brokerages, underwriting, merchant banking, derivative boutiques, are what have made the ideas of Douglas-Orage more important than ever before.

"'Problems occur when the banking system operates according to its own agenda, with the requirements of the consumer a secondary consideration. Unlike the social reform business, the banking business is immensely powerful, talks very little, acts quickly, knows shat it wants' (Douglas, 1922b). 'The quantity of money is dependent upon the power of the banker's pen. Banks create new money which ranks equally with legal tender as a means of exchange. Although credit is more properly regarded as common property, it is administered by the banker primarily for the purpose of private profit' (Douglas, 1923, 1919b). According to orthodox theory, money, equivalent to the price of every article produced, exists in the pocket, or in the bank, of somebody somewhere in the world. It is assumed that the collective sum of wages, salaries and dividends distributed in respect of the articles for sale at any given moment is available as purchasing power at the same moment. Some persons may have more money in their pocket or bank than they wish to spend on consumable goods. By abstaining from consuming, they form a fund which enables capital goods such as tools, plant and factories, to be paid for, and therefore to be produced. Crucially, the money which they 'use to spend or invest is constantly created and destroyed by the banking system for its own financial advantage' (Douglas, 1924a).

"Real credit is the 'effective reserve of energy belonging to the community.' Its administration has fallen to the banking system and financial institutions generally. Consequently the 'creative energy of mankind' becomes subject to artificial restrictions which bear no relationship to the realities of everyday existence' (Douglas, 1919b). The potential real wealth of society is communal in origin and should therefore be subject to the control of the entire community. Financial credit is administered by the banking system 'primarily for the purpose of private profit' (Douglas, 1919b).

"The Douglas/*New Age* texts note that banking originated as a private venture, observing that at the time the Bank of England remained a private institution. Nevertheless, the guild socialists did not consider that a politically controlled central bank would be truly independent of private banking interests. Just as state capitalism, i.e., a socialist government under the existing economic conditions would produce wage slavery as effectively as private capitalism, so too would state banking continue the *status quo* in terms of financial control over industrial policy.

"Hence Orage's derision of the Labour Party, on its rejection of the Douglas/*New Age* scheme. History has confirmed his judgment, but it is, however, important to remember the international campaign of the Bank for International Settlements in the 1980s to declare the independence from their governments of all central banks. Given what it had in the works, the world banking community clearly needs all the safeguards and secrecy it could get."

Finance Rules the Rulers of Kingdoms

"The creation of 'financial credit' ensures that 'industry becomes mortgaged to the banking system' (Douglas, 1924a). 'Appreciation of the role of finance in initiating economic activity was noted in *The National Guilds*' edited by Orage (1914) and originally printed as a series of articles by S.G. Hobson in the *New Age* in 1912-13. 'A great financial network covers the world, operating on an informal but highly centralized basis. It rules the rulers of kingdoms.'

"At this point, Hobson and Orage went no further than suggesting that the (industry-based) guilds would have to become their own bankers, working through a national clearing house."

At this point Douglas formulated his "A+B theorem," which focused on an aspect of financing production quite different from what economists and accountants had even considered.

"In 1908 he had been in India in charge of Westinghouse's interests in the East. One of those concerned the survey of a large district with a view to installing hydro-electric equipment. The prospects were good. On his return to Calcutta, however, it became clear that there was no money to proceed with the project. At the time labour was plentiful in India and the manufacturers in Great Britain were short of orders. Furthermore, prices for machinery at the time were very low indeed. Douglas recalled having been taken into the confidence of the Comptroller – General of India in Calcutta on the matter of 'credit.' He was told of the trouble he experienced with the Treasury officials at home in England, and with their departments in India, in regard to the extraordinary operations they undertook melting down rupees to deal with the exchange. This was done with regard to 'what they called the quantity theory of money.' The Comptroller-General concluded that 'money and currency and the silver rupees, etc., have almost nothing to do with this situation. It almost entirely depends on credit. Silver and currency form only a very small part of financial operations. Douglas noted this for future reference.'

"Some years later, before the outbreak of World War I, Douglas states he was employed by the British Government at home to design and ultimately construct a railway which runs underneath London from Paddington to Whitechapel. Despite the absence of physical or engineering problems and a plentiful supply of labour, the project could not be completed. Finance lay at the root of the problem. However, as soon as the war commenced, money was available for practically anything.

"After 'an interval' Douglas 'was sent down to Farnborough, to the Royal Aircraft Factory, in connection with a muddle into which the institution had got.' Douglas concluded that the only way to ascertain how work was being allocated 'was to go very carefully into the costing which took place.' The existing costing system produced 'admirable information about what happened three years and two months before, but that was not of any use to me.' According to Douglas, he introduced very early computers – 'tabulating machines' used on the London and North Western Railway. Information was punched on to cards and the cards were put into the machine that processed them. One day it occurred to him that by the end of the week total wages and salaries were not equal to the value of the goods produced during the week. The fact of this happening in every factory across the land *at the same period of time* meant that the purchasing power distributed in the form of wages and salaries will not be sufficient during any week to buy the product unless extra money is being injected into the system each week."

That was the origin and significance of the notorious A+B theorem. It was not enough to point out, as did many including myself, that the discrepancy was because many items produced both as intermediate goods as manufacturing parts, buildings, engineering projects would be useful over many years and would be financed until they were fully depreciated years later. That is exactly what he wished to free society from – dependence on the financial institutions. Hence he brought in the concept of a social dividend representing the contribution of society over generations in creating the institutions, the inventions, the scientific and technical discoveries that made the productive potential of our world possible. It would include, too, the unrewarded labour of slaves, the contribution of martyrs and prophets that made possible the social and legal framework for modern society and its productivity. That could be allotted to all citizens and it would fill the gap and free society from servitude to financial capital.

Instead of patenting scientific discoveries, even genes, for speculative investors to collect a rent on them, the social dividend would contribute to gear down the drive to maximization of the financial sector. It would encourage alternate life styles that would cultivate other goals than the consumption of highly promoted items of little or negative usefulness.

The contribution of Douglas-Orage to the incorporation of the non-market sectors of the economy – health, education, social security, the environment – is crucial. The power-grab of the banking system that Douglas and his associates identified almost a century ago, have come into a lethal flowering. In the long-overdue reassessment for what passes as economic science, their ideas will require careful attention. The Hutchinson Burkitt book is mandatory for preparing ourselves for the task.

William Krehm

Antidotes to Addictions

T HE BURDENED SOUL, unable to bear what it perceives as reality, turns to some behaviour which soothes and comforts. We call it going on vacation. If the "vacation" is unduly frequent, however, we may call it "a problem." If the problem behaviour becomes destructive or counterproductive, then it is probably addiction. The word is certainly being thrown around a lot lately, what with joggers addicted to "runner's high", or North Americans addicted to oil, or my cousin George addicted to food. On the economic front, too, there seems to be an addiction to "growth." And some, otherwise normal citizens are unmistakably addicted to shopping. Think, too, of those who get twitchy if they miss their daily eight hours of TV. Finally, there is Joel Andreas' "illustrated exposé," *Addicted to War* (rev. 2003).[1]

This book is subversive. General Electric, or the Pentagon, or perhaps the Canadian Council of Chief Executives should be buying up all copies of it, as the Church of England in the mid-sixteenth century bought up copies of William Tyndale's English translations of the Bible. (Their purchases gave Tyndale funds to bring out an illustrated edition of his next book of the Bible.)

This book is subversive. It gives a listing of American foreign military campaigns since the War of Independence. For example, "Between 1898 and 1934, the Marines invaded Cuba 4 times, Nicaragua 5 times, Honduras 7 times, the Dominican Republic 4 times, Haiti twice, Guatemala once, Panama twice, Mexico 3 times and Columbia 4 times," in addition to China, Russia and North Africa; and "during the Cold War, Washington intervened militarily in foreign countries more than 200 times."

This book is subversive. One of its conventions is that anything in quotation marks is a real quotation. For example: 1991 Henry Kissinger "Oil is much too important a commodity to be left in the hands of the Arabs." 1894 Senator Orville Platt: "I firmly believe that when any territory outside the present territorial limits of the United States becomes necessary for our defense or essential for our commercial development we ought to lose no time in acquiring it." 1945 President Harry Truman: "We pray that God might guide us to use [the bomb] in His ways and for His purposes."

General Smedley Butler of the US Marines is quoted extensively. Butler was recruited by anti-democratic elements in the 1930's to raise a force of 450,000 ex-soldiers to take over Washington and depose Franklin D. Roosevelt. He declined to complete the assignment. "I spent 33 years and 4 months in active military service…. And during that period I spent most of my time as a high-class muscle man for Big Business, for Wall Street and the bankers. In short, I was a racketeer, a gangster for capitalism…. I helped purify Nicaragua for the international banking house of Brown Brothers in 1902-1912. I brought light to the Dominican Republic for American sugar interests in 1916. I helped make Honduras right for American fruit companies in 1903. In China in 1927, I helped see to it that Standard Oil went on its way unmolested."

This book is subversive because it is funny. Interviewer: "Just how many lives can these new high-tech weapons save, Colonel?" After a summary of US attacks on Cuba, we are given the American President on the telephone getting "serious" about terrorism, "Listen Jeb, You're going to have to cough up the terrorists or we start bombing Miami tomorrow!"

This book is subversive because it gives only simple statistics: the US "defense" budget amounts to a million dollars a minute.

Above all *Addicted to War* is subversive because it is in comic book form! That is correct, in comic book form. That means it is within the reading capacity of at least half the American population. Even those addicted to TV might get partway through it; the segments are way shorter than the 30-second limit for episodes in soap operas. Of course, unlike TV, the print medium does allow the reader to pause to grasp what is meant.

So its 70-odd pages might take a little longer to read than a couple of hours of TV.

Lest the naïve reader might see it as a celebration of 200 years of glory – in the style of the late-night war movie – a well-supported subordinate theme makes it clear that when the elite go to war, it is the ordinary people who pay the fare, in taxes, lives lost, security shattered. Actually Andreas' elite do not personally go to war; they stay home and chortle all the way to the bank. Their sons say, "My daddy told me I could serve my country better by going to law school." *Addicted to War* is definitely subversive stuff. Its last panel is captioned, "Kick out the war junkies!"

But there are other addictions associated with militarism. How revealing it was shortly after 9/11 to hear the US President giving people his answer to the question, what can I do to serve my country? He said – to put it in the simplest terms – shop. Don't let a little thing like the WTC collapse interfere with your responsibilities as consumers.

Fortunately for the economy, shopping addiction is widespread. It would, in fact, be an economic catastrophe if everyone curbed their shopping and attempted instead to pay down their mortgages. Less stuff and less debt: now that could be a very enticing goal. But if all that money were drawn out of the real economy and poured back into the already over-stuffed financial sector, what would the result be? Probably, for a very short time, it would puff up the stock market. What else could the banks do with the money but buy securities? They could, of course, try to take on more and more risky loans. But reality, and deep depression, would soon set in.

The "laws" of our economic system are strange indeed, when a general action as benign and seemingly sensible as reducing one's debt and curtailing the flow of new "stuff" to be dumped into backyard storage sheds and public landfills, would bring on economic collapse. Like the addiction to war, that bears some thinking on.

Maybe we need to replace our private debt-based monetary system, with a public non-debt system, with the Bank of Canada fulfilling its statutory mandate to "regulate credit and currency in the best interests of the economic life of the nation, to control and protect the external value of the national monetary unit and to mitigate by its influence fluctuations in the general level of production, trade, prices and employment, so far as may be possible within the scope of monetary action, and generally to promote the economic and financial welfare of Canada." (Preamble to the Bank of Canada Act). That might well mitigate the destructive effects of our addiction to "growth."

Gordon Coggins

1. Andreas, Joel (2002, 2003). *Addicted to War: Why the US Can't Kick Militarism.*

Did Lincoln Actually Speak the Lines on Money Creation Attributed to Him or "Just" Put Them into Practice?

MY HUNT for the origins of "Lincoln's Monetary Policy" led me to what is probably a more important question.

To refresh your memory, several current Money Reform sites on the Internet publish a brief statement under the above title, and some of them go so far as to cite as a source "Senate Document 23, 1865" and embellish it as something Lincoln wrote himself just before his assassination – which was, they say, the act of his real enemies, the international bankers (e.g., Michael Rowbotham in his book, *The Grip of Death*) I did find the actual author of the statement, a Canadian politician of our grandfathers' generation who was a vehement and articulate promoter of money and banking reform (a cartalist as I have come to understand the term) and also a great admirer of Lincoln. Gerald Grattan McGeer, of Vancouver, [once mayor of the city and then its member of parliament]. His book, *The Conquest of Poverty*, was published in 1935. The by now widely circulated statement of "Lincoln's Monetary Policy" is very clearly acknowledged there to be his own inference from reading Lincoln's writings and recorded speeches. He leaves no room for doubt that he is putting words into Lincoln's mouth, albeit with full confidence that he is right about the Great Emancipator's intent. The currently published versions of the statement provide rather obscure or perplexing source references, but they do point to two twentieth century politicians, Jerry Voorhis of California and Robert L. Owen of Oklahoma. I haven't yet seen a copy of Voorhis' book, *Out of Debt, Out of Danger*, published about 1943 as I recall, but I have gotten hold of Owen's *National Economy and the Banking System of the United States*, published in 1939 as Senate Document 23, 76th Congress, 1st Session (108 pages). On page 67 Owen says this:

"Lincoln thoroughly understood the constitutional right of Congress to exclusively create money and to regulate the value thereof. An abstract of his views is given by McGeer in *Conquest of Poverty*." The views of Lincoln are of surpassing importance. "McGeer's abstract will be found in the appendix."

And so it is, exactly as I have read it in McGeer's book.

It is reassuring to get Owen's affirmation, because on reading the McGeer book I am not impressed that the quotations he provides from Lincoln really add up to an inference of the man's views that is as unmistakable as McGeer would like his readers to believe. Owen's book is impressive; a well-marshalled argument for what he alternately terms "modern monetary science" and "stable money." I have a collection of small books and pamphlets which manifest a movement of the 1930s in the US and other English speaking countries that Owen identifies as the "Stable Money Association under the leadership of some of the greatest leaders in finance and industry." The first named of these is Owen D. Young, chairman of GE, and the list includes several prominent economists of that era. An interesting coincidence I located Robert Owen's book in the "Owen D. Young Library" at St. Lawrence University in Canton, NY. The librarian told me that Young had been an important sponsor of the University.

"Now the puzzle. I have seen enough to be assured that there was indeed a significant movement for money and banking reform in the Depression era, which can be generally described as consistent with what I understand to be cartalism – and also with the Social Credit idea of an annual citizen's dividend. The list of people in Owen's book who were supporters of the Stable Money Association is very impressive – the kind that cannot at all be dismissed as fringe players or cranks: Alfred P. Sloan, Charles Evans Hughes, Elihu Root, John L. Lewis, Bernard Baruch, Henry A. Wallace, John R. Commons, Wesley Clair Mitchell, Pierre S. DuPont, George Eastman, Irving Fisher. Owen's presentation is seductive. Had I read it before tackling Zarlenga's *Lost Science* I would have had a vastly better understanding of what is at stake in the latter.

"The great puzzle to me is why Owen's name is not better known among our generation. As one of the first two senators from the then new state of Oklahoma, he drafted the Senate version of the *Federal Reserve Act* of 1913 and was thereafter prominent as a critic or commentator on banking affairs. Nevertheless, he rates virtually no mention in economics literature of the post-war era. Carter Glass gets plenty of mention, but the only place I could find mention of Owen in a shelf of books on money and banking is a footnote in F&S's *The Great Contraction* where he is described as a banker and lawyer before being elected to the Senate and being chairman of the Banking and Currency Committee when the *Federal Reserve Act* was passed. He is quoted there as testimony before the House Banking and Currency Committee in 1932.

"More important than the puzzle is the question of what happened to this apparently influential (?) movement for Stable Money in the aftermath of War II? I re-read Chapter 3 in *Super Imperialism* and see that it reinforces the notion that the New Deal team was more interested in domestic policy than in internationalism. Owen has a late chapter on "International Stabilization Impracticable." On the last page of his main text he notes his belief that a majority of the House in the 75th Congress "were in favor of congressional control and regulation of the volume and value of money. The matter is being debated on the hustings throughout the United States. Study clubs throughout the country are giving attention to this matter." I have in front of me two small books written expressly for the latter purpose.

What happened during the War and its aftermath to bury all this interest and initiative, I wonder? Its progeny seems to have turned very snarly and full of the great conspiracy theory when resurrected after 1950.

Keith Wilde

EDITOR'S NOTE: I remember Bill Hixson when working on his fine little book *It's Your Money* telling me that he had tried tracking down the statements attributed to Lincoln supporting his Greenback issue, and, being convinced that they were not authentic, avoided using them. That in no way invalidates the significance of Lincoln's issuing the Greenbacks to finance the Civil War, rather than borrowing from private banks at usurious rates. In most times of major crises prejudices tend to be laid aside to ensure society's survival. That takes conviction, even if the theory may not have been elaborated or published. That is what happened during the civil war and again to a limited extent under Roosevelt during the great beggaring of the world in the 1930s. And it continued in the financing of World War II and the subsequent reconstruction. That explains why so impressive a list of politicians of every hue and even powerful industrialists espoused money creation backed only by state credit. The credibility of the banks, after all, was in the gutter, and many leading industrialists faced with bankruptcy were open-minded for a way out of the mess.

The comeback and subsequent conquest of the economic universe by finance capital has been so well-organized that many reformers have enough to snarl about. Money backed by nothing but the credit of the state made it possible to abolish slavery in the US. Today Globalization and Deregulation is well on the way of bringing it back. The suppression of all information on money creation and its background in economic history, is complete in our universities.

Had this happened during the Depression of the Thirties, we would never have left the Depression behind, and Hitler would probably have won WWII. Go to any second-hand book store and seek out university text books on economics published before 1991, and the chances are that you will find an explanation of how the banking system created nine times the statutory reserves of legal tender – i.e., federal government credit – that it kept with the central bank. Today with the banks' newly acquired brokerage, underwriting, merchant banking firms, and derivative boutiques, that multiplier in Canada hovers around 380 to one, and there is no reference to money creation in our university texts. And our hyperactive deregulated banks are exposed to every stock market bubble. Of course, the two phenomena are closely connected. *W.K.*

TAX CUTS AND THE BUSH DEFICIT

"Secure Location" to Earth: Deficits Don't Matter

A RECENTLY PUBLISHED BOOK not only reveals the extent to which the tax-cuts took centre-stage in Washington's policies, but the extent to which the president is manipulated by stronger wills in the administration. *The Price of Loyalty* is written by former *Wall Street Journal* reporter, Ron Suskind, based partly upon a series of interviews with former Treasury Secretary, Paul O'Neill, and partly upon access to documents that include some almost verbatim reports of Bush cabinet meetings.

After the mid-term elections in 2002, O'Neill, concerned about the growing deficit, argued against a second round of tax cuts. Cheney's answer to O'Neill was, "You know, Paul, Reagan proved that deficits don't matter. We won the mid-term elections, this is our due." O'Neill was flabbergasted by this rapacious attitude.

Shortly afterwards, the tax cuts were decided upon at a meeting in the White House. Cheney participated by video-link from his "secure location." Everyone expected Mr. Bush to rubber stamp the new big tax cut designed for the wealthy once more to get most of the benefits. O'Neill alone voiced opposition. But, uncharacteristically, the President had some second thoughts. "Haven't we already given money to rich people? This second tax cut's gonna do it again." Now, somebody said, "Well Mr. President, the upper class, they're the entrepreneurs." The president first goes along with this, but then returns to his apprehensions. "But, shouldn't we be giving money to the middle, won't people be able to say, You did it once, and then you did it twice, and what was it good for?"

A Lesson Learned

Was Bush already grappling with the possible impact of too one-sided policies would have on the approaching elections? With the President vacillating, political advisor Karl Rove jumped in: "Stick to principle. Stick to principle." This he repeats over and over again like a mantra. "Don't waver." With that, Bush sputters out and the matter is settled. A week later Cheney called O'Neill and told him he was out.

Since this meeting, Rove must have had Bush under intensive coaching in the art of staying on message. Whenever he pops up on a TV screen these days, one can be sure that, the tax cut message will be woven into his speech. However, there is now a difference: the focus is not on new tax cuts. After all, tax cuts implemented this far have lowered federal revenue to roughly 16.5 percent of GDP, the lowest level since the 1950s.

This time, the main goal is to make the tax cuts permanent, canceling the existing sunset provisions. However, such a change will once again upset the deficit forecasts.

Staking the elections on making the tax-cuts permanent confuses the issue, so that the average Americans don't realize the high costs they are being tagged with. They have already been confronted with rising local taxes and user fees, while in many areas services have been deteriorating.

Forgotten: The Propensity to Consume

On top of all that the employment situation has been bleak. Thus far, the tally is 2.5 million jobs lost. That threatens to make Bush the first President since Hoover with a term of net job losses. And the return to high job growth that is constantly touted remains elusive: The number of jobs created in February was only 21,000. Since 75,000 new jobs monthly are considered necessary just to keep up with demographic growth, the recovery is still essentially jobless.

A main avenue for achieving the necessary obfuscation has been to try equating tax cuts with growth. This would paint democratic attempts to hold the tax cuts in check or even roll them back as a sure road to diminished prosperity.

An advisor to Bush has claimed that all economic textbooks state that tax cuts lead to growth. This comment was, of course, nonsense. No serious economists, even of the most neo-liberal brand, would make such an unqualified connection. This is a good example of how spurious "economic laws" more and more are being invoked in defense of socially unbalanced policies.

Had our good economic advisor leafed a bit further into his economic textbooks, he would have met the concept of propensity to consume. When a sagging economy receives a tax cut, how it actually translates into boosting the economy depends on the recipients' propensity to consume. That shows how people divide a marginal disposable dollar (that is, an extra dollar either earned or retained because of a tax reduction) between consumption and savings.

Low and middle incomes naturally have considerably higher propensities to consume, sometimes even reaching 100 percent, while high incomes have low propensities to consume. Since most of the money accruing from the Bush' tax cuts went to the rich, relatively little of it has been pumped back into the economy through consumption. Thus, while the Bush tax cuts may have helped the stock market to recover, their impact on the real economy was not significant. They might quite possibly have held the economy back even in the short term, and certainly in the long term, when the deficit starts to take its toll in earnest.

Meanwhile, Bush has his friends he can count on in a tight spot. So on bad days when the disappointing job numbers dominated the news cycle, Steve "Flat Tax" Forbes sprang into action. There is still room to push taxes even lower, he intoned over the air waves. There is no alternative to Bush's policies if continued prosperity is the goal. And, happily, we are still the world's leader in creating economic growth.

With his statements Steve Forbes showed that besides being the perennial champion of a flat tax, he is, in fact, living in a flat world. In it there only exists one dimension which can be used to measure growth: whether or not the assets of the "rich" are going up in value.

The reality is that growth has many dimensions. The income of middle-class families, for instance, whose incomes in real, inflation-adjusted terms has been stagnant since the Reagan years. Only during the last Clinton years did they experience a mild bump upwards. Exacerbating their problems is the spectre of unemployment and spiraling down into the pool of unskilled or wrong-skilled workers, when their current jobs are offshored. For such families, it is not a good economy, no matter how many billionaires have been added the most recent list in Forbes magazine.

The almost religious belief of neo-conservatives that the United States is the world's undisputed leader in economic growth, is once again a view seen from the perspective of a flat economic universe, where only value measures defined by the Americans are valid.

The Myopia of American Neo-conservatism

However, there are other factors defining the picture. The United States has a growing problem arising from its disdain for public institutions. The Bush slash-and-burn policies towards all public institutions (except the military, of course) have not helped. Development of infrastructural networks and maintaining social services, that only can be properly done in the public domain, are increasingly neglected.

Traditionally, the European Union core states have had both considerably higher tax levels and a more activist conception of government than the United States. Therefore, besides straight money-valued GDP comparisons, there are other important factors to be considered, that the American neo-conservatives refuse to acknowledge. First, the value of public goods and services are calculated at costs, which means that nations with higher levels of public goods and service creation will show GDP figures undervalued by standard measures. Second, the European nations with an activist public role, have been better at controlling the negative "externalities" created by the production and transport activities of industrialized societies. Third, they have been better at preserving sensitive nature and heritage areas, and promoting a more widespread access to art and other cultural activities, in contrast to the American, "make money or die" attitude.

As such, the international statistics are closer aligned to the American concept, making it look better than its reality is. The apparent wealth of American economy increasingly is due to a rising number of unpaid bills, that sooner or later will knock on the door.

Dix Sandbeck

"So Near to the United States, So Far from God"

IN A SEEDY DISTRICT alongside the old University in Havana stands a touching cluster of memorials to a batch of medical students who had taken up arms in the early 1870s against Spain, and were executed on this site. With characteristic Cuban bite, the figures falling before the firing squad are shown not in bas relief, but concave, scooped out as were their lives. It could allude as well to the later kidnapping by William Randolph Hearst and Teddy Roosevelt of the fruits of Cuba's three-decade struggle against Spain or to the lot of so much of Latin America. Symbolism within symbolism, when I chanced on it, a humble citizen was relieving himself against the memorial.

Mexico in particular came to mind, the land that under Lazaro Cardenas in the 1930s had stood up to Washington as Benito Juarez had to France before.

And consider how low Mexico has fallen, degraded to the land of the maquiladoras that pollute its northern frontier. Above all with respect to its banking, the institution that has come to dominate the world. *The Wall Street Journal* (17/03, "Political pressure builds on Mexico's foreign banks" by John Lyons): "When Mexico's top bankers gather tomorrow for their annual meeting in Acapulco, everybody from President Vicente Fox to former US Treasury secretary Robert Rubin will show up for the lavish ritual. But actual Mexican banks will be in short supply."

A Warning for Canada?

"Nearly a decade after a Mexican financial crisis all but wiped out the world financial system, the foreign banks bought up the remains of Mexico's banks, and now dominate the domestic market. World powers such as Citigroup Inc. of NY, Spain's Santander Central Hispano SA and HSBC Holdings PLC of Britain, control 85% of local banking assets, the highest ratio of foreign ownership in Latin America.

"These banks are turning gigantic profits. They also face growing resentment and political pressure that may make the operating environment tougher in the years to come. An increasingly vocal group of executives and public officials say the banks have betrayed the public trust by failing to lend to individual borrowers and small and mid-size businesses.

"Lawmakers, already pressing banks to return some funds received in the 1995 bank rescue, plan to call bank executives to formal hearings on why lending has lagged behind other Latin nations, says Representative Francisco Suarez y Davila, secretary of the lower house Finance Committee. The hearings may lead to closer regulation of banking fees or new laws to lower borrowing costs and increase competition among lenders.

"A long-time friend of the banks, Guillermo Ortiz, who in a previous post oversaw the privatization of the state-owned banking system, has publicly opposed plans by Spain's Banco Bilbao Vizcaya Argentaria SA to purchase all the outstanding shares in its Mexican unit and remove it from the local stock exchange. That would undermine the equities market and shroud Mexico's largest bank from scrutiny of financial analysts, he says.

"The prospect of congressional hearings, new banking regulations and a move to audit the terms of the nine-year-old bailout threaten to alter the framework of a financial system that has been fortified with international management, new technology and more than $20 billion (US) of foreign investment since 1999. If they materialize, the changes may limit profits and prompt lenders to delay investments in the $600 billion economy, banks say.

"As yet, foreign banks show no sign of backing away from Latin America's biggest economy, also seen as back door into the growing US Hispanic market.

"BBVA's $4.1 billion tender offer for the outstanding shares in Grupo Financiero BBVA Bancomer will write one of the closing chapters in the transformation of the banking system. The transaction, which has regulatory approval and will go forward despite Mr. Ortiz's concerns, will leave only one of Mexico's top five banks, Grupo Financiero Banorte in local hands.

"Acquisitions have paid off for the foreign banks. Citigroup's Banamex unit contributed $1.45 billion, or about 8%, to the world's biggest financial services company's bottom line. Europe's largest lender cited its acquisition of Grupo Financiero Bital SA as a major reason its profit rose 41% last year. Profits at Bancomer equal about a quarter of the income earned by all of BBVA.

"Still, executives complain that instead of providing credit to companies that could become engines for economic growth, banks profit by expensive commissions for services such as credit cards and filling loan portfolios with government bonds.

"Mexican commercial bank loans to the private sector equal about 15% of gross domestic product, central bank figures show. That compares to about 67% in Latin America's other big investment-grade economy, Chile, and 36% in Brazil, according to UBS Warburg."

Washington's Revenge for the Oil Expropriation?

The loss of 85% of their banks to foreign ownership has been particularly humiliating to Mexicans, for whom the nationalization of their oil fields in 1937 is still a principal anchor of national self-respect. In 1982 Mexico's banking system was on the verge of collapse, the first major victim of the unbridled speculation brought on by the neo-Con free market faith imposed on the world by the US. Wedded to Mexico's endemic political corruption, the unbridled powers entrusted to the free market could have no other outcome. Paul Volcker's mad attempt to impose a flat price level with screechingly high interest rates on a world that was rapidly adopting higher technologies, and urbanizing, was the final blow. The Federal District of Mexico with a population of some 35 million is one of the three largest urban spreads in the world, and that means a lot more tax money must be spent on the most basic services. The precipitous fall of oil prices added to the disaster, as did the heads stuffed with free market theology that Mexican advisers brought back from their studies at US universities. In 1982 to forestall the collapse of the Mexican banking system, the banks were nationalized.

For a decade the Mexican banks operated under government ownership along relatively conservative lines. In their absence from speculative areas, the stock market took over most of the unofficial money creation. Financial and political power shifted from the old corrupt political bosses and trade union leaders to a new group of daring stock market operators who soon had a lock-hold of the entire economy. Only the banks were missing in their tool-kit. That was made good under Carlos Salinas de Gortari who assumed the presidency in 1990. Eventually the unbridled boom that resulted was to haunt the US itself.

Mexico's financial hyper-inflation spread to Eastern Asia and to Russia, and came back to Washington's doorstep. Early in its regime the Salinas government retained C.S. First Boston as General Counsel to advise the government on the privatization of the banks. It was hardly a happy choice. The reputation of C.S. First Boston was founded on its aggressive prominence in the field of mergers and privatizations.

For one thing it reversed the order of things throughout much of the world. In Canada and the US, following upon the stricken banks' bailout of the early 1990s, the banks were further deregulated to take over the stock markets, and just about every other engine of money creation. In Mexico, with the banks nationalized, the new wave of hyperinflationary money creation began with the stock market and the new group of speculators that dominated it. These mated a proficiency in handling the new speculative tools such as derivatives with the old Mexican tradition of financial rot. Once they had amassed fortunes a digit or two higher than that of the old bankers, they

took over the banks that were privatized again in 1991.

During this period the rise in speculative activity against the Mexican peso, exceeded anything known before. With the reprivatization of the banks largely by their sale to foreign conglomerates, all this overflowed into the financial markets of the world. And with the flight of Mexican speculative capital out of the peso, the Mexican government began issuing debt denominated in dollars.

Mexico's financial system was hollowed out. And its misadventures spread to the Far Eastern countries, to Europe, Russia and the United States itself. The threat to the world financial system was so great that Clinton Government took the initiative in setting up a $51 billion emergency fund to prevent a worldwide financial collapse. The chapter – which would have been unthinkable without the US imposition of Globalization and Deregulation on the world – has been described as the first large crisis of the 21st century. It left Mexico crushed under a burden of US-denominated debt.

Mexican big players seem to have reconstructed their own financial system as a huge accordion, It gambled the capital of the domestic banks into insolvency, and at that point, the government at a vast cost to the nation, nationalized the banks. And then when they had been brought back to a degree of health, they were sold to foreign and the odd domestic stock market tycoon who had used the period of nationalized banks to shift the stock market as the major vehicle of unbridled credit creation. And the "Washington Consensus" guaranteed that the world would dance to the irresistible rhythms streaming out from Mexico. It poisoned further the relations of Washington with Latin America. It was hardly a helpful backdrop for Washington's Iraqi adventure.[1]

Latin America Talks Back to Washington

Thus *The New York Times* (8/01, "Latin America is Speaking Up" by Christopher Marquis) informs us: "Latin American leaders say they are newly pragmatic in their relations with the United States. They are also unafraid to challenge Washington, even in the face of considerable pressure. In the United Nations Security Council, Chile and Mexico opposed a resolution authorizing force in Iraq, and only 7 out of 33 Latin American and Caribbean nations supported military action.

"When Roger Noriega, the assistant secretary of state for Latin America, criticized Argentina's warming relationship with Cuba, the reaction from Buenos Aires was swift and indignant, with one cabinet official declaring that the days of 'automatic alignments; with Washington were over.'

"When Brazil led nations in insisting that American farm subsidies and steel protections be included in trade negotiations, Robert B. Zoellick, the US trade representative, lashed out at what he terms 'won't do' nations. But Brazil held its ground on a watered-down agreement that set aside the most sensitive issues."

The Wall Street Journal (12/02, "Latin America Grows Poorer Despite Boom" by Joel Millman) informs us from Lima, Peru: "On paper, Latin America is enjoying boom times. Surging commodity prices for everything from copper and iron ore to soya beans and fish meal, have powered growth in gross domestic product, almost entirely owing to swelling demand from China. Currencies are stable and low US interest rates have made borrowing inexpensive. GDP has grown an average of 4% across the region for the last three years, nearly triple the average in the 1990s.

"Yet a gloomy undertone permeated the annual meeting of the board of governors of the Inter-American Development Bank last month. The reason: even under such promising conditions, Latin America is getting poorer.

"'It may surprise you to learn that during the past decade Latin American and Caribbean governments increased social expenditure, in real terms, by about 58% per capita,' Enrique V. Iglesias, the president of the Inter-American Development Bank, told delegates in his welcoming speech. Yet the results were dismal. 'After a decade of higher social spending,' he said, 'there are many more poor people now than in 1900,' with at least 20 million new poor slipping below the poverty line since 1997."

That should not be surprising, even beyond the serious misrepresentations built into the GDP statistic wherever it is used. The vast processes of urbanization under way throughout Latin America replaces many of the supports of pre-market economies ignored by the GDP, that are lost when people flock into large cities.

"Meanwhile, Latin America's debt problem is worsening. Despite billions of dollars raised through the privatizations of state assets such as telephone companies, iron mines and railroads, Latin America's overall debt-to-GDP ratio has risen to 51% of GDP in 2002 from 37% in 1997. Foreign investment has plunged by 20% in that same period. Unemployment was up to 15% in 2002 from 10% in 1997.

"If all this is occurring in good times, many at the meeting wondered, what can Latin America expect when borrowing rates begin to rise again, as they must as soon as US rates go up? Historically, every rise of two percentage points on US rates has translated into upticks of five percentage points or more in Latin America, Mr. Iglesias warned."

That is readily understood. As rates go up, the quality of Latin American debt deteriorates, and a premium is tacked on by lenders. It should be noted that credit card debt is being pursued avidly not only in Latin America, but in Eastern and South Asia and Eastern Europe. It provides the growth that has replaced all Ten Commandments as the condition for survival in today's world.

Even without Washington's military adventures the outlook for the world is unsmiling.

William Krehm

1. My source for the details of the Mexican bank nationalization in 1982 and its reprivatization of 1991, is a magnificently detailed study, "La Singular Historia del Rescate Bancario Mexicano de 1994 a 1999 y el Relevante Papel del Fobaproa," ("The Unusual history of the Mexican Bank Bailout of 1994 to 1999 and the Lender of the Last Resort"), by Francisco Javier Vega Rodriguez, Biblioteca Plural, Economia, Finanzas y Politica, Mexico, 1999. The parallel with Canada's bank bailout, e.g., the suppression of the banks' statutory reserves and much else is striking. We will review this imposing work in detail in our next issue.

BOOK REVIEW

Light from Mexico

La singular Historia del Rescate Bancario Mexicano 1994-1999 (The Amazing Bank Bailout of Mexico 1994-1999) by Francisco J. Vega Rodriguez, Biblioteca Plural Economia, Finanza y Politica, 1999, Mexico, 780 pages)

THE EVIDENCE that Globalization and Deregulation was not working has piled up so high that it is toppling over on all continents. Crowning interest rates as sole "tool" for enforcing the unenforceable – a flat price level in a world undergoing undreamt of urbanization and technological revolution – has split the world into murderous camps. The Koran after all condemns to eternal hell-fire those persisting in charging interest, let alone making usury the cornerstone of statesmanship. Historians like the late Ferdinand Braudel long ago caught the point that a developed urbanized society implies vastly more public services and thus a growing layer of taxation in price. Yet the point still eludes economists.[1]

So I decided to celebrate my 90th year sampling some of the "heterodox economic conferences" springing up across the world. The 1930s had been a period of black despair, but at least there was a substantial degree of free enquiry even in Washington. Without that, the world could never have groped its way out of the Depression. Even high executives of some large corporations espoused heterodox views on money creation. A Utah banker. Marriner Eccles, was Roosevelt's Secretary of the Treasury, largely responsible for the reform of the monetary system along "Keynesian" lines without having heard of Keynes.

Keynes not only rethought much basic economic theory, but gave due credit to the great independent thinkers in the field – Karl Marx, Gesell, Douglas. Resistance to such rethinking came less from governments than from academic economists. In Oxbridge it was his colleagues who restrained the otherwise unrestrainable Keynes from going public with his ultimate conclusion – "Equilibrium [theory] is blither."

A Back Door Left Open for the Bank Comeback

The urgencies of the war and reconstruction provided the framework for the emergency work to be done. But the language of "official" economists remained that of equilibrium theory that assumed a self-balancing "pure and perfect market." And that left the back door open for a comeback of the financial sector, when it finally got out of the doghouse. Banks had been severely separated from other capital pools, such as insurance and the stock market, precisely because of their money-creation powers. Ceilings had been set on what interest they could pay or charge. But left flying on the flagpole, marginal theory proclaimed that stable prices will result from a "free and perfect" market that in a stunning bit of circular reasoning was itself

defined as one that keeps prices stable. All actors are posited of such tiny size that nothing any one does or doesn't do can affect the market. However, when the immense public investment got underway to repair the neglect of 10 years of depression and six of war, when price controls came off (just in time for the Korean war!), prices moved up jauntily. And that set the stage for a *coup d'état* behind President Truman's back. The Treasury and the Federal Reserve had been negotiating for weeks about adjusting interest rates to the price movement. In his memoirs Truman tells of his surprise in learning that his own Treasury had double-crossed him, and surrendered the interest-rate peg as such. In the long run that empowered the banks to throttle and choke.

The book that we are reviewing begins by establishing that the "free and perfect market" is something that never existed. It goes on to show that Deregulation and Globalization, blasting in from Washington, combined with Mexico's rich tradition of corruption to give rise to crises that just missed bringing down the world financial system.

In 1981 Mexico's banks were in such bad shape that the government nationalized them as a "more economical way of avoiding their bankruptcy than bailing them out." The dean of specialists on the international economy, Robert Triffin of Yale, on analyzing the venerable institution of the gold standard, concluded that the textbooks describe what never existed. Similarly, the existence of a respectable, orthodox banking tradition in Mexico before the banks' nationalization is a fiction created by those who lost their power. Legislation had granted immense discretion to the private bankers. In the late 1960s and early 1970s the merging of banks was allowed and a banking monopoly resulted. Special privileges took the form of anonymity of bank stockholders, preferential tax treatment, and the prohibition of bank employees' unions. The Bank of Mexico, the central bank, was a limited society, with private bankers prominent on its board.

"The structure of the banking system shielded speculators from undesirable obligations of ownership so ingeniously as to attain sheer beauty. The banks could advance funds to economic agents (corporation treasuries, and exchange and stock market operators) having ties to bank shareholders. The latter in turn were able to buy dollars against nominal guarantees. And when speculation approached its peak, the wealthiest of these could secretly divest themselves of their equity, and deposit the proceeds in *offshore* banks. Such scams continued long after the reserves of the central bank had vanished and devaluation was inevitable.

"Such practices made the economic elite particularly arrogant in their dealing with government functionaries who knew that they would shortly be shorn of office. That is basic to the crisis psychology that accompanies the installation of a new president every six years. The nationalization of the banks in 1982 was not a response to populist pressure. It resulted in a lack of mediation between the incoming and outgoing elites.

"In addition, during the 1981-2 deficit, Mexico's foreign balance of payments suffered from a dramatic fall in oil prices, and the explosion of international interest rates due to the madcap monetarist experiment of the US Federal Reserve under Paul Volcker in the name of prudence. The Mexican market experienced an acute shortage of both domestic and foreign currency. Between 1977 and 1981 four fifths of the deficit in the current account was due to financial services. The financial deficit, amounted in 1982 to 16% of the NDP. The collapse of the economy was imminent.

"The government of Jose Lopez Portillo responded with what has been considered the 'first macroeconomic readjustment since the oil boom of 1977-1980. This consisted of a combination of orthodox and heterodox remedies. Its main components were:

"Devaluation of the currency, with rate changes for successive quarters of 8.4%, 10.7%, 12.4%, and 16.4%. Import controls. Increasing domestic interest rates. A projected domestic budget reduction of 8%.

Mexico's Debt Becomes Dollar-denominated

"Only the circle around the President failed to see that the projected devaluation would lead to a panicky flight of capital. Between 1980 and 1981, $10,915 million left the land. By October, 1981 inflation had shot up to 100%, the federal debt doubled to $12,544 million. Bank liabilities had become dollar-denominated. The debt of firms exploded in peso terms. Deregulation and Globalization prevented any barrier to the free exchange of currencies. In February,1982, the free float of the peso advocated by Milton Friedman was brought in.

"Reintroducing import controls.

"Increasing export subsidies.

"Increasing domestic interest rates.

"A projected reduction in the annual budget of the public sector of 8%.

"The policy pursued after February 19th was the usual orthodox macroeconomics. The 1983 budget showed a reduction of 3% over that of the previous year; domestic interest rates were raised; restrictions on imports were removed; users' fees were increased in the public sector; and confirmation issued that Mexico would respect international commitments. An onerous increase in private debt resulted from both the higher interest rates and the devaluation. This led to labour disputes and threatened the liquidity of large Mexican corporations. By June Mexico was no longer able to obtain foreign credits without special guarantees. There was nowhere to go but nationalize the banking system. Only under government guarantee could Mexico hope for more credit.

"The outgoing president Lopez Portilla began negotiations with the IMF. This paved the way for a new era of austerity under his successor, President de la Madrid. The central bank authorized the banks to receive deposits that could be withdrawn at pre-established dates, the withdrawals being denominated in so-called Mex-dollars. Like the *tesobonos* – dollar bonds issued

by the government – they left the economy vulnerable to further shocks. No margin remained for further flights of capital. Nationalization of the banks and general control of all currency change alone could stave off total disaster. The American press and even the banks, temporarily set aside their prejudices against nationalization.

"Under cover of the technological and financial revolutions, centuries of experience went into the dust-bin. It was proclaimed that only a free market could guarantee order and progress. And its key weaponry was the new derivative products: futures, options, swaps. The resulting experiments encroached on the state domain. Denationalizing the currency was part of the program. Money creation was to be shifted from public to private firms."[2]

Bank nationalization left the stock market with a virtual monopoly of speculative money creation in Mexico. This reversed the sequence in Canada where the control of money creation had been shifted from the central bank to private bankers; and then by further bank deregulation, to a stock market that banks, drawing on their annual entitlement under their bailout, had been able to take over to a growing extent.

"In Mexico the elevation of the stock market elite to control had to do with the explosion of government debt. The main component of this were the 'CETES' distributed by auctions on the stock market. This deprived the nationalized banks of the lucrative business of placing the government's swelling debt." The new stock market elite grew fat and imperious. For sheer cheek, it even outstripped what happened in Canada where our banks, freshly bailed-out, were then deregulated.

In either case, the Bard put it best: "Thrift, Thrift, Horatio, The funeral baked meats did coldly furnish forth the marriage tables."

Not all Bubbles come from Clay Pipes

The bubble on the Mexican Bolsa de Valores was without precedent. In 1982 there had been only 66,000 investors trading on that stock market, but by September 1987, this had risen to 4.17 million. Many folks mortgaged or sold their houses and automobiles to plunge into the game. On October 5, a day after the inauguration of President Salinas, shares traded were up 26,677 points during the first hour. Two weeks later, this had become "Black Monday." Panic took over. Everybody wanted to sell, but no buyers were around. More than 180 thousand investors lost their money at a single stroke. Multi-millionaires suddenly found themselves penniless, but the brokerage houses overnight acquired huge fortunes. A new financial elite had replaced the banks which, due to their nationalization, were absent from the orgy.

"The euphoria culminating in this crash, the devaluation of the peso, and the subsidence of inflation all resulted from President Miguel de la Madrid's obstinate insistence to pay off the debt. It had grave consequences on income distribution, employment and production. The magnitude of the transfers for interest payments abroad were compared with the tribute paid after a lost war. It brought on the break-up of the old government party, the PRI, after more than a half-century in power. In the 1990s. the 'technocratic' takeover produced an armed revolution in the southern state of Chiapas, and rocked the economy.

"When Carlos Salinas de Gortari took over the presidency, after the most questioned election since the war, he proposed bringing the economy back to health by an ambitious program of privatization. It was to take place in fields as diverse as telecommunications, mining, food production, and above all the banks. And it led to the free trade treaty (TLC). On top of that he staged a series of political coups (the jailing of trade union leaders, and notorious functionaries and promoters) that won him some popular support. Few suspected that all this would lead to the most devastating Mexican crisis since 1910.

"A radical rethinking of the role of the state began. No longer were growing powers of government over the economy seen as progress. Throughout the world an anti-statist counter-revolution had begun.

"It was with a touch of mourning, that the general directors of the nationalized banks met at the Mexican president's residence, Los Pinos, on May 2, 1990. They had already been notified that their banks were to be privatized. Despite their economic persuasion, heading a government bank had bestowed on them all sorts of influence. However, as usually happens in Mexico, the Minister of the Interior had already summoned the members of the ruling party in the national legislatures and among the state governors and informed them of the position to take. None of them, including the minister himself, was without misgivings. The nationalized banks, with PRI members occupying key positions and sharing information to which only banks are privy, had its advantages. Virtually only the party of the left, the PRD, founded by Cuauhtemoc Cardenas, son of the president who in 1936 had nationalized the petroleum industry, opposed the privatization. What would be next? The national oil company itself?

The Vast Booty of Privatization

"Yet the booty for insiders was vast – 18 bank corporations, 4,500 branches (40 abroad), 200,000 employees not allowed to organize trade unions. Stock brokers, the business tycoons and financiers of Monterrey, and the former bank owners competed for the quarry."

Canadians should be interested in the detail that one of the advantages offered bankers by the privatization was the replacement of statutory reserves in legal tender (encaje legal) with a liquidity quotient of 30% of the banks' liabilities. This corresponded to the abolition of the statutory reserves in the 1991 Canadian Bank Act revision slipped through our Parliament in 1991. Both in Mexico and Canada these moves allowed the banks far greater leverage in their operations. "The concept of 'liquidity' is difficult to confirm in the real banking world." Instead of "cash," the ghost-like concept of "liquidity" became the yardstick of bank soundness. In Mexico, for a tiny portion of the going rate on Wall St., you could get an accountant to swear that a bank's liability was "capital."

Government bonds, proclaimed "risk-free" by the Bank for International Settlement's *Risk-Based Capital Requirements*

guidelines brought in shortly before, actually lose value whenever the central banks push interest rates on new bond-issues higher than the coupons of the old ones hoarded by banks under the new dispensations. And higher interest rate to "lick inflation" had become holy script to central banks. In Canada it made it possible for banks to quadruple their holdings of federal debt without putting up money of their own. The effect in Mexico was similar. It paved the way for the Mexican bank crisis of 1994 that almost brought down the world financial system.

"After the banks were privatized, the 'liquidity coefficient' was wholly suppressed. This was the main factor flaring Mexico's credit bubble. The so-called 'L' bond series was introduced that allowed holding companies to acquire liabilities and to merge with other financial companies in highly leveraged transactions."

"The belief took over that the unfailing mechanism of the market would itself ensure order. A new bumper harvest of 'derivative' products were contrived to serve the experiments in globalization and deregulation: futures, options, swaps. This moved in step with the proposals of the most radical neo-classical thinkers like Professor Hayek who advocated the closing down of central banks and denationalizing the currencies. Money creation was to be entrusted to private enterprise." Mexico was marching to a world bass drum. Since the early 1970s no other legal tender existed in the world than the debt of government. Government, from "the lender of the last resort," was overnight transmuted to the donor of the first resort. In this way the multiplication of government debt was brought about by the very monetarists who professed to loathe it.

"In choosing C.S. First Boston as advisers for the bank privatization, the outgoing Mexican president, Carlos Salinas, passed on a time-bomb to his successor, Ernesto Zedillo. In its report First Boston, true mercenary, emphasized the rise in the stock market index – 69% and 37% in dollar terms during 1989 and 1990. Citing the relative low ratio of prices to earnings compared to that of most markets in the world, it presented the Mexican market as the most liquid in Latin America, and the best serviced. On the market crash of 1987, and the financial scandals that led to jail sentences, it was mum."

"[Instead] the rapidity with which privatization was carried out and the handsome prices obtained for the banks were interpreted as a sign of the Salinas administration's success." Obviously no small part of the expertise of First Boston was its skill in misleading markets. A few months later, in the elections for the deputies of the Assembly, the official party, the PRI, swept in victoriously, without need for fraud. Between June 7, 1991, and July 3, 1992, every single bank was taken over by private buyers.

"But trouble loomed. To straddle the gap between the dollar and the peso and cover the banks' losses, the government had issued *ajustabonos*, middle- and long-term debt in dollars. But another canyon suddenly yawned deep and wide. To lick 'inflation' once and for all Paul Volcker, head of the Federal Reserve in the United States, was shoving up interest rates, without thought of the effect on banks that had loaded up with totally leveraged debt as the means of their bailout. As the international interest rates continued rising, the market value of earlier debt with lower coupons plummeted. A single bank, Banamex, was absorbing 200 million of old pesos lost in *ajustabonos*, and the plight other banks and brokerage houses was similar. The National Banking Commission, the National Securities Commission, and the Bank of Mexico had no clue of these losses. A special futures market in these instruments papered over the evidence. This black-out of reliable information had been critical for the privatization success taken as a sign of the soundness of Mexican banks. Only much later was it revealed that they had unloaded *ajustabono*s and other low-yield securities onto their trusting clients to earn handsome commissions and lighten their own exposure."

First Boston's Expertise in Misleading Markets

And on top of it all was the swarm of new derivatives, some hardly understood even by their authors on Wall St., and completely beyond the ken of the Mexican market. The lights simply went out in Mexico's hour of trial. And from this witches' brew a miraculously self-balancing market was supposed to emerge!

"Not until 1994, three years later, did the government make even a pretence of bringing in rigid capital requirements for the banks."

It is a remarkable feature of the Vega book that for each of the great bank scandals the author breaks down the complex frauds coming together from all directions – Wall St. and Pancho Villa traditions, derivatives and political bagman smarts. And in doing so the book, published in 1999, was able to anticipate many irregularities similar to those Eliot Spitzer exposed years later. The major role in all this of blind faith in the self-balancing market is laid bare – something absent in Spitzer's otherwise spectacular performance. In both the US and Europe, piety warns off research as it approaches ground consecrated to burial rather than disinterment. There the Canadian record is the most dismal – near-total absence of investigations that might embarrass Bay St.

Take for example, what Vega calls "Typical operations of bank treasuries and money shops based on private intermediation.

"The present market and bank treasuries in Mexico allow significant trades of bank and government securities outside the market through simple off-record agreements. This is known as 'private intermediation' that by-passes licensed brokerages and banks. One of several examples:

"The promoter in a brokerage or bank attracts clients by offering loans at yields varying from 0.25% to 2.5% below market. The brokerage or bank then places the loans directly on the interbank market or through the intermediary. The yield is guaranteed.

"The promoter receives the commissions of the brokerage or bank as profit arising from the differential in the yields agreed upon. Taxes are paid. The net profit of the promoter is shared amongst all those involved. Brokerages in particular succeeded in contriving commissions amounting from 20 to 60%. In this variant the longer term loans are the most profitable and most sought after."

The play here is attracting borrowers with lower rates, and then creeping up on them with exorbitant ongoing commissions. Something similar is practised in Canada and the US – abusing innocent customers with initial low rates.

"Those who work this strange market, carry out different combinations [involving differentials not only of interest rates, but of currency exchange rates]. Some prefer small returns in yield so that the quotes don't differ markedly from market and the game is less likely to be unmasked. Profits though small are constant. Other operators prefer adhering to normal practice and then surprising the victim from time to time with substantial divergences. Whatever the route chosen, the result can be a substantial transfer of wealth. It can work only in a highly concentrated market as to location, complexity of financial instruments available, an intimate buddy-system, and the existence of private intermediation, controls feeble or absent. Mexico satisfied all these requirements."

Derivatives, still unregulated, help immensely in keeping such deals off balance-sheet, and capitalizing the lack of transparency. They permit the unrecorded sale and even the shorting from an original equity position while still peddling the stock to clients. This happened with at least of two of the largest Canadian banks in Enron partnerships, and earned them a huge fines plus public-relation black eyes.

There has never, of course, been a better laboratory for studying scabrous financial practices than Mexico And to not a few of these its great northern neighbour has generously contributed.

"Early in 1996 the Mexican National Commission on Banking and Securities issued a report on a series of typical operations on the local financial market over the previous decades. The report concluded an underground network had been created in just two decades made possible a vast accumulation of private wealth that transformed the very political and economic structure of the country.

"Mexico's financial bubble had been blown up to such outlandish proportions, that the question arises, how could it have been unchallenged? Vega addresses the question, and draws heavily on the warnings of John Kenneth Galbraith who had certainly sounded his magic whistle forewarning of the busts of 1987 and 1994 – to little effect. Rudiger Dornbusch of MIT had conducted a campaign pointing out that Mexico had to devalue its currency by 20% to reduce its commercial deficit and its dependence on foreign credit. The entire apparatus of the Mexican state reacted by satanizing Dornbusch as 'a dangerous man.' Speaking engagements were cancelled. Mexican economic policy became entangled with the marketing needs of New York financial houses, as well as with those of the new elite at home."

The argument of *The Wall Street Journal* and others was that the since the commercial deficit arose from the expansion of the private sector it was not dangerous but necessary. Besides Mexico's growth rate was nowhere near that of Singapore! But the money borrowed abroad was not invested in building factories. Instead, it covered the short-term borrowing of the government, and the flight of capital from the country. Agustin

Carstens of the Bank of Mexico defended "a monetary policy that was strictly anti-inflationary, and cited the econometric doctrine of "Monetary Neutrality" of Robert Lucas, that was supposed to prove that the monetary variables had no real economic effect "in the long run." Lucas was the Nobel Prize for Economics laureate of 1995.

Sitting in the Soup

Since the notion of a "level playing field" is basic to equilibrium theory, let us examine this Monetary Neutrality theory in its light. The different actors, and the different social classes are affected in quite different ways by the unlimited "long run" that the "free market" may take to work its supposed magic. Financial institutions are consoled by ever higher interest rates during the long wait. Their income becomes richer en route. That is hardly the case with those thrown out of jobs to bring in the "natural rate of unemployment." Even the formulation of such a model, let alone bestowing a prize on its authors, is an insolence.

However, it was on these grounds that the Bank of Mexico rested its case for doing nothing about the peso's overpricing:

"The deficit on current account is simply the counterpart of the positive balance in the capital account.

"The existence of perfect financial markets proves that there can be no such thing as an overvalued currency.

"The exchange value of the peso is determined by real factors, and it cannot be affected in a lasting way by any monetary or exchange rate policy."

During the Russian Civil War of the early 1920s, the great Russian satirist, Isaac Babel, wrote a powerfully mordant account of the atrocities of both sides in his "Red Cavalry." This drew a sharp rebuke from the legendary Soviet cavalry chief Marshal Budyenny, who made much of the fact that comrade Babel (who also happened to be a Jew) served in the commissariat and took no part in the actual fighting. To this Lenin is supposed to have replied, "Comrade Budyenny, to be a good cook, you don't have to sit in the soup." Sometimes, however, that does help. And that was the case of Mexico on the receiving end of just about every swindle that Wall St., the US academe, and its own gifted financiers could devise.

"Denting these dreams of equilibrium, imbalances grew severe enough to trigger disastrous political effects of serious economic consequence. Thus the Zapatista rebellion broke out in southern Mexico. The assassination of two leading figures of the Mexican official party – were clear indications that the old alliances of different social groups reaching back over sixty years were crumbling. The sense of well-being created by the prospect of the *Free Trade Treaty* suffered. Mexico lost $10 billion of its $28 billion cash reserves. By the end of 1994 the outstanding *tesobonos* that little more than a year before had amounted to $1.3 billion touched the $20 billion figure. To make matters worse, in November the US Fed raised interest rates by 0.75%.

"The full toll of the depression became clear in 1995. The GDP dropped by 6.2%, construction was down 23.5%, private investment by 31.2%, total investment by 29%, imports by

15%. In January, the US congress turned down a bill presented by President Clinton for $40 billion of credit guarantees for Mexico to forestall the further collapse of the peso. The full danger of the crumbling of Mexico's economy reached the ears of Leon Panetta, the head of Clinton's cabinet on a cold afternoon on January 30. He was silently contemplating the dozens of possible solutions presented by Robert Rubin and Larry Summers for the greatest financial rescue in history to convince Michel Camadessus, the stubborn president of the International Monetary Fund. At 8 p.m. a call reached him from the new Mexican Minister of the Economy, Guillermo Ortiz, announcing that the Bank of Mexico had used up its foreign exchange reserves, and Mexico was on the verge of chaos. A second call from Senator Gingrich, head of the Republican majority, announced that there would be no support for a further credit to Mexico. That meant that President Clinton alone would have to assume the entire responsibility for such a loan. There was no other recourse, but to go back to the IMF and ask that it increase its support from $7.7 billion already committed by another $10B. Faced with the alternative, Camdessus, suspending the monetarist faith of a lifetime, consented. By the next morning President Clinton was able to announce that with the help of the IMF, the World Bank, and the Canadian government, he had succeeded in putting together $51 billion in aid to Mexico, even without the consent of Congress. Camdessus hailed the coup as an answer to the first great crisis of the 21st century." Without, of course, mentioning the deeper implications of that statement.

Pontius Pilate in the Guise of a Mexican Economist

"In its annual report for 1995 the Bank of Mexico stated its position on the seismic happenings of the previous months: 'The crisis, the report argued, was not the consequence of policies adopted. Instead, what was to blame was the adverse movements of the economic variables: reversed capital flows, devaluation, expectations of greater inflation, the rise of interest rates and the drop in aggregate demand.'

"No reason was given for the accumulation such a tremendous amount of foreign capital, without the government becoming aware of the dangers of such a situation. There was no explanation of the self-deception that 'takes for granted' that monetary neutrality prevails, the accepted doctrine of the Bank of Mexico. According to this creed monetary variations do not affect the real equilibrium of the economy!

"Up to 1994 the exchange rate of the currency was taken to be the anchor of the economy and the central bank undertook to keep the exchange rate of the peso within an acceptable band. Monetary policy was subordinated to keeping prices within the national currency in a determined range. The effectiveness of such a regime depended on the monetary authority being able to fend off speculative attacks against the local money.

"Under the new regime, the nominal anchor of the system was the monetary base and domestic and foreign credit. These are the variables assigned the main role. This doctrine led to the following policies:

"Strict limits imposed on the net growth of domestic credit.

"A floating exchange rate.

"An average zero statutory reserve set for the banks.

"Limits were imposed on the positive balances of credit institutions, to be calculated by monthly averages.

"In auctioning credit, the rate of interest for financing was kept free.

"Limits were set on the borrowing by commercial banks from the central bank. The new policy adopted was based on quantitative limits of monetary control, and *on a zero average of the banks statutory reserves*." [My emphasis.] In the opinion of the Bank of Mexico this was of exceptional importance The monetary authorities affirmed that such a policy permitted it to control the economy at the lowest possible cost. (The central bank did not include unemployment amongst such costs.)"

The Fiction of Market Efficiency

"Two important officials of the central bank, Agustin Carstens and Alejandro Reynoso set forth the monetary policy of Mexico as follows: 'In the first semester report of the Bank of Mexico in 1997, the two ideas formed the central content of the document: firstly, the neutrality of its counter-cyclical monetary policy; and secondly, the role played by liquidity in the development of the financial markets in support of long-term growth.'

"The doctrine of monetary neutrality holds that nominal variations cannot affect the real equilibrium of the economy. Their only effect is to alter the rate of inflation.

"Monetary equilibrium, according to this doctrine, rests on the view that the key variables of the economy are the interest rate, the exchange rate, the wage rate does not have a 'natural' level, but each of these are governed by conventional motives of a psychological nature. When Alan Greenspan warns against irrational bubbles of speculation as the cause of financial crashes, and when George Soros pleads with authorities to impose restrictions on speculative flows when these become destabilizing, they are asserting that the aforesaid variables (interest rates, exchange rates, etc.) have no centre of gravity, i.e., a 'natural rate' towards which the system tends.

"This conventional view of the interest rate and the exchange rate explains why the system does not automatically generate full employment, since its volatility is unable to compensate for the fluctuations in investment.

"Such a view is tantamount to the recognition that private investment is an extremely volatile factor, related as it is to expectations of future profits. That is why it is subject to surprising fluctuations having nothing to do with the level attained by the interest rate. In such a context, monetary policy to be effective, would have to resort to very substantial changes in interest rates, to the point where these would have negative effects on the economy. This means that monetary policy alone is incapable of stabilizing the economy. This idea was dramatically borne out in the 1994-1999 period. According to the neoclassical doctrine of the neutrality of money, the economy can be stabilized through the flexibility of the prices and wages throughout the system if the money supply is held to a fixed rate of increase. The central bank economists tend to forget in their rigid fundamentalism, that monetary equilibrium can be reached at any level of employment. The doctrine of monetary neutrality tries forcing a complex capitalist system with highly developed bank and financial sectors to behave like a simple monetary economy where money is just another commodity, in which the flexibility of variables leads automatically in the longer term to full employment.

"Contrary to neoclassical doctrine, it is not true that floating exchange rates and perfectly flexible interest rates promote an efficient distribution of resources, and an optimal rate of capital accumulation and stable employment. The hidden variables are manipulated by our central bank, and a menu of other measures are used by the government to try stabilizing the economy."

This careful analysis should finally lay the notion of the neutrality of monetary policy to rest.

"The cost of this adventure to Mexico was eventually $70 billion, when the peso finally collapsed. as the President finally revealed in February 1995.

"The vicious circle of credit speculation had been made possible by the banking and monetary deregulation, *especially the disappearance of the statutory reserves*" (p. 352). (Our emphasis is for the attention of Canadian readers.)

There is a further neglected area, vital to economic analysis, that the Vega book brings to the fore.

"The centralization of political decisions in the hands of the Mexican president seemed an advantage in the massive introduction of market reforms. [However] in the midst of so much goodwill and misplaced confidence in Mexico on world markets, Salinas overreached himself in political initiatives. He undertook key unacknowledged borrowing from the programs of the opposition – the rightist agenda of PAN and even some concern for human rights from the leftist PRD. This helped him to a resounding electoral victory in 1991. But [mistaking political strength for economic soundness] he ignored the vulnerability of the economy, and tried bringing inflation below its double-digit level. Salinas depended on the Free Trade Treaty to help him deal with the collapse of his economic and political positions." And overnight his apparent strength turned to dust. "Jeffery Frieden of Harvard has documented the idea that the exchange rate of currencies is essentially a political variable. Frieden's theory helps draw attention to the obscure ties between the fundamental economic variables and the political processes in which they are embedded. Salinas was intent on avoiding the short-term costs of a traumatic devaluation of the peso, since that would have cost him popularity amongst the middle and working classes." The anti-inflation obsession of Salinas resulted in a 45% depreciation of the peso in 1994.

The Role of Social Institutions in Determining Economic Well-being

In the light of this, Vega gives prominence the ideas of an American economic historian, Douglass North, Nobel Prize for Economics laureate in 1993. In his early work he used neoclassical tools and econometrics, but arrived at the realization that he had need of Marx's analysis to reach an understanding of social institutions. That is particularly relevant in Canada. Our 1991 banks' bailout, followed immediately by their further deregulation, wrecked the reigning Progressive-Conservative Party. And the surrender of most of our money creation to banks was continued with hardly a burp by the Liberals who succeeded them. Now the Liberals seem faced with a similar fate for the same reasons as the Conservatives before them. The broad social alliance that both the "Red" Conservatives and the Liberals espoused after World War II lies dismantled. When an important shift occurs in the distribution of the national income, the old distribution of political power amongst stakeholders becomes outdated. It is like the geological drift that converts seabed into mountain chains.

Canadians may wish to call this "the Brian Mulroney syndrome" since the surrender of money creation with attached interest was achieved under his reign. Mexicans would call the disastrous surrender of their financial system to their new stock market elite "the Salinas syndrome." The British may end up talking of "the Thatcher Syndrome."

While seeking secret "weapons of mass destruction in Iraq, and itself aspiring to them in outer space, the "Washington Consensus" has suppressed the economic understanding dearly bought by the West in the 1930s. This increases the prospect of an eventual military clash with China that could wipe out humanity as we know it. *The Globe and Mail* (22/05, "China Feasts on Canada's Resources" by John Heinzel) contains this significant passage: "In a bid to prevent the bubble from bursting China's central bank has raised reserve requirements for banks."

Canada however, did away with such reserves in 1991 without debate or press release. That was the defining measure of the "Mulroney Syndrome." The United States and the UK retain them but make little use of them as a matter of deep dogma. That gives China a crucial advantage over the West in any future armament race. And the disadvantage that imposes on the West can only encourage China to move aggressively to solve its own vast internal problems. No need to seek foreign spies for having deprived Western governments of the use of government credit for its survival needs. It was the drive to exponential growth of the financial sector that carried out that unqualifiable blow to the world's security.

In its well-documented indictment of the Washington Consensus the Vega book is a powerful tool for society's defence.

William Krehm

1. Krehm, William (1975). *Price in a Mixed Economy – Our Record of Disaster.* Toronto. Krehm, William (May 1970). "La stabilité des prix et le secteur public." *Revue Économique.* Paris.
2. "In the neo-liberal excitement, the misgivings concerning the self-balancing market" of one of the great creators of marginal theory (A. Cournot) to another (L. Walras) were forgotten: "I shudder – Cournot wrote to Walras – when I note that your curves of intensive and extensive utility would lead to pure Laisser Faire, that is, to the equivalent in domestic economies to the deforestation of the globe, and in the international economy, to the suffocation of plebeian races by the privileged ones as per the theory of Mr. Darwin" (Vega Rodriguez, p. 167).

Dr. Griffith Arthur Vincent Morgan

O N MAY 7, 2004, Dr. Griffith Arthur Vincent Morgan, retired professor of family studies and clinical psychology at the University of Guelph, passed away suddenly while engaged as a volunteer guiding a group of visiting students. Born (1925) in Pontardwe, Wales, he studied at Cambridge and London Universities. He came to Canada in 1971 and after a distinguished career kept busy in his retirement in social causes. For years, he was a member of COMER, and will long be remembered as gentle as a Welsh song. Our condolences to his wife, Vi, and family.

The New Class Society

B Y THE END of the Second World War America had emerged as undisputed leader of the Western capitalist states. The defining moment came when the Bretton Woods' economic conference in 1944 rejected Keynes' proposal for a post-war reserve system based on a new supra-national currency.

Alongside the exhausted European allies, the Americans called the shots at Bretton Woods. Roosevelt, a novice in hard-hitting international geopolitics, had at first supported Keynes' plan, but eventually some of his advisers convinced him that the plan by the wily Brit was about to rob the United States of the greatest possible spoil of the war: the dollar's ascendancy to a position of undisputed international reserve currency. A reserve currency serves the same basic functions on an international scale as normal currencies do nationally: A, as a medium of exchange in trade between nations; B, as a safe medium of liquidity preference; and, C, as a transnational store of wealth. These functions all create seigniorage for the country issuing the reserve currency. With gold reduced to a symbolic role (and even that came to an end in the early 1970s), this created a critical advantage for the United States. Furthermore, this advantage has grown sharply in recent decades mainly due to a rising demand for dollar reserves held as a store of wealth in the tax-havens.

The Keynesian Years

While Keynes' plan for an international reserve currency lost out at Bretton Woods, many of his general ideas were widely accepted in the post-war period. Governments, left and right, all called themselves Keynesian and implemented his ideas about economic policies where public expenditures played an important role by automatically counterbalancing market-driven instability.

An integral part of these policies was to redistribute incomes through progressive income taxation and public social programs. This heightens the aggregate propensity to consume, a key measure in the Keynesian system, where it is a main determinant for the force of automatic stabilizing levers.

Many have considered the "closing of the gold window," the right other central banks had to exchange dollars holdings for gold (which often in practice meant the a pile of gold bars was rolled from one corner of a vault in Fort Knox considered "United States," to another corner considered, say, "the Netherlands") and the subsequent collapse of the system of fixed exchange rates as the end of Bretton Woods. These changes, in fact, only meant that a restrictive contradiction within the system was cleared out. Bretton Woods' main outcome, elevating the US dollar to the role of the primary international reserve currency, not only remained in place, but in fact acquired much new force in an environment of floating currencies and policies of financial deregulation.

The Neoliberal Surge

Under the changed conditions, a new international doctrine, later to be known as the Washington Consensus, arose claiming international economic conditions also should be governed by the neoliberal laissez-faire principles. The best way to foster general growth, and assisting true progress in the developing world, was to get government out of economic activities and fully unleash free market forces. But many governments in the 1970s continued to follow the Keynesian policies. These had to be pushed aside and replaced by governments embracing the neoliberal principles, which happened when Reagan became president in 1980. His economic policies were based on neoliberal doctrine, including reversing the Keynesian-period policies of income redistribution. Instead, taxes were cut with most of the cuts going to the rich, and income inequalities were allowed to soar once again.

For the American multi-national corporations and the elites controlling them, these policy shifts were good news. First of all, they made it much easier to take advantage of investments opportunities on a global scale, and draw in raw materials and products produced by cheap labour in the developing countries. All this was done on exchange terms very favorable to the American corporations, partly because of the dollars strong position and partly because the growing globalization saw their ability to control economic and other social conditions rise to new heights of asymmetry. Furthermore, the corporate elite's opportunities for maximizing disposable incomes and wealth holdings were also enhanced. That even included down-sizing oversight authorities such as the IRS, making tax evasion a much easier and almost risk-free sport. To this was, of course, added the many new possibilities for rerouting surpluses to offshore tax havens.

Unfalsifiable Fundamentalist Views

Neoliberal populist economics has been called market fundamentalism, since like other forms of fundamentalism, it rejects evolutionary explanations. Especially, it appears to consider the central economic institution of the market to have descended to the world-creationist style – in full and perfect form. In common with all fundamentalist movements, it is unable to grasp the simple epistemological fact that a belief in creation is founded on individual existential experience. As such,

it is not in opposition, but complementary to an evolutionary interpretation of the phenomena that we can observe and gain common knowledge about.

Evolutionary claims and theories, if they are properly conceived, can be subjected to Popperian falsification tests. Fundamentalists happily avoid such stringent requirements with their absolutist postulates about the existence of perfect markets, red swans and other mythical creatures. Even though nobody has ever seen any of these, the unqualified form of the postulates makes it impossible to get rid of them by scientific argument. In line with this, neoliberals view current conditions to be an absolute arbiter of economic efficiency. For example, neoliberal logic considers it efficient to export toxic waste to LDCs (Less Developed Countries), because when it kills a person there the productivity loss is smaller than if it had killed a person in the industrialized country that exported the waste.

Essentially, this claims that if we can ascertain current differentials adjusted for eventual transaction costs to be positive when expressed in money values, we have an absolute reason for endorsing it. Even considered on its own premises the logic is faulty. The deciding factor can never be to compare persons earnings in static wage costs alone, but must include the rate of marginal productivity growth that their labour resources create. Thus, while an engineer in a less developed country probably has a considerable lower wage than, say, a minimum-wage unskilled Wal-Mart "associate" in the United States, the engineer's specialized labour resource, which is extremely scarce in a LDC, has high rate of marginal productivity growth for the economy of which he is a member. Therefore, the comparison must first ensure that the respective persons, between which the toxic exposure is transferred, has comparable rates of marginal productivity growth. However, seen from the view of evolutionary, situational economics a more serious question is raised by the fact that efficiency can only be measured against prior established reference points, to which they stand in a path-dependent relation.

A Predatory Interpretation

This refutes the neoliberal assumption that any current path-dependent economic condition, by its own very existence, automatically is a proper reference point for efficiency judgments. Neoliberalism abdicates all responsibilities for, and even interest in, how the current conditions are the outcomes of past political and economic developments. That, for example, the developing world has low incomes and the industrialized countries high ones is, at least in part, an outcome of the Western worlds' colonial expansion based upon superior weaponry. Similarly, the United States's economic dominance owes a lot to the dollars' role to as a reserve currency. All these facts are, in the neoliberal view, irrelevant. What counts is that, today, my life is worth more than yours, simply because God, firearms and capitalism enables me to make more money.

The basic mistake is, of course, that economic reasoning can only prove that if we take A for initially given, then B might be a possible efficiency outcome. But it cannot prove why A should be considered a reasonable initial assumption. To answer this questions other factors must be brought into the picture, including an understanding of how previous political and economic developments have shaped present distributions of wealth and power. When the neoliberals ignore the path-dependency of current conditions, it is not only a non-scientific approach, but also a morally bankrupt one, which sacrifices the possibility for a balanced development in the name of a predatory interpretation of economics and politics.

I-make-more-money-so-I-am-more-worthy-than-you attitudes, justified by the false neoliberal paradigm, proliferate today. A standard economics textbook, for example, thinks that the following is what students ought to learn: "It is sensible for the retiree, living on a modest pension and having ample time, to spend many hours shopping for bargains." Well, welcome to the modern version of class society, where hunting for bargains in the drab world of look-alike discount stores offering a diminishing variety of look-alike products is what the neoliberal economic models deem ordinary people to be worth! Whether they are retirees, or workers whose job have been outsourced to third world workers squeezed from the other side, or simply average families still dreaming of giving the two kids an education that, however, slowly is slipping out of reach as it becomes impossible to square the circle between falling real incomes and rising education costs.

Meanwhile, it still all looks very nice up in the sky for the new elite, zipping past in private "cost savings" jets (the cost saving accruing from the fact that their time is so much more worth, even when they play golf). As they move around between lavish houses on the Riviera, in the Caribbean, or in the Malibu Canyons, their main problem is to figure out how keep up spending the enormous windfalls that the new corporate economy has thrown to them.

Seigniorage is defined as the differential between the cost of creating money and the purchasing power it commands when issued. In the case of modern monies with no intrinsic value, the seigniorage is essentially equal to the full face value.

The example is not fictitious but taken from a 1991 internal World Bank memo, the main part of which reads: "...a given amount of health-impairing pollution should be done in the country with the lowest cost, which will be the country with the lowest wages. I think the economic logic behind dumping a load of toxic waste in the lowest wage country is impeccable and we should face up to that." A recent recapitulation of this conviction occurred on March 13, 2001, in the *Boston Globe*: "Harvard Students Rip New President Lawrence Summers on Toxic Waste Memo."

Dix Sandbeck

Those who Bury the Past are Condemned to Relive It

THROUGHOUT THE WORLD there is a problem with the anticipated rise in interest rates. I don't know whether the executioners who operated the guillotine during the French revolution asked the condemned whether he/she was comfortable when slid beneath the blade. But I suspect that question would have been considered irrelevant. The same can be said of the slew of articles in the media asking whether the coming higher rates will add to the sense of well-being of investors.

Take as an example (*The Globe and Mail*, 14/05, "Banks in unique position to weather rate rise" by Sinclair Stewart): "Banks and interest rates have always had a pretty simple relationship: when rates go up, the banks take a beating. In other words, if you own bank stocks, now might be a good time to sell.

"Or maybe not.

"Despite predictions that the US Federal Reserve will increase rates this summer, some observers believe for the first time, banks are in a unique position to weather the storm."

The word "storm," however, is like a gleam from the axe about to fall. Yet the tone is one of determined reassurance.

"For one thing, the sector has never witnessed such a period of low, cellar-dwelling rates."

But the origin of those low interest rates is never mentioned. It had to do with the bail-out of our banks from their crushing losses in their oil, real estate, and stock market gambols in the 1980s. The gimmick for achieving this was so crooked, it couldn't bear the light of day.

Accordingly, the bill for the decennial renewal of our *Bank Act* was slipped through Parliament without debate or press release. In that revision the statutory reserves that our banks had to put up on a non-interest-bearing basis with the Bank of Canada were done away with. These were a redeposit with the BoC, usually from 8% to 10% of the deposits they took in from the public in chequing accounts. At the same time the debt of Canada and other OECD countries was declared risk-free, thus requiring from the banks no additional capital to acquire more of it. In this way our banks were enabled to quadruple their holdings of federal debt by another $60 B without putting up a penny of their own. That was no one-shot bailout, but an entitlement. recurring year after year. The government began paying in interest on the increased federal debt held by the banks anywhere from $5 to $8 billion, depending on how high the BoC had screwed up interest rates.

And to make matters worse, the Mulroney government went on to deregulate the banks that they had just bailed out so liberally, to allow them to take over in Canada and abroad, stock market brokerages, underwriting, merchant banking, credit card institutions, selling and themselves using the most complicated derivatives that in complex ways not fully understood by their very designers allow anonymous participation in the wildest leveraged gambles. That raises some questions:

How could a government that had just bailed out our banks to the tune of a capitalized amount of at least $100 billion, go on to deregulate them to engage in such a variety of activities? It is rare enough for a bank to bail out a client who had lost most of his capital. But to bail out the banks and then at once allow them to enter fields so incompatible with banking allows only one explanation: the banks had acquired near dominant power over our government. That changed the nature and the morality of public life in Canada. It is, in fact, the hidden dead rat under the floorboards that ever since has polluted our political scene. It accounts for most of the $300 billion of the federal debt increase since it happened. On page 16 of this issue of *ER* we explain the details.

It is important to note, as well, that banks today, with deregulation, have become a tangle of businesses in the stock market including, of course, stock brokerages. And to any business dependent on the stock market, higher interest rates are poison. They are also involved up to their shoulders in gambles with complex derivatives that allow wildly leveraged gambles, and afford the illusion of "managing risk" whenever it can even better disguise risk. Instead of the simple, upright establishment, the model of honesty, prudence and candour for the entire community, a bank these days has become a monster of many stomachs, many heads, and a shrunken conscience. You need only read the 9- and 10-digit settlements that New York State Attorney Elliot Spitzer is obtaining from the largest banks to grasp the point.

William Krehm

COMER is Not Connecting

WHAT DOES IT TAKE to get COMER's message out? I am beginning to feel like I have some horrible social disease because whenever I mention the Bank of Canada – are people actually running away when I mention Bank of Canada or is it just my imagination?

Why is the CCPA not talking about it?

Why doesn't Linda McQuaig talk about it?

Why aren't other journalists talking about it?

Use of the BoC to finance public capital projects would provide many thousands of jobs, so why does the CLC ignore it?

On March 5/04, Chris Watson, Federal Secretary of the NDP, stated in reply to a letter about "The Mother of All Scandals" that the draft NDP election included a proposal to bring some of Canada's national debt under the control of the Bank of Canada. Apparently this did not get across to Sandra Cordon of the Canadian Press in Ottawa who, after interviewing some senior members of the NDP on March 5, reported that the NDP platform talks about "high bank charges," "pocket-book protection," "balanced ledgers" and so on, but no mention of the Bank of Canada. She also commented that the NDP is "trying to shed its spendthrift image."

Good Lord! The NDP has never been in power federally. Liberal and Conservative governments created the $590 billion federal debt, 94% of which was due to interest, not program spending. The NDP had nothing to do with it. Why don't we hear the NDP attacking the Liberals and Conservatives for creating this monstrous debt and spending hundreds of billions of dollars on unnecessary interest payments while unmercifully chopping programs and services. *COMER's message is not getting out!*

I wrote to Chris to say the election platform is very good news and asked if COMER had been invited to help draft the proposal to bring some of Canada's national debt under the control of the Bank of Canada. Then I learned that Chris didn't know about COMER. Obviously, *COMER's message is not getting out!*

COMER's message, if heard at all, is not getting the support it needs to effect necessary changes in the way the Bank of Canada is used. John Hotson, Professor of Economics, Waterloo U, seemed to be making some headway, but his untimely death in 1996 put a stop to that.

The CCPA used to refer to the Bank of Canada when it prepared the Alternative Budget, but has not done so for a few years.

The Canadian Labour Congress, while recognizing that "monetization of debt is an important policy tool," is "not convinced it needs to be used right now."

The Federation of Canadian Municipalities does not support using the BoC even though municipalities are "starving" for lack of funds. This is not for lack of communication, though, so something else is influencing their decision.

A Hot Topic Put into the Freezer

Nevertheless, there is a lot of interest in this question. For example, a letter was sent to the CBC Fifth Estate requesting them to do a program on the subject, a copy going to COMER members across Canada suggesting that they show support for such a program. Within 48 hours a letter was received from the Fifth Estate stating that their "mailbox had been inundated with e-mails from people suggesting the same story" and asking that people "refrain from sending additional messages." It is a hot topic.

At the same time, it is not getting the support it needs from some economists. Jim Stanford (CAW economist), Andrew Jackson (chief economist with the CLC), Hugh Mackenzie (economist and CCPA research associate), Ellen Russell (CCPA's senior staff economist), Armine Yalnizyan (economist with the CCPA) and others comment in the April issue of the CCPA Monitor on Paul Martin's goal of smaller government and the privatizing of public services and assets. They point out that the deficit justification for slashing programs was a fraud, using tax dollars to pay down the debt was unnecessary and the tax cuts primarily benefited the wealthiest among us. No mention was made, however, of the role the Bank of Canada played in the accumulation of the huge debts, or the role it could play to reduce the interest bearing debt by assuming part of it on a gradual basis or how it could finance investment in public infrastructure – the most crucial point of all.

They say, correctly, that the deficit and the debt to GDP ratio would have decreased without the severe program slashing because revenues increased. This overlooks the fact that we spend huge amounts every year on unnecessary interest ($65 billion for all levels of government) which reduces the funds available for public programs, and the fact that the government continues to use the cost of interest to justify spending its surplus on debt reduction – an argument that many Canadians seem to support. Ms Russell speaks of the 2004 AFB proposal for the establishment of a Canadian Infrastructure Financing Authority (CIFA) to raise federally-guaranteed credit to finance infrastructure projects when the Bank of Canada is already established and could do this at zero interest cost to the government.

COMER's message *is* heard at CCPA, but the lack of support for it there may be one of the reasons why others, who look to economists for direction in these matters, are not acting on it. Can we expect politicians, who may not be well informed on monetary matters, to take a strong position if there is a perceived split among the "experts"?

In Kingston, as in many other communities, we have had monthly meetings, special public meetings with guest speakers and written letters to the local papers, but the level of understanding has remained low, although it does seem to be increasing. However, the rate of increase is so small I fear that I will be dead before I see a great change. So, with this in mind letters were written to CBC programs – *The National, The Current, Counterspin*, Rick Mercer's *Monday Report, The World This Weekend*, Anne Medina, Michael Enright, Don Newman, Wendy Mesley, Brian Stewart, and *The 5th Estate*. Rick Mercer's office replied to say that he would not be available until September. *Counterspin* replied to say that their program was to be discontinued. The only other program to respond was *The 5th Estate* which said that our suggestion to do an investigative report on the misuse of the Bank of Canada was being considered, and that should they decide to proceed someone would be in touch with us. To date I have heard nothing more.

How can COMER get its message out? William Krehm states in a reference to *The 5th Estate* that for years the CBC has used every trick conceivable to keep the issue out of the purview of our national broadcaster. "Now it is time to brandish the new medium, e-mail," he said.

One of the tools in the e-mail toolbox is mouseland (www.ndp.ca/mouseland), a discussion group for NDP members, which could be used a lot more than it is for discussion of economic and monetary policies. Another is Vive le Canada – organized by Mel Hurtig); its mission is "to involve Canadians in grassroots efforts to protect and improve Canadian sovereignty" by encouraging comment, debate and discussion.

There is "meetup.com" which "allows people to organize informal, in-person meetings simultaneously in numerous locations across the country and the world once a month."

Vive le Canada has just set up a Meetup for people interested in discussing Canadian sovereignty. Just visit http://canadiansov.meetup.com to get all the information.

Then there are the newsletters put out by political parties and social action groups, some of which are interested in carrying information on monetary matters and the Bank of Canada. The CAP_PAC Newsletter (www.canadianactionparty.

ca) comes to mind.

Lastly, in addition to group discussions and newsletters there are petitions which can be tabled in the House of Commons. An example is the one organized by the NDP to "stop the war." Why not have a petition to use the Bank of Canada to finance public capital expenditures?

As William Krehm said, to get the COMER message out it is time to brandish the new medium, e-mail. It is a major challenge for the COMER board of directors to organize.

Richard Priestman

Like a Miracle of Medieval Faith — Washington Learns to Say "I'm Sorry"

LIKE A MIRACLE of medieval faith – say a divine lily shooting out from granite rock – Messers Bush and Rumsfeld have sprouted a conscience. A single whistle-blower in the US army shocked by the murderous violence applied to Iraqi prisoners in Baghdad's Abu Ghraib prison, passed on some photos to the American press, and may have brought down the administration's urgent plans for an early pull-out from Iraq. Incredibly, that has elicited a belated apology from the lips of Bush and Rumsfeld. *The Wall Street Journal* (10/05, "Prisoner Abuse Could Undercut US Credibility" by Greg Jaffe, Carla Anne Robbins and Robert Thurow) offers us the stunning implication of this: "Evidence of widespread prisoner abuse in Iraq is raising concerns that the war on terrorism has fostered a broader culture of impunity to international norms that could undercut US overtures to allies and increase risks for its troops.

Nothing New About US Abuse of War Prisoners

"Before the Iraq war, US allies in Europe expressed strong concerns about President Bush's decision to bypass international agreements by removing the US signature from the International Criminal Court treaty and declaring that the Geneva Conventions governing warfare didn't apply to the fight against Al Quaeda.

"The publication of photos showing prisoner mistreatment in Iraq could bolster charges the US has set itself above the law. That has some US and international officials worrying about practical consequences. That could, for example, make it harder for the US to persuade other countries to send troops to Iraq. Legal experts say that governments that signed onto the International Criminal Court now may balk at turning over prisoners captured in the war against terrorism to US custody because of concerns that they won't be treated according to the Geneva Conventions. Some legal experts in the US military also worry that by weakening the Geneva Conventions, the US lost leverage to restrain others from torturing American soldiers. 'The US does set an example in the world for what it means to be a democratic, law-based nation,' said Antonella Notari, a spokeswoman for the International Committee of the Red Cross in Geneva."

A confidential report of the ICRC, reviewed by *The Wall Street Journal*, charges that US forces committed a "number of serious violations of International Humanitarian Law, at several prison camps throughout Iraq. The violations – including holding prisoners naked in empty cells and firing from watchtowers at unarmed detainees – suggested ill-treatment of detainees that might be considered a 'practice tolerated' by US forces.

"Human rights groups say similar abuse has been committed in Afghanistan. The death of two prisoners at Bagram air base in December 2002 after apparent beatings were ruled homicides by US military doctors and an investigation was launched.

"Retired Major Gen. Robert Scales, a military historian, says there is nothing new about abuse of prisoners of war at US hands, citing prison riots on Koje-DO Island during the Korean War and alleged atrocities against prisoners in 'Tiger Cages' by the US-backed South Vietnamese government. Still, in this case the impact is magnified by the rapid distribution around the world of graphic digital pictures of the abuse and details of an internal Army investigative report by Maj. General Taguba. 'The report is damning, but it doesn't carry the shock value of the pictures,' said General Scales.

"The disclosure of the abuses undermines the army's central goal: to win the trust of the Iraqi people.

"Critics trace the prisoner scandal back to Mr. Rumsfeld's order in early 2002 that fighters captured in the war on terrorism wouldn't be designated prisoners of war under the Geneva Conventions. Instead, the Pentagon came up with its own new category, 'unlawful combatants,' whose rights would be determined solely by their American captors. After widespread international outcry, the White House pledged that the prisoners would be treated humanely in a manner 'consistent with the Geneva Convention.' But the administration still denied key protections, including limits on interrogation and the right of legal representation.

"'Mr. Secretary, in January 2002, when you publicly declared that hundreds of people detained by US and Allied forces in Afghanistan do not have rights under the Geneva Convention, that was taken as a signal,' Sen. Hillary Clinton told Mr. Rumsfeld at Friday's Senate Armed Service Committee hearing.

Flirtation with the Geneva Conventions

"The Geneva Conventions are rooted in 19th-century discussion and were signed in 1949. They were updated in 1977 after various wars of independence and internal armed conflicts. The International Red Cross is the monitor of the conventions.

"'The Bush administration has said it considers the Geneva Conventions to be in force for the war in Iraq, and soldiers there are following them,' Mr. Rumsfeld told the Senate panel Friday.

"Still Mr. Rumsfeld acknowledged that the conventions weren't followed in the cases of abuse. And that could cause further problems. The abuse reports could imperil US efforts to further internationalize the Iraqi occupation. Many potential coalition partners lack the manpower to run large-scale interrogation facilities. If they send troops to Iraq, they would have to turn over prisoners to US forces. The International Criminal Court, however, precludes ICC signatories from turning over prisoners to countries known to be in violation of the Geneva Conventions. If they do, their commanders could be held criminally or civilly liable for abuses suffered. In May 2002, President Bush withdrew the Clinton administration's signature from the treaty, insisting the US could be trusted to uphold basic human rights."

The US is not only an imperial power striving to bring even the cosmic spaces into its missiles' range. It is also a land of a litigant culture, with an oversupply of lawyers back home greater than its under-supply of troops in Iraq and Afghanistan. That means that any brave ally in Micronesia that ventures to send troops to the "coalition" in Iraq may find themselves the defendants in lawsuits. Launched where? Why in the good old United States of America.

Thus "the repercussions could also sway the US Supreme Court, which now is considering three high-profile cases challenging the indefinite detention, without hearing, of 600 foreigners in Guantanamo Bay, Cuba, and two US citizens held at a military jail in South Carolina. All have been deemed enemy or unlawful combatants."

What we have is a crumbling of the institutional infrastructures from an explosive expansion of military power in the service of deregulated finance. This has upset the previous existing alliances between the various sectors of the economy and what respect previously existed amongst different cultures. Such respect calls for breathing space between cultures, not the destabilization of their economic bases by Globalization and Deregulation. More remarkable than the failure of the CIA and the FBI to foresee the Twin Tower attack has been its persistent blindness to the contribution to Muslim terror of the Washington Consensus's elevation of interest rates to "the sole blunt tool" to fight inflation. Islam, whether Shiite or Sunni, considers even simple interest, let alone usurious interest, if persisted in, a crime punishable by eternal hell-fire. Surely, rather than torturing prisoners, Washington should pursue this obvious lead. Or did Bin Laden have a surreptitious finger in designing the Washington Consensus?

William Krehm

"Help Students Not Banks"

THESE DAYS two themes hog the headlines of the US media. The deficit is leading the major parties to invoke "fiscal responsibility" as the last surviving principle of morality; and the prowess of Attorney General of New York State, Eliot Spitzer, in tracking down high corporate fraud. Canada's political leaders, on the other hand, while matching the concern about "the deficit" south of the border, have shown little taste for investigations of white-collar crime in high corporate places at home. Instead, we are still being drilled to nurture, cherish, and deregulate our huge banks to compete head-on with their biggest rivals abroad, and bring laurels back home. The logic is,

I suppose, that having only five or six monster banks, they must be cuddled like near-only children.

But there are problems with this one-string morality. How can you aspire to "fiscal responsibility" while leaving accountancy out in the cold? Accountancy is basically a simple thing. It sorts out the movements of money into two columns – one for assets, values that we own; and liabilities, values that we owe. Between "owe" and "own," stands a single final letter. If you have a huge balance on the "own side" of these columns you are one of the Lord's anointed. If the huge balance is under the "owed" heading however, you are in great trouble. Confuse those two columns and you are a candidate for the poor-house or even the penitentiary. Nobody, but nobody, should be allowed to monkey around with the last letter of these tiny words!

But where there is a will to complicate simple matters, there is always a way. What, for example, happens when a private individual buys a house or a corporation a building that will last for a generation or two? To begin with, the ground beneath it, if well located, will probably gain rather than lose value. The house sitting on that land is "depreciated" over its likely useful life and its residual value carried on the books to contribute to the individual's net worth. And the debt to the mortgage company is "amortized" to a maximum of the residual usefulness of the asset. The common root of "amortize" and "mortgage" tells the tale of such accountancy. That Latin root, *mors, mortis*, means "death" and should refer to the loan, not to the borrower. This system is known as "accrual accountancy" or more popularly, as "capital budgeting." If they didn't apply such book-keeping in the private sector, the mortgage companies and the mortgage departments of banks would be out of business, for they couldn't keep track of the collateral securing their loans.

However, when the government purchases a building, or makes other investments that are likely to retain their usefulness for decades, this simple accountancy principle is violated. Governments have always bought services and commodities that are wholly consumed in the year of their purchase (e.g., paper clips, soap for the wash-rooms, and most services). But as society developed, far more durable acquisitions by the state became necessary: roads, bridges, railways, schools, education, prisons, harbours. These required spending vast amounts of money, that would come back gradually as the debt for financing such facilities could be discharged. That means that over the period of its usefulness it paid for itself through the discharge of the principal part of the financing. The two columns "owe" and "own" had to be considered singing a duet, not a solo.

As the Clank of Sword on Armour to War-Horse

But to bankers the very mention of debt is like the clang of sword on armour to a war-horse of yore. At once nostrils flare and palms start itching. When money was silver or gold, countries without mines could run out of the stuff. But for over thirty years even the pretence of gold or silver backing the world's currencies has disappeared. Money today is nothing more than the credit of the central government. If the necessary human skills, materials and equipment are at hand, or can be imported, governments can always finance a socially necessary project. Historically, their powers to do so reaches back to the monopoly of the ancestral monarch in coining or clipping the currency by recoining it. The difference between the cost to the king of the coin and its purchasing power was known as "seigniorage," and the rate of seigniorage has grown wildly, since the gold standard was abolished, and the computer came in the physical cost of creating money and transmitting it across oceans was reduced to pennies. The resulting explosion of seigniorage opened intoxicating vistas of a near-total seigniorage: profits on money that was not theirs but merely deposited with them or borrowed. And opportunities especially come during election time when politicians pay for all those costly TV ads. Opportunity not only knocks on the door but replaces it with an open archway. So in 1991 in Canada a major bailout of our chartered banks from their gambles in gas and oil, real estate, and much else, was smuggled through parliament. The MPs hadn't a clue of what they were voting for, nor were they encouraged to ask. This bit of legislation – alongside the Bank for International Settlements' *Risk-Based Capital Requirements* – shifted the powers of money creation from the central bank to the private bankers.[1] The government's money needs, *though money had become entirely government credit*, came to be borrowed increasingly by the government not from its own bank at a nominal cost, but from the private banks. These as a group have been bailed out by the same governments about once every ten years.

Smuggling Accountancy into the US Government Books

Banks long ago found out that when they receive deposits instead of letting the money lie inactive in their vaults they can lend out most of it, retaining only enough to cover cheques likely to be written by the account-owners in favour of a client of another bank. In normal times they know from experience what cash holdings are likely to be needed to meet such withdrawals from short-term accounts. Other banks who receive the cheques from the payee written on the first bank do the same. They keep enough of such deposits to take care of withdrawals and lend out the rest. And the same process goes on from bank to bank: similar proportions are held by each in "sterile" cash to honour claims for the deposits.

To make sure that the private banks do not lend out too much of the funds deposited in short-term accounts, central banks used to require that a small proportion of such deposits be redeposited by the banks with the central bank where it usually earned no interest. That not only gave the government the free use of such money within the existing constraints. In addition the arrangement allowed the central bank to fight perceived inflation without relying entirely on raising interest rates. Combined with the *Risk-Based Capital Requirements* guidelines issued by the Bank for International Settlements shortly before, the end of the statutory reserves allowed Canada's chartered banks to quadruple their holdings of federal debt to $80 billion. The interest the banks received from the government on this increase in the government debt they held amounted to anywhere from $5 to $8 billion annually, depending upon how high the central bank had driven up interest rates.

Though in the US accrual accountancy was brought in incognito at the beginning of 1996 where physical investments of government are concerned, its even more productive investments in human capital – education, health, and social services – have not even been mentioned. And yet in the 1960s, Theodor Schultz was awarded a Nobel Prize for Economics for his work proving government investment in human capital – health, education, social services – to be by far the most productive investment that society can make. Immediately after WWII Schultz was one of many young American economists sent by Washington to Japan and Germany to forecast how long it would take for them to reemerge as competitors on the world market. In retrospect he marvelled at how wide of the mark their predictions turned out to be. His conclusion: their mistake was concentrating on the physical destruction of factories and infrastructure and overlooking that the highly educated, motivated populations that remained intact.

From that he concluded that human investment is the most productive of investments. Even though the immediate results of these investments are lodged in private heads and bodies rather than in the public domain, the increased productivity that results will expand the government's tax base and hence qualify as a capital asset of government. Today his work is completely forgotten.

However, in their haste to head off one bank crisis, BIS and the Bank of Canada had unwittingly hit on a complex of bad policies that guaranteed the next bank bust. This is explained in our footnote.

When COMER finally disinterred the details of the 1991 bailout, the banks in chorus protested that the statutory reserves had been an "unjust tax." In fact, quite apart from harking back to ancestral monarch's monopoly for coining of precious metals, it represented part payment for costly current services of our government to the chartered banks. To begin with there is the role of government's central bank as "lender of the last resort." In every bank crisis, there is need for some institution of unquestionable solidity to come forth to lend the funds that will prevent a bank-run. Runs on banks plagued banking from time to time, right up to the 1930s, when 38% of the thousands of banks in the US had shut down and a moratorium on all banking was proclaimed by the time F.D. Roosevelt took over the presidency. We no longer experience runs on banks in the First World because our government steps in at once to stave them off. The cost to the government both as lender of the last resort and through its deposit insurance agency has been enormous.

Today all major parties are under a compulsion to promise not only that they will balance the budget, but even retire the debt. However, since the only legal tender – i.e., the only cash – has since the early 1970s been central government debt, what money will our politicians pay the debt with since all cash money today is government debt? Notes of a different colour? And deficits, as we have seen, can result from overspending for current needs, or they can be contrived by cooking the books, entering as current spending the cheques written for infrastructure that will last for decades.

Do we Need Higher Education for our Excess of Talent?

With that background, we can examine the latest US scandal arising from the misapplication of cash flow accountancy where it has no place. Students who need help in financing their university education are less and less getting it. The problem exists in Canada to the same extent. The world is being globalized and deregulated and useful production is being outsourced to other countries for the greater profit of the financial community. That development has an unrecognized corollary. Much of the education and training that was recognized as a good investment essential for those in power a generation ago is coming to be regarded as redundant when ever more high-tech production is being outsourced to cheaper countries.

Let me cite a recent editorial in *The New York Times* (25/04, "Help Students, Not Banks"): "Faced with soaring tuition and dwindling aid, record numbers of students who would excel at college are no longer applying. If the trend persists, this country could easily return to the time when the poor were locked out of higher education and college was hardly a given for middle-class families.

"To help prevent this, the aid programs contained in the federal *Higher Education Act* of 1965, which is due to be reauthorized this fall, need to be updated. The top priority should be increasing the amount of the Pell grants which covered more than 80% of the public-college tuition a quarter-century ago but only about 40% today. Congress also needs to revise the federal college loan program so that more money flows into the loan program itself instead into the coffers of the banks.

"The government offers two basic college loan programs. The direct loan system, developed under Clinton, allows students to borrow from the government through their schools. It actually makes a small profit by cutting out the banking middlemen.

"This program competes with the Federal Family Education Loan Program (FFELP), under which private banks receive generous federal subsidies to make student loans guaranteed by taxpayers.

"The Clinton administration wanted to expand the direct loan problem, and phase out the FFELP. [But] the banking industry blocked the move in Congress and declared all-out war on the direct-loan program. The banks have benefited, as have politicians more interested in pleasing the banking lobby than in helping the largest number of students at the lowest possible costs."

Ripe for Political Picking

And *The Wall Street Journal* (5/05, "Student Loans Take Political Stage" by June Kronehole) adds: "All that is making political fodder out of a 30-year old federal entitlement that has helped about 50 million people through college. Any student is entitled to a loan, and for low-income families, the government defers interest on that loan while the student is still at school."

But those loans don't stretch as far as they once did. A freshman can borrow a maximum of $625 at a record low 4.25% interest this year, but that's only enough to pay one-quarter the cost of tuition and room and board at the typical state university. That loan limit hasn't budged since 1986. Though President Bush proposed raising it to $3,000 in his 2005 budget, the White House hasn't mentioned the idea since.

"The student-loan program is so rich for political picking because it involves banks, a dependable Republican ally, and middle-income students who must borrow to pay their way through school, a potential Democratic constituency.

"In the past school year, students and recent graduates held $181.3 billion in outstanding loans, and added to that by borrowing $52B this year. About a third of those loan dollars now come directly from the US Treasury. The government sets interest rates slightly above its own borrowing costs, and when students repay the loans, the government keeps the profit, which it predicts will be $500 million in the next school year.

"The rest of the loan money comes from commercial banks, which charge students the same government-set interest rates. But because the government reimburses the banks if the student borrowers default and also sets a guaranteed return, the Treasury says these loans will cost it $7 billion next year. Mr. Kerry, most congressional Democrats and some Republican leaders want less of that money going into corporations and more of it used for loans. Public-college tuition rose 14% last year, but if the government were to raise the student loan ceiling by as much, the cost of the loan program would soar.

"Banks put up a ferocious fight when President Clinton proposed cutting them out as the student loan middleman in 1993 and keeping all the profit for the government. The banks argue that they deserve federal guarantees because student borrowers have no credit history."

Are the young voters turning their backs on the polls? Raise the student-loan scandal as an issue and that could change on the double-quick.

William Krehm

1. The Bank for International Settlements (BIS) was founded in 1929 as a technical body to handle the conversion of German WWI reparation payments into strong currencies. These were to be syndicated as bond issues, and marketed abroad. That never came to pass because the great Wall St crash of 1929 intervened. At Bretton Woods in 1943, Resolution Five was passed calling for BIS's liquidation at the earliest possible moment, because it had surrendered the gold reserve entrusted to it by Czechoslovakia as soon as Nazi troops marched into Prague. Because of the low-profile BIS cultivated under the shadow of that hangman's noose, it came to serve as the ideal secret bunker for planning the world-wide take-over of money creation by the private banks. The essence of its *Risk-based Capital Requirements* guidelines was to shift the criterion for banks' solvency from their cash holdings to their reserves of "capital." But the "capital" of banks is rarely held as cash, because cash in their vaults earns no interest. It gets put out as loans totalling many times the deposits taken in. And – under the bank deregulation also sponsored by BIS – it gets invested in brokerage houses, insurance companies, and every form of stock market gambols that are usually booked at their original cost, not their current market values.

So hastily had the Guidelines been improvised to deal with the world banking crisis created by deregulation, that BIS overlooked that these guidelines were bound to bring on another banking collapse. They declared the debt of OECD (the most industrialized. countries) "risk-free" and hence requiring the banks to put up no additional capital to acquire. But at the same time the BIS was pressuring central banks to enforce "zero inflation" with higher interest-rates In this BIS had overlooked a detail that COMER did pick up and tried bringing to our government's attention. Whenever interest rates go up, the banks' hoards of government debt purchased on the cuff shed value. If you can get, say 10% annually on a newly issued bond, pre-existing bonds with lower coupons, will fall below par. And if the terms of the debt are long enough, and the amount of bonds held by the banks big enough, a new bank crisis will ensue from their very previous bailout.

That indeed is what began happening. And that is what caused the Clinton government to introduce accrual accountancy on-the-sly and, carrying the adjustment back several years, to pick up a trillion dollars of Washington's physical investments that had been written off in a single year rather than depreciated. This new bigger figure replaced the old incorrect one in the Department of Commerce's business statistics as of January 1996. But Clinton's Secretary of the Treasury, Robert Rubin, a brilliant hard-hitter recruit from Wall St. – listed it not as "investment" for it is an article of faith of the right that governments cannot invest money, but only waste it. So instead of "investment," which such neglected assets of the government were since they consisted of buildings, schools and penitentiaries, they were listed as "savings." That suited Clinton's political strategy of avoiding alarming the ideologists of the right. It left the lights turned off on the nature of that improved statistic. By its grace, however, the bond rating agencies, interested only in the bottom line, raised their quality-appraisal for government bonds and brought interest rates down. That allowed the economy to start booming once again until its next crash.

Canada had no Robert Rubin in its federal cabinet. We did profit by the lower interest rates brought in south of the border. However, when it came to bringing that broken shard of sensible accountancy into our government's books, everybody in Ottawa was out to lunch. The issue arose, however, in 1999 when the Auditor General withheld unconditional approval of two years' balance sheets of the government unless it agreed to bring in capital budgeting. Such a measure had been advocated to no avail by three royal commissions during the previous four decades and innumerable Auditors General. However, the current one, Denis Desautels, dug his toes in, to the point of accusing that the government was "cooking its books." Though that remark was not without news value, it was not reported by the media. Our troubles are not confined to accountancy.

Straightening Out our Government's Farm Policies

AT COMER's recent conference Milan Sojak, a retired academic and COMER veteran, distributed a remarkable document of the National Farmers Union (Canada) "The Farm Crisis, Bigger Farms and the Myths of 'Competition' and 'Efficiency'" (20/11/03). For its grasp of the issues involved, it is in striking contrast to the output of Ottawa analysts.

Let me pass on the gist of this remarkable document:

"Governments and agri-business transnationals have a plan for Canadian farmers. *Driven by competition and aided by technology, farms must become larger and more efficient, though less numerous.*

"The assumption is that open, deregulated, globalized markets will drive our farms to higher levels of efficiency, raising income for farmers and lowering prices for consumers. A key part of this plan is to increase farm size. And that will require a decrease in the number of farmers. (While governments have recently been less explicit about reducing the number of farmers, they were formerly very explicit indeed, as the report will show.)" From the four pages of quotations from government and farm-supply corporations to this effect I will, select only two from the famous 1969 Federal Task Force on Agriculture report, *Canadian Agriculture in the Seventies:*

"Individual farm enterprises must continuously expand and improve efficiency to maintain or increase incomes. Unfortunately, many farmers have too small earnings to be able to save or justify borrowing in the competitive race, even though they make some improvements in productivity. Those who fall behind tend to receive declining real and relative incomes and may either become part of the rural poor or be forced out of agriculture altogether (p. 21).

"Increased mobility out of farming helps to achieve a higher per capita net farm income for those left in farming while at the same time obtaining better paid employment for those who leave agriculture (p. 32)."

There is no thought given to family farming as a desirable, "alternate" way of life, less destructive to the environment than migration of farmers to the cities.

"In a 1981 report, the Canadian Department of Agriculture and Agri-Food again returned to the themes of efficiency and competition:

"Part-time farmers and those soon to retire generally may not be willing to leverage their operations to the same extent as the more technically advanced producer. A number of farms fail to achieve the optimal level of efficiency. It appears, however, that there is sufficient transference of farm ownership to facilitate long-term adjustments" (Agriculture and Agri-Food Canada, *Challenge for Growth: An Agri-Food Strategy for Cana-*

da, July 1981, p. 83).

"All the above statements contain the same basic prescription: Competition (facilitated by globalization, free trade, open markets, and deregulation) combined with technological innovation will lead to higher efficiency and fewer but larger farms.

"Myth 1: Farmers need to become more efficient.

"The graphs below show that the prices farmers receive have not increased over the past 25 years (not adjusted for inflation). Farmers' ability to continue producing without a price increase for 25 years – despite rising rices for fuel, fertilizer, and other inputs – suggests a high degree of efficiency. General Motors, Shell Oil, and Coca-Cola cannot today make and sell their products for 1975 prices."

We haven't the space to reproduce the graphs, but here are the figures. [The price of] one bushel of wheat (Saskatoon) remained approximately unchanged from 1975 to 2002, but the retail price of the bread made from that bushel rose from $30 to well over $90.

One kilo of corn (FOB Chatham, Ont.) stayed the same between 1976 and 2002. A kilo of corn flakes, however, rose from $1 per kg to well over $6.

Hogs: dollars/pound (Ontario index 100 hogs, dressed), while pork chops rose from about $2.00/pound (Canada average).

Figures for barley and beer prices tell a similar tale.

"Myth 2: Farmers will become more efficient as farms become larger.

"Economists point out the benefits of 'economies of scale': larger operations – because of specialization, division of labour, optimized equipment, access to capital, etc. – can produce goods and services more cheaply than smaller operations. For many government and corporate leaders, it is an article of faith that giant international corporations are far more efficient than our relatively small family-run farms.

"To understand the economic position of the family farm, one must understand its context within the agri-food chain. At one end of the chain are fuel, oil, and natural gas companies. At the next link, fertilizer companies turn natural gas into nitrogen fertilizer. Next come chemical and seed companies, machinery companies and banks. In the middle sits the family farm. Continuing down the chain we find grain companies and railways, packers and processors, retailers and restaurants, and, perhaps not coincidentally, every one of these links is characterized by large profits.

"Consider a simple bread production chain made up of farmers, a grain miller that makes flour (such as Archer Daniels Midland (US-based), it owns 47% of Canada's flour milling capacity), a baking company such as Maple Leaf's 'Canada Bread' subsidiary) and a food retailer (such as Weston's 'Superstore'). The retail price of a loaf of bread has risen from 75 cents in 1975 to $1.39 today. Since farmers have received none of this increase, the large and allegedly efficient corporations that do the milling, baking and retailing must have tripled the amounts they charge for their services. Assuming that the price increases reflect costs and, thus efficiency, this indicates that the largest firms in the bread chain are the least efficient. The graphs on pork chops, cereal and beer indicate that farmers may be the most efficient links in those chains as well. While it contradicts economic doctrine, this evidence strongly suggests that Canada's family farms are the most efficient firms currently operating in the entire agri-food chain; perhaps in the entire economy. The evidence also suggests that if farms expand and adopt the corporate model, we can expect lower efficiency and higher food prices.

"Myth 3: Farmers will benefit by becoming more efficient.

"Will farmers themselves benefit if they enlarge their farms and become more efficient? By expanding, will farmers escape the chronic farm income crises?

"To answer these questions we have decades of experience to draw upon. Farmers *have* expanded their farms. Where there were 300 and 600-acre grain farms a generation or two ago, today we often see 3,000 and 6,000-acre grain farms. Dairy, potato, vegetable, cattle and hog farmers have similarly doubled and redoubled their production. A generation ago, a big tractor had 100 or 200 horsepower; today a big tractor has 300 or 400. Total acreage, acreage per farm, animals per farm, production per acre, production per farm, and total production are all up, and Canada's agri-food exports have doubled in the past decade. But getting bigger and more efficient has not helped farmers. Instead, most are struggling with the worst farm income crisis since the 1930s.

"Over the period 1969-2003 per farm production of grains, oilseeds, and special crops has doubled from under 150 tonnes per farm to nearly 400. But net income from grain per farm has fallen from just over $15,000 to just under $15,000." Similar figures are shown by hog farms, cattle, vegetable, dairy and other farms.

"Moreover, Realized Net Farm Income is not the same as profit. Corporate net income (profit) is calculated after everyone – workers, managers, and the CEO – gets paid. In contrast, net farm income is calculated before any allowance is made for labour and management contributions of family farm members.

"Myth 4: Economies of scale are the only way to gain efficiency.

"When retail bread prices rise, the reason may be that transnational millers, bakers and retailers are becoming less and less efficient as they get larger. Alternatively, the reason may be that the large size of these companies and the low levels of competition they face may allow them to take ever-larger profits and management salaries from the revenue streams within the agri-food chain. It would appear that one or the other of the preceding explanations must be true. Both cast doubt on the naive faith in automatic benefits from economies of scale.

"Economists confirm that as corporations merge and become larger, there is not just one effect – increased efficiency due to economies of scale – but also a second and countervail-

ing effect: increased oligopoly power. These researchers note that when increases in efficiency are smaller than increases in oligopoly power, prices will rise. Given the opportunity to charge less, but also the power to charge more, corporations will act predictably.

"Researchers Rigoberto Lopez, Azzeddine Azzam, and Carmen Liron-Espana have studied 32 US food-processing industry including meat packing, cereal production, soyabean milling, and coffee roasting. They calculated the magnitude of the efficiency effects and the oligopoly-power effect that would result from mergers and increased concentration. They conclude: 'Although cost-efficiency effects from concentration are important in one-third of the industries, in nearly every case the oligopoly-power effects dominated, resulting in higher output prices.'

"Why should we destabilize our farm families, ceaselessly pushing them toward ever-larger economies of scale, making them live in insecurity and worry, breaking farms and emptying communities, if, in the end, any efficiency gains will simply be pocketed by the transnationals?

"Myth 5: Technology will make farmers more efficient and prosperous.

"Farmers' gross revenue, net income and technology adoption 1947-2002.

"The new technologies have helped Canadian farmers double their (inflation-adjusted) gross revenue – from about $17 billion in the late 1940s to over $35 billion today. Farmers' net income, however, fell. Net income fell in the 1940s when many farmers were buying their first tractors and electrifying their tools, pumps and barns. It fell as farmers doubled and redoubled their fertilizer use. It fell as farmers adopted new chemicals to control insects and weeds. While there are fewer farms today among which to share the net income, even on a per-farm basis, net income is far below its 1940s level. On a per-farm basis, adjusted for inflation, farmers' net income today is far below its 1940s level. On a per-farm basis, adjusted for inflation, farmers' net income has been lower than at any time since the 1930s. To stay on the land, most families must now rely on off-farm jobs.

"The preceding dismissal of technology as a farm-income enhancer is not a Luddite position. Nor is it a blanket condemnation of technology. Most Canadian grain farmers do not want to go back to using hoes or oxen. Despite the romance, the majority of cattle farmers do not want to go back to spending long days on horseback and nights under the stars. This report's intent is that everyone should move beyond the simplistic assumption that the financial benefits of technology-enlarged production will automatically flow to farm families.

"While farmers retained (in net income) about one dollar out of every two that they generated in the late 1940s, today farmers retain just one dollar in ten. While new technologies and inputs have helped farmers increase production by about $18 billion (from about $17 billion in the 1940s to about $35 billion today), the corporations that sold those inputs and technologies to farmers not only swallowed up the entire $18 billion in increased production revenue, but an additional $8 billion as well – driving farmers' net income *down*. Over the past fifty years, for every dollar that the new technologies have contributed to farmers' revenues farmers have been made to pay $1.44.

"Dr. Martin Entz is a University of Manitoba plant scientist. He also leads the Glenlea Long-Term Crop Rotation Study. For twelve years, Entz and his team have used test plots to compare costs and yields for conventional, low input, pesticide free, and organic crop plots to compare costs and yields for conventional low input, pesticide-free, and organic crop production systems. Their findings: farmers achieve their highest net returns per acre when they use no purchased crop inputs – when they farm organically – even if they do not take advantage of premium prices for their organic crops.

"Agricultural technologies and purchased inputs *could* help farmers increase their net income, but not when corporations that sell those products use their overwhelming market power to price according to what the market will bear.

"During the first half of the 1990s, wheat prices rose and fertilizer prices tracked those increases. In the second half of the 1990s, wheat prices fell and, with a lag, fertilizer prices tracked wheat prices downward. In 2001, wheat prices again began an ascent, as did fertilizer prices. When grain prices rise, fertilizer companies raise their prices to snatch any additional revenue right out of farmers' pockets. Such pricing tactics are impossible in markets with real competition.

"**Myth 6: The rest of the economy is seeking efficiency through competition.**

"Of all government policies, the ones that most affect farmers' competition levels and the levels within the rest of the agri-food chain are the global integration and so-called 'free trade.' As trade and investment agreements have torn down the economic barriers between nations, these agreements have thrust all the world's farmers into a single, hyper-competitive market. At the same time, globalization and trade agreements have spurred the dominant transnationals to merge into ever-larger, less numerous mega-corporations. Globalization and trade agreements have increased competition levels for farmers – driving down farmers' prices and profits – and the effects for the dominant agribusiness transnationals have been just the opposite."

"**Myth 7 – Farmers are producing too little…and *too much*.**

"Governments are telling farmers: Technology and efficiency contribute to overproduction and declining prices; and declining prices necessitate more technology, higher efficiency, and increased production. While absurd, such a stratagem might have a tiny chance of success if powerful transnationals were not poised to skim off any benefits farmers might gain from increased production. As the system is currently structured, farmers are just the hamsters in the wheel that powers an expanding agribusiness empire. And government's solution to the farm crisis is for the hamsters to run faster.

"**Myth 8: Canadians will be better off if farmers compete, become more efficient, and become less numerous.**

"Even if farmers could achieve perfect efficiency and deliver food for free, routine price increases by processors and retailers would erase any such savings within a few years. An illustration of the disconnect between farm gate and retail prices came in 1988. That year, the federal government terminated Canada's Two-Price Wheat Program. As a result, the price that Canadian millers paid farmers for wheat fell from about $7 a bushel (under the Program) to about $5. Bread prices rose.

"**Myth 9: We are actually pursuing efficiency.**

"In the face of accelerating climate change and binding Kyoto commitments, is it efficient to drive farmers off the land and replace them with increased carbon-fuel use? In the face of polluted rivers and dead zones in our oceans, is it efficient to uproot third-generation farm families from their homes and replace them with megatons of nitrogen and phosphate fertilizers? With expanding slums of unemployed and starving people already encircling many cities in the developing world, is it efficient to displace several hundred million farmers in poor countries and replace farmers with tractors, Roundup, and genetically-modified crops?

"That we are pursuing real efficiency – in our food system or in our larger economy – is a myth. Economists merely create the illusion of efficiency by refusing to factor in resource depletion, bio-diversity loss, habitat destruction, water use, pollution, climate change, the degraded nutritional value of some foods, and a host of other 'externalities.'"

The more sophisticated publications in the United States from time to time deal with individual fragments of this grim picture, without, however, assembling it into the fullness of its message. There was something portentous when Columbus, having discovered America, honestly believed he had come to India. Ever since, our governments in the US and Canada have been prone to confusion where continents are concerned. Too readily do they impose as benefactions overseas what they occasionally recognize as evil back home.

The Wall Street Journal (27/01, "Bully Buyers – How Driving Prices Lower can Violate Antitrust Statutes" by John R. Wilke) informs us: "As most of the world's market become dominated by a few big companies, a rare form of antitrust abuse is raising new concern when corporations illegally drive down the prices of their suppliers.

"On the coast of Maine, blueberry growers alleged last year that four big processors conspired to push down the price they pay for fresh wild berries. A state-court jury last year awarded millions in damages. In South Carolina, International Paper Co. faces a lawsuit that it conspired with its timber buyers to depress softwood prices in several states. In Alabama and Pennsylvania, federal antitrust enforcers last year targeted insurance companies that imposed contracts forcing down fees charged by doctors and hospitals. The insurers abandoned the practice."

However, the same government has pushed through globalization that seeks to level all barriers that prevent the ever fewer large corporations from organizing to keep prices low. It has also mobilized the international monetary bureaucracy – the International Monetary Fund and the World Bank – to increase Third World countries' export of staples – no matter at what prices – to service their debt. Thus it is servicing debt rather than the interplay of supply and demand that increasingly determines prices on world food markets. At the same time other features of Globalization and Deregulation make local government liable for damages if they outlaw advantages already enjoyed by foreign corporations that have proved ruinous to the environment and society.

There is a fancy Greek name for buyers conspiring to drive down the prices paid to producers – oligopsony. But nowhere else have I encountered so thoroughgoing an analysis of how oligopoly – concerted purchasing power of sellers to up the prices of components they sell to producers – can combine with oligopsony – to squeeze life blood out of the same producers, while the government cheers on the process.

The model developed to explain the plight of our family farms, can be generalized on a world scale to understand the destructive effects of Globalization and Deregulation of entire economies. It begins with a harmless technique of infinitesimal calculus on which the supposed mathematics of "the pure and perfect market" is based: all actors in the market drama are assumed of such tiny size, that nothing they can do individually will influence the market and its prices. But the conglomerates that have taken over today as the suppliers of farmers or the distributors of their crops don't remotely fill that bill. On the contrary: growth and merger, the patenting of modified and unmodified genes, the relentless bullying of the little guy is the basic code of their behaviour. The constant climb of the price of their stock market shares is the one measure of their success and survival. That imposes upon them a model of conduct that resembles the mathematical process of integration rather than differentiation. The prestige of mathematics is thus purloined to cover up a degree of illiteracy that would get a freshman kicked out of any science course.

A prevailing way in which this shows up on a world scale and throughout the economy, is the competition of Third World countries to entice transnational corporations through tax-exemption deals to set up branch plants in the soliciting lands. The same game is played by the smaller jurisdictions in competition with one another within the provinces of the same country or between municipalities. And with the same ruinous results: tax exemptions are disastrous to their budgets faced with new responsibilities arising from the very success of their bid for branch plants. Thus they will never have the resources to educate their work force, and move up towards the next notch of "progress" as an "emerging" country. In short the host country attracting branch plants of international conglomerates is in exactly the position of our farmers squeezed between powerful oligopolist suppliers and equally oligopsonist customers, that is so well analyzed in the National Farm Union report.

William Krehm

Deficits and the Neoconservative Agenda

Starving the Beast

The new Canadian Conservative Party under Harper clearly owes much of its ideological baggage to the old Alliance and not much to the more centrist Progressive-Conservatives that it swallowed up. Canada's political and economic questions are viewed in a neo-conservative perspective, according to which all social and economic questions boil down to narrow efficiency measures. These purport to gauge whether they promote short-term maximization of individual wealth holdings.

The main ingredients of the neocon agenda are implementing tax cuts, reducing the size of the public sector, and ignoring investments in environment protection and infrastructure development. The US has been following such policies for more than two decades, only slightly dented by the more centrist concerns under Clinton. However, during his last six years, Clinton was left with little room for maneuver, faced as he was with a Republican Congress dominated by neocon ideologues such as Newt Gingrinch, Dick Armey and Tom Delay.

One result of that has been a dramatic widening of American income inequalities, raising the income share of the richest one percent of the population from 7.5% of national income in 1979 to 15.5% in 2000.

Neocons are always faced with the problem that their agenda, in reality, only serves the interests of a small minority of voters. One way around this is to focus the voters' attention on non-economic issues. But sometimes this is not enough, and consequently the economic agenda has to be packaged so that its real consequences become unclear especially for the voter-rich middle group. Increasingly, therefore this group is robbed of its of its fair share of society's productivity growth.

Thus, reducing government spending on identified social programs would be risky. So, instead, the neocon strategy of "Starving the Beast" was devised to overcome this hurdle. The term, "starving the beast," reputedly originated among some of President Bush's economic advisers. It refers to a strategy where the government's coffers are starved by reducing its revenues with large tax cuts, while at the same time raising spending on the military and other conservative pet programs. When "unexpected" deficits then emerge, this can, at a later stage, be used as a justification for the original intention of cutting back the public sector or privatizing large chunks of it.

That a policy of "starving the beast" is deliberate was confirmed when President Bush during a press conference in 2001 called the looming deficit "incredibly positive news," because it would produce "a fiscal straitjacket for Congress."

The costs of financing tax cuts by running deficits will in the long term dwarf the initial modest tax increases that fall to most voters. When the starving beast begins to bite, costs for health care, education and other social services will go up, as, chunk by chunk, they come to be privatized. Then different service levels will be adjusted to risk analysis and prospective patient-customers' ability to pay. For lower and middle income groups this process will once again squeeze the real purchasing power of their stagnant incomes. Conversely, the rapidly growing disposable income of wealthier strata, benefited, both by the tax cuts and privatization, will more than offset their higher user fees.

Incredibly Positive News

An example of how the structure of social services can be expected to look soon, is a recent development in the US health care system, where a new type of family doctor is appearing. For their patient base, they have only a limited number of wealthy individuals, who are charged high yearly fees. A reported case was US$20,000 a year. In return, these patients have the right to access the doctors at any time around the clock, including even being visited by them if need be.

In Canada, there have been a long standing debate about preserving our health care system as a universal system, and avoiding the two-tier system, commonly identified as typical of health care in the US. But the above shows that the discussion with reference to the American two-tier social system is outdated. Instead, Bush's America is now developing a three tier system, where the needs of the super-rich at the top are personalized and highly resource-intensive options provided.

Meanwhile, the middle class is being caught in a squeeze of rising costs for deteriorating services, while the lowest income groups without any abilities to pay the user fees demanded by for-profit providers are fighting to hang on at a bottom with only access to spotty and chronically resource-starved public systems. This is not only the case for health care, but also other major sectors of social services and infrastructures, such as the education system and public transport. Thus, for example, in the transport sector the three tier options start with the spotty and under-funded public services for the poor, clogged highways for the middle class, and – as the new third tier – expensive privately owned toll highways leading to the suburbs where the gated communities for the rich are concentrated.

That is the unholy trinity that is taking over our essential services.

Supply-side Obfuscations

To hide their plan to lead Canada down a similar path, the Harper Conservatives have been putting forward the usual economic half-truths, notably the old supply-side claim that all tax cuts will heighten economic activity to a tune where the tax cuts will pay for themselves. This is designed to convince the voter-rich middle class that it has nothing to fear from its slash-and-burn tax policies.

The supply-side claim rests on two functions. First, people raise spending when their disposable incomes go up. Second, if income taxes are lowered, people will respond by working more, thus creating more income to be taxed. Such effects do exist, but hardly to the extent claimed by the neocons.

Thus they ignore the well-known fact that households on different income levels will spend new disposable income differently. Poor households, always struggling to get by, will spend almost the entire amount on buying essentials that they are almost always short of. This means that the demand stimulation of extra disposable incomes among lower income groups is strong. However, as we have seen, most of the neoconservative designed tax cuts give very little to these income groups. On the other hand, high-income households will spend less on new consumption and more on private savings, which in modern economies are mostly channeled into financial instruments rather than directly productive assets. Thus, contrary to the claim, their effect of tax cuts on jobs and real economic activity can often be quite limited. Under some circumstances, raising wealthy households disposable incomes might even have negative effects for the economy by fueling asset inflation and speculative bubbles.

The second supply side claim ignores that wage work seldom is available in incremental steps, leaving ordinary wage earners with limited ability to adjust their work to changes in taxation.

The large deficits that developed during the Reagan presidency and now again under Bush clearly underscores that the supply-side claim, when put to practice, does not work. When the Conservatives before the election based their calculations on distorted to make them look reasonable, they inadvertently acknowledged that they are well aware of the fact that tax cuts seen in isolation will create deficits.

The Costs of a Free Lunch

Some have countered that deficits in modern economies do not matter as much as traditional theory assumes. Thus, the US apparently has gotten away with running large deficits relatively unscathed. Why shouldn't Canada join the free lunch?

As the Maestro himself, Alan Greenspan, recently acknowledged during a Congressional hearing, even he hasn't figured out how to invent a free lunch. One could add what America is enjoying is not a free lunch, but one partly paid for by others. Due to the US's pivotal role in the world, which includes the use of its dollar as the main international reserve currency, it can bend international economic relations to its own narrow economic interests.

This allows it to run deficits and consume more than it produces by sending part of the bill to other countries in the form of dollars and IOUs. Especially the amount of IOUs (American debt) that is held outside of the US has created a throwing-good-money-after-bad-money effect, which works to the American advantage. Few want to see the dollar tank, as this would sharply reduce the value of their own wealth portfolios, heavy with American IOUs; and destroy the American market capacity to absorb their exports. That is, except for Chirac and Schroeder, the political godfathers of the Euro, and their enthusiastic follower Saddam Hussein. Until, of course, he ended up in a hole near Tikrit, he was planning convert Iraq's foreign trade and portfolio holdings to Euro-denomination. Was that the real axis of evil that the Americans lashed out against?

Canada is, in fact, one of the countries that chip in substantially when the world pays for part of the American bills. One third of its production is sold to the Americans, and besides the official reserves maintained for such transaction purposes, many companies also hold dollar amounts privately outside the foreign reserve statistics. In consideration of the volume of trade, the obvious solution would be to create a Euro-style currency union between the two countries, which would distribute the seigniorage gain caused by nominal growth in trade reserves equally between the two nations. But does anyone expect that the Americans would accept that? We can adopt the American dollar if we want (as indeed some conservative Canadian economists have proposed). This, of course, would not only abdicate all chances of recovering the trade related seigniorage, but on top of that, also abandon the seigniorage that the Canadian government gains as a result of money expansion in the local economy.

The harsh reality is that Canada cannot expect any free rides on the international markets. On the contrary, they quickly would punish the reemergence of deficits by pushing the currency down and demand higher interest rates for Canadian debt.

Thus, behind the neocons' rosy picture of self-sustaining tax-cuts there lurks a very different reality. Such policies, if implemented, would set in motion a spiral of rising economic and social costs. These, furthermore, would be distributed very unequally. That could only lead to a more divided country, American-style.

Dix Sandbeck

From Lakeshore News, Wednesday, June 23, 2004

AT THE URGING of a group of residents, Lakeshore Council is pushing the federal and provincial governments to abandon the current system of property assessments and reinstate loans from the Bank of Canada for municipal infrastructure projects.

Council passed two resolutions at a recent meeting, the first asking the province to abolish the current system of property value assessments carried out by MPAC, and the second petitioning the federal government to instruct "to instruct the Bank of Canada to buy securities issued by municipalities to pay for necessary infrastructure and other capital works projects and to refund to municipalities any interest paid."

Andre Marentette, a local resident who chaired the delegation, said the current system of having properties reassessed through MPAC was proving too burdensome for taxpayers and insufficient to finance municipal infrastructure programs.

"Our municipal tax system is in trouble," he said.

Municipalities across Canada have long struggled to keep their expenses under control while attempting to meet ever expanding needs. In recent years, municipalities have become unable to meet the responsibilities they face."

Gordon Coggins, a retired professor from Brock University, said a better program could be set up through the Bank of Canada, which is chartered to create money and lend it to all three levels of government.

Coggins explained that the Bank of Canada is one of only

three nationalized banks among the world's rich nations. As a publicly-owned bank, it can make loans to government at lower interest rates than private banks. However, lobbying by private financial institutions has led to the marginalization of the Bank of Canada over the past half-century.

The reason for that marginalization, he said , is fear mongering over inflation.

"Bankers and their spokespeople always get edgy when anybody breathes the idea of money creation by government. They always warn of the horrors of inflation," Coggins said. But since the total money supply would remain consistent under such a program, Coggins argued that inflation isn't what the private banks are really worried about.

"The real motivation for this objection is pretty obvious. If municipalities can borrow from the Bank of Canada, they won't borrow from the private banks."

Deputy Mayor Tom Bain said he likes the sound of the delegations' resolutions.

Although County Council issued resolutions of their own earlier this year, the new ones were more straightforward, he said.

"The Council resolution asks the province to review the current assessment system; this one asks them to abolish it."

Copies of the package Marentette presented to Council are available from Lakeshore Community Services for $1.39.✻

Helping Us Diagnose Society's Fatal Illnesses

TO LEARN FROM our successes and failures is one of the purposes of history. It helps us identify threats to our survival as a species. However, our economists pay little attention to the performance data of past policies. When our paleontologists find life forms that survived only in primeval rocks, the first questions they ask are "when and why?" Even in more recent records of some government departments, the evidence is carefully collected for its possible usefulness. In matters of economic policy, however, such enquiry rarely take place.

That is why a recent front-page article in *The Wall Street Journal* (14/06, "They Go Through the FDA's Closet Looking for Treasures" by Anna Wilde Mathews) should be a polestar for befuddled economists searching a way out of the world's current mess.

Institutional Alzheimer

"Rockville, MD – In the windowless basement conference room of a Food and Drug Administration building, two agency officials hunted in dusty boxes for valuables.

"Before long, they unearthed a Dalkon Shield, the notorious birth-control device tied to several deaths in the early 1970s; a 'Waist Whittler' belt for plump women of the 1960s who wanted to trim inches without exercise; and 'Acupuncture pants' underwear, with a strategically placed magnet that supposedly increased male potency.

"Dr. Junod, and her associate, John P. Swann, are historians of the FDA. Part of a little-known fraternity of historians who work at government agencies, the two provide historical context for FDA regulatory and legal decisions and publish original research about the agency's past.

"They also serve as custodians of the FDA's collection of historical objects. Because the FDA is where remedies get approved, the scholars find themselves at the centre of American medical ingenuity and controversy, from the dangerous early patent medicines to the debate over silicone breast implants.

"Not all the issues are so weighty. One day recently, Dr. Junod and Dr. Swann pondered a thumb-sized plastic cylinder and wondered: Why would anyone want to use something called the 'Hemorr-Ice?' The package said the gadget was a method of treating hemorrhoids through cryotherapy. 'Most people, said Dr. Junod to her colleague, 'would have sat on an ice cube.'

"Many federal agencies have historians to preserve and interpret their pasts, though their purposes vary widely. At the National Aeronautics and Space Administration, historians advise movie makers, release CD recordings of famous missions and preserve relics viewed by millions of museum visitors.

"'We perform the function of an institutional memory,' said Dr. Junod. 'Issues of interest to consumers re-emerge – vitamins in the 1950s, dietary supplements in the 1960s.'

"As part of their jobs, they track down additions to the collection. One acquisition: an original bottle of a treatment called 'Elixir Sulfanilamide' that killed 107 people in the 1930s before the FDA seized all the medicine, which contained a deadly solvent."

Now just imagine what similar historians retained to preserve the knowledge of our past economic policies could achieve!

A deregulated stock market in the early 1930s led to hundreds of thousands of deaths, more than Elixir Sulfanilamide – if you include brokers jumping out of skyscrapers and the millions who expired from various forms of undernourishment and starvation, and the toll in twisted lives and broken families in those days of breadlines four abreast encircling entire New York blocks.

Dozens of heads of huge corporations like General Motors, and General Electric, Thomas Edison, Henry Ford and many others espoused various forms of monetary reform that are usually dismissed as "off the wall." Surely that is a detail worth preserving to warn of the costs of deregulated speculation. The same conditions superimposed on the legacy of the lost World War I gave rise to the Nazi movement in Germany and to World War II. Or how the tight separations of the four Pillars of finance – banking, insurance, the stock market and mortgage-lending, prevented the compounding of the various sorts of financial leverage (money-lending and money-creation powers). Instead, governments themselves through their central banks took to creating more of the money directly. That not only guaranteed that when the market system had broken down under the weight of its greed and corruption, the state could step in to fill the resulting gaps.

Not only do we lack official historians to conserve our past, but for three decades we have had a campaign to hide the failures of globalization and deregulation. Instead, each disaster has led to a stepped-up dosage of the failed policy. After all, hadn't it been called "the pure and perfect market"? To enforce that obvious bit of nonsense, thousands of university professors have been given early retirement, and even more have been refused tenure. There is little room in our mass media for any mention, let alone serious examination, of failed economic doctrines, or even of the public policies that worked well in the past.

Sitting on the Volcker Glacier as a Cure for Piles

The FDA historian compared Hemorr-Ice to sitting on an ice cube to cure hemorrhoids. Similarly US Federal Reserve Chair Paul Volcker converted the American economy into a vast artificial glacier for the US to sit on to cure what he took to be "inflation." That of necessity had to be abandoned, but a truthful account of the experience has never been carried in the official record. Right-thinking economists if they refer to the crippling experiment at all are like to do so in terms of praise – Volcker's "victory over inflation." The parallel case in Canada was the experience of Governor John Crow of the Bank of Canada, who even pushed interest rates five points above those attained by Volcker in the US.

Or the nonsense sent out by the Bank for International Settlements (BIS), the central bankers' private club in Basel, Switzerland, that repeatedly broadcast the grim warning that if even a smidgin of "inflation," i.e., rise in the chosen price index, were allowed, it would inevitably lead to a repeat of the German hyperinflation of 1923. That warning implied that if interest rates had been pushed up high enough in Germany in 1923, there would have been – by a retroactive miracle – no WWI for Germany to lose, no occupation of the Ruhr, the German industrial heartland by the French army to collect the reparation payments in foreign currency that the Germans could only pay in their currency that nobody wanted. It would also have to be assumed that there would have been no general strike to protest the occupation of the Ruhr, supported both by the left and right parties, that no virtual civil war took place, no assassination of the German foreign minister who had signed the treaty with the Allies. That nonsense, however, was repeated by government spokesmen, and the media, and even by economics professors worried about getting early retirement if they questioned it. Where are the historical displays to remind us of all that?

"He who forgets his past is condemned to relive it." It is in fact far worse than that. What has taken over is the control of a financial system that can survive only by incorporating into the present value of stock portfolios the rates of growth to higher powers already attained into the indefinite future, and using such valuations as collateral to finance further such valuations. What results is in fact an exponential curve – the mathematics of the atom bomb. Not only is such a growth rate unsustainable, but the merest shortfall of that growth already embodied in the collateral that supports the boom, can bring on a bust of equal momentum. Students in economics courses who spend so much time on the mathematics of the "pure and perfect market" (on which all actors are of such infinitesimal size as to make irrelevant what each does or does not do individually), should be carefully instructed in the nature of the exponential curve. It is not just the cumulative effect of compound interest. Compound interest deals with the same rate of interest applied to higher powers. In an exponential progression the rate of growth of the rate of growth, to ever higher powers to infinity moves upward in step with the value of the function itself. That is why the historians of deregulated finance, that has removed the firewalls between banks, stock markets, and mortgage institutions, would have to include a chapter on the atom bomb and trace the processes that link it to the our derivative-driven economy today.

William Krehm

COMER Conference Exudes Promise

BY NASAL COUNT the COMER Conference held in Toronto on May 29, was modest enough – attended by between 50 and 60. However, an election campaign was gearing up, and a well-advertised international conference questioning the Bush government re the Twin Tower attack had come to town. But in other respects it was full of promise.

COMER, of course, is not a political party, but a think-tank particularly concerned with the blocking of information vital to our democratic rights. In our ranks we have members and sympathizers of many democratic parties. On this occasion, we had invited a host of organizations to state their concerns, but then to tell us how they proposed to answer "Where will the Money Come from?". Of official representatives of political organizations, only Canadian Action Party (CAP) turned up officially and answered that question convincingly: by making use of the Bank of Canada for the goals for which it was founded and nationalized (1935 and 1938 respectively). These are still to be found the *Bank of Canada Act*. They made it possible for this country to begin groping its way out of the Depression of the 1930s, finance our part in WWII at low interest rates through the BoC; catch up with sixteen years of neglect and destruction of our physical and human infrastructures; assimilate a vast, penniless immigration. And at the end of the war, the ratio of Canada's federal debt to its Gross National Product was 170%.

Yet, by the mid seventies, after achieving so much, our ratio of debt to GNP had been brought down from 170% to less than 25%! Today. however, our government claims that we cannot afford to maintain the infrastructure that we managed to build in those lean, heroic years"! How was that possible? By increasing the proportion of the federal debt financed through the Bank of Canada from some 16% at the height of the war to 22% in the mid-1970s. How was that possible? By increasing the portion of its borrowing from its own bank on a near-interest-free basis. Today that ratio hovers around 5%. But wasn't that funny money? On the contrary it was achieved through good capital-

ist institution: dividends. The interest paid on its loans from the central bank returned to the government substantially by that channel.

A positive feature of the conference was the appearance not only of Paul Hellyer, the retiring leader of PAC, and Deputy Prime Minister of Canada under Trudeau, but of his successor in that post, Connie Fogal. The gathering gave Paul well-earned applause for holding high the memory of those better years. Connie laid out not only CAP's adhesion to the use of the Bank of Canada for its intended purpose, but the importance of bringing capital budgeting (accrual accountancy) into the government books. For if you write off government investments like bridges, buildings in the year that they were made rather than depreciate them over their useful lives, you show only the liabilities incurred for their acquisition. And that exaggerates your net debt. By booking such capital assets starting with year two at a token dollar, you also set the stage for the privatization of government investments carried on the books at one dollar for a ridiculous fraction of their real value.

That is the message that Connie is carrying into the current electoral battle.

Bill Krehm dealt with the perverted metric that COMER must face: the more views that COMER fought for since its founding that are being adopted piecemeal and in stealth, the more thoroughly those views are being suppressed in public discourse. The have been removed from university texts; professors teaching them are given early retirement.

A new phenomenon must be recognized, identified by a "structural economic historian", Douglass North: all political regimes are based on compromises allowing an alliance of different economic forces. If for purely political interests, a regime indulges in too headlong a redistribution of the national revenue, it destroys these alliances and undermines economic stability. That happened in Canada in 1993, in what we might call the "Mulroney syndrome." that reduced the Progressive Conservative Party to a couple of parliamentary members. Britain had its "Thatcher Syndrome", that cut the Conservatives off at the knees. More drastically, Mexico in 1994 went through its "Salinas syndrome" that brought back the period of rule by political assassination, and just stopped short of bringing down the world financial system. Visibly something of this sort has happened with Paul Martin's soaring ambitions.

Other speakers were Gordon Coggins, Richard Priestman, Herb Wiseman, Bob Campbell, Keith Wilde, with adequate discussion and debate from the floor. Another issue that was discussed was how complete a statement of our common positions can be ventured without frightening off aspiring parties. The prevailing view was that key positions are not subject to compromise. Otherwise we could be collaborating in the suppression of vital information indispensable for sound law-making.

W.K.

Poor Mr. Greenspan and His Impossible Task

OUR GLOBALIZED and deregulated world has become ever more complicated, and unless we take into account the conflicting interests involved, we will never learn to manage it. For that we must have complete freedom of information and that has not been forthcoming. The article of James Grant, editor of Grant's *Interest Rate Observer*, on *The New York Times* oped page (16/05, "Low Rates, High Expectations") illustrates the point. Mr. Grant writes: "Why the Fed decided to propagate inflation, after having so long battled against it, is a story that begins with the return to common usage of an old word. Late in 2002, officials began to warn of the danger of 'deflation' or broadly falling prices. Everyday low prices are well and good, the central bankers allowed. Yet if prices steadily and predictably fell, people would stop buying things. They would stay home to wait for tomorrow's guaranteed lower prices."

If matters were really that simple! The sudden rediscovery by the Fed and the Bank for International Settlements, after years of fanatical espousal of "zero inflation," that not only inflation was not necessarily always a bad thing, but that up to some two percent, inflation was "good." "Good inflation" so belatedly discovered, is apparently essential to lubricate what has been termed a "pure and perfect market" that in fact, never existed, and was thus never open to the Popper test, not being disprovable. However, grant that and what assurance have we that is falls short of perfection and purity in yet other respects: perhaps its axles are broken, its tires flat, and the drivers are cooking the books showing its fuel efficiency?

The Popper Test Goes Pop

Fortunately, however, we can use our imagination to summon up an emergency substitute for a "pure and perfect" Popper test.[1] Today when genes and even species are subject to patents producing "rents," imagine what would have happened had Isaac Newton been able to patent the law of gravity, so that whoever used it had to pay a rent. Or Einstein, who came to America as a privileged refugee with a $35-a-week job, had not neglected to "lock in" his rights to a rent on his relativity and quantum theory discoveries. That would have required other impecunious scientists who wished to make use of them to pay him a rent It would certainly have done wonders for the GDP, but would it have helped licking inflation? Worse yet, suppose that the theory of relativity had been suppressed, so that other physicists could write oped letters to *The New York Times* decades later unaware of its existence.

It is no secret that during the 1980s the deregulation of the banking systems of this continent had led to the banks losing much of their capital in gambles in gas and oil, real estate, and mergers and acquisitions. To bail them out in Canada and Mexico, the statutory reserves were abolished. These the banks had had to redeposit with the central banks as a modest proportion of what they took in as deposits in their chequing accounts. In the US and the UK, though such reserves remain on the books,

their use has sunk to insignificance. Such statutory reserves had provided central banks with an alternative to raising interest rates to rein in perceived "inflation." Interest rates, as sole blunt stabilizing tool, however, have the disadvantage of hitting everything that moves in an economy that grows by piling up debt in both the government and private sectors. Reducing the quantity of available credit to control perceived inflation rather than raising interest rates permitted more selective targeting of anti-inflationary policy. And the interest paid by the government on its debt held by the central bank reverted substantially to it by virtue of the ancestral monarch's right of seigniorage – his monopoly of coining precious metals. In countries like Canada and the UK where the government is the sole shareholder of the central bank the mechanism is simpler – minus an overhead charge, all profits of the central bank find their way to the government as dividends. A good old capitalist institution, remember? The use of the non-interest-bearing reserves thus afforded the federal government a near-free use of credit within the existing constraints.

A little earlier the Bank for International Settlements had brought in its *Risk-Based Bank Capital Requirements* guidelines that declared the debt of OECD countries "risk-free" requiring no additional capital for banks to acquire. This shifted the monitoring of banks' solvency from cash reserves to capital. Banks do raise capital as cash – either by selling shares or through retained earnings – but only a minimal portion of such capital increases is allowed to remain as cash. For cash earns no interest. It gets invested, and most banks enter such investments on their books at historic rather than at market value.

But what was overlooked in the urgency to cast a life-line to the banks floundering from previous indiscretions, was that the combined effect of these two measures was certain to bring down the banks once again. They certainly contributed to the Mexican monetary meltdown of 1994 that, were it not for the $51 billion standby put together by President Clinton, the IMF and Canada, would have crashed the world financial system. This has been documented brilliantly in a remarkable study by Francisco J. Vega Rodriguez (*La Singular Historia del Rescate Bancario Mexicano, 1994-1999*).

Ruthless Progeny of Policy Gaff

But a policy gaffe, if buried rather than learned from, begets a ruthless progeny. Throughout the Americas and to an extent the world, the mad drive to flatten prices through high interest rates under Paul Volcker created damages that this neglected Mexican book compares to the cost of a lost war. By allowing the banks to accumulate government bonds entirely on the cuff, the terms of the banks' bailout left them vulnerable to any interest rise that would devaluate their bloated bond hoards. The chosen cure thus became a guarantee that the disease would break out in still more virulent forms.

But how to bring down interest rates without eating crow, a proscribed diet for those in charge of our monetary affairs? That would reveal the unspeakable secrets of both the banks' bailout and their inexcusable further deregulation. The latter led them to multiply their speculative credit creation to acquire brokerages, merchant banking, insurance underwriting activities, both as marketers and as principals in complex derivative deals executed in deep shadows. The answer came apparently from Robert Rubin, Clinton's Treasury secretary, a brilliant alumnus of Wall Street. Accrual accountancy was brought into the government's books to reveal the true depreciated value of physical capital assets that had been totally written off in the year of their acquisition, while their cost remained on the books to swell the government's deficit and debt. Of course, the resulting budgetary imbalance drove up the interest rates the government had to be pay on its debt, shifted largely from the Fed to the private market. By correcting the one year write-off of assets that would last for decades and carrying the correction back several years, the Fed's balance was improved by approximately 1.3 trillion dollars. But since President Clinton was determined to hold the political centre, this could not be named for what it was: "government investment." By the neo-liberal faith governments are not supposed to be able to invest. The foregoing can be verified by consulting the *Survey of Current Business* for January-February, 1996, p.13, of the Bureau of Economic Analysis, and the *Federal Reserve Bulletin* table A-40.

It should be noted that these corrections still leave untouched the distortions of government accountancy that ignores the vast investment of the federal government in human capital – education, health, and social security, that was recognized in the 1960s by Nobel Laureate for Economics Theodore Schultz and others as the most productive investment a society can make. Economic historians like Ferdinand Braudel have emphasized that the higher price level in cities over that in the countryside in large part reflects the higher living costs of urbanization due to the indispensable services that only large cities provide. Nobody who moves from a town of 10,000 to New York City expects his living costs to stay the same. How then can we when humanity has been making just such a move? All that is lost in the simplistic version of Mr. Grant.

While one aspect of Mr. Alan Greenspan is seen as the secretive sage who reads the future from the murky crystal ball of "inflation, both good and bad," in another he is the poor fellow on whom has been downloaded the impossible job of deducing solutions to an ever more complicated problem by contemplating his navel and the single variable dear to bondholders and their spokesmen.

William Krehm

1. Karl Raimund Popper was an Austrian-born, British philosopher who developed the notion of "testability" essential to proving a thesis correct. This consisted in being able to present the opposite, i.e., the negative of the scrutinized proposition in a form that could be disproved. Thus you cannot prove that angels don't exist, because no one has ever seen one, but that merely leaves the question of their existence open. Likewise, the existence of a "pure and perfect market."

Ruminations on the Number Three

THREE is the number of the Trinity: Father, Son and Holy Ghost; though the Third Party has had his mediaeval moniker somewhat degraded by a million trick-or-treaters and is now better known as the "Holy Spirit."

In Renaissance numerology three is the number of marriage, where one plus one makes a third.

In classical logic three is the number of parts to the syllogism, where Major Premise plus Minor Premise produces Conclusion. For example:

1. Economics is the master science. MAJOR PREMISE.

2. The proposal to run 10,000 trucks a day through the middle of the city of Windsor is an economic decision. MINOR PREMISE.

3. Therefore the proposal to run 10,000 trucks…is a master scientific decision. CONCLUSION.

The conclusion follows logically from the premises. To refute the conclusion, it is necessary only to prove that one on the premises is not true. In this example, that is not difficult.

Three is also the number of the Hegelian dialectic, where thesis vs. antithesis brings forth the new synthesis. For example:

• Thesis: capitalism
• Antithesis: Marxism
• Synthesis: liberal democracy

Sometimes the flow of history needs a little touch of revolution to hasten it to its end. There are three stages in the making of a successful revolution: (1) seizing political control; (2) controlling the media (e.g., state, or corporate TV); and (3) shaping public education to keep the next generation on the right road. Perhaps there is a fourth stage, deification of the ruler, of which more later.

The Solipsism of Technology

There are, on the other hand, three stages to the response of a ruling elite to revolutionary criticism: (1) Pretend they have not heard the criticism. If it becomes too raucous, (2) discredit the critics ("poor benighted anti-globalists; they just don't understand"), and (3) if the criticism still persists, smash the critics, and thus silence the voice of criticism. The heavy police response to anti-globalization and anti-war demonstrations looks like evidence of a shift to stage three, of which perhaps more later.

In the major media, particularly American, we are told, *ad nauseam*, that "9/11 changed everything." Three books from the previous decade that I have recently read or re-read suggest, rather to the contrary, that "Plus ça change, plus c'est la même chose."

This is not a book review, but a rumination on:

Thomas Frank: *One Market under God: Extreme Capitalism, Market Populism, and the End of Economic Democracy* (2000).

Neil Postman: *Technopoly: the Surrender of Culture to Technology* (1994).

Francis Fukuyama: *The End of History and the Last Man*

(1992).

Frank traces the history of business rhetoric over the last two or three decades as it has attempted, with considerable success, to assimilate "democracy" into the worship of its great god, "The Market."

Postman reaches back as far as Plato and Aristotle, but his focus is contemporary America, where, he argues technology has invaded our thought to the extent that we are effectively ruled by and live in "technopoly" (Gr. polis, city, and techne, practical skills – what Plato calls "mere knack"). Technopoly tends to block all other thoughts but its own. Its three pillars are: (1) bureaucracy, whose guiding principle is efficiency, without regard to collateral consequences; (2) expertise, which is ignorant of any human concern lying outside of its own area.; and (3) technical machinery misapplied to human issues. As examples of the last Postman cites "IQ tests, SATs, standardized forms, taxonomies and opinion polls."

Fukuyama's book is the most ambitious of the three, because it aims to be a definitive philosophy of history. The fate of Karl Marx's similar attempt comes to mind. Fukuyama develops, with an impressive but eclectic assembly of historical and philosophical data, the extraordinary thesis originally proposed in his 1989 essay "The End of History," that the acme of human social achievement had been reached with [particularly American] liberal democracy and unrestricted market capitalism. (He has no doubt contributed to the tendency of many Americans to treat those two terms as synonymous.)

When Arnold Toynbee wrote his great *A Study of History* (1934-61) to refute Oswald Spengler's bleak tomes, *The Decline of the West* (1918-22), his best compromise with the Splenglerian doctrine of the inevitable decline of civilizations was carried in the metaphor that the rise and fall of civilizations is cyclical, but cyclical like the turning wheels of a carriage which itself is on an upward course.

Fukuyama is of Toynbee's camp, but with a new twist; he resists the idea of the inevitable decline of liberal democracy and unrestricted market capitalism, but he does conclude the book with his own wheely metaphor, likening the various societies of the world to wagons in or on the road to the final settlement site. "Rather than a thousand shoots blossoming into as many differing flowering plants, mankind will come to seem like a long wagon train strung out along a road," its final destination the *polis* of liberal democracy and unrestricted market capitalism.

Obviously, Fukuyama's blind side is a tendency to see contemporary United States in Dr. Pangloss' terms – a society where "all's for the best in the best of all possible worlds." It is the unchallenged launching pad of this "Study of History."

The argument depends on the concept of a three-part division of the human soul: (1) reason, which gives us science and technology; (2) desire, the impetus to satisfy practical needs; and (3) Plato's *thymos*, the desire for recognition. The greatest of these is *thymos*, which takes two routes, depending on whether you are a master or a slave: *megalothymia*, which leads to a desire to dominate; and *isothymia*, which leads to a desire for equality. "The problem of human history," he says, "can be

seen, in a certain sense, as the search for a way to satisfy the desire of both masters and slaves for recognition on a mutual and equal basis; history ends with the victory of a social order that accomplishes this goal."

Revisiting his thesis post 9/11 in an article in *Policy* (Winter, 2002), he writes: "More than ten years ago, I argued that we had reached the 'end of history'…that History understood as the evolution of human societies through different forms of government had culminated in modern liberal democracy and market-oriented capitalism. It is my view that this hypothesis remains correct, despite the events since September 11." He confidently asserts that "Western institutions are like the scientific method, which, though discovered in the West, has universal applicability." They operate through a three-stage mechanism. (1) Economic liberalism creates a middle class. (2) The middle class demands political democracy. (3) Cultural convergence follows. But if one perceives that two events in Fukuyama's own backyard – the "hollowing out of the middle class" that the statistics on wealth distribution suggest is taking place, and the unbridled *megalothymia* of the American elite – one is inclined to suspect that a fourth stage is already emerging. The "end" may turn out to be just the beginning of another cycle, as the great god, Market, further exposes his clay feet and ruthless spirit.

Gordon Coggins

The Dead Rat under the Floorboards that Poisons the Political Air

THIS YEAR of untimely wars and weather, seems to be confusing Santa Claus like the rest of us. For though the flowers are out in their glory, that fat old gent seems stuck on his way down the chimney, giving the world a bad case of smoke in the eyes. No, it is not a second Xmas, just election time, the season of fake miracles and empty promises. And the centre of the stage is occupied by our political super-marketeer, Paul Martin. When the Liberals were elected in 1994, he had promised as future finance minister to repeal the Goods and Services that had knocked the wind out of the budgets of our most defenceless citizens. For they, too, have budgets that must be balanced, good years or bad, which is not really the case with the federal government. Nor have they a chance of cooking their books.

Elsewhere we have explained in detail how our banks were bailed out by the Mulroney conservative government in 1991 from their immense losses gambling in gas and oil, real estate in the US. And having achieved that in secret, Mulroney went on to remake the banking laws that had been brought in during the Great Depression to make the banks stick to banking – rather than pretending they were master gamblers playing in their own casinos.

That is important stuff, but a little hard for the average voter. Especially when the details of how this was done is the best-suppressed secret of the land. Today I'm going to approach the problem in an easier way for people who haven't time to go into all the technical details with the election practically upon us.

What marks out this election is the deep disillusionment of voters with the two major parties. One, the Conservatives, had so completely sold out, that a decade ago its leaders didn't even bother running for reelection. They simply retired to lucrative jobs in the service of large corporations that they had served too well. Today their successors, the Liberals, are almost in the same predicament. The air, heavy with unspoken secrets of how the postwar world not only promised but delivered so much that was suddenly loused up to resemble the plagues of Egypt rather than the promised land.

The Redolent Rat under the Boards

The big unspoken secret at the bottom of all this, the dead rat under the floorboards, is forcing its way to the surface. For example *The Globe and Mail's* Business section (June 3, "Tories' financial savvy an unknown quantity" by Heather Scoffield) has this revealing passage:

"'A Conservative election would be problematic for financial markets,' said Rob Palombia, analyst at Standard and Poor's. The core of likely candidates to carry the economic load – names such as Monte Solberg, James Moore, James Rajotte, Jason Kenney and John Williams – have been impressive as party critics on some of the key files, but don't have the credential or cachet to assuage Bay St. worries. There would be a testing period, Mr. Palombi said.

"Ultimately, the Conservatives will need to groom some talent from deeper down the party bench, and from parts of the country outside Alberta and British Columbia, to provide comfort to the business community."

What, we must ask, is troubling Bay Street? There is no lack of economic Ph.D.s around, and graduates of business faculties trained to present the case of business. Or civil servants to instruct fledgling cabinet ministers. But obviously it is the dead rat under the floorboards that troubles them, the secrets of past bailouts and deregulations that can't bear the light of day. Their sense of this explains the deepening disillusionment of the voters today. There is a sense of secrets that require special handling – rather like the password that opens the vaults of a bank.

Why are Governments Suppressing the Records of our Most Successful Years?

After ten years of depression and six years of war, Canada emerged with a debt equal to an estimated 170 percent of the Gross National Product. It caught up with the neglect and mayhem of those sixteen years, housed and brought up the post-war generation, and assimilated an unprecedented flood of mostly penniless immigrants to standards undreamt of before. On top of that by the mid-1970s the government had reduced that ratio that we hear so much about from Mr. Martin, that of federal debt to the GNP, to about 22% from 170%.

How did our parents manage that when, according to Mr. Martin, we cannot even afford to *maintain* the infrastructures that were created in those happy years. This relates to something

basic in economic reasoning that has been buried out of sight. It simply has to be disinterred, if our democracy is not to become a bad joke.

Obviously, with his rich experience in twisting the facts during his ten years as Finance minister, such a whopping secret is catching up with Mr. Martin.

Thus *The Globe and Mail* (26/05, "Mr. Martin's big pledge: $9 billion for health"): As Mr. Martin unveiled the platform at a hospital in Cobourg, he had to fend off allegations that he created the problem by slashing federal health-care transfers to provinces in his 1995 budget.

"'The fact is that we had to do that,' he responded. 'And I don't back down from that one bit. If we had not taken the action that we did in 1995, we would be Argentina today.'

"Mr. Martin insisted that tax increases would not be required to pay for the health-care plan and that the program would fit inside current government surplus projections."

But what he doesn't mention is that the previous Auditor General, Denis Desautels, in 1999 had to carry on unpleasant arguments with Finance Minister Martin for weeks, and even accuse him of "cooking the books" before he was able to get investments like roads, bridges, buildings, treated as the investments that they are, rather than written off in a single year and carried on the books at a token dollar. At the same time the debt incurred to acquire them was fully booked on the liability side of the ledger. This violated the basic principle of double-entry bookkeeping, one of the great achievements of humanity some 1,000 years ago. And even so, the government still writes off investments in human capital – education, health, and social security as a current expense though they are the most productive of all investments.

Had economists not been educated to the need for anti-cyclical budgeting – running up a deficit during recessions and a surplus – after observing double-entry bookkeeping – in boomtimes, we would still be in the Great Depression of the 1930s.

Paying Off the Debt in Bills of a Different Colour?

But instead of double-entry bookkeping, Mr. Martin practices his old-wives' prudence of salting away a few billions of revenue "for a rainy day" so that he can meanwhile slash social programs and precipitate recessions to please his sponsors. To understand the extent of the deception you need only note that the only legal tender today is the credit our central government, backed by the human and physical resources that are the tax base. Gold and silver are no longer money.

Today, the only collateral for the government's credit is the brains, brawn, and training of our population and the nation's physical resources. If you do not maintain those, you are undermining the collateral of the government's debt which is its tax base. This is nothing to be gambled with, either by our deregulated banks or politically by the Mulroneys and Martins. The credit of our government lies not in its cash holdings (for the only cash is in the federal government's debt!), but in the productivity of the nation.

There is in fact an immense load of unspoken and unspeakable secrets between that Mr. Martin as Finance Minister kept with the banking community – the details of their bailout at the expense of the social services of the country, followed by the subsequent deregulation of the Banks that allowed them to take over a crucial part of the financial system.

The moral rot of our public life is sensed by the frequency of the financial scandals that have occupied the regulatory authorities in the US, in which three of our largest banks (CIBC, RBC and TD) have been fined as much as $80 million US, with possible class actions in the offing. Significantly, there has been a marked absence of similar investigations of our financial institutions in Canada. That makes all the more disturbing the power over government that our banks – through the very nature of their bailout of 1991 and subsequent further deregulation – have acquired. That is the dead rat under our floorboards that has polluted the very political air we breathe. Democracy without information is unthinkable. That is why after the Mulroney-Martin information-controls, this country of ours must move on to proportional representation. Only that will give the electorate the real facts concerning our history and our politicians' escapades.

William Krehm

The NDP's Important First Step towards the Essential Use of the Bank of Canada

WE ARE INDEBTED to Richard Priestman for the following note: "Some of you may be interested to know that the NDP platform contains a statement on using the Bank of Canada to carry public debt. It happens to be the very last statement of the very last section, "Clear Choices on Debt Reduction." We quote:

"Jack Layton and Canada's NDP will give Canada clear choices on debt reduction by bringing some of Canada's national debt under the control of the Bank of Canada, as it used to be, and paying the interest to ourselves as opposed to chartered banks.

"We haven't heard Jack talk about this as yet. I hope he will soon and show how using the Bank of Canada in this way will make it possible to finance hospitals, schools and other infrastructure and still balance the budget as he has promised to do. While the savings in interest are substantial, even greater savings could occur by depreciating capital projects over their expected life, thereby reducing the annual payments of principal.

"The platform is a 65-page document which you can access at www.ndp.ca."

Our congratulation to the NDP for this important step, but to it we must attach a caution:

The return to the use of the Bank of Canada as originally intended is not an option, but a stark necessity. Without it the speculative bubbles on which the end of the statutory reserves and their further deregulation have made possible will lead this country to the most devastating financial bust yet experienced. In addition to making it possible to finance essential government investment in physical and human capital, it would bring our banks back to responsible banking which the country stands in need of.

Once before COMER warned an NDP government in good time that the proper use of the Bank of Canada was not an option but a dire necessity. Under date 21/10/91, Premier Bob Rae, at the time when the Ontario NDP was at the height of its prestige, replied to John Hotson and myself as follows:

"In your letter, you suggest the Bank of Canada should follow a regional policy, by buying bonds issued by the governments of provinces suffering economic hardship. Our government would prefer federal-provincial transfer programs continue without successive reductions and formula overrides. In any case, your proposal would not deal with the high cost of credit faced by private borrowers through the financial system."

It would be a tragedy for Canada, if the NDP gave us an encore to Bob Rae's blunder.

W.K.

The Hipshot Fiction of the Self-balancing Market

SET YOUR EYE, if it is not of glass, for a close-up view of just about any aspect of the "pure and perfect market" that is said to watch over our destinies, and you will recoil in shock. Who could have dreamt up so crude and colossal a swindle, and imposed it on a society aching to get on to other planets, perhaps because we are so well on the way to lousing up so definitively the one we're on.

We live in the age of the SUV but our world automobile industry, unconcerned about what is to be used to fuel them, and who is to pay for the vastly over-expanded auto industry, seems to have found a solution: forcing the subcontracting firms to outsource to China and slash their costs by circumventing their own obligation to their workers and taxpayers. Probably in the fullness of time, this cute "derivative" outsourcing will be patented by accountants or some corporation employing it.

For the details let's tap *The Wall Street Journal* (10/06, "Chain Reaction – Big Three's Outsourcing Plan: Make Parts Suppliers Do it" by Norishko Shirouzu): "Global trade and American labor are creating a quandary for the Big Three auto makers. Facing intense price competition, they want to take advantage of the plunging cost of manufacturing in China. Yet their labor agreements at home make it hard to shift jobs overseas.

"Now the auto giants have hit upon an unusual strategy. Push their suppliers to do their outsourcing for them. Consider the case of Superior Industries International Inc., a big aluminum-wheel-maker in Van Nuys, Calif. For years, President Steve Borick dismissed Chinese manufacturing. The quality of Chinese wheels didn't impress him. The logistics of shipping thousands of rims across the Pacific seemed too complicated.

"Then Mr. Borick started getting a blunt message from General Motors and Ford with whom Superior does 85% of its $840 million a year in business. Match the prices they were seeing at Chinese wheel suppliers. If Superior didn't agree to new terms, both auto makers said separately they could go directly to the Chinese or turn to a North American wheel-maker that would.

"'This is the price we are getting for this product. You either match that or the auto-maker will look elsewhere. The message is: "Close the gap no matter how."' In Superior's case, that meant cutting its profit margins – and finally deciding to make its own wheels in China. Both GM and Ford acknowledge that Chinese auto-parts suppliers now serve as global 'benchmark' for quality and price for certain components such as electric-wire cables, radios, speakers, small motors, and even brakes, suspensions and aluminum wheels. The prices reflect China's average wage costs of 90 cents an hour compared with $22.50 in the US, according to Roland, Berger Strategy Consultants of Troy, Mich."

Muddled-up Comparative Advantages

Talking of wooden horses, even the location of the consultant spills the beans.

"'It's Economics 101, Adam Smith,' Ford President Nick Scheele says. 'It's the law of comparative advantage." In fact he got that, like so much else, all wrong. "Comparative advantage" was the brain-child not of Smith, but of David Ricardo, and it referred to natural advantages like favourable climate, soil, and so forth, not how low wages could be squeezed. There is nothing natural about that. Rather it is the result of a social system that is filling the world with SUVs beyond even the available gasoline to run them, provided that the buyers can come up with the credit to show off their privileged position. That has to do with the folly of those in power. Nature in fact seems to be preparing her own grim rejoinders.

"He says the benchmark component prices Ford is asking suppliers to match these days represents 'optimal,' and come from anywhere in the world including China." Including the United States, if wages are driven down to Chinese levels there as well. And to that must be added that Chinese wages, as low as they are, are still on their way down.

"Ford opened its China purchasing office in Shanghai in 2002 and is aiming to buy billions of dollars of components in the country, a good portion of which would end up in cars built in Ford's North American assembly plants. US suppliers say the pricing policy leaves them scrounging to close a cost gap as wide as 20% to 40%, even after taking into account the costs caused by the distance between Asia and North America.

"Detroit's preoccupation with China goes back to the late 1990s, when the first wave of GM executives began coming home from the auto maker's joint ventures in Shanghai. The intensity of the auto industry's interest in China increased markedly in the months after Sept. 11, 2001, terror attacks. With cash discounts and no-interest loans, the auto industry managed to keep itself afloat despite a darkening economic picture. The price war has continued even as the economy recovers.

"With their own moves constricted by job-protection restrictions built into their pacts with the United Auto Workers, the Big Three began leaning on suppliers to help with cost cutting. The Big Three say they are still a long way from fully exploiting China's potential as a source of parts. Less than 5% of the components Ford uses to build vehicles in North America come from off shore, says Ford spokesman Paul Wood.

"At GM, only one-tenth of materials and parts the company uses in North America come directly from China – though some parts from suppliers might contain sub-components from China and other low-wage countries, says Tom Wickham, a GM spokesman.

"Overall, China last year exported $1 billion of components to the US, up 32% from 2002 and more than double the 2000 level, according to Commerce Department data. Still, China trailed far behind Germany and Japan, which shipped to the US $2.2 billion and $7.3 billion of components, respectively, in 2003.

"At Superior, the pressure to cut costs has been relentless. During the fourth quarter of last year, Mr. Borick says Superior agreed to cut prices of products shipped to GM and Ford. 'It was a matter of survival,' he says.

"Superior has a 38% share of America's market of 40 million wheels a year. To protect that position, the California manufacturer had to accept a big hit to its profit margins. In this year's first quarter, Superior's margins are expected to fall to 5.5% from the 8%-to-8.5% range last year. A few years ago they were as high as 12%. Superior has seven US plants in Arkansas, Kansas, Tennessee and California. When the company starts producing wheels in China and adds a third plant in Mexico over the next few years, Mr. Borick says Superior will 'reassess some of [its] existing North American operations.'

"If the company eventually shutters its Van Nuys, California, plant it would represent a major blow to the town that once thrived as the Detroit of the West. GM produced Camaros and Firebirds in Van Nuys until 1992 when it decided to shift production to Canada. 'California is tough,' Mr. Borick says. 'It is the highest cost state to manufacture in. California is going to keep losing its manufacturing base."

Such are the ashen realities of Globalization and Deregulation.

William Krehm

The Busy Underground High in the Sky

HIGH IN THE SKY there is a busy underground thumbing its nose at the official suppression of information vital for the management of this planet. An agent, whom we shall refer to by the code name "Lucky Eye," spends much of his time keeping tab on this seditious retrieval of our own history. With his special talent for sorting out the authentic from the make-believe, he has sent out this most recent report:

"The commentary by a veteran British banker seems to parallel some of your positions on policy, but what do you think of his forecast re automation and its implications? Chris Meakin is a colleague of Michael Hudson in his 'gang 8' discussion.

"Any possibility that Economic Literacy has taken root among the leading central banks is rapidly being dispelled. Yesterday the Bank of England pushed base interest rates back up to 4.5%, and in doing so returned to the bad old ways of Voodoo Economics – the antithesis of economic literacy.

"Here is the Bank's own announcement in full:

"The Bank's Monetary Policy Committee today voted to raise the Bank's repo rate by 0.25 percentage points." (The repo rate is the rate at which the Bank advances money for the purchase of securities under contract to resell them to the buyer on set terms.)

"The global recovery is continuing in the UK. Official data and business surveys suggest that growth remains around or above trend. Household spending, public consumption and investment have all grown strongly and the housing market is buoyant. The labour market has tightened further.

"Consumer Price Inflation has been below the 2% target, but pressures are rising. As indicated in the May Inflation Report, a diminishing margin of spare capacity means inflationary pressures are likely to continue building. Against that background, the Committee judged that a further increase of 0.25 percentage points in the repo rate to 4.5% was necessary to keep CPI Inflation on track to the target in the medium term.

"The minutes of the meeting will be published at 9.30 p.m. on Wednesday 23 June.

"The BoE statement is much too long on non sequiturs for any of us to feel comfortable. The saddest is the notion that raising interest rates will reduce inflationary pressure. There has never been one iota of evidence to show why raising interest rates ever does anything of the kind. So we are left with Voodoo or Knee-Jerk Economics.

"The very day before the Bank made its move, at least one British newspaper ran as its front-page headline the statistic that borrowing in the UK has just topped one trillion pounds. Given the free-for-all in shoving credit card borrowing down people's throats by rapacious banks and retail groups…is anyone surprised by that statistic for even a microsecond?

"Yet if the objection to high levels of individual borrowing is concern about people's ability to repay, what possible purpose is served by arbitrarily pushing up the cost of repayment? If the concern is that people have borrowed too much, then the economically literate response would be to lean on the greedy financial houses which are encouraging them to do so. By raising interest rates the Bank is in fact doing the opposite. If you want to stamp out drug addiction, you chase the drug pushers, not the drug addicts."

Chasing the Addicts Instead of the Pushers

"The Bank of England has still not realized after 310 years in the business, that interest is a transfer payment not a price or a tax. It is a transfer payment from borrowers to lenders. So every time the Bank raises interest rates, it impoverishes borrowers such as mortgagors and manufacturing industries. but at the same time it enriches lenders (such as banks) and savers such as the elderly.

"If a central bank:

1. Permits an unseemly free-for-all in stuffing huge quantities of borrowing down the throats of people the length and breadth of the land;

2. Then increases the rewards to the institutions that have been doing the stuffing;

3. It can only encourage and strengthen more such stuffing!

"An economically literate Bank of England would look for some evidence that the big lending institutions will respond to its rate hike, not by raising their own rates, but by cutting the amount they intend to lend. They will wait and wait and wait for that until – as in the old Russian proverb – the lobster whistles on the hill!

"But that complete absence of any rational, useful, positive response to the Bank's rate hike will not deter it from pushing up rates by another quarter percent, and then another quarter percent, in the forlorn quest for something which interest rate hikes on their own cannot possibly deliver.

"And why? Because back in 1997 the British Chancellor of the Exchequer, Gordon Brown, told the Bank of England its job was to manage the rate of inflation and the only management tool it was given was the rate of interest. That 'ducking out from under' manoeuvre, helpful though it was in preventing the even crasser Treasury from trying to manage interest rates, asked the Bank to keep its eye on a single index which ought to be the concern of others, and gave it but one inappropriate (and even counterproductive) weapon with which to keep bashing the index.

"The only reason the BoE has got away with it since 1997 is that forces far, far greater than central banks have been controlling the rate of inflation. Computerization and automation of manufacturing processes all over the world, but most notably in China have been bringing the price of manufactures crashing down for over a decade now.

"President Clinton claimed credit for that himself, Chancellor Brown has been doing the same. Neither of them ever realized the shift in the inflation rate is caused by the 'automation factor'; and is a once-for-all shift, not a new and different economic mechanism, of their own creation. What have they ever done to create it?"

"Once all the knock-on effects of the global 'automation factor' have worked their way through the system (such as cheaper and cheaper computer kit making it economically viable to computerize more and more industrial activities) then the system will revert to its time-honoured balance between inflationary and deflationary pressures. At that point ancient control techniques, those Green Goddesses of the economic emergency service which have been languishing awhile in a never-never-land of atrophied economic logic, will be shoved back into service and the economic 'sages of governmentland' will then have the shock of their lives.

"As was predicted right here on Gang of Eight way back in the late 1990s!"

It is good having free discussion, and from the above you at least have a devastating job done on the use of high interest to stabilize prices. However, we must avoid carrying over the bad habit of seeking any single cause and hence a single simplistic solution for the increasing complexity of an economy that has resulted not only from globalization and deregulation, but from the development of an urbanized high-technology since War II. Few things have a single cause, and least of all what we call "inflation." If quite distinctive causes may be at work, they must be identified, distinguished by a fitting nomenclature, and their interaction studied. For that you need systems theory, i.e., a view of interlocking subsystems of the economy, all of which must be kept in functioning order for the economy and society as a whole to work. That excludes the notion that one subsystem and its particular revenue is dominant, i.e., determines whether the whole is in functioning order by the growth of its revenue real or fictional.

The Automation Factor Isn't Automatic

This is far from saying that computerization is caused by "the automation factor" and that once [that] has worked its way through the system (such as cheaper and cheaper computer kit making economically viable to computerize more and more industrial activities) then the system will revert to its time-honoured balance between inflation and deflationary pressures. Computers are a specific technology. That could be used for quite opposite purposes than those for which it is presently employed. It could for example help tracking down the deterioration of our environment, the effects of that on planet warming. Surely the outsourcing of most simple operations to the third world in a constant quest of cheaper labour, and fewer social and environmental standards is not making the host countries or those who purchase virtual slave labour products "more stable." Factoring into the GDP the debt run up through negative conservation, or the decline of educational or health programs is the work of the devil rather than of the archangels. Nor can it be blamed on the innocent computers who have their own list of sins to answer for. If I may say so, that narrow view of the computer's effect on society appears seen from a bank executive's suite, an enlightened bank executive, to be sure, on the matter of interest, but obviously not too interested in what is afoot in China with the unemployment and underemployment of a cut of population of the same order as the total number of inhabitants in the USA.

Keep up your excellent vigil, Lucky Eye, thank your enlightened banker on our behalf for his analysis of the high interest scam, but urge him to broaden his researches to take in the rest of the Globalization and Deregulation beat.

But before you let him go, ask our banker friend whence comes the notion "of the time-honoured balance between inflationary and deflationary pressures." The *solidus* in Roman imperial times was a valuable gold coin that was used only in major transactions amongst governments, conquerors and conquered. The middle class used only silver coins and *hoi polloi* copper ones. The descendant today of the golden *solidus* is the French sou (the name comes from *solidus*). Today, the sou, I believe, is not even a coin any more – its value down the ages has fallen so steeply. Economic historians like the late Frenchman Fernand Braudel emphasized that living costs in great cities like Venice were always dearer to live in, because of their higher level of services and culture. The key trouble is the assumed trend of

prices toward equilibrium. Or taking all price movement to be "inflation," i.e., an excess of demand over available supply. Part of it is obviously due the deeper layer of taxation in price that reflects the urbanization of the world and the high technology which calls for higher educational, health and social standards to protect the vessels in which society's most productive investment – education and skills – are contained. That was realized by economists in the 1960s, when Theodore Schultz was awarded a Nobel Economic prize for his studies on the rapid recovery of postwar Germany and Japan, entirely unforeseen. Though the cities and factories of the defeated powers were devastated their highly educated, and culturally motivated population survived almost intact.

We've got to get away from simplistic self-equilibrating models, no matter what the one privileged factor advanced may be.

You must have read all this in almost the same words in our publications a boring number of times. My apologies for the repetition. I am interested, moreover, in what any open-minded person has to say. And I think that e-mail despite its spam and much else is probably the one great last chance of society recapturing the free flow of information that its survival depends upon.

Bill Krehm

The Unlearned Lessons from Nortel

WHILE MYSTICS may ponder and reponder the question of an after life, the stock market has enacted a second *death* – with the rider of a second, and why not a third and fourth with heady moments of resurrection in between? Would it not be a more efficient way of keeping the big game going than having to dream up new jazzy company names all the time?

But let's present the Nortel record. For the purpose we draw from *The Globe and Mail* (29/4). So sensational was Nortel's resurrection followed so soon by a second death, that no less than eight separate articles were needed to handle the black miracle. "Owning Nortel stock is like a bad habit," "Nortel aces CEO and senior officials" "Mired in a genuine crisis of confidence," "Former US Navy Admiral takes helm." (This can be interpreted as a commitment to get the immortal company of many deaths afloat again.) "Lucky fund managers read the tea leaves" "Unravelling the turmoil of the numbers," "Firings another blow to staff morale."

But we will begin by quoting from yet another article, "A very immodest company" by Gordon Pitts: "At some point Nortel Networks Corp. quit being an engineering-dominated company and was gripped by a high-flying culture of finance, acquisition, and compensation."

Revelation on a Ten-Lane Toll Road to Damascus

"The supremacy of science gave way to celebrity CEOs and option-enriched executives, who led the telecommunications giant to a massive stock run-up, outrageously expensive take-overs and a stunning fall from grace as the bubble burst." From a top price of $124.50 a share to penny-stock status.

"With the firing of Frank Dunn over financial-reporting issues, three of the past four Nortel CEOS have left under a cloud – an ignoble record for a once proud company that was deemed to hold Canada's telecom future in its hands.

"Nortel still boasts strong technical expertise among its remaining 35,000 people, said Robert Ferchat, a former Nortel senior executive in the past decade, "It has been facing towards Wall St. rather than facing customers. It is also a danger culturally and personally when you start to believe your own press clippings.

"But Jean Monty, who was an effective Nortel CEO in the mid-1990s, argued that the company has been led more by innovation than stock markets. He pointed to pioneering work in digital switching, fibre optics and wireless technology.

"Mr. Monty, who went on to head BCE Inc., Nortel's then sister company, feels the company's recent plight reflects the bubble-and-burst times more than an internal culture change.

"These contrasting views on Nortel's culture are embodied in John Roth, the CEO of the late nineties to fall, 2001. He is a talented engineer, but his legacy will be as the $135 million man, who collected a fortune from stock options before Nortel's crash wiped out many small investors' savings.

"In replacing Mr. Roth with Mr. Dunn, who had been chief financial officer, the board hoped to move quickly on a recovery path by installing someone who knew the company. It appears that the appointment reinforced the cultural dysfunction that had taken hold.

"The leadership of Nortel has been a huge and constant lightning rod in Canada because of the company's status as the country's chosen instrument in technology markets.

"Yet the company's origins are quite American. It started life as the Canadian branch of US telephone giant Western Electric but was cut loose in the unbundling of Western's parent company, AT&T, under US anti-trust pressures.

"Left to its own devices, what was then Northern Electric depended heavily on innovation that was streaming out of its Bell Northern Research labs in Ottawa. But it also enjoyed favoured status as equipment supplier to giant Bell Canada, the monopoly subsidiary of BCE.

"'Nortel has always been a technological powerhouse,' said Edmund Fitzgerald, the US businessman who became chairman and CEO of Nortel in the 1980s. He represents another deep strain of Nortel senior management – the US connection.

"'My charge was to globalize the company,' said Mr. Fitzgerald. This drive to globalize also led to the appointment as CEO of a company director, Paul Stern, a brash US executive with a rich Rolodex of contacts around the world, including the higher echelons of the US administration. Mr. Stern's appointment in 1990 was an unqualified disaster. While he led the company to record profits, he damaged morale, alienated customers and cut away at the research and development that had underpinned Nortel's success.

"One observer who knows Nortel well sees disturbing parallels between the appointment of Mr. Stern, as Nortel board member, and yesterday's emergency appointment of director William Owens as CEO. Once again, he said, the company is turning to a director in response to fast-unfolding events and the need for a quick fix."

A Quick Fix from South of the Border

Nortel may, in fact, be taken as an example of the shadier side of the absorption of Canadian companies by American conglomerates. With this comes an overriding focus on maximising stock market valuations and the rewards of the higher executives. Could it be that the extravagances of Nortel and other US firm-controlled firms in Canada can be traced to a servility towards US interests? Our mind turns to that nagging line in our national anthem: "O Canada! We stand on guard for thee!" The heck we do! No more than Vancouver authorities do over the fate of the ladies of the night in the seedier parts of that great town.

"The task of finding out just what's gone so wrong at Nortel speaks to Canada's loss of economic sovereignty, as US regulators continue to take the lead in investigations into Canadian companies. Nortel announced in early April that Washington's Securities and Exchange Commission had launched a formal probe. It was revealed only about a week later that the Ontario Securities Commission, the domestic market watchdog, was investigating the Brampton, Ont.-based company's bookkeeping. The RCMP also are taking a close look at the situation.

"The OSC has done a lousy job of staying ahead on the regulatory curve. The OSC is going to likely lose the only Bre-X case it's ever brought forward. The SEC took the lead on Nortel, just like it took the lead on Conrad Black and Hollinger," a money manager said.

Could that be because American regulators feel more at home in dealing with most of our large corporations than Canadian authorities do?

William Krehm

AMSTERDAM, JULY 9, 2004

Address to the Global Conference on Business and Economics

THROUGHOUT THE WORLD an inverted metric has taken over. The more events confirm the need for policies that saved society in the past, the less the freedom to even mention these. Money-creation has been shifted from central banks to the private banks. The steps by which this was achieved is the best kept of secrets. As entry fee for earning a living as economist, journalist, or politician, you must respect that great hush-up. Because of this perverse metric, our success or failure must be measured not by counting noses at our conferences, but by the surreptitious, fragmented adoption by governments of much that dissidents have been proposing for years.

At this point let me introduce a key low-profile player: the Bank for International Settlements (BIS) located in Basel. It is a private club of central bankers, whose stock you can buy on the Paris exchange. No elected public official may attend its sessions. It was established in 1929 as a technical agency to syndicate Germany's WWI reparations as strong-currency bonds. The Wall Street crash upset that mission.

At Bretton Woods in 1944, Resolution 5 was passed calling for its liquidation at the earliest possible time. Reason: its past favours to the Nazis. In the shadow of that noose, BIS cultivated a low profile. And that low profile commended it as ideal bunker for directing the undoing of the banking legislation brought in by Roosevelt that had spread throughout the Western world. That legislation made possible the Allied victory in World War II, and the reconstruction of the world.

Throughout the1980s and much of the 1990s, BIS drummed into our heads that the slightest rise in the price level, unless repressed with punitive interest rates, would lead to hyperinflation as that of Germany in 1923.[1] That hyperinflation had arisen through the loss of a world war, the occupation of the industrial heartland by the French army to collect reparations, a general strike backed by the entire German nation, right and left, and the outbreak of a virtual civil war. Suggesting any similarity between that hyperinflation and the rising prices in the Western world in the 1990s, was charlatanry. It implied a great retroactive miracle: had interest rates been pushed high enough in 1923, there would have been no lost war, no occupation of the Ruhr, no general strike, no civil war. Yet academics who knew better joined in spreading that nonsense. The penalty for questioning such nonsense was early retirement.

Let me quote from a work of Frances Hutchinson, and two collaborators, *The Politics of Money* (Pluto Press, 2002): "In the

US there is evidence of a purge during the 1990s of non-neo-classical and non-mathematically orientated economists from university faculties. This has been described as a 'stalinization' of the profession with history of economic thought particularly targeted."

When their inflation theory proved lame, right-thinking economists proclaimed it a mystery: "stagflation." However, COMER identified a new factor in price behaviour.[2] In the post-war, the neglect of ten years of depression and six of war was caught up with. Housing, hospitals and schools were provided for one of the greatest refugee movements in history Inevitably this led to a deeper layer of taxation in price. This I called the "social lien." When even an economist moves from a town of 10,000 to New York City, he is not fool enough to expect his living expenses to stay the same. How then can he expect the living costs of the nation to do so when it makes a similar move? Try to squeeze out of existence with higher interest rates the resulting price rise having nothing to do with an excess of demand over supply, and you only steepen this "structural price gradient." For it shrinks the tax-base while increasing the need for more government services.

In 2002 – a mere 32 years later – the US Federal Reserve and BIS took to speaking of "good inflation" – up to 2% and 3% or even 4% – and "bad inflation" beyond that. For that there was a reason.

In 1991 the bailout of the banks from their huge losses in gas and oil, real estate, and the stock market, allowed them to load up with government debt without putting up money of their own.

The Secret of Seigniorage

The statutory reserves were abolished in Canada and Mexico. In the US and the UK they were left on the books but fell into virtual disuse. These reserves had required a modest portion of the chequing account deposits the banks received to be redeposited with the central bank. These redeposits earned no interest. They gave the central bank a second tool against perceived inflation and thus lessened the government's dependence on interest rates for the purpose. High interest rates hit everything that moves. Raising the statutory reserves limited the *quantity* of credit banks could create on a given intake of deposits. They also gave the central government more elbow room for borrowing from the central bank within existing constraints.

When a government borrows from its central bank, almost all the interest paid on that debt returns to it – as dividends in Canada or Britain where the government is sole shareholder of the central bank. But even in the United States where the central bank is owned by private banks, roughly the same proportion of its profits go back to it – as seigniorage, an echo of the ancestral monarch's monopoly in coining precious metals. The bailout of the banks shifted the bulk of the borrowing previously done by the government from the central bank to private banks. These kept the interest paid by the government on its debt they held. That was in its very essence of the bailout of the banks from their gambling losses. And it was no one-time affair. That interest flowed in from their bonds every year. Inevitably, it left the federal government with a huge hole in its budget. The use of high interest rates to "lick" the growing layer of taxation in price further devastated the economy.

The suppression of what had been learned at crushing cost in the 1930s has brought back the dogma that created the Great Depression. In both the US, Canada, the UK and the EU, a balanced budget is considered by all major parties as the major goal of political process.

Since interest is the revenue of a group needing no encouragement to become parasitic, this involved a major redistribution of the national income. And the Koran condemns as a mortal sin not just usury, but any interest – "riba" – in the event of relapse punishable by eternal hell fire. This massive redistribution of the national income in the West has done nothing for its relations with Islam. Why have the numerous US investigations of the roots of the Twin Towers attack avoided so much as a mention of this unnecessary provocation of Muslim religious principles?

To make possible the bailout of the banks in the early 1990s, it was also necessary for the BIS to bring in its *Risk-Based Capital Requirement* guidelines. These declared the debt of developed countries risk-free, needing no additional capital for banks to acquire. Between the abolition of the statutory reserves and the BIS risk-based capital requirements, Canadian banks were able to take on another $60 billion dollars of government debt without putting up a penny of their own. Depending on how high the central bank screwed up interest rates, this amounted to an annual entitlement of anywhere from $5 to 8 billion a year.

The banks in fact elbowed out the neediest citizens from the relief lines. Worse was to come. The banks were next deregulated further to enable them to acquire brokerages, underwriting and merchant banking houses, interests in insurance companies, and derivative boutiques.

Compared to Derivatives, Las Vegas is a Convent

What are derivatives? If I may risk a metaphor, they are arrangements for dealing not in roses, but in the mere scent of the rose, freed of thorns and the hard work of caring for the bushes. You buy or sell not a security, but bet on the change in its yield or the change in the value of the currency of its denomination. And since you merely bought the fragrance and not the whole flower, you can manage gambling on a far greater quantity of that aspect of the rose.

Derivatives permitted George Soros to outgun the Bank of England and bring down the pound with a profit of a billion dollars or so and then go on to shoot down the Italian lira and other currencies. Since derivatives are unregulated to this day, they permitted three of Canada's six large banks to take part in the trading partnerships organized by Enron executives. The banks were fined by US regulators as much as $80 million US each for these illegal gambles, and still face possible class ac-

tions by investors who feel bilked by them. These large banks used unregulated derivatives to avoid reporting that they had unloaded their own interests in the Enron partnerships onto their clients to make a killing at their expense.

And then came the talk of "good inflation" – an official acknowledgement of COMER's "social lien" but in a way that cut off rather than encouraged serious analysis. "Good inflation" is, it seems, necessary to lubricate what is termed "the pure and perfect market." But surely this is evidence the market is less than "pure and perfect." Imagine what the state of medicine would be if we called medicine "good poison."

But there is another important change that is being introduced secretly in fragmented form by the very people who resisted it for decades.

When a government builds a building or a bridge, it has until recently treated that investment as a current expense. It was written off in a single year like the soap for its wash rooms. If private firms practiced such "accountancy" they would all be undischarged bankrupts. Instead, they carry forward their assets at depreciated value to offset the mortgages that financed their acquisitions. This is known as "accrual accountancy" or "capital budgeting."

In Canada three royal commissions and successive Auditors General had recommended accrual accountancy. To no effect. The apparent deficits and debt that result are used to propagate the view that governments are incapable of "managing money," unless, of course, they are building penitentiaries, preparing for war, or bailing out banks.

This makes it necessary for government out of the current year's revenue to raise taxes higher to cover the cost of buildings and other infrastructure in a single year. Governments then can put up for sale assets carried on their books at a token dollar at say five percent of their value, book a profit, and apply that profit "to reducing the debt." Then promoters can go public with the assets acquired for a song. They make a huge profit, and leave the public paying through the nose for user services from assets which they had already paid for in taxation.

Which in turn gooses the growth of private corporations. And once achieved, these growth rates are extrapolated into the far future and incorporated into present stock market prices. The pricing of a stock as a result shifts from its sustainable earning power to the capitalized rate of growth of its one-time scams or miracles, on the assumption that the rate of growth and the rate of growth of the rate of growth – the derivative of the second degree – will be sustained. You need only turn to the financial pages and see the chart of the latest stock market wonder. Its graph starts out horizontal plotting its market price over time but before you know it is standing erect like a Viagra ad.

That is the pattern of the exponential curve when an infinite growth rate is achieved. And, once established in share prices, any shortfall from this capitalization brings down the whole house of cards. Essentially what you have here is a deal with the devil. Whatever growth rate you reach in a single year you extrapolate into the future and capitalize the result in your current share price. But on one condition: that you maintain that growth rate. If you fail but a single time, the whole exercise collapses. That drives corporations and their accountants to end up cooking their books. To maintain their success they had to not only cover up their past dodges but continue them on an ascending scale.

The High Art of Cooking the Government Books

No room is left for morality, or democratic process. Fewer people bother to vote. The expensive cost of political advertising on TV prime time completes the picture.

The furtive adoption of bits and pieces of what was learned at a staggering price in the thirties is proof that our government is at its wits' end. It has basically no place to go. It is important for humanity to confront the great storms already upon us that some of us cup the flame that alone can offer mankind access to its own history.

We should consider the remark in his final book *God & Golem, Inc.* (1964) of Norbert Wiener of MIT: "The success of mathematical physics led the social scientists to be jealous of its power without quite understanding the intellectual attitudes that had contributed to this power. Just as primitive people adopt Western modes of denationalized clothing and of parliamentarism out of a vague feeling that these magic rites and vestments will at once put them abreast of modern culture and technique, so the economists have developed ideas in the language of infinitesimal calculus." The time has come to mobilize all available resources to break this deal with the devil.

The history of economic thought must be scoured for leads to solutions to save our society.

A good beginning of such an enquiry has already come from what may have seemed an unlikely source. By the nature of his very genius Major Douglas owed little to other great economists. Even his terminology was original and difficult for those raised within the concepts of standard accountancy and mainstream economic theory. It is a hopeful sign that one of the most fruitful essays of reviewing the record of economic thinking should come from his heirs.[3] It revolves around the notion of a social heritage earned by the contribution of countless generation of prophets, martyrs, slaves, scientists, saints, and lawmakers that must be recognized in the form of a social dividend to permit a variety of alternate life styles to remove the pressures from the environment and what economists choose to call "externalities." This would help answer the concern with effective demand that requires constant ramping up of the scale of production, no matter how artificially drummed up the usefulness of many of the products.

Every precedent for packing our real needs within a smaller gross production should be seized upon and studied. In sciences there are many such principles that have been completely ignored by economists too busily maximising their GDP and peddling Globalization and Deregulation. There is dimension analysis introduced by Galileo pursuing the lead of Archimedes. Noting that certain forces depend on the three dimensions – for example mass and weight, while on the other hand resistance to such forces usually depend on two dimensions – the cross-sections of human limb or sustaining surface. From that Galileo concluded that by increasing the scale of a building design

but retaining all relative proportions, a point must be reached where girders must crumble and structures collapse.

Physicists have long worked on the principle that nature prefers the path of least rather than most action. Some of these I develop in a book of mine, *Towards a Non-Autistic Economy – A Place at the Table for Society* (2002).

William Krehm

1. The strongest statement that effect can be found in the BIS statement for 1991 of its then general manager Alexandre Lamfalussy.
2. Krehm, William (May 1970). "La stabilité des prix et le secteur public." *Revue Économique*, Paris.
3. Hutchinson, Frances, Mallor, Mary and Olsen, Wendy (2002). *The Politics of Money: Towards Sustainability and Economic Democracy.* London and Sterling, Virginia: Pluto Press.

REVIEW OF A BOOK BY JOHN K. GALBRAITH, HOUGHTON MIFFLIN COMPANY, BOSTON AND NEW YORK, 2004. HARD COVER, XI + 62 PP.

"The Economics of Innocent Fraud"

YET ANOTHER DASH of sly but affable invective from Galbraith, calling our attention to conventional wisdom that isn't. And although participants in most of these frauds may be innocent, the phenomena he ridicules are not. They are more accurately described as euphemisms for what adds up to a serious package of misconceptions about "the economy." The first few do sound as if they might be inconsequential, even trivial, but as they accumulate, the consequences compound. Many years ago (before I had color television), I watched Galbraith participate in a debate with Wm. F. Buckley, Jr., before an audience of students and professors at Oxbridge, taking the affirmative side to the assertion that "The Market Is a Snare and a Delusion." To my surprise, the audience vote came down in favor of Buckley – a portent of Thatcherism and the content of *The Economist* magazine in recent decades. As I set fingers to keyboard for this review some 35 years later, the mental effort to encapsulate *Innocent Fraud* brought back that earlier phrase as the perfect candidate.

The most striking in breadth of the fraudulent euphemisms is the shift in the subject matter of economic investigation and analysis from *capitalism* to "the market system." *Capitalism* had to be expunged from polite discussion because of the bad flavor it acquired after Marx identified it. "Free enterprise" was promoted as a substitute, but its defensive tone was a reminder of the cogency of its critics and the distortions in economic performance between the world wars.

The succeeding "Market System" has the aura of something natural, impersonal and objective that can be explored and analyzed, in contrast to an *ism* or political structure that powerful people are trying to impose in their own interest. It is still fundamentally the same system, evaluated by much the same techniques for most of the 20th century, but defects in its operation which used to be attributed to individual actors in the system (the monopoly power sought by greedy capitalists) are now discussed as if they were the sputtering of a gasoline engine and therefore subject to fine tuning by wizards in central banks, IMF and BIS.

No longer is it wicked capitalists who are responsible for economic ills. They have been replaced by ourselves, the sovereign consumer. On the production side, writers of economics textbooks still permit the impression that the economy is a competitive collection of small farmers, shopkeepers and service providers (with an exceptional few large industrial corporations that provide context for a following chapter about optimization policy under conditions of monopoly and oligopoly). The economic machine is operated by expert managers who take their orders not only from consumers as the ultimate authority, but also from wise and alert boards of directors. The latter class of philanthropists assures that managers take the decisions that will make all of us wealthy as we put our savings into shares of the corporations they oversee. Ergo "pension fund socialism," brought to us by the followers of management guru Peter Drucker. Fraud!

The Hidden Realities of "The Market System"

The "market system" is in fact a world dominated by giant corporations, most of which operate in supra-national disdain for would-be government regulators and incur a very large share of their expenses in the process of manipulating their "sovereign masters" – whether the latter be conceived as consumers, share-holders, parliaments, or regulators. Economists used to spend a lot of time studying and tut-tutting about the malign consequences of monopoly power, but despite frequent bouts of merger mania over recent decades, anti-trust actions are rarely heard of since the "discovery" that consumer-share-holders are the sovereign beneficiaries. (What happened to that federal department called Consumer and Corporate Affairs, and the Foreign Investment Review Agency? Oh yes, Industry Canada.) We no longer gnash our teeth about the unseemly fortunes of "capitalists" or "captains of industry," but marvel instead at the high value attributed to "corporate managers" in the kingly salaries and other compensation awarded by perceptive and grateful boards of directors. (A phenomenon that is an admitted mystery to analysts of managerial compensation.)

Analogous to the managerial compensation fraud is the fiction that all kinds of activities for which payment is made constitute "work." The fact is that real work is very poorly compensated compared to the rewards of what Veblen called "the leisure class" whose members are paid handsomely for what they would otherwise do for entertainment or other personal gratification.

The corporation is a bureaucracy. This fact has to be smothered by a fraudulent denial, however, because bureaucracy is a disease of government – believed to be an unnecessary impediment to getting the world's important work done. This denial is an element in the fraudulent distinction drawn between "private" and "public" sectors of the economy. The unavoidable refutation of this myth is the American military-industrial complex, which features control of an immense part of the economy by Pentagon bureaucrats and has gotten to the point where even soldiers are in the employ of corporations. (For a striking confirmation of this point see the Paul Krugman column "Accounting and Accountability" in *The New York Times* (23/07), which suggests that billions of dollars authorized by Congress for reconstruction in Iraq are being misappropriated in favor of American oil companies.)

While the tragedy of war and its associated miseries are the climax implication of *innocent fraud*, readers of ER will be especially interested in Galbraith's comments about economic and financial analysis of "the market system." Belief in the forecasting acumen of Wall Street analysts is a manifestation of successful fraud, he says, for it is simply not possible to be confident of forecasts in a domain that is subject to even more vagaries than the weather. "Our most cherished, and on examination, most evident form of fraud…" is the conceit that "…quiet measures enforced by the Federal Reserve are…the best approved, best accepted of economic actions. They are also manifestly ineffective."

Keith Wilde

Questioning the Rule Books of Banking in our Day

THE CRISIS currently engulfing the world doesn't just concern the GDP and our stock markets. As it develops it is bringing to the fore issues long banished from public attention. Not least of these is the relationship between high finance and the real economy.

In its remote origins money was essentially a measure of value and a medium of circulation. In those capacities it was a handmaiden of trade. Only later did it become primarily a store of value. Most recently it has become a highly speculative game in itself. The process that effected this ultimate apotheosis was begun in the early 1950s, and received its final touches, when money creation was "privatized" and increasingly removed from the control of central banks. Today, it feasts on rather than serves the real economy. The effect on society has been devastating.

On a single page (C1) of *The Wall Street Journal* (C1) every headline speaks with ashen tongue: "Questioning the Books – Tweaking Results Is Hardly a Sometime Thing. Many Firms May Play with Numbers," "Ripples from Enron Rock Bond Market," "Enron Official Failed to Warn Participants of 401(k) Plan," "More and More, Mergers of '90s are Becoming Today's Spinoffs," "Investors' Mood is Blue Leaves Indexes in Red."

Several factors and stages can be identified in the process that eventually led to the Enron phenomenon. Historically, in both the United States and Great Britain, the reigning rule of banking had been that the central bank could lend only against the security of "real bills," i.e., drafts and notes of exchange arising out of actual commercial transactions usually with a maturity of not more than 90 days. "The real bills idea of money responded to a body of theory that limited the paper 'eligible' for discount to that generated in trade. It specifically excluded stocks and bonds, because of a conviction that left to their own devices, the banks would misdirect the credit resources of the nation to speculation. Until the 1920s, nationally chartered banks in the US were not permitted to lend on the security of real property, though state-chartered banks or trust companies usually were able to do so." Monetary policy of the government and the role of central bank were seen as essentially passive. The Fed discounted eligible commercial paper brought to its "discount window" to release the banks' capital for further financing. For years even government bonds were not acceptable as collateral for loans that were the money-base on which further loans were pyramided. If the Fed bank wanted the banking system to do more lending, it lowered its discount rate below the interest rates in the local market. This encouraged business people to increase their volume of transactions. Gold movements also played its part. It was only later that government bonds under normal circumstances were accepted as collateral.[1]

The discount window was passive – it depended upon what discountable paper was brought to it by the banks. But the local Fed banks could play a more active role, seeking out paper to discount through the Fed's Open Market Investment Committee. In the early Fed years they were driven to do so to cover their expenses and pay dividends to the banks who held their shares. Bankers' acceptances (paper endorsed by a bank) and government bonds were the collateral most prized by the banks and the Fed.

All this suggests that commercial banking saw its role as serving the productive economy. In our day the reverse has become true.

Creating a Class of Money Jobbers

Highly important in the this transformation was the creation of a short-term money market that was encouraged to set a discount rate that would keep the economy on an even keel. Persistently the Bank of Canada resorted to various inducements to create a class of jobbers in short-term government debt. It conceived them immaculate, nursed them from breast and bottle until they took over the entire show. In effect the central bank fashioned the god of clay to whom it could surrender the determination of short-term interest rates – the "young men in red suspenders" who terrorized the business world and shot down the British pound, the Italian lira, and the Canadian dollar from their high perches in the fall of 1992.[2] In Canada this required a dogged effort on the part of the central bank, though the final result "the money market" has been held up as a masterpiece of nature itself.

Eventually the Bank designed the repossession arrangements by which the securities it accepted as collateral for financing the brokers' short-term debt inventory could be purchased from it by the jobbers at predetermined price.

The emphasis on short-term loans ruled out not only many long-term investments in the private sector when money grew tight, but restricted the ability of the government to finance its own longer term investments through the central bank. When the BoC holds federal debt it is at a near zero-interest rate:

over 95% of the interest the government paid on the debt held by the BoC would revert to it as dividends. For since 1938 the federal government has been the sole shareholder of the Bank of Canada. However, in recent decades the BoC holds only around 5% of the federal debt. In the mid 1970s that proportion was well over 20%. To bail out our chartered banks from their crushing speculative losses in the 1980s, they were relieved of their obligation to deposit on an interest-free basis an average of around 4% of the public deposits they took in. That, and the deregulation of what they could invest in, allowed them a leverage in their current gambles that has risen from 11:1 in 1946 to as much as 400 to 1 in more recent years. Part of the credit they have created went into financing some of Enron's shadowy partnerships.

With the availability of bank financing to productive industries and consumers restricted by a monetary policy that favours speculation, the ability of banks to service brick-and mortar investments was curtailed. Monetary policy, surrendered largely to "the market," became a wedge inserted between central and commercial banking and the needs of the real economy.

This alienation of banking from the real economy reaches back to the adoption of marginal utility theory which replaced value theories that had linked economic analysis to the real economy. These had made a sharp distinction between the last transaction price of a given commodity on the market price and some more significant and enduring value. One of these theories that was replaced was the labour theory of value that had attained its most refined form in the work of David Ricardo and related the value of a good to the amount of "average labour" needed for its production. This had been taken up by Marx and other socialists to support their views for restructuring society in a way that would have curled the hair on Ricardo's head. It certainly had become increasingly unacceptable to the propertied classes in the raw 19th century capitalism when the anti-capitalist movements were acquiring a strident voice. The other was the cost-of-production theory of value, that added up the average costs of entrepreneurs in producing a commodity plus a reasonable profit. It is not irrelevant to note that this theory of value which resembles in broad terms what accountants are supposed to be up to, would have helped keep Andersen, the accountants of Enron out of trouble. Instead marginal utility, dealt entirely with price, and concentrated on the movement of the price of the most recent transaction reflecting the balance or imbalance of the supply and demand "on a pure and perfect" market. The reader will note: (1) To have their price model taken seriously the founders of marginal utility theory had to restructure – notionally of course – society beyond recognition. Everybody, from the unemployed to the most successful bankers were regarded wholly as traders, each intent on maximizing their satisfactions. The unemployed for example, stayed unemployed because having compared the satisfactions between accepting work at the wage offered and the delights of leisure in their parlors, their choice had alighted on the latter. All actors in the economy were of such tiny power and importance, that nothing that they did or decided not to do individually could influence price. That provided the smooth curves necessary for applying the infinitesimal calculus that the authors of the model mistook for scientific method – the high-tech of the day.

Leaving it All to the Allures of Marketing

For this model to fly, as the volume of production rose, the costs per unit rose. This was essential to provide the points of intersection between cost and price curves that provided the equilibrium points to which the prices and everything else would be brought on such a "free and perfect" market. (2) If it were simply a matter of increasing demand over available supply to raise prices which are identified with value, then the techniques and allurements of marketing could take care of that. All that would be needed was to contrive enough demand to push up prices to arrange for a glowing future for a company. The reader will note that "marginal utility" signifies that value was identified with the rate of increase of price – a purely market phenomenon – rather anything pertaining to value already attained. Notable, too, is that the "first derivative" the *rate of growth* is the same term and, indeed, the same concept as the financial instruments used in hedging to control the risk of changes in price of financial securities (or commodities).

By hedging against unpleasant surprises by buying futures to cover losses if the prices of the security held, or the exchange value of the currency in which they are denominated, or the weather, or just about anything else, the illusion is created that risk is "managed." But these charming and allegedly benign people-friendly derivatives, are kept off the hedging company's books. The underlying notion of a hedge is that the costs of getting a third party to guarantee you against the adverse movement of any of these risk factors, will be balanced by what you will pay for another philanthropist agreeing to accept your security at an agreed price if the market has gone against you. Were that so, that would leave you enjoying the interest paid by the security that is the basis for these derivatives. But philanthropy, on this planet at least, has not become so widespread that there will be investors who knowingly will agree to assume your risk on such a gamble and leave you free to pick up the profit. At best he will have miscalculated. That means that as the figures run into enough digits to come to resemble an astronomical statistic, your counterparty is likely to have evaporated, and is no longer there to perform.

All this can be summed up by observing that though the significant detail has escaped economists and enquiring reporters, the very name "derivatives" of these infernal instruments stems from marginal utility theory. That indicates that our present nightmare is deeply rooted in our basic price theory which turns its back on the sphere of production, i.e., the real economy to concern itself with a highly idealized version of financial markets.

W. Krehm

1. *Federal Reserve Act* as amended, section 13(2) quoted in Mayer, Martin (2001). *The Fed – The Inside Story of How the World's Most Powerful Financial Institution Drives the Markets* (p. 148). New York: The Free Press.
2. "For several years the Bank, in trading treasury bills, had progressively widened the spread between its buying and selling levels to create an incentive for the chartered banks to look elsewhere for buyers. These efforts had met with little success and in early 1953 a number of new steps were taken. The objective was to broaden the market for treasury bills and other short-term paper by encouraging some of the larger investment dealers to act as 'jobbers,' i.e., to hold an inventory of short-term securities and to stand ready to buy or sell. The Bank of Canada undertook to provide investment dealers prepared to take a jobber position with an alternative means of financing inventories of short-term Government securities through the Purchase and Resale Agreements (PRA).The Bank would, if required, provide dealers with short-term accommodation by purchasing treasury bills and/or short-term Government bonds under an arrangement to resell the securities at a pre-determined cost to the dealer. Initially these facilities were made available to 'approved' dealers at a rate lower than that charged by the banks for call loans, but it was hoped that a true call loan market would develop and that the Bank would become a lender of the last resort." The shift of the central bank policy to short-term government paper as the medium of control, and that left largely to "the market," elevated to the position as a natural phenomenon despite the Bank's arduous labours in setting it up, widened the gap between the real and the speculative economy. What is most important for the real economy is the availability of long-term financing. Speculators, however, are interested in quick predatory assaults on the productive economy.

New Deal for Municipalities

"*VIRTUALLY all ideologues, of any variety, are fearful and insecure, which is why they are drawn to ideologies that promise prefabricated answers for all circumstances. Every society contains such people. But they can exert considerable power only when they control public purse strings.*" – Jane Jacobs, Dark Age Ahead *(2004)*

Two COMER members were recently asked to address the Town Council of the Municipality of Lakeshore in southwestern Ontario on the subject of the Bank of Canada loans to municipalities. The following is the text of their address.

There is no reason why the Bank of Canada cannot make loans to municipalities for major projects.

There are three things you need to know about the Bank of Canada. (1) It is owned by the Government of Canada. (2) It has the sovereign power to create money and lend it; in fact 3-5% of the Canadian money supply is created by the Bank of Canada. (3) There is provision (1938) in the legislation that set up the Bank of Canada to make loans to the Federal government, loans to the Provinces, and loans to the Municipalities. Whether it does so or not, is totally a matter of government policy.

Let us elaborate a little on these three points.

1. The Bank of Canada is one of only three central banks among the rich nations *which is owned by its national government.* An earlier private Bank of Canada was nationalized by the Mackenzie King government in 1938. Since then, all 100,000 shares of the Bank are held by the Minister of Finance for the Government of Canada. Further, the *Bank of Canada Act,*

Article 14, provides that the Governor may be dismissed by the government if he does not comply, as James Coyne was by the Diefenbaker government in 1961.

2. Although the Bank of Canada now creates only 3-5% of the Canadian dollar supply, that, too, is a government policy decision. The bulk of the Canadian money supply is now created by the chartered banks. And – something else you need to understand – *they do it only by making loans.* That is, over 95% of our money supply is created by and loaned to us by the chartered banks, and we pay rent to use it. That has been a government policy decision, implemented bit by bit, over the last 50 years.

The Legislation

3. Article 18c of the *Bank of Canada Act*, 1938, says the Bank "may buy and sell securities guaranteed by Canada or any province."

Article 18j says the Bank 'may make loans to the Government of Canada or the government of any province."

Accompanying that 1938 Act was Bill 143, called the *Municipal Improvements Assistance Act.*

That act provided for:

1. Loans to any city, town, incorporated improvement district and even unincorporated districts administered by a province.

2. For such things as the renewal of a municipal waterworks system, a municipal gas plant, a municipal electric light system, or other municipal project."

There were two provisos:

1. "Provided, however, that the project...will be a self-liquidating project." That means that it will earn money sufficient to pay the loan. Under these terms a sports complex, which was designed to charge for use until the loan was paid off, would qualify, or a sewer line, if it was to be paid for by a levy on the users, and

2. Provided that the government of the Province backs the loan.

That *Municipal Improvements Assistance Act* has since been rescinded. Its specific details would be obsolete today anyway. But *there is no reason that a new Municipal Assistance Act,* in some form or other be re-instated, if the government chooses.

The Opportune Time

Now is a very good time to try to get this policy re-instated. The municipalities have been starved for nearly a decade. During the election, at least two of the major parties talked about "a new deal for the cities." They promised that specified taxes – on gasoline, or on cigarettes, or the GST – could be transferred to municipalities. But direct loans from the Bank of Canada would be "revenue-neutral." That is, the government would not be giving up any tax revenue. Because the government owns the Bank of Canada, the Bank's profits are returned to the government. So interest rates for loans to municipalities could be set low enough to cover only the costs of administration, and it would cost the government nothing. That is a very persuasive argument.

The Obstacles

So what are the obstacles to municipalities getting Bank of Canada loans?

There is only one.

Private bankers and their spokespeople always get edgy when anybody breathes the idea of money creation by government. They always respond by warning of the horrors of inflation. So you can be sure that any Finance Minister who wishes to use the Bank of Canada to make loans – even for such a good purpose as building municipal infrastructure – will get a lot of pressure in private from lender lobbyists. And the public – that's you – will hear a great deal about it being inflationary!

The real motive for this objection is pretty obvious. If municipalities can borrow cheaply from the Bank of Canada they won't borrow from the private banks.

Tailoring the Argument

You do need to understand, however, *why* Bank of Canada loans in such a case are, in fact, *not* inflationary. If it is merely a substitution of Bank of Canada loans for what would otherwise be private bank loans, the *total* money supply will remain the same. That is not inflationary. The history of the Bank of Canada supports that.

So what can a municipality do?

1. Remind the party leaders of their pre-election promises. Insist that the government re-establish Bank of Canada loans to municipalities.

2. Do what other municipalities are doing, such as Toronto, Kingston, Squamish, BC. Forward to provincial and federal governments municipal council resolutions urging the practice of Bank of Canada loans for capital projects.

(And, we would add, in your resolution or covering letter be sure to emphasize two things: (1) that such loans will *not* be inflationary; and (2) that they will be revenue neutral for the government.)

The Bank of Canada does have the power under the Act to make loans to municipalities, and, whatever anybody may say, it is totally a government decision whether they can do it or not.

This simple presentation, which is not ideological, apparently made sense to the Lakeshore councillors. They passed a resolution petitioning the federal and provincial governments "to instruct the Bank of Canada to buy securities issued by municipalities to pay for infrastructure and other capital works projects; and to refund to municipalities any interest paid."

The request is a reasonable one. In the two-thirds of a century since the founders of the Bank of Canada devised this simple, practical mechanism for assisting in a small way the country's cities and towns, Canada has undergone a vast urban transformation. Reinstatement of the policy of Bank of Canada loans to our revenue-restricted municipalities is now timely and practical. It remains to be seen whether ideology and interest will yield to logic and public need.

Gordon Coggins and George Crowell

In Memoriam – James E. Potts

IN HIS 94TH YEAR, Jim Potts has left us. But only after his legendary courage and unfailing good humour in adversity had come through great trials with flying colours. At no time did they dent his wit, nor his concern for how the world was being spun.

I first knew Jim in the mid-1930s when he was a student at Western University, he played the college football team, contributed to his tuition by giving a hand with the university books, and still found time for activism as a CCFer. Every week I would hitch-hike to London to conduct a study-class on anti-Stalinist socialist theory organized by Jim.

On at least one occasion it took place in the class-room of Jim's economic course at Western with the participation of the professor. For freedom of discussion in the thirties tended to be surprisingly the real thing. Without it the world could never have found the way out of that nightmare.

In the seventy years that followed, Jim remained Jim. On retirement he was ever an activist in some social cause, whether organizing the marketing of handicrafts for aborigines in the Maritimes, or as a volunteer with CUSO in Mexico and Central America. Always, too, he remained in complete control. When he left us, it was by his decision that he decided that he had lived a full life.

W.K.

PART 1 OF A REVIEW OF A BOOK BY F. HUTCHINSON, M. MELLOW AND W. OLSEN, LONDON & STERLING, VIRGINIA: PLUTO PRESS, 2002

"The Politics of Money: Towards Sustainability and Economic Democracy"

TIME THERE WAS when Social Credit spoke its own arcane language not easy for outsiders to understand. That is no longer so. Anybody seriously concerned with money sooner or later must come to terms with Major Douglas; and in that respect the Social Crediters are meeting the rest of us more than half way. This is the second excellent book co-authored by Ms. Hutchinson that not only unrolls Major Douglas's ideas, but presents him in the context of other great thinkers such as Karl Marx and Thorstein Veblen. That is an immense help, since, like Marx, Douglas has not been happy in some of his followers. Particularly was that the case in Canada.

Douglas devised his idiosyncratic tools because he felt he needed them to pursue some penetrating observations of his own. Money and its creation he identified as the root of much of society's troubles – much as Freud did sex. While many orthodox economists dismiss money as "neutral" and attribute importance only to the "real" factors of production, they in fact call to mind the attitude of Victorians towards mating. Though

supposedly practiced only in holy marriage and there only for procreation, from Gladstone to Oscar Wilde, sex played an obsessive part in their lives.

So, too, with the "neutrality of money." "Of the total international transactions of a trillion or so dollars each day, 95% are purely financial. Globalization is not about trade; it is about money. Global trade as a percentage of national output is very little different to what it was at the end of the nineteenth century – around 40% (1999). Investors no longer put their money into factories or merchant ships but, instead, into a plethora of overlapping 'financial products' such as futures, derivatives, hedge funds or currency speculation."

And corresponding to the institution of marriage, "there is also a theoretical assumption that economic activity is organized within an orderly circular flow. People sell their resources (labour, land, capital) so that tangible goods and services can be produced. In exchange they receive money. That money they take to the market place and buy the goods and services they require. This completes the circle. The assumption is that, left to itself, the circle will meet all economic needs. No one will produce more than can be sold, no one will be left without. If everything is not in order, the money and interest rates may need to be adjusted so that the quantity of money does not exceed the quantity of goods available for exchange. Next, economists distinguish between wants backed by money (effective demand) and needs that may exist but do not register as economic 'facts.' Economists also tend to assume that money prices have a natural equilibrium, e.g., an equilibrium exchange rate, as does the interest rate.

"Academic economists are judged by their publications in a 'Diamond list' seen as representing the best international journals constructed by Peter Diamond, an orthodox economist. The Diamond list concentrated on journals which espoused orthodoxy, such as the *Economic Journal* and omitted several important heterodox journals, such as the *Cambridge Journal of Economics*. In the US there is evidence of a purge during the 1990s of non-neo-classical and non-mathematically oriented economists from university faculties. This has been described as a 'stalinization' of the profession with history of economic thought particularly targeted."

The Ultimate Pollution of Nature — Proclaiming Capitalism a "Natural" System

"Central to the definition of orthodox economics as a science is the assumption [that] capitalism is the natural system. Its essence is the money/market system. There is no alternative, because the 'free' market is the only route to political freedom.

"Within the classical theory which underpins conservative macro-analysis of the self-sustaining economy, money is purely a measuring device having no influence on economic outcomes. Commodities exchange for commodities, while money merely facilitates the exchange. There are two key ideas within this view: first that money is neutral and without history – it simply exists as a technical resource; secondly, a circular model of the economy."

"People are seen as utility-maximizers in all aspects of their life. Politics is taken out and replaced by economics. The irony is that economics itself is what Hazel Henderson has aptly termed 'politics in disguise.'

"The non-existence of time is directly related to the non-existence of capital within the circular flow model. The study of economics postulates three physical factors of production: land, labour and capital. The owners of each factor receive a money reward (rent, wages or interest) for the 'disutility' of allowing the factor to be consumed in the production process. Abstinence, the failure to consume, normally considered the source of physical capital is a logical impossibility. Once the circular flow is established, the productive forces of land and labour sell in exchange for consumption goods. Whether the goods produced are 'producers' goods' or 'consumers goods' is immaterial.

"In each period the real services of labour and land are exchanged for consumption goods produced in the previous period. Each good sees two periods, the one in which it is produced, and the one in which it is consumed. 'Capital' cannot be stored up because there are no gaps in the continuity between the process of production and the process of consumption. Counting abstinence as a legitimate cost would involve counting the same item twice (Schumpeter)."

Shockingly, the neo-classical circular model holds even many of the great rebels in thrall. Keynes's final rebuttal of the self-balancing model [at least in public] still adhered to its basic paradigm. Despite Karl Marx's astounding anticipation of the most involved curves that the contemporary financial sector can pitch, "many 20th century Marxists have followed the orthodox path of erasing finance from the study of economics (Alan Freeman). For Freeman, capitalist power stems from the *financially* based institutional constructs of legally enforced contract and sale. Unfortunately, Marx's labour theory of value has been interpreted from the neo-classical simultaneous methodological standpoint, in which the profit rate is everywhere actually equal, technology does not change, and the market always clears during each act of circulation, and money is a pure *numéraire*. In this analysis money and time do not exist.

"The model of orthodox economics fuses and confuses wealth production with money making. Within a capitalist economy production would not occur if there was not a product. The starting point for establishing an alternative framework must be to question the construction. Separating production from wealth creation follows an old tradition that can be traced back to Aristotle. Daly and Cobb define *chrematistics* as the branch of political economy relating to the manipulation of property and wealth to maximize the short-term monetary exchange value to the owner. By contrast *oikonomia* is 'the management of the household to increase its use to its members over the long run.' Mainstream neo-classical economics has not only fused chrematistics and oikonomia, it has concentrated on the former to the exclusion of the latter.

"The fossilization of economic thought renders economists increasingly incapable of offering coherent explanations of economic phenomena. It would appear that the aim of neo-liberal economic theory is to dominate all other theories, just as the aim of market capitalism has been to eclipse all value systems beyond those of the money economy."

Why the Spartans Outlawed Money

"Evidence of the use of money dates back to 3000 BC, and the earliest writings were statements of accounts. There is evidence that communal grain stores were used as a banking resource in ancient Egypt with what were effectively cheques exchanged between depositors. However, until modern times the use of money to settle everyday social obligations was virtually unknown. Money was used in exceptional circumstances, in times of famine, hard times generally, for travel and warfare. What is new is a society driven by money, banking and credit. With Marx we agree that the role of money in acquiring the means of sustenance is the critical feature of modernity. Concern about usury in the Old Testament also shows that the idea of lending money for interest is very old and religious laws against that were carried into both Christianity and Islam. Usury is still against Islamic law."

Indeed, it is the very taking of interest ["riba"] rather than just "usury" that is proscribed in the Koran. Profit from risk-taking was on the other hand allowed. Venice, whose trade was to a large extent with Islamic lands, devised risk partnerships between traders who accompanied their goods and the financiers who stayed behind that were acceptable to the Muslims Venice dealt with.

"The Lydians of Greek Asia Minor are credited with the invention of money as coin. In the seventh century BC they were striking coins from electrum, a gold-silver alloy occurring naturally near their capital Sardis. Their King Croesus became a symbol of the accumulation of riches. The distrust of money led to its being outlawed in Sparta. Aristotle records the marginal status of bankers in Athens.

"For James Buchan 'since money is a purely social construct it is of concern that trust in money displaces other values like a cuckoo in the nest.' This is the victory of money that Margaret Thatcher infamously celebrated when she said there was no such thing as society, only individuals and their families.

"What money does is enable things to happen. Money is not a neutral instrument within trade. It creates the very potential of trade. Control of, or access to the creation of money is vital to social and political power. Evidence for this exists in the 'John Law' phenomenon, an aspect of economic history which James Buchan argues has been largely hidden from mainstream economics.

"Law was the son of a goldsmith/banker from Edinburgh born in 1671. After a rakish youth (including killing someone in a duel) he tried in 1705 to get Scotland to issue paper money to get out of an economic crisis. Law argued that what was needed was 'stimulatory paper currency.' He based the issue of paper money on the future productivity of land and rejected more traditional options such as exchange controls, coining plate, 'raising the Money' (devaluation), or a sovereign loan (viz. Bank of England).

"Still with an English warrant on his head, Law had to leave Scotland after the Act of Union in 1707 and continued promoting a 'bank of issue' in Paris. He was expelled from the city. Law's last chance came to put his ideas into practice in Regency France, bankrupt after years of war and court extravagance. In 1715 Law opened a private bank which operated with only one-sixteenth of its equity in coin. The bank's paper became highly valued and by 1717 was used to pay taxes. By 1718 the bank was effectively nationalized and used to capitalize the state of Louisiana. John Law became effectively Prime Minister and all national debt and credit was taken on by him. He converted *rentes* and *billets* into a national commercial venture and the entire liquid capital flowed into the company. The word 'millionaire' was coined for him as he owned a lot of France and half the present US. As Buchan points out, effectively the entire nation became a nation of traders.

"In many ways Law's speculative ventures would have been at home today. He tried to buy into the English Indies market by selling short, but the market carried on rising and he ended up paying £372,000 for stocks contracted at £180,000. To maintain liquidity he increased money supply; this led to inflation. By 1720 it was all over and, in final irony, London and Amsterdam crashed not long afterward with their own bubbles.

"Schumpeter argued that the 17th century 'cowboy' experimenter in banking Law fully realized the business potentialities of the discovery that money – and hence that capital in the monetary sense – can be created.' James Buchan agrees with Marx that he was a mixture of swindler and prophet.

"For Schumpeter when money has no intrinsic value it is possible to *manage* the quantity of money, paving the way for 'management of currency and credit as a means of managing the economic process.' Recognition of this destroys the concept of the equilibrating circular flow. Law observed that once a commodity like silver and gold is used as money in coinage, its value changes. And once such a commodity like silver is used almost exclusively as money, it can easily be replaced by one that has no commodity value at all like paper. Law saw money as 'pure function' and attacked the bullionists like John Locke who argued for a gold standard. Buchan goes on: 'Law believed money was a distillation of human relations and might be turned to create a prosperous and just society and he damned near pulled it off.'

"Thereby lies an irony. While, as we have argued, money values are social, or at least relative rather than natural, the presumed 'naturalness' of the economy justifies extreme inequality even to the present day. It is taken for granted that there is no *economic* basis to question what 'the economy' is doing, whether making weapons, trafficking in women, enslaving children, using environmentally destructive productive methods, or trading in drugs. The will of the people can only be expressed through the cash register.

"Before Adam Smith it was assumed that bankers were intermediary lenders of other peoples' money. However, economic outcomes are affected when such sums are lent out again and again *before the first borrower has been repaid.*' It would be logically possible for a cloakroom attendant at a restaurant to hire out the coats of diners while they were eating. But it would be impossible for two people – the owner and the hirer – to wear the same coat at the same time. However, that is exactly what happens when a banker makes a new loan. It changes the quantity of money in existence. 'While I cannot ride a claim to a horse, I can, under certain conditions, do exactly the same with claims to money as with money itself. In short, the institutions of banking and finance create the money supply through a range of mechanisms ultimately endorsed by statutory authority.

"Real goods and services are created by labour's use of the natural resources of the planet. Money, the defining element within the formal economy, is created by financial institutions. [However], banks and financial institutions need to stay in business and the statutory framework is constantly adapted to take account of changing practice. With the development of off-shore financial havens (*not* tax havens), the legal loopholes are increasingly difficult to police, while international finance has become a law unto itself.

"When a bank issues a loan, it needs reserves of some kind to guard against the whole value of its outstanding commitments being presented at the same time. These fractional reserves may take the form of cash and coins held by the commercial bank, together with the bank's deposits with the central bank. In theory the government/statutory authority, through the central bank, can regulate the money supply by manipulating reserves and reserve requirements. [Such] evolving financial practice is progressively endorsed by the statutory authority.

"Although the banking system as a whole creates 97% of new money as loans, it was, until very recently, assumed that the money creation process was regulated by a central banking authority through its ability to regulate the issue of notes and coins. However, the money created by banks is not the same as notes and coins, which have a tangible existence. We could call the former 'bookkeeping money' and the latter 'pocket money.' Pocket money, when used by ordinary people for their everyday transactions is normally regarded as real, tangible money, 'as good as gold.' Bookkeeping money has no existence outside a bank or financial institution. To use bookkeeping money one needs a bank account. Bookkeeping money determines the quantity of cash in the economy."

The Credit Card Takes Over

"Since the 1980s in the US and the UK money has been increasingly issued into the economy through credit card borrowing, giving rise to 'credit card capitalism.' Credit cards were originally issued as a company currency. The first Diner's Club of 1949 was issued by oil companies to create brand loyalty and a symbol of creditworthiness. VISA issued by the Bank of America in 1958 is now a network of 20,000 banks, and the largest mutual company in the world of up to 600 million card-holders. The important change with the widespread use of credit cards is that the responsibility for the issuing of debt money into the economy and thereby ensuring its vitality now rests with consumers." A form of economic democracy? "That ignores the role of advertising and the problems of those burdened with consumer debts. Credit cards also make a mockery of the idea of a control of money issue in an economy where nearly every store now has its own credit card. The non-bank financial markets have their own deposit banks, money-market funds, that can be lent repeatedly (multiplied) without limit. Lending to the financial sector – up 40% since 1998 – is a turbo-charged credit machine into financial assets and corporate balance sheets."

William Krehm

The second instalment of our review of this valuable book will be carried in our next issue.

Rectification

OUR APOLOGIES to Bob Campbell for failing to mention his having introduced us to the remarkable document of the National Farmers Union, "The Farm Crisis, Bigger Farms and the Myths of 'Competition and Efficiency.'" We found particularly interesting the analysis of the plight of the Canadian farmer – sandwiched between oligarchic high-tech suppliers and distributors of his products who have enlisted his own government to impose the debasement of his products. We shall continue applying the relevance of this sandwich model to other areas here and abroad.

Spencer and Modern Market Fundamentalism: The Institutional Aspect of Economic Activity

IN A THEORETICAL SENSE, the modern version of neo-classical economics considers the influence of institutions on economic activities relatively unimportant. Instead, it continues to uphold the central role of laissez-faire markets, seen as self-correcting mechanisms in which the economic agents respond to price signals in a fully rational way.

However, if we think a little about the economic situations that we meet in everyday daily life, different institutional forms obviously create very different conditions for market activities. Take for example one of the many farmers markets that spring up during summer weekends at parking lots at the malls' backsides. In these markets, items such as greengroceries, fruit, bread and similar items are offered for sale by small independent producers who themselves bring the produce to market.

Thus, when a consumer buys foodstuffs at a farmers market, he or she will in most cases interact directly with the producer. Furthermore, most items are displayed in the open, so that it is easy to compare prices and qualities between the different suppliers in the specific market location. Quite often there is also room for price bargaining.

If one instead goes across to the other side of the mall where the discount outlets are found, one will encounter an entirely

different market form, in which up to four or five links will separate one as consumer from the primary foodstuff producers. In the discount outlets, everything is pre-packaged and pre-priced, leaving no room for a close inspection and price bargaining. Price and quality comparisons between competing outlets offering similar products are also difficult.

Modern economic theory ignores that such highly divergent institutional market forms, which furthermore represent different evolutionary stages, still exist side by side. The different levels of asymmetry that they may project are not always understood. For example, a student buying a CD in a corporate chain store or a cup of lemonade from a fellow student turned temporary street vendor may make no distinction between the nature of these exchanges.

Commonly, Adam Smith's invisible hand is considered the origin of modern economic laissez-faire. However, many of the modern laissez-faire economists, notably Hayek and Friedman, owe a big debt to the English social philosopher, Herbert Spencer, a contemporary of Darwin who was a major figure developing what came to be known as social Darwinism.

Spencer didn't focus on economic questions in his writings, but on general principles of social development. In parallel to the ideas that Darwin worked out for biology about evolutionary adaptation, he formulated principles for the evolution of social organisms. "Societies, like living bodies, begin as germs – originate from masses which are extremely minute in comparison with the masses some of them eventually reach." Increase in the size of units is invariably accompanied by an increase in the complexity of the structure, which is a process of integration. Integration in its turn is accompanied by a progressive differentiation of structures and functions, which must be so if the organism or the societal unit is to remain viable – that is, if it is to survive in the struggle for existence.

Spencer's analysis also included a an early example of a formulation of the principle of path-dependency: "The average opinion in every age and country, is a function of the social structure in that age and country." Furthermore, he recognized that the evolutionary progression is an aggregate trend over time; in the case of individual societies at specific moments, regression and even extinction is not only a possibility, but in fact, a fairly common one.

But though breaking important new ground, Spencer's conclusions turned into a capitulation to a barren social philosophy of a "survival of the fittest," the now famous term that he is believed to have originally coined. This led him to conclude that governments, and in a wider sense all public activity, should be reduced to a narrow set of minimalist tasks, mainly connected to providing security. The state has "the duty not only of shielding each citizen from the trespasses of his neighbors, but of defending him, in common with the community at large, against foreign aggression." Everything else was to be left to the free initiative of individuals making contracts and agreements with one another.

The intervention of government in social affairs, Spencer argued, will distort the necessary adaptation of society to its environment. Once government intervenes, the beneficent processes that would naturally lead to man's more efficient and more intelligent control over nature will be distorted and give rise to a reverse maleficent process that can only lead to the progressive deterioration of the human race.

This led Spencer to come strongly out against government regulations that were starting to appear in the British society of his times, counterbalancing the excesses of the early industrial age. The Poor Laws and regulations aiming at enhancing workplace safety, protecting child labour, and, finally, laws regulating working hours, all were things that Spencer pointed to as examples of government interference in the beneficent working of natural social processes which would guarantee the survival of the fittest. With a surprising virulence Spencer held that such interference only "encourages the multiplication of the reckless and incompetent by offering them an unfailing provision," disturbing "the natural order of things [according to which] society is constantly excreting its unhealthy, imbecile, slow, vacillating, faithless [sic] members."

Spencer and Neoclassical Minimalism

During the last three decades of the nineteenth century Spencer's writings became immensely influential, rivaling even Darwin's. Especially in North America, in the days of the robber barons. His vision of a minimalist government offering no social services, coupled with the concept of survival of the fittest, were eagerly welcomed. It provided the capitalists with a world-famous social scientist's approval of their unbridled and rapacious version of capitalism.

The period was also the formative period of neoclassical economics, and while there is no evidence of Spencer having direct influence on the works of the neoclassical economists, it seems fair to assume that his ideas had become such an important part of the general intellectual fabric, that they wielded a considerable indirect influence.

However, the way Spencer defines the roles of a minimalist government, which essentially are identical to modern proponents of extreme laissez-faire, such as Milton Friedman, contains some serious inconsistencies. First of all, with regards to the government's role in providing external defense and internal security, if we look upon these social functions from a historical perspective nothing appears to be especially compelling about the division he makes. Thus, during the medieval age, providing military services was a decidedly entrepreneurial activity typically organized by some lesser noblemen, who specialized in raising and maintaining mercenary armies that in time of war were rented out to the highest bidder among the warring kings and princes.

It is true, that from the French Revolution onwards, governments have raised national armies, which have dominated warfare. But we appear to be at a turning point where the trend is reversing toward a renewed importance of entrepreneurial involvement in military activity. Corporate warriors – i.e., specialists providing soldiering, intelligence, and diverse logistical services – are hired by private corporations, which rent them out as a service package to governments engaged in wars or low-level conflicts. After a modest start in the sixties in Africa, where several governments were overthrown by coups resulting from such entrepreneurial market services, corporate warriors have become a booming business, as their engagement in America's recent wars prove.

With regards to protecting personal safety and property, privatization is also an obvious trend. Private security services are not only increasingly employed to keep teenagers and other loafers with no shopping intentions out of the malls, but are also seeing growing employment in securing that the rich can sleep soundly behind the walls of their gated communities. They need not fear that misguided Robin Hoods will try to sneak off with some of their wealth.

With no compelling reasons for the scope of a minimalist government that Spencer and the modern laissez-faire economists argue for, the concept collapses. The whole discussion about whether the "greatest happiness for the greatest number of people" is best served by a minimalist government, or by the opposite contention of a maximalist government held by the Marxists, leads down a blind path.

Spencer himself gives us some clues of this riddle. An example: "It inevitably happens that in the body politic, as in the living body, there arises a regulating system. As compound aggregates are formed, there arise supreme regulating centers and subordinate ones and the supreme centers begin to enlarge and complicate." And: "Differentiated states in which parts become dissimilar. Moreover, once parts have become unlike, they are mutually dependent on each other." These statements clearly envisages that in response to the growing complexity of social organism, regulating and coordinating functions will also grow in complexity.

But Spencer, as do the modern market fundamentalists, fails to incorporate two important aspects of social development. The evolution of social forms not only creates rising complexity and differentiation, but also rising tendencies to asymmetric alignments of the facets that define a society, including technological capabilities, information dispersion and regimes of institutional control.

In a modern complex society, the reality is that in order to provide efficient social feed-back loops, rising levels of both coordination and entrepreneurial activity will be part of the social fabric. Cybernetics, a modern addition to evolutionary theory, explains how control and feed-back loops works in the adaptive processes occurring in biological and social organisms. Incorporating the understanding of cybernetics, the discussion should not be whether the government should be minimalist or maximalist. The focal point should be how best build up efficient social feed-back and coordinating loops in response to actual conditions. Sometimes this means more government and more regulation of entrepreneurial activity, sometimes the reverse will be the case. But, importantly, the response should weigh which actual mix best serves the population's current needs and desires. The factors to be considered include not only how to shield the population and their property from physical threats, but also from the adverse effects of the growing tendencies of complex societies to adhere asymmetric patterns.

Dix Sandbeck

Prying into the Affairs of the Privileged

HEDGE FUNDS up to now have been a privileged class of investment around which regulating authorities moved on tip-toe. They are open only to very rich investors, supposed themselves able to assess and manage their risks. And just in case they cannot, the funds rely strongly on fancy derivative instruments that supposedly take care of exposure to high hazard.

A few years ago, however, there was the case of the Long-Term Capital Management Fund directed by an economist awarded a Nobel prize for Economics precisely for his work on derivatives supposed to exorcise risk. Yet that fund got into big-time trouble – to the point where Washington felt obliged to stand-by with a fistful of billions lest it bring down the finances of the world. So important had the funds become – if not precisely for what they had been intended. But the beauty of official beliefs – if well-enough sponsored-is that no matter how often they are proved false, they go on as gospel. Such matters get decided by wallet-linings rather than brains or conscience. All mention of their performance record is hushed up, like the burp of an important guest seated well above the salt.

Since then the stock market has not lacked its unpleasant surprises, and hedge funds have lowered their sights. Today they are receiving with open arms plain vanilla millionaires rather than insisting on billionaire credentials. Incorrigible optimists might take that as a symptom of a healthy democracy. The fact, however, is that when whales or even cod are in poor supply, fishermen do take a second look at sardines and minnows.

And, one thing leading to another, in the fulness of time we come across the headline in *The Wall Street Journal* (1/07, "SEC Pushing Proposal to Regulate Hedge Funds" by Deborah Solomon): "Washington – Securities and Exchange Commission Chairman William Donaldson is pushing ahead with a proposal to regulate hedge funds, despite stiff opposition from critics both inside and outside the agency.

"On July 14, the SEC plans to formally propose a rule requiring hedge-fund advisers to register with the agency. If adopted, the rule would give the SEC power to look into hedge funds – private investing pools for the wealthy and institutions that often use leverage to bet on global markets – to see if they are keeping adequate records and appropriately valuing securities, among other things."

Heck, if the big guys can't have their own way in valuing securities "among other things," what was the use of all this globalization for a better version of Las Vegas without having to leave Lower Manhattan?

"Mr. Donaldson said yesterday that the $650 billion hedge fund industry has grown so large that the SEC needs to know more about the funds' operations to avoid significant investor losses. The SEC's proposal would allow its examiners to identify risks if there's a problem. Mr. Donaldson said he has no 'vendetta' against the fund industry, but that the time is ripe for regulation." Indeed that has been an oft-repeated conclusion in

many quarters for over a decade, since hedge funds operating with derivatives shot down the British pound, the Italian lira and other currencies seriatim for the greater glory of really big operators. Not to mistake the really big guys with the miserable margin accounts of brokers that can be preyed upon whenever the broker feels he need some spare cash and is in a mood to pick up some timely bargains. Besides isn't seeing that participants in the hedge funds are not taken advantage of only one part of the problem? Shouldn't the SEC be making sure that the hedge funds not only do fine by their investors, but don't abuse the public at large? Is the record of shooting down major currencies with high-powered derivatives to become acceptable because the booty may have been distributed equitably among those within the cabal?

The Resistance to Regulating Derivatives

"The SEC's plan has run into resistance from some powerful forces, including Federal Reserve Chairman Alan Greenspan, the head of the Commodity Trading Commission and two Republican SEC commissioners.

"Opponents of the plan say it is not necessary to regulate an industry dominated by a relatively small number of wealthy investors who understand the risks. Critics also say the SEC's plan would divert resources away from the mutual fund industry where many more Americans invest money and which is suffering from a scandal that has hurt investor confidence.

"Opinions within the hedge fund industry are mixed. About 40% of the hedge fund advisers are already voluntarily registered with the agency, and some hedge funds say they welcome regulation to help make their business more sound. But others see it as an unnecessary intrusion that could lead to more invasive regulation down the road.

"The SEC is expected to vote 3-2 on the proposal, with Mr. Donaldson and the SEC's two Democratic commissioners supporting the role."

Jack Gaine, president of the Managed Funds Association, which represents hedge funds, said registration isn't necessary since hedge-fund investors know the risk they are taking when they invest. Under current rules, hedge funds can accept only investors with a minimum net worth of $1 million or whose income has been above $200,000 for at least two years."

From what Mr. Spitzer has been digging up, that would seem pretty small potatoes in the world of high finance.

The subject remains a gnawing one, and by 22/07 the *WSJ* ("High-Flying Hedge Funds Face Tougher Scrutiny by Regulators" by Ann Davis) returned to the theme.

"Regulators have stepped up their policing of the brokerage firms market and service hedge funds, the secretive and largely unregulated private investment pools. The SEC is shaping a proposal that would require hedge funds to register with the federal regulator and allow it to examine their activities. In April the agency sent a lengthy questionnaire to many big Wall St. firms seeking extensive information about potential conflicts of interest involving hedge funds. Meanwhile, a number of smaller brokers have been hit with civil charges by the National Association of Securities Dealers, the self-regulating body of brokers, for allegedly using misleading marketing with hedge funds.

"Barry Goldsmith, executive vice-president of enforcement at NASD, says brokers have begun recommending hedge funds as some investors sour on mutual funds in the wake of scandals. In a turbulent market, the appeal of hedge funds – private, often-risky investment partnerships for institutional investors and wealthy individuals – has soared, with a growing number of pension funds and endowments signing on in hopes of higher returns. Since the end of 2000, hedge fund assets have swelled to $845 billion from about $400 billion, according to Charles Gradante, managing principal of Hennessee Group LLC, an adviser to investors in hedge funds. Hennessee estimates that there are 7,000 hedge funds, up from 4,800 at the start of 2001 and 1,840 a decade ago.

"Hedge funds are estimated to generate more than $10 billion annually, or 7% of total revenue for Wall St. securities firms. Of that, roughly $7.5 billion comes from stock-trading services, says Richard Strauss, a brokerage industry analyst at Deutsche Bank AG. Hedge-fund trading activity in bonds, commodities, currencies and options adds roughly another $2 billions to $3 billions in annual revenue."

Bringing Hedge Funds Down to the Common Millionaire

"In return, Wall St. firms are helping hedge funds get off the ground, from providing free or discounted office space to throwing soirees at swank hotels to introduce them to potential investors.

"Given that regulators currently lack the authority to walk in and examine hedge funds directly, they are making use of powers they already have to regulate Wall St. brokerage firms. In the case against UBS, settled last month but not yet announced, the firm was censured and fined $85,000 for distributing sales literature to high-net-worth individuals that lacked 'adequate risk disclosure.' The agency faulted UBS for citing a fund's 'target' return without giving clients enough information to determine if the goal was reachable.

"Last year, the NASD also censured and fined a broker-dealer, Allegris Investments Inc., for allegedly failing to disclose risks of hedge funds that were highly speculative and leveraged. For instance, it said, one piece of research called one option 'an ideal fund for conservative investors. Both the NASD and SEC also are probing whether the prime brokerage divisions of big brokerage firms, in return for linking hedge funds with investors, seek payback in trading commissions and loans. Brokers claim this matchmaking service, known as 'capital introduction,' doesn't equate to endorsing the investments. But regulators argue that if a securities firm believes a client could be a big fee generator, it has an incentive to recommend funds that may not be right for the investor.

"Morgan Stanley, Goldman Sachs Group Inc. and Bear Stearns Cos. have long been leaders in prime brokerage, collectively holding more than a 60% market share, says Mr. Strauss. In a sign of other firms' interest, Merrill Lynch & Co. a month ago hired away David Barrett, Morgan Stanley's capital-introduction head, to start a group that explicitly raises money from investors for hedge funds.

"But brokerages aren't just acting as middlemen. An array of brokers has provided seed capital to start-up hedge funds through 'incubator' arms. Bear Stearns has invested in one hedge-fund incubator partnership with Mestrow Advanced Strategies Inc. To provide investment capital and consulting services to early-stage hedge-fund managers. J.P. Morgan Chase & Co. has an incubator arm of its own that invests seed capital with hedge funds. Citigroup Inc. now has four internal hedge funds with $9 billion in assets under management. Deutsche Bank formed DB Advisors to seed hedge funds for traders to keep them from leaving.

"Hedge-fund managers welcome the attention. Many can get heavily discounted or free office space, with computers and wiring intact, from prime brokers. They effectively use clients' money to pay for such perks via trading commissions, despite getting management fees of 2% of assets and 20% of returns.

"The concern is that people will quickly latch on and say, 'Look, this will give me a return of 15%,' says Samuel Israel, an NASD enforcement attorney. UBS declined comment.

However, if it is "hedge funds" that you are talking about, at once the black magic of George Soros should spring to mind. His use of derivatives enabled him to shoot down the British pound with one hand behind his back, before going on to mete out the same fate to the Italian lira and other currencies.

However, the regulators miss the crucial point: the belief in a risk-free hedge-fund investment vehicle is rooted in the self-balancing "free and perfect market" doctrine devised to impose the view that an unregulated market is by nature self-balancing. Towards that end the differential calculus was enlisted, but it was necessary to assume a market in which all actors were of such infinitesimally small size that nothing done or left undone by them could possibly influence the market "in the long run." Unless the premises you assume really correspond to reality, anything you prove will be not only irrelevant but misleading. Our neglect of that basic principle by most tenured economists has raised "Globalization and Deregulation" above the possibility of sin. No need then to worry about such externalities as the environment, social services, unemployment. The differential calculus, once the above assumption is made, leads you directly to the equilibrium points you are seeking. Once that is assumed, a bit of high-school calculus will reveal equilibrium points that will "in the long run" show money and credit to be neutral. If you have this faith, market equilibrium translates into a flat price level, and if this doesn't happen, you make it happen with interest rates "high enough to do the job," i.e., to enforce the "self-balancing" market. Whoever questions this article of faith, is simply refused tenure on university staffs, or publication in the peer press. In the name of "science" buttered with a daub of self-interest, what can't one do? Note, too, the class of financial instruments known as derivatives are an extension of the growth rate concept of various degrees used in differential calculus. And that another extension of their use gave us the exponential curve that is the mathematics of the atom bomb. And who says Hedge Fund implies "derivatives" that covers the whole field of risk, from the imaginary "pure and free market" right to the atom bomb. Hedge funds thus can offer many investors, and indeed society itself results more reminiscent of the Hiroshima bomb than of 15% returns.

William Krehm

Will General Electric End Up Running the Metropolitan Opera?

THE NATIONAL FARM UNION (Canada) report that we summarized in our last issue has gone on resonating to suggest some startling analogies in the world economy. We noted that Deregulation and Globalization (D&G) "seeks to level all barriers that prevent the ever fewer large corporations from organizing to keep prices low in their purchases from the family farmers and the prices of their sales to them at the highest possible levels, leaving them with net revenue that has remained static for decades." We noted, too, that "the International Monetary Fund and the World Bank have been mobilized to increase the Third World countries' exports – no matter at what prices – to service their debt." Thus it is the debt burden rather than the interplay of supply and demand of the commodities exchanged that increasingly determines prices on world food markets. The model developed to explain the plight of our family farms can thus be generalized on a world scale to better grasp the destructive effects of D&G.

And all this began as a harmless exercise in price theory to create the model of a "pure and perfect market," on the mistaken assumption that incorporating a bit of calculus into your equations qualifies them as serious science. But to do that the assumption has to be made that all actors in the economy are of such negligible size that nothing they do or don't do can affect prices. Yet the conglomerates that have taken over today as suppliers of farmers and as distributors of their crops and livestock don't remotely fill that bill. On the contrary: growth and merger, the patenting of genes, the relentless drive of mega-transnationals to bully the little guy and enlist the government in their own interest rather than that of the farmer is the basic code of their behaviour. That imposes on them a conduct that resembles the mathematical process of integration rather than differentiation. The prestige of mathematics is thus purloined to cover up a degree of illiteracy that would get a freshman kicked out of any science course. It is thus that the fate not only of the family farm, but of humanity itself is being sealed.

And now *The New York Times* (18/07, "The Conglomerate will see You Now – Is what is Good for G.E, Good for Health Care?" by Reed Abelson and Milt Freudenheim) lights up a similar process at work between the mammoth suppliers of medical diagnostic technology and the health care system.

"Imagine a small town where one person not only owns the hardware store, but is also the banker and the doctor's most trusted adviser. In a sense General Electric is trying to play such

a role in the nation's $2 trillion health care industry.

"New York – Presbyterian Hospital, one of the country's largest academic medical centers, is among the hospitals making a bet on GE's move toward one-stop shopping. Last fall it announced a seven-year $500 million agreement that calls for GE to offer advice – and discounts – on technology, as well as ways to increase efficiency. Also options for financing.

"Dozens of GE-trained 'black belts' and 'green belts' – experts in a data-driven management method called Six Sigma – are already wandering the hospital's halls, looking for things to improve.

"And if New York – Presbyterian needs light bulbs, GE will supply those, too.

"With $14 billion in sales, GE's health care business is among its fastest growing and most profitable units, central to the vision of its chief executive, Jeffrey R. Immelt. Mr. Immelt rose to the top job after running the company's medical systems unit.

"'We run the business to make a buck for investors; we run the business to help our customers,' he said recently at the company's headquarters in Fairfield, Conn. 'GE knows a lot in this space and could be helpful in public policy.'"

What's Good for GE is Good for Nation's Health

"Some critics ask, however, if what is good for GE is always good for the nation's health care. Medical technology, the company's specialty, is a leading contributor in runaway health costs, and some medical professional and consumer groups say the conglomerate's growing influence among hospitals and doctors raises issues about how scarce dollars are being spent.

"'Very few people would want GE to run the Metropolitan Opera,' said Dr. Robert Michels, a former dean of Cornell University's medical school, now affiliated with New York – Presbyterian. Providing quality care is much more complicated than making cathode ray tubes in X-ray equipment, Dr. Michels said. And it is unclear whether it saves money.

"GE is famous for its sophisticated diagnostic imaging equipment. Using new CT scanners, doctors can take an image of the heart in five beats, to check for a narrowing of the arteries. Or they can perform a 'virtual colonoscopy' without the invasive procedure patients find so unpleasant. And GE's ultrasound system, 4D, lets expectant parents view extraordinarily detailed, nearly real-time images of a developing fetus.

"Diagnostic imaging, a crown jewel in GE's businesses, is regarded as a way to enter other fast-growing and profitable health care businesses. 'It's important to be big in big markets,' says Mr. Immelt, who has identified health care as one of the richest opportunities in an aging America. Spending is forecast by about a percent a year, as far as the eye can see.

"*Policy analysts, however, say that this rate of growth is being driven in large part by the very technology that companies like GE are promoting. Doctors and hospitals are eager customers of the latest machines as they increasingly turn to diagnostic tests as a source of additional revenue. Doctors, in particular, are looking for new income as insurers have squeezed payments for traditional office visits.*" [Emphasis ours.]

"In health care supply creates its own demand,' says Christopher J. Queram, CEO of the Employer Health Care Alliance Cooperative, a non-profit purchasing group in Madison, Wis., who is concerned about the proliferation of magnetic resonance imaging machines in doctors' offices.

"Advances in technology – a special MRI machine to take pictures of a knee, or digital mammography to screen for breast cancer – do not always result in better health, these analysts say, and there is little hard evidence that some of this equipment can cost more than $1 million is worth the cost.

"Says John C. Rother, policy director for AARP, the lobby for older Americans, 'In this country we have no systematic way of evaluating technologies for cost effectiveness.'

"GE's pitch is aimed squarely at a doctor's desire to make more money from doing more tests. In selling an exam table that doubles as a device to measure bone density, GE trumpets the system's potential revenue: $30,000 a year if a doctor sees five patients a week.

"As the hospital market has slowed for equipment like MRI's and as care is increasingly delivered outside hospital walls, GE is turning its attention to doctors in their offices. This year it bought a company specializing in financing doctors and dentists.

"Said John J. Donahue, CEO of National Imaging Association, a consulting group based in Hackensack, NJ, 'GE distinguishes itself by masterfully leveraging the entire GE family.'

"Critics say the results can be too much equipment and too many tests. The Medicare Payment Advisory Commission, which advises Congress on the Medicare program, has also raised concerns about the spread of medical technology, has questioned whether some doctors are using the equipment appropriately.

"As one of the nation's largest employers, GE knows a lot about rising health care costs. It spends almost $2 billion a year to cover 400,000 employees and their families. Dr. Robert Galvin, director of global health care at GE, leads the Leapfrog Group, an advocacy group representing more than 150 public and private organizations providing health care benefits; it has been pushing hospitals to install computerized systems to cut down on mistakes in ordering drugs and tests."

Resistance to being "Leapfrogged"

"Illustrating the sometimes complicated currents buffeting a giant like GE, many hospitals, including GE's potential customers, have resisted some of the initiatives pushed by Leapfrog. GE has also taken heat for the way many doctors use some of its products. A few years ago it and others successfully lobbied Congress to authorize higher medical payments for digital mammography for routine breast cancer screening. Digital mammography, which costs much more than older technologies that use X-ray film, is widely approved for women who have already had suspicious tumors detected, but experts say there is no evidence to justify the extra expense of digital for routine screening.

"The company has identified another need among hospitals: sophisticated computer systems that can keep track of a patient's medical records and give doctors ready access to infor-

mation about how to treat certain diseases. In this market, however, GE trails many competitors. Rather than match the large hospital-wide systems offered by its competitors, GE focuses on building its business by computerizing specific departments, like radiology or cardiology.

"In other areas, GE is being more aggressive. Mr. Immelt, for example, agreed to buy a British biosciences company called Amersham last October for about $10 billion, giving GE expertise in biology to bolster its traditional prowess in physics and engineering; GE hopes to use Amersham's knowledge to help it develop technology that lets doctors diagnose diseases on the molecular level.

"But, critics add, the unfettered use of technology can also be problematic. 'Medical technology is creating a greater set of quality management challenges every day than the day before,' said Dr. Arnold Milstein, a senior health care expert at Mercer Human resource Consulting. 'It is both a blessing and a curse.'

"From most patients' point of view getting a hospital bed and professional attention in good time in the case of a heart attack or some other crisis of survival is the crucial concern. Due attention to that might not be precisely what preoccupies GE in its conquest of the medical care market."

Much like the focus of the fertilizer and the genetically modified seed people in their influence of government agricultural policy!

William Krehm

A Most Special Bank in a Most Special Town

WASHINGTON is the capital of the United States and beyond that of much of the world as well. Banks, for their part, wherever they might be, have in recent years come to cast a deep shadow over the rest of the economy. Into their broad bosoms they have gathered stock brokerages, underwriting establishments, merchant banks, insurance companies, derivative boutiques, and any surface horizontal or tilted upon which dice can be cast. When it comes then to a Washington-based bank, we would naturally expect something special.

And it was precisely that that was found in the case of Riggs Bank. *The Wall Street Journal* (15/07, "Riggs Bank Draws Harsh Criticism – Congress Report Says Firm turned 'Blind Eye' to Data Showing Wide Corruption" by Glenn R. Simpson): "Washington – Riggs Bank, under intense regulatory scrutiny for months for its work within Saudi Arabia, 'turned a blind eye' to evidence of massive corruption involving US oil companies and an African autocrat, a new congressional report alleges. The bank also allegedly helped former Chilean dictator Augusto Pinochet hide millions of dollars from US and European authorities.

"The federal bank regulators charged with overseeing Riggs fell down on the job, the study says, failing to guard against conflicts of interest and neglecting to punish a unit of Riggs

National Corp. for egregious violations of money-laundering rules until earlier this year, 'Million-dollar cash deposits, off-shore shell corporations, suspicious wire transfers. alteration of account names, all the classic signs of money laundering and foreign corruption made their appearance at Riggs Bank,' said Sen. Carl Levin, a Michigan Democrat who led a Senate inquiry into the institution. 'When a bank operates with such reckless abandon and federal regulators are so ineffectual, it does little to inspire confidence in the country's determination to stop money laundering.'

"The panel's findings could give impetus to calls on Capitol Hill to strip bank regulators of their authority to enforce money laundering regulations. Allegations Riggs hid information from regulators and enforcement officials – and possibly facilitated corruption – raise questions about whether any of the bank's current or former executives might face criminal charges."

"Major oil companies made millions of dollars in questionable payments to the government of Equatorial Guinea or the country's top officials, often through about 60 different accounts at Briggs. ExxonMobil Corp. and Amerada Hess Corp. are in business with members of the first family of Equatorial Guinea and buy security services from the president's brother, investigators found. Marathon Oil Corp. and ChevronTexaco Corp. allegedly made other questionable payments such as tuition for the children of top government officials.

"'Prior information had already been reported regarding the bank's failure to report tens of millions of dollars in suspicious transactions by diplomats for the government of Saudi Arabia' said Washington criminal defense lawyer Bruce Zagaris. A federal grand jury is probing the Equatorial Guinea accounts, from which Riggs, says a former bank executive, improperly diverted more than $1 million.

"The report could also cloud a potential sale of Riggs, which some investors have been counting on as a way to solve the bank's woes. Riggs, known as the bank of presidents for the special status it has enjoyed in Washington for decades, is controlled by billionaire Joe L. Allbritton and his family. It has been hit with a $25 million fine for a range of money-laundering violations related to accounts held by diplomats."

The Miracle of Corporate Resurrection

What does a bank caught red-handed in such a mess do? It pays the fines imposed, fires the high officials who may have received prison sentences, capitalizes the net profit after deducting the cost of these adversities, and merges or sells itself to another bank perhaps at a good net profit. Such is the miracle of corporative personality that exceeds personal resurrection proclaimed from more conventional pulpits. Something of that

sort may be underway in the case of Riggs.

"As a result, Riggs which for years had fiercely resisted take-over overtures despite its strong position in the Washington, DC, retail-banking market, has been discussing a sale with several suitors. At 4 p.m. on the Nasdaq Stock Market, shares of Riggs were trading at $22.50 up $1.05 or nearly 5%, and significantly higher than the $15 level at which they traded in February.

"The Senate investigators' concerns focused in large part on the way in which Riggs handled Equatorial Guinea's dozens of accounts. Riggs handled deposits of that government of $400 to $700 millions at a time 'with little or no attention to the bank's anti-money-laundering obligations, turned a blind eye on numerous suspicious transactions,' the report states.

"Investigators found that more than $35 million in oil receipts were withdrawn from official E.G. Government accounts and wired 'to companies unknown to the bank and had accounts in jurisdictions with bank secrecy laws.' At least one of the firms appeared controlled by the President of E.G., the panel said.

"The tiny, poverty-stricken West African nation of 500,000 has vast oil reserves and a history of dictatorship and corruption."

"Internal Riggs memos led investigators to other discoveries, such as oil company lease payments connected to President Obland [of that land]. An ExxonMobil subsidiary called Mobil Equatorial Guinea Inc. leased a 50-acre compound from the president's wife (and later, a company controlled by the president) for more than $150,000 annually. ExxonMobil also leased a house from the agricultural minister and paid for by contract labor supplied by the interior minister. The company is also in a joint venture with one of the president's companies involving oil distribution.

Riggs's deals did not have to stink of oil. The smell of blood seems to have sufficed as well: "Riggs sought out Augusto Pinochet's business in 1996, while he was still in control of the Chilean army. The bank 'served as a long-standing personal banker for Mr. Pinochet and deliberately assisted him in concealment and movement of his funds while he was under investigation and the subject of a world-wide court-order freezing his assets.'

"The panel also alleged that an Office of the Comptroller of Currency examiner, R. Ashley Lee, took steps to prevent information on the Pinochet account from being placed into Riggs' supervision files. Mr. Lee later went to work for Riggs, where he allegedly worked with the bank on OCC matters, 'ignoring post-employment restrictions on OCC contact,' the report alleges."

All in all it sounds like one big, happy family.

William Krehm

The Pressure Mounts

Our Unasked and Unanswerable Questions

This is an unusual issue of *ER*. It is an attempt to understand why so many unanswered, and indeed, unasked questions are leading the world where it does not choose to go. The most astounding answers are coming out of the woodwork.

We were all shocked by the last US presidential vote recount that placed a candidate with the minority popular vote in the presidency. But didn't Clinton-Gore do something not dissimilar when the world financial system was saved in stealth by a limited unacknowledged introduction of capital accountancy that responsible accountants and economists had been advocating for generations? Instead, the universities were cleansed of tenured help who advocated the proper keeping of the government's books at the very time that the groundwork for bigger and better Wall St. scams was being laid. The result: the mega scam of Globalization and Deregulation that has made its contribution to the Iraq adventure. In the present and recent election campaigns on either sides of our border, the two major parties haven't dared question the mandatory goal of balancing budgets that cannot and should not be balanced.

When are we going to learn the lesson that we cannot come clean only on matters that we *choose* to come clean on; that it is the issues that we choose not to face on which governments take the fatal turns? And these are kept under wraps because they may lose the political centre for our professional politicians. And the political centre – defined as what will enable parties to pay for prime-time advertising on the boob-tube – is the surest pass to hell.

From the most sophisticated business press, we have chosen a mere handful of suppressed issues that are coming out of the closet with an ominous force that simply will not be denied. Rationed openness, at a time like this, becomes tantamount to betrayal.

Documentation

July 28, 2004
City of Kingston

Mayor Harvey Rosen and Council,

There is another choice for financing municipal infrastructure other than borrowing at commercial rates or entering into public private partnerships as suggested in the *Whig* newspaper report, May 26, but it would require the co-operation of the federal government. For several years municipalities across Canada (including Kingston and Toronto in 2001) adopted resolutions asking the federal government to allow them to get financing from the Bank of Canada.[1] Financing public debt through the Bank is not a new idea. The government did this for 35 years – 1939 to 1974 – during which time we fought a war

and afterwards built houses, water lines, hospitals, universities, sewer systems, roads and other infrastructure. Except for the war period, debt never grew very large because the government financed part of it through the Bank at very low cost (as low as 0.37%).

Because the federal government owns the Bank of Canada, any interest paid to it comes back to the government as a dividend minus the cost of administration. If municipalities were allowed to borrow from the Bank of Canada they would benefit not only from low rates, but also from a long amortization period which could and should be set at the expected life of a given project.

For example, a sewer costing $50 million with a life expectancy of 50 years would be amortized over 50 years at an average cost of $1.6 million a year including a 1% cost of financing. If funded through a public-private-partnership the cost would depend on the terms of the contract, but would likely be higher than either of the other methods of financing because on top of the cost of money there would be the added cost of profit.

Municipalities have sent their resolutions either directly to the government, as Toronto did, or to the Federation of Canadian Municipalities (FCM), as Kingston did, FCM in turn forwarded them to the federal government. However, the government refuses to return to the way the Bank was used prior to 1974, taking the position that using the Bank of Canada to finance government debt would be inflationary, in spite of 35 years of evidence to the contrary. In fact, inflation only became a serious problem *after* the government reduced its use of the Bank to finance long term debt. During the '50's inflation averaged 2.4%; during the '60's it averaged 2.5%; during the last half of the '70's the average climbed to 8.9% and peaked in 1981 at 12.4%. Today it is low again. The simplistic view that using the Bank of Canada to finance government debt will cause inflation does not hold water. There are other factors at work.[2]

The decision to reduce the Bank's holdings of government securities had other devastating effects. To begin with, because the government was financing long-term debt after 1974 almost entirely through the private sector, its debt ballooned when interest rates went through the roof in 1980 and '81 and again in 1989-90, reaching $588 billion in 1997. Interest on this debt amounted to between $40 and $50 billions all during the '90's and is still around $35 billion per year. On top of this is the interest paid by provinces and municipalities amounting to as much as $32 billion a year.

It is because of this interest that there is not enough money for infrastructure – or anything else. It is a deep hole out of which our governments will never climb unless they make use of our national bank by gradually transferring to it at least some of the public debt.

Municipalities have had heavy responsibilities dumped on them as a result of the decision to reduce the use of the Bank for long-term financing, and would be justified in demanding that the government allow them to get financing from the Bank of Canada for capital expenditures. No one is saying that it will be simple, but we have the competence to do it and we should.

There has been enough shilly-shallying, procrastination and disinformation. Municipalities should act *now!* The financial system is sucking us dry. Kingston could provide leadership through the new group of small city mayors, Municipalities United for a New Deal, headed up by Mayor Rosen. If municipalities do not act in their own interests to get financing through the Bank of Canada, it is quite clear that no one else will do it for them.

We would be pleased to provide more information or come before Council to answer questions if that is your wish.

Richard Priestman, President, Kingston Chapter, Committee on Monetary and Economic Reform

(Inflation averages were provided by Garth Rutherford.)

Priestman to the Honourable Ralph Goodale

August 16, 2004
The Honourable Ralph Goodale
Minister of Finance
Government of Canada

Re: The suggestion that governments borrow funds directly from the Bank of Canada to finance public capital expenditures in Canada.

Dear Mr. Minister:

Thank you for your letter of June 14 replying to my earlier correspondence with the Honourable John Gerretsen, Minister of Municipal Affairs and Housing for the Province of Ontario.

I regret to say that I am deeply disappointed, even shocked by your statement that using the Bank of Canada to finance capital expenditures of Canadian governments would be inflationary, a position which is contradicted by our history. I expected that our Minster of Finance would be better informed. This misinformation is hurting Canadians by supporting a system which is draining $65 billion a year from their pockets in unnecessary interest – money which could be used for much better purposes.

For 35 years, 1939 to 1974, Canada used the Bank to finance a significant portion of its debt, and during that time inflation never got out of control. For example, in 1952 the inflation rate was 2.4%, and while it rose and fell over the years it was never very high, being only 3.2% in 1971. Mortgages of 25 and even 35 years were obtained, indicating a stable dollar. After 1974, Canada's use of the Bank to finance long-term debt for public capital expenditures was reduced, yet inflation was severe, increasing from 6.8% in 1978 to 11.4% in 1980. Today it is low again: the simplistic view that using the Bank of Canada to finance government debt will cause inflation does not hold water. There are other factors at work.

The Committee on Monetary and Economic Reform would like to see the Government support use of the Bank as it previously did for 35 years, and encourage provincial and local governments to use it as well. The savings which would ensue could then be used for health, education, infrastructure and other essential needs.

I have attached a letter recently sent to Mayor Harvey Rosen of Kingston, and information prepared by William Krehm of Toronto, Committee on Monetary and Economic Reform.

Respectfully,

Richard Priestman, Committee on Monetary and Economic Reform, Kingston

cc: The Honourable Paul Martin, Prime Minister; The Honourable John Gerretsen, Minister of Municipal Affairs and Housing, Province of Ontario; Mayor Harvey Rosen and Council

Note from Richard Priestman: Congratulations to Gordon Coggins and George Crowell for their presentation to the Town Council of the Municipality of Lakeshore. Also to be recognized is Andre Marentette who helped to get them on the agenda by connecting their presentation to his on the Municipal Property Assessment Act *(MPAC). If your municipality has not yet passed a resolution in support of using the BoC to finance municipal capital projects, maybe you can help them to do so. Let's keep the ball rolling.*

1. Resolutions passed by Kingston and Toronto:
   Kingston, April 3, 2001
   (A) The City of Kingston request the Government of Canada
   (i) to instruct the Bank of Canada to buy securities issued by municipalities and guaranteed by the Government of Canada to pay for capital projects and/or pay off current debt;
   (ii) to refund to municipalities any interest paid by municipalities to the Bank of Canada;
   (B) That a copy of this motion be forwarded to the Federation of Canadian Municipalities, the Association of Municipalities of Ontario (AMO) for circulation to other Municipalities within the Province of Ontario with a population over 50,000, to the local M.P. and M.P.P., requesting their support and endorsement.
   Toronto – April 23 – May 2, 2001
   The Policy and Finance Committee recommends that:
   (1) The Federal Minister of Finance, in conjunction with the Province of Ontario, be requested to provide low cost, below prime, long-term loans to municipalities, such as through the Bank of Canada; and
   (2) A copy of this request be forwarded to the Federation of Canadian Municipalities and the Association of Municipalities of Ontario.
2. One of the other factors which helped to avoid inflation was the system of statutory reserves by which the government was able to require the commercial banks to put some of their cash in reserves with the Bank, thus reducing the amount of credit *they* could create and therefore the total amount of credit money in circulation. These reserves were abolished by Brian Mulroney in 1991 and would have to be reinstated.

China Once More to the Fore

IT IS AN ILLUSION that after all its murderous writhing, the world will fall back into its old familiar patterns. While everybody is wondering how Washington is ever going to wriggle out of the Afghan-Iraqi mess, the next great reshaping of the planet's pecking order seems under way. And here, too, Washington is doing much to bring its coming problems upon itself. The culture that gave us the "End of History," is about to be engulfed in another chapter of that imperious companion. Just as Fukuyama was penning the US's great dream, Cleo was turning several sharp corners.

Ted D. Fishman in the cover story of *The New York Times Magazine* sounds an autumnal note (4/06, "The China Bind – The global economy is not likely to be led by the US forever. Is this the beginning of the End?").

Suddenly it is becoming recognized that with the Americanization of the world, the US may in special cases actually be breeding its competition. Nations fall into a variety of categories. There are those who are primarily a source of cheap labour, initially to support their own hierarchies, and later to allow Americans to outsource their less skilled operations. But China cannot be locked in that niche. They are a people with an immensely rich cultural background, inventors of paper and gunpowder, and responsible for much of the world's pioneering in ocean navigation. With a background like that the cheap labour that so bemuses American corporations is readily internalized at low cost for their own exports. Labor in China today is so cheap and so efficient that Central America and Mexico are losing much of their *maquiladora* industries to it. From their long history of staving off unwanted intrusions on all points of the compass, they have developed a genius for turning relationships with the West around and inside out. Listen, for example, to this passage from the Fishman piece on the Wanfeng automotive factory outside Shanghai.

"Ten years ago, Wanfeng was hammering out motorcycle wheels by hand in a Chinese garage; a few years later it was No. 1 seller of aluminum-alloy motorcycle wheels, first in China and now in Asia. It soon became a top national and global seller in alloy automobile wheels as well. It now turns out about 60,000 vehicles a year that, if you squint just a little, appear remarkably like Jeep Grand Cherokees. They come with every luxury, including leather seats and DVD video systems, and purr when driven.

"Yet Wanfeng's factory itself is a bare-bones machine. Tellingly, there is not a single robot in sight. Instead, there are hundreds of young men, newly arrived from China's expanding technical schools, manning the assembly lines with little more than large electric drills, wrenches and rubber mallets. Engines and body panels that would in a Western, Japanese or Korean factory move from station to station on automatic conveyors are hauled by hand and hand truck here. That is why Wanfeng can sell its hand-made luxury versions of the Jeep (to buyers in the Middle East mostly) for $8,000 to $10,000. The company isn't spending money on multimillion-dollar machines to build cars; it's using highly skilled workers who cost at most a few hundred dollars a month. Factory wages in the country's booming east coast cities can be $120 to $160 a month and half that inland, according to Merril Weingrod of China Strategies, an affiliate of Kurt Salmon Associates, a consulting firm."

Labour Cheaper than Robots

"Wanfeng is hardly the first to mobilize Chinese labor as a stand-in for machinery. Mao Zedong believed that China could leapfrog other developing countries in the late 30's. He exhorted the Chinese to build backyard furnaces to melt down their iron implements, all in service of his goal to have China outproduce Great Britain in steel and surpass the British economy in size in 15 years. Instead, the people were left without the few tools, pots and pans they had started with. And they starved. The Great Leap Forward, the direct cause of the famine that killed 30 million people, [ranks] among the deadliest man-made disasters in history."

Mao failed to recognize another great asset of China – its rich cultural tradition that has made it possible for Chinese émigrés and even some of those who stayed at home to sop up Western science and technology.

But all the while, even if they did not know it, the Communists "were priming China for capitalist successes to come. They exercised complete control over the deployment of labour – determining, for example, who moved out of the countryside and into the cities. Prasenjit Duara, professor of history at the University of Chicago, acknowledges the paradox: The Marxists made the work force docile and organized labor a work force that could be continually mobilized. An obedient labor force keeps management costs down too. [Today] the ranks of managers who supervise enormous numbers of workers in Chinese factories are remarkably thin by Western standards. Despite the enormous numbers, you might see 15 managers for 5,000 workers, an indication of how well-managed they are. And culturally, the Chinese put a very high premium on not losing face. In manufacturing that translates into not making mistakes on the production line. 'If you look just at low wages, you overlook the talents of Chinese manufacturers to drive their costs down,' Weingrod says.

"By now most of us know that China is the factory floor of choice for the world's low-road manufacturing: it assembles more toys, stitches more shoes and sews more garments than any other nation in the world. But moving up the technological ladder, China has also become the world's largest maker of consumer electronics, like TV's, DVD players and cell-phones. And climbing higher still, China is moving into biotech and high-tech computer manufacturing. Behind China's rapid economic ascendancy over the past 25 (and especially last 10) years is her huge population. China is home to close to 1.5 billion people, probably. That would make the official census figure of 1.3 billion too low by an amount equal to roughly the population of Germany, France and the UK combined.

"China is not home to the cheapest work force in the world. Even at 25 cents an hour, Chinese workers cost more than laborers in the poorer countries of Southeast Asia or Africa. In the world's miserable corners, children carry rifles and walk mine fields for less than a dollar a day. China is the world's workshop because it sits in a relatively stable region and offers manufacturers a reliable, pliant and capable industrial work force.

"The other great contributing factor is the migration of hundreds of millions of peasants from the countryside now that the government insists that the farmers fend for themselves and is all but evicting peasants from the land. The plots allotted to farm families are on average 1.2 acres, but can be as small as one eighth of an acre. Average city incomes, according to the government, are $1,000 a year, three times what they are in the countryside. The disparity has set in motion the largest human migration in history. By 2010, nearly half of all China's people will live in urban areas."

The result: "The productive might of China's vast low-cost manufacturing machine, along with the swelling appetites of its billion-plus consumers, have turned China's people into probably the greatest natural resource on the planet. That will shape our economy (and every other economy in the world) as powerfully as American industrialization and expansion did over the last hundred years."

"We have Created a Monster."

"[Our] framing of the debate over where the world's companies choose to exploit low-cost manufacturing implies that American consumers and businesses have strong choices. However, increasingly, what Chinese businesses and consumers choose for themselves determines how the American economy operates.

"The experience of Motorola, the US telecommunications giant, offers a lesson in how China's size changes most rules. Every month five million new subscribers sign up for mobile-phone service in China. The country's 300 million mobile-phone users make China by far the largest such market in the world. It gives them a chance to grow at a time when the big European and US markets are saturated. China is also the most competitive and protean market in the world. New manufacturers appear out of nowhere; new phones materialize daily at big-city stores. There are 800 current handset models to choose from. Young urban consumers change phones on the average after only eight months – they sell them to someone else or pass them to family members.

"And this mobile phone market in China is one that Motorola invented.

"For Robert Galvin, the company's former CEO, China in the early to mid-1980s promised to more than make up for Motorola having been foiled in Japan for years. But first the company had to develop a top-drawer telecommunications infrastructure. At a dreary state ceremony, during a tour of the country, Galvin turned to the minister of railroads and asked whether he wanted to do a good job as minister and be done with it, or to create a world-class society. In doing so, he tapped a thick vein of economic patriotism.

"Motorola's deep and open company archives show that Galvin knew that eventually the transfer of technology would sow formidable Chinese competition. Nevertheless, Motorola decided that the best strategy was to get into China early."

Let us pause here to note that those archives at this point disclose the Achilles' heels of the Globalization and Deregulation model: that deal with the devil imposes the need of growth rates that have already been incorporated into stock prices. The slightest hiatus in observing that commitment will bring its share price crashing. And that can bring down the whole structure of further financing for which those shares have served as collateral. And as support for executive option values. It is this deep vulnerability of the model that imposes the need to conquer the world that the Chinese are riding so well. And you cannot suppress the thought that their background in Marx, no matter how ossified, has left them with a keen sense of the West's vulnerabilities. Thus they lassoed, and brought into their corral the most tip-top infrastructure of communications technology – in some senses out front of the US itself.

In this way the curtain arose over the most incredible theater of the absurd – the one-sided duel between David and Goliath, with "little" David the heavier and by far the brighter of the two.

As a result China's "mobile communications network calls get through to phones on high rises, subway cars and distant hamlets – connections that would stymie mobile phones in the US.

"What no one at Motorola foresaw was that the Chinese market would become the most competitive of all. Nokia and Motorola now battle for market share in the Chinese handset business. German, Korean and Taiwanese makers figure strongly enough. And all these foreign brands are now facing intense competition from indigenous Chinese phone makers.

"'Competition goes through a cycle in China,' says Ziru Tian, at Insead, the French business school. 'At first foreigners can make things at much lower cost than the Chinese. But as local companies come along to supply the multinational companies, the supply network expands very fast. Then local manufacturers can start to source their parts in China and drive the prices of their products far lower than the multinationals.'

"One of the biggest challenges facing Motorola and other global manufacturers is that Chinese suppliers are getting too good. Their quality, low-priced parts have helped create new, homegrown and extremely aggressive competitors. More than 40% of the domestic handset market now belongs to local companies. One of the many, Ningbo Bird, will produce 20 million handsets in 2004 and is likely soon to nudge its way into the ranks of the 10 top mobile phone-makers in the world. Yet Motorola can't exactly exit the Chinese market. If it did, says Jim Gradoville, Motorola's vice-president of Asia Pacific government relations, the Chinese companies that emerged from the crucible of their market would be the leanest and most aggressive in the world, and a company like his would not know what hit it. So Motorola stays. Already the largest investor in China's electronic industry, Motorola plans to triple its stake there to more than $10 billion by 2006."

Trap or Opportunity?

But what is not clear whether that is a trap or an opportunity. The same may be said of the long-term effects of Globalization and Deregulation.

"China's crazy quilt of state-owned, village-owned, private and hybrid businesses was stitched together over 25 years of rocky reforms. Peasant entrepreneurs, opportunistic officials, government planners, new urban sophisticates and foreign investors all created operations that best fitted for the moment they stepped into the evolving market economy. But one overwhelming fact stands out. 90% of everything made in China is in oversupply; nearly every manufacturing industry has excess capacity. And instead of using cheap labor to push their profit margins higher, Chinese companies use cheap labor to drive down prices.

"A Chinese family can live a life comfortably close to that of the American middle class for a fraction of the cost. Though China claims urban per-capita income is $1,000, 'the government numbers on incomes don't tell the whole story on the consumer class, especially not in the eastern cities,' says Merrill Weingrod. 'People in industrial centers tend to have two and three jobs with many taking in short-term assignments here and there. Annual real income in Shanghai, for instance, is close to $2,500 per capita, $5,000 per household. The Chinese can, on average, buy nearly five times in goods and services per dollar that an American can with the same dollar in the US. Chinese urban incomes approach the buying power of Americans making $12,500 a year – for working couples $25,000. You can understand why Shanghai looks as prosperous as it does and everybody seems outside shopping all the time. China has now 100 million people who are comfortably middle class. The allure of China's market is that huge volumes of potential sales mean that even products with the most modest margins can earn lots of money.'

"'Look, China is the most exciting place in the world right now to be a manufacturer,' says Mark Wall, president of the greater China region for F.E. Plastics. His operation sells the plastic pellets used to make everything from DVDs to building materials. Wall, who came to China from G.E. Plastics, Brazil, describes a country in love with manufacturing like no other, where engineers come in excited and readily work long days. Where university students clamor to get into engineering and applied sciences. Wall talks about working in China with the delight that young computer whizzes felt when they found Silicon Valley. There is no going to a cocktail party and then trying to talk around the fact that you make things in factories. G.E. has every plan to capitalize on the local zeal for manufacturing. It recently opened a giant industrial research center in Shanghai that by next year will employ 1,300 people in its Chinese labs.

"The government is pouring resources into creating the world's largest army of industrialists. China has 17 million university and advanced vocational students (up more than threefold in five years). China will produce 323,000 engineers this year. That's five times as many as in the US, where the number of engineering graduates has been declining."

That should not be surprising. Precisely since those early 1980s in North America, the financial sector took over the economy, and industrial firms were reduced to mere gaming chips for its greater profits. That was reflected in the huge disparity between the rewards of stock market and high financial executives and mere industrial CEOs. And in the number of trained engineers who ended up financial CEOs and even featured in some of our greatest financial scandals.

There remains the rickety state of China's banks loaded with debt to state and private firms of dubious quality. Obviously with both the politics and the economy in a state of rapid transition, with private fortunes being made, that is a factor that could well lead to a major setback for China and her economy. But there too she is no longer frozen in dogma as the West happens to be. In respect to banking policy it would be more enlightening making comparison with the North American policy of the latter 1980s than with that enthroned there today. At that time the banks of the United States and Canada were dangerously loaded with the dubious financing of the late oil and real estate booms, the mess of the US Savings and Loans and in Canada the financing of an Ottawa developer's shopping spree in the US for retail store chains.

To bail our banks out from the losses from those follies, our government did away with the statutory reserves that the commercial banks had to leave with the central banks as security for a modest portion of the deposits they had received from the public in their chequing accounts. Those deposits earned the banks no interest, and moreover, provided an alternative tool that could be used by the central bank to combat perceived inflation. Shortly before the Bank for International Settlements in Switzerland – a technical body that allowed no elected representative of a government to attend its sessions – had introduced its *Risk-Based Capital Requirements* guidelines. This declared the debt of developed countries to be risk-free and thence requiring no additional capital for banks to acquire.

That was a bad blunder, because at the same time BIS was advocating eliminating any increase in the price level with the sole remaining blunt tool of higher interest rates. The incompatibility of the two policies contributed to the Mexican monetary crisis of 1994 that spread both to Eastern Asia and Russia with devastating results. That had by then been made still worse by the deregulation of the banks that followed their bailout and that allowed them to acquire brokerage houses, underwriting and merchant banks, derivative boutiques, and overturned the pillars that had been established by the Roosevelt regime to prevent the recurrence of the Wall St. crash that ushered in the Depression of the 1930s.

Is China Avoiding Surrendering Money Creation Wholly to their Banks?

All this is frightfully relevant today when interest rates are being turned around to climb once more in a world economy that has been loaded to the rafters with debt to keep the economy from collapsing.

Those higher interest rates will disadvantage Western industries in their competition with China. That is particularly so since China has declined to depend on higher interest rates for restoring its banks to liquidity. Instead, as of September 21st last, it raised the statutory reserve that commercial banks must hold against the deposits received from 6% to 7%. This decreases the multiple of the credit they are free to create in loans for their clients rather than raising interest rates. Higher interest rates reduce the competitive price advantage of its exports by strengthening its currency. If in fact, on top of the multiple advantage that the Fishman article outlines, there is a further competitive advantage arising from China and Washington pursuing their diverse ways with respect to interest rates. The result can be utterly catastrophic for the West and humanity as a whole. It would formally mark the refusal to relegate Chinese industry to the happy hunting ground of finance, as happened in the US in the 1990s.

William Krehm

ER Mail Bag

Dear Mr. Krehm,

It was absolute pleasure in having a private conversation with you on the world economy at the Third Global conference in Business and Economics July 9-11 Amsterdam. I was particularly intrigued by your comments regarding the possibility of impending correction of the global economy.

While I am not a economist by discipline I see the globe through strategic eyes and formulate my analysis of the environment on strategic tools. My humble view is that the economic state of the globe is largely based on false media driven perception often used to drive the speculation in a particularly desired geo-political direction. My humble analysis seems to suggest that we have a fragile global financial system with hairline cracks which would eventually crumble leading to severe economic crisis. I do not profess to be an expert and have a lot to learn from scholars of your stature. I would therefore like to exchange ideas with you if you have time. I fully realize that a scholar of your stature specially a scholar who bring a great deal of honesty in their views would be highly in demand. I would be honoured if we can keep in touch from time to time.

Warmest regards and best wishes,

Dr. Shahid Yamin
Senior Lecturer in Strategy
Australian Graduate School of Entrepreneurship,
Swinburne University of Technology

Dear Dr. Yamin,

I will be delighted to remain contact with you, and hopefully we will meet again at Atul Gupta's conference at Oxford next year. I should point out that I am not an academic and that accordingly the title "professor" with which you adorn me is inappropriate.

All best,

Bill Krehm

REVIEW OF A BOOK BY JOEL BAKAN. VIKING CANADA (PENGUIN GROUP), TORONTO, 2004

"The Corporation: The Pathological Pursuit of Profit and Power"

T HE PERSPECTIVE of a law professor adds just enough new material to give a fresh and compelling interpretation to issues and events familiar to anyone who has paid modest attention to economic policy fashions over the past half century. This book is a serendipitous complement to *The Economics of Innocent Fraud.*[1] A review of the latter work appeared in the Financial Times on August 12, 2004 under the title of "deceptions for which no one can be held responsible." After reading this exposition on the corporation a reader may be less than willing to agree that no responsibility can be assigned for the deceptions. Bakan brings a degree of precision without identifying individual malefactors. He manifests no disagreement with Galbraith's observation that "the corporation…is an essential feature of modern economic life. We must have it." His book is rather an expansion on the next sentence: "It must conform, however, to accepted standards and requisite public constraints."

Not So Innocent Fraud

The critical, core concept here is the *person* status with which the corporation came to be endowed, especially in U.S. law, as the 19th turned into the 20th century. Bakan provides a tour through the legislative and judicial history of the corporation to show that much of the popular economic dogma impaled as *innocent fraud* by Galbraith is traceable to the success of corporate promoters in persuading politicians and judges to give them privileges that are effectually denied to real persons.

The corporation is not a person, of course. It is instead a socially created institution, quite recent in origin, utterly insensitive to the moral codes and principles out of which laws affecting interpersonal behaviour have evolved. The *person* parallel emerged from judicial decisions after agitation by corporate promoters had expanded the scope of its legislated privileges. A few decades of experience with the consequences prompted a more apt metaphor in a 1933 decision by Supreme Court Justice Louis Brandeis, who characterized the corporation as a Frankenstein monster. "Corporations, like the monster, threaten to overpower their creators." Monsters need to be kept on a chain to keep them from causing harm. Since corporations are created by acts of sovereign governments, those governments must regulate them to protect the interests of the people (who are the supposed sovereign in democratic nations). The corollary of the corporation's birth in a legislative act is that it can also be killed through the same process. That is not a notion that appears often in newspapers, but Bakan's references demonstrate that legal scholars are thinking and writing about it as an important policy option.

Graphic accounts of corporate misbehaviour are abundant

these days, even as we enjoy the apparent fruits of corporate "efficiency" in the production of a rising flood of abundantly affordable "stuff." Although we wouldn't want to give up the corporation in principle, the good work it does for us comes at a high social cost, for the corporation does all it can to reduce expenses by forcing others to pay them. The "others" include employees, customers, suppliers, innocent bystanders, even shareholders and corporate managers in their roles as citizens and inhabitants of the common biosphere. Abuses of these kinds have long been addressed in economics literature as "externalities." The difficulty of evaluating their magnitudes to facilitate parallel comparison with internal money savings has made it too easy to dismiss them as "mere" – even if the word is not voiced. In this book, and especially in the film *The Corporation*,[2] Bakan has provided impressive documentation of the high costs we all pay (and that future generations will pay) for the internal efficiencies of the corporation. As Milton Friedman is fond of saying, "there's no free lunch."

Bakan demonstrates by extensive presentation of judgments against corporate abuses that they seem virtually immune to condign punishment, even though the penalties imposed might be expected to deter *real* persons from repeat offenses. Fines and damage awards are accepted as a cost of doing business. The managers of corporations are required by law to make money for shareholders. The list of judgments illustrates the cold-blooded risk analyses that corporations make in determining how many customers and employees they can kill and maim and still come out ahead on a comparison of likely penalties to the known savings afforded by cheap design and lax administration of safety procedures. Executive spokesmen manifest no personal shame in these instances, for it is in fact a requirement of their job. Peter Drucker is quoted as saying that a manager with a social conscience must be fired immediately. It is only when managers defraud *shareholders*, as in Enron, that they get sent to jail.

Traits of Psychopaths

In support of his sub-title, Bakan calls on a specialist in psychopathy to witness that the corporation's institutional character manifests most of the traits of human psychopaths. Fundamentally, that means a focus on the self to the exclusion of all others. Identifying symptoms include *irresponsibility* – they put others at risk in order to reach their own goal. They are *asocial* in *refusing to accept responsibility for their own actions* and are *unable to feel remorse*. Like human psychopaths they are *manipulative* and *grandiose* (we're the best), relating to others *superficially*, for "their whole goal is to present themselves to the public in a way that is appealing…. Human psychopaths are notorious for their ability to use charm as a mask to hide their dangerously self-obsessed personalities." Corporations present a façade of social responsibility, but it goes only so far as the consequences are good for the bottom line. This behaviour is an inevitable consequence of the corporation's institutional structure, which impels managements to seek ever more powers by telling ever more lies about the corporation's aspirations and performance. Even when they undertake "good works" for

public relations, a cost-benefit calculus is required. There must be a reasonably foreseeable pecuniary reward.

Government was not always so toothless against corporations as it appears today. The first corporations emerged in England in the late 16th century and by the early 18th had left a trail of scandals and corruption that climaxed in the South Sea Bubble. That event goaded Parliament into passing the *Bubble Act* of 1720, "which made it a criminal offense to create a company 'presuming to be a corporate body,' and to issue 'transferable stocks without legal authority.'" That prohibition lasted for more than a century. But the industrial revolution was coming on, and the new opportunities for application of non-animate power for transportation and urban infrastructure called for greater pools of financial capital than had hitherto been contemplated (outside of warfare). Railroad building was the activity that vaulted the corporation into the form and dominance it has manifested for the past 150 years. The critical step in that evolution was the granting of *limited liability*, which became entrenched in English corporate law in 1856 and in the various American states over the remainder of the nineteenth century. The process speeded up in the two decades at the turn of the 20th century as states began to compete for the corporate charter business by offering attractive privileges, such as no longer restricting the charter to a specific range of activities and permitting mergers. Those "reforms" sparked a mushrooming in the scope of corporate organizations and spawned a new industry in shares trading and acquisitions and the financing of these activities. Between 1898 and 1904, 1800 corporations were consolidated into 157, and "the US economy had been transformed from one in which individually owned enterprises competed freely among themselves into one dominated by a relatively few huge corporations, each owned by many shareholders. The era of corporate capitalism had begun." (And Karl Marx had already been dead for 20 years!)

An important consequence was that shareholders had lost control of the corporations they owned. "Unable to influence managerial decisions as individuals because their power was too diluted, they were also too broadly dispersed to act collectively." This created a problem for the law, for someone had to act and be held accountable if the corporation was to be able to buy, sell, own and engage in physical acts of creation and destruction. By various legal decisions over time, therefore, the corporation emerged as a legal "person." "By the end of the nineteenth century, through a bizarre legal alchemy…the corporate person had taken the place, at least in law, of the real people who owned corporations…. Gone was the centuries-old 'grant theory' which had conceived of corporations as instruments of government policy and as dependent upon government bodies to create them and enable them to function." Gone also the rationale for restrictions on corporate behaviour. "The logic was that, conceived as natural entities analogous to human beings, corporations should be created as free individuals… protected by…rights to 'due process of law' and 'equal protection of the laws.'"

With that kind of legislative and judicial backing, the corporation was off and running. It was nonetheless nagged by the "robber baron" image of ruthless monopoly capitalism, and for a long time manifested an attitude of being persecuted by unfriendly governments. Corporations undertook campaigns of public relations to develop an image of themselves as friendly and even benevolent. Excesses nevertheless came in for a considerable share of blame for the Great Depression, and the New Deal initiated an era of reforms that included not only more strenuous regulation but also macroeconomic management by government. The latter innovation was motivated by the conviction of Keynesians that laissez-faire had been given sufficient rope to prove that "equilibrium is blither" (*ER*, November 2003).

The Invisible Hawk has No Grip

In other words, "the market is a snare and a delusion," and the "invisible hand" has no grip. In the period of post-war prosperity that ensued, labour unions forced better wages and working conditions, and then there was the sixties wave of "new social legislation" – environmentalism, human rights, worker and consumer safety (Nader!), culminating in the LBJ campaign promise of a Great Society. That was the low point in the government-business relationship so far as the corporations were concerned, and they mounted a counter-offensive in 1972, setting up the Business Roundtable to co-ordinate a lobbying campaign.

Since then there has been a profound change in business-government relations. All major companies now have offices in DC. They won the right to finance elections under freedom of expression provisions of the US Constitution – an extension of the "person" metaphor. Corporations have subsequently effected a near-complete takeover of the electoral process (102-3). This is the end-point of a long struggle to gain freedom from democratic control. They have managed to cut funding to regulatory agencies, gutting enforcement mechanisms, and have succeeded in effecting repeal of several (especially environmental) regulations. "Corporate welfare bums" are frequently seen to threaten governments openly – "give us what we want or we'll take the relocation bonus you already gave us and leave, taking our jobs with us."

Consequently, it is no surprise to read that "the attitude that business is a victim is basically disappearing," and that "today corporations essentially feel that they're partners with government…not adversaries of government…(107). This is a dangerous notion," says Bakan, "for partnership implies equality. If corporations and governments are indeed partners we should be worried about the state of our democracy, for it means that government has effectively abdicated its sovereignty over the corporation" (108). Deregulation takes away the democratic right of "the people" to control corporate behaviour. The PR campaign against government seems to have persuaded citizens these days that they are unlikely to get effective help from that source, so prominent social activists (he cites Naomi Klein) aim their efforts directly at corporations (150). This is a flawed strategy because it concedes to corporations "all the coercive power and resources of the state, while citizens are left with non-governmental organizations and the market's invisible

hand – socialism for the rich and capitalism for the poor…." (151). Quoting Noam Chomsky: "Whatever one thinks of governments, they're to some extent publicly accountable…. Corporations are to a zero extent. …One of the reasons why propaganda tries to get you to hate government is because it's the one existing institution in which people can participate to some extent and constrain tyrannical unaccountable power" (152). The bottom line: "Without the state, the corporation is nothing. Literally nothing" (154).

Citizen action to reassert democratic sovereignty is inhibited by the success of a cultural campaign over many decades in the past century to demean and denigrate the utility of government action. The issue is summed up in a statement by Friedman to the author: "The big difference is whether you are really willing to accept the idea that civil servants are pursuing the interest of the community at large, rather than their own self-interest. That's the big divide. That's the divide between Galbraith and myself" (117).

Keith Wilde

1. This statement from John Kenneth Galbraith's *Innocent Fraud* was quoted in my review of the book (*ER*, August, 2004).
2. Reviewed by Gordon Coggins in *ER* this past spring.

Two Unsucculent Sandwiches

COULD A BENIGN GOD be writing out the message in letters of petroleum crude, so that we can no longer miss it?

The Wall Street Journal (6/08, "Russia Revokes Access to Bank Funds" by Guy Chazan) gives the background: "Moscow – "Russian authorities invoked a decision allowing OAO Yukos to use its bank accounts to pay day-to-day operating expenses, raising fresh fears its oil exports might be disrupted and help push oil prices to new highs.

"The government's about-face, which reversed a decision made just the day before, ended a fragile reprieve that would have eased pressure on Yukos as it struggles to pay a potentially crippling 99 billion ruble ($3.9 billion) back-tax bill for 2000. Yukos, Russia's biggest oil producer, warned two weeks ago that it would run out of cash by mid-August if the accounts remained frozen, forcing it to stop production.

"A Yukos spokesman said the company hadn't received official notification from the Justice Ministry and assumed the accounts were still unfrozen.

"The government flip-flop created jitters in a market already worried that world demand for oil may be overtaking production capacity. September crude-oil futures rose $1.58 to $44.44 a barrel on the New York Mercantile Exchange."

Those impossible Russians!

However, let's shift to other articles in the same issue of the *WSJ* to see how Russia's erratic handling of its oil politics has some disturbing parallels with the Western central banks' management of their benchmark interest rates ("Fed is Unlikely to Reverse Plans for Increasing Interest Rates" by Greg Ip). "Fed officials say that their main concern is that today's extremely low level of interest carries a high risk of fueling inflation years down the road, and that outweighs concerns about damping the expansion [of the economy] by gradually raising rates to a so-called neutral level between 3% and 5%.

"That perspective suggests the Fed is almost certain to raise its target for the federal funds rate, charged on overnight loans between banks to 1.5% from 1.25% on Tuesday. That also means that, barring a significant reversal in the economy, it likely will raise rates in September and at one or both of its meetings in November and December."

Then comes a suggestion of doubt.

"The decision may not seem straightforward. After all, economic growth slowed sharply to a 3% annual rate in the second quarter from 4.3% in the first. Terrorism fears and tight global capacity also have pushed oil prices above $44 a barrel, a record, which could crimp consumer spending and confidence. Higher petroleum prices already are eroding stock values. Indeed, some Fed officials have trimmed their projections for economic growth in the second half of the year."

And that, we feel, is the message that Somebody above the clouds has been trying to get across to Mr. Greenspan for some time now. That Somebody might reason "If that fellow presumes to act for Me, he should at least lend an ear to what I am trying to tell him."

For isn't the last quoted passage from the WSJ proving to us that using high oil prices exactly as the Fed for decades has used its benchmark interest rate, highlights the absurdity of raising interest rates for cranking up multiple disasters throughout the world?

Comparing the Benchmarks in Oil and Banking

Why, for example, be troubled about oil above $44 a barrel, "crimping consumer spending and confidence," or, "eroding stock values"? Wasn't that what Volcker's 14% rates for overnight loans achieved throughout the economy where it was translated into rates in the mid-20% range for most producers? Couldn't higher oil prices contribute to decreasing the number of SUVs on American, European, and now Chinese roads, and thus help the environment and keep our health bills down a bit?

"But softer growth and easing inflation aren't likely to convince the Fed that it can hold off tightening rates. Right now, Fed officials believe that keeping interest rates below the level of inflation – meaning that there is a negative 'real cost' cost of borrowing – invites higher inflation down the road even if there is not yet a sign of it in the data." Couldn't the same be said of oil prices over $44 a barrel? If that over-night rate of 1% doesn't cover the real cost of interest if you note the rate of inflation, what happens if you apply the same test to $44 a barrel oil? Allow for the movement of the Consumer Price Index since 1980, apply it to $44 crude and you come up with a far lower "real" price for oil than in 1980. Nevertheless democratically elected regimes were overthrown in Iran and in Venezuela and in other oil producing countries to *prevent* oil prices from catching up with the cost of living.

Moreover – the most important point – the $44 per barrel is the actual market price of oil today, while the 1.5 % benchmark rate is just a benchmark, that tells us very little about the actual market price of credit. Very little money gets loaned between banks at that benchmark rate. More and more of the credit created in our society is created by credit cards on which delinquent accounts pay as much as 26%. And a front-page article in the same issue of the *WSJ* ("New Group Swells Bankruptcy Court: the Middle-Aged" by Surin Hwang) informs us: "Many of today's bankrupt baby boomers simply weren't as frugal as their Depression parents. But the increase in middle-aged people filing for bankruptcy is also attributed to soaring medical costs, an unstable job market, *and years of aggressive credit-card marketing.*" [Emphasis ours.]

"Increased family obligations play a role too. The so-called sandwich generation often bears financial responsibility for both their children and their parents, because people are living longer, middle-aged Americans are now eight times as likely to have a living parent as previous generations. And since many parents waited to have children later in life, tuition bills come later as well.

"Ben B. Floyd, a personal bankruptcy trustee for the past 30 years, says he is now seeing people 'who obviously had a white-collar background. They come in looking lost.' 'They didn't take their credit cards to Atlantic City,' says Gabriel Del Virginia, a New York bankruptcy attorney. 'It's largely because people lost their jobs or had a catastrophic illness.'

"Until last year, Charlene Freeman, a 48-year old in the Boston area, worked at home doing technical writing on a contract basis. As the family's primary earner, she was earning $150,000 a year. She had a perfect credit record and a spacious home with a pool. Her husband is an independent computer technician.

"Then her long-controled kidney disease turned into kidney failure, halting her income while her medical costs mounted. Although she paid $725 a month to insure herself, her husband and child, Ms. Freedman wasn't insured for the numerous drugs prescribed to her. Although Ms. Freeman has disability insurance, it wouldn't insure anything related to kidney problems because it was a pre-existing condition. To pay the bills while she battled her illness, Ms. Freeman drained the couple's retirement savings, her home-equity line, and tapped her son's savings accounts. She used 10 credit cards. What she didn't realize was that her husband was using checks sent to them by credit-card companies. These checks, sent unsolicited, have no grace period: interest begins to accumulate on them as soon as they hit the cardholder's account. Before long the couple had accumulated $115,000 in debt. She plans to file for bankruptcy in the fall.

"In recent years the credit-card industry has grown increasingly aggressive in raising interest rates for certain consumers. Interest rates can go up when a person's payments are late, or when their debt passes a specific limit. Six months ago, Ms. Freeman realized that Bank of America had raised her interest rate on its card, citing the total debt her family owed. Other credit card issuers soon followed suit. Today 9 of her 10 cards are charging her 25.9% instead of the 11% she previously paid."

So much for Mr. Greenspan's 1.5% benchmark rate. The

point is that the entire economy depends on this ultimate usury since the financial sector has taken over control. From China to South Korea to the US and Europe everything depends on credit card usury, to keep the compulsion of the exponentially-driven expansion of the economy seemingly on track.

In our economy there are benchmarks and benchmarks – on central bank over-night inter-bank rates set by the central bank and there is the real credit rate upon which the system depends. Oil prices are similarly judged by a benchmark price that officially is considered not only fair but inevitable. It is the distribution of power that determines the gap between Mr. Greenspan's 1.5% benchmark and the real interest rates that the empowered depend on for their survival. The contrast between the gap in oil prices between benchmark and reality in interest rates and the zero gap between benchmark and real oil prices has to do with the contrasted power distribution in these two fields. On two occasions that changed the course of history, Washington overthrew democratically elected governments – in Venezuela and Iran – for their part in organizing the original OPEC to bring oil prices in better line with oil costs. On the other hand economic policy and even the economic theory taught in our universities around the same time came to be twisted to attribute the high interest rates and the restrictions on public spending to the free and independent market that must not be interfered with.

The late French economist François Perroux formulated a theory of the "dominant revenue" that shows how in every particular social form the revenue of a particular group becomes identified with the welfare of society. Even the memory of Perroux and his theory have vanished since his death in the latter 1980s, but history has fleshed out his theory in the bloody chasm that has opened between much of Islam – whose faith condemns all interest-taking, not just usury. Clearly, it is the crucial gap between the respective benchmarks and the realities that they are supposed to govern that must be considered in appraising events in Iraq, Afghanistan and the world economy. Incredibly as it may seem to Washington, the retrieval of production costs of oil – a wasting resource – is quite as important to oil producers as having enough oil to slake the thirst of the SUVs on our roads.

William Krehm

An Open Letter to the Minister of Finance

August 16, 2004

The Honourable Ralph Goodale
Minister of Finance
Government of Canada

Dear Mr. Minister:

Regarding your letter of June 11th to Richard Priestman, who had written to the Honourable John Gerretsen, Minister of Municipal Affairs and Housing for the Province of Ontario,

suggesting that the Government use the Bank of Canada to finance a substantial amount of public capital expenditures of all three levels of government, which is still provided for in the *Bank of Canada Act* (18c,h).

When this is done, as it was under the Federal governments right into the 1970s, the interest paid on the government debt ends up substantially with the federal government in the form of dividends. For though the Bank of Canada was founded in 1935 as a bank owned by private shareholders, in 1938 a Liberal government fulfilled its election promise to nationalize the Bank. That more than anything else made it possible not only to finance the Second World War at minimal interest charges, but to catch up with a decade of neglect and six years of war in renewing our infrastructures and assimilating a vast, mostly penniless immigration.

Canada's shame today is that our federal government claims that we cannot afford to maintain the infrastructure that the proper use of the Bank of Canada made possible to create under the most difficult conditions. On top of that, by making proper use of the central bank, Canada was able to reduce the ratio of our federal debt to our annual gross domestic product from the record 170% in 1946 to less than 20% in 1973. Those figures were obtained from the Bank of Canada Review. (Though they deal only with the funded debt, since the ratio of funded debt to GDP was being rapidly brought down, those figures probably understate the achievement if we included the unfunded federal debt).

You write, "The Bank holds a portion of the Government of Canada's debt on its balance sheet as assets to offset its liabilities of currency in circulation. If the Bank were to finance expenditures of Canadian governments, it would hold the governments' debt as assets on its balance sheet, resulting in a significant increase in its liabilities and hence in the money supply. The expansion of the money supply would be inflationary. The resulting inflation would ultimately hurt the economy, increase interest rates and reduce the standard of living of Canadians."

This is a tangle of distortion. First of all, Mr. Minister, since double-entry bookkeeping came in some seven centuries ago, every liability incurred by anyone including our government should have an asset to balance it. Only in the event of scandals of one sort or another is this not so. However, the assets acquired fall into categories – some are for current needs, others are for long-term investment. In proposing to use the Bank of Canada as it was used for almost four decades of its existence, we are talking entirely of capital investments, not of current expenditures – of bridges, roads, hospitals, schools, and health, not of paper clips and floor-wax.

Canada Year Book as Witness

A nationalized central bank could provide near interest-free loans to the federal government, which would hardly be inflationary since the unemployed labour forces and the physical means are abundantly idle. It is a matter of mobilizing such wasting resources for social benefit. But to bring that to pass requires that the credit of the central government – which today is the only legal tender, i.e., the only Canadian money in existence – be available at affordable rates for essential capital purposes. This would cover the services that have been systematically loaded down from the federal government to the provinces without the funds to pay for them. The provinces in turn have passed them to the municipalities on the same impossible terms, and the municipalities have been left holding the bag.

Let me refer you to a description of the facilities still in the *Bank of Canada Act* today, but are rarely if ever mentioned in public. Accordingly, I will cite them from the Canada Year Book of 1973 (page773), along with the explanation of their purpose given in the same source.

"The provisions of the *Bank of Canada Act* enable the Central Bank to determine the total amount of cash reserves available to the chartered banks as a group and in that way to control the rate of expansion of the total assets and deposit liabilities of the banking system as a whole. The *Bank Act* which regulates the operation of the chartered banks, requires that each chartered bank maintain a stipulated minimum average amount of cash reserves, calculated as a percentage of its Canadian dollar deposit liabilities, in the form of deposits at the Bank of Canada and holdings of Bank of Canada notes. The minimum cash reserve requirement, which came into effect under the legislation beginning February 1 1968, is 12% of demand deposits and 4% of other deposits. The ability of the chartered banks as a group to expand their total assets and deposit liabilities is therefore limited by the total amount of cash reserves available. An increase in cash reserves will encourage the banks as a group to expand their total assets (which consists chiefly of loans and marketable securities) with a concomitant increase in their deposit liabilities; a decrease in cash reserves of the chartered banks will bring about a decline in their total assets and deposit liabilities as they seek to restore their cash reserve ratios.

"The chief method by which the Bank of Canada alters the level of cash reserves of the chartered banks over time, and through them the total of chartered bank deposits, is by purchase and sale of government securities. Payment by the central bank for the securities it purchases in the market adds to the cash reserves of the chartered banks as a group and puts them in a position to expand their assets and deposit liabilities. Conversely, payment to the central bank for securities it sells causes a reduction in the cash reserves of the central banks and requires them to reduce their holdings of assets and deposit liabilities.

"The influence the Bank of Canada exerts on credit conditions (i.e., on interest cost and other terms of borrowing in financial markets) stems from its ability to limit the growth of bank credit and of the community's holding of bank deposits and currency." In short, at the time this and similar passages in later Canada Year Books were published (right into the latter 1980s), it was not only the Bank's benchmark interest rate that was used as 'the one blunt tool' to enforce a supposedly self-balancing market, but the ability of the central bank to expand or curtail the power of chartered banks to create further credit. Indeed, official dogma is that banks do not create credit as a multiple of the base-legal tender, i.e., federal debt, they hold, but rather merely act as intermediaries of what they themselves borrow from the market.

What Happened to Zero Inflation?

You write: "That is why the Bank of Canada and the Government of Canada agreed in 1991 to adopt an inflation-targeting regime. The target range was reduced to between 1 and 3 percent and was extended several times..." That is being less than frank; the goal dictated by the Bank for International settlements was "Zero inflation," and the attempt was made by the Mulroney government to put that in the constitution. Only the refusal of the finance committee caucuses of all three major parties stopped that.

The Bank of Canada under Governor John Crow was preaching the nonsense that if the slightest amount of price rise were tolerated, it would end up as the sort of hyperinflation that hit Germany in 1923. But Germany had lost a war, and the French army occupied its industrial Ruhr heartland to exact reparations for that war in strong currency that Germany did not have. What ensued was a general strike and virtual civil war. To suggest any similarity between that hyperinflation and the slight amount of price rise in the 1990's was charlatanry. What was targeted in 1991 was not a goal based on any serious economic theory, but the interest of the speculative finance capital that had gambled and lost big in the 1980s in gas and oil, in real estate like London's Canary Wharf, and builder Robert Campeau's sudden passion for collecting merchandising *chains* in the US.

In 1991, with neither debate nor even explanation in parliament or the media, the government began phasing out the statutory reserves that were described in the 1973 Canada Year Book and as the very essence of controlling inflation or deflation as the need may arise by encouraging or discouraging the chartered banks to create more or less credit without shooting down anything that moves in the economy. Toward the end of 1990 the Bank's benchmark interest rate rose to 14.5%, which means that businesses were paying rates in the mid-twenty percent rage.

In addition to helping to bail out overstretched banks throughout the Western world by the phasing out of the statutory reserves, the Bank for International Settlements' *Risk-Based Capital Requirements* had already declared the debt of the developed (OECD) countries to be risk-free, requiring no additional capital to acquire. Between these two measures, Canada's overstretched chartered banks were able to take on another 60 billion dollars worth of federal debt without putting up any money of their own. And that was not just capital that they were relieved of having to put up, but *cash*. Banks raise their capital as cash, but leave no more of it in that form than is strictly necessary because cash is lazy, sterile money that earns no return.

A return to the use of the Bank of Canada for municipal and provincial financing, with an arrangement for the provinces and municipalities to get some of the interest that would end up with the federal government, could serve to get agreement on the adoption of federal standards and head off the eternal bickering between Ottawa and the provinces.

William Krehm
Committee on Monetary and Economic Reform

PART 2 OF A REVIEW OF A BOOK BY F. HUTCHINSON, M. MELLOW AND W. OLSEN, LONDON & STERLING, VIRGINIA: PLUTO PRESS, 2002

"The Politics of Money: Towards Sustainability and Economic Democracy"

"THE IMPORTANCE of the enclosure of land as private property is that many of the resources communities held would have been in the form of common land. Common resources are those which have no deeds of ownership but are regularly used for farming or harnessing subsistence. Under these conditions most people would have gathered, hunted, gardened and herded, growing and preparing their own food. The emergence of capitalist market society together with industrial patterns of resource use including agricultural production has broken down the direct relationship between people and the source of their subsistence for at least two-third of the world's population. Self-provisioning has been replaced by waged labour contractually engaged 'through a network of society-embracing markets.' It was this compulsion into waged labour, ironically described as 'free,' which Marx argued made capitalism a unique form of exploitation.

According to John Locke (1632-1704), although God gave the land to be held in common, it was the duty of individuals to improve [it] with their own labour. Where the land is made more valuable and profitable, common possession must give way to private property. According to this theory, land has value in itself. Hence when an individual encloses waste or common land, and labours to improve it, they add to, rather than take away from communal welfare.

"Such improvements enabled the individual household or firm to produce commodities for sale for money in distant markets. In the process it created the illusion that unsustainable practices could be escalated indefinitely.

"The process of absorbing the commons into the market system continues apace today. Forest people in particular are struggling for the retention of the commons of tropical rain forests from Sarawak to the Amazon. Across the globe indigenous peoples are launching anti-globalization campaigns.

"Equally, the state can guarantee the rights of the international, global capitalist elite class to plunder the social and ecological commons, placing the short-term profit of powerful individuals and corporations before the common good. In the eyes of many people organizations like the World Bank, IMF and WTO are just that, agents of property regimes that seek to transfer all resources into capitalist corporate regimes.

"Capitalism is the enclosure not only of land but also of tools and knowledge for the purpose of private financial gain. As Veblen has argued, all invention is based on the common cultural inheritance built up over countless generations. Although the fencing of land is commonly portrayed as a means of introducing more 'efficient' farming methods, it entailed far more than mere fencing. Loss of subsistence access through enclosure, exclusion or patenting leads to a loss of social inheritance and knowledge.

"Intellectual property has now become an important aspect of world trade. The patenting of seed in particular is causing a loss of species as well as denying poorer people access to their traditional plants. Often this is because the seed has been hybridized and patented. What this might mean in the longer run is that hardy species developed over millennia to resist salination, drought or low temperatures, or forage animals that can live in difficult terrain, will be lost forever."

Enclosing Intellectual Property

"To live people must do paid work or find a source of money income. The entire edifice of economic theorizing has been built upon the false premise that *things* exchange for *things* and not for *money*. That was why Marx was so outraged at the argument put forward by Jean Baptiste Say that in every sale there is a purchase, and in every purchase a sale, exactly as in barter. Marx is quite clear that money, not commodities, is the focus of the market economy.

"Only if money is eliminated is it possible to regard 'capital' as the *commodities* or 'things' comprising a necessary element in the productive process: hence the common misapprehension that ownership of the *physical* rather than the *financial* means of production is the key issue in the control and production of wealth. It is also possible to be drawn into the debate on booms, slumps, inflation, stagflation, unemployment and the general tendency for a falling rate of profit without challenging the conceptualization of a formal economy which is assumed to be providing for universal welfare through the production of *things*.

"According to Freeman and his colleagues the study of economics which ignores the central role of money in the economy has also invaded Marxist economics. Economics must be situated in real time and the real world."

Striving Towards Exponential Growth

That is far truer than Alan Freeman seems to realize. Not only have money prices and money profits replaced the prime role of commodities in the economy, but the rate of growth of the profit already obtained by public corporations in a single year, is by grace of an alleged knowledge extrapolated into the remote future and then discounted for present value and incorporated into present price. The knowledge of such items is supposed available from equilibrium points located with "derivatives." The result: market prices of successfully promoted stocks strive towards the exponential curve which is the mathematics of the atom bomb.

Man shapes his theories under the influence of his technology. Marx's view of the society's future, was obviously inspired by the railway-building age in which it was conceived: its course was plotted via foreseeable stations to the socialist terminal. This is what Veblen identified as Marx's "teleological" aspect (Hutchinson et al., p.106). With our contemporary economists, the major influence is the split atom. It is the model not only for the stock market but for the entire economy.[1]

Veblen laid a finger on the vulnerable "romantic" side of Marxism ("a sequence of theory"). "Capitalism relies on two basic mechanisms of cultural conditioning. First, the conditioning of 'chronic dissatisfaction' associated with emulative consumption (consumerism) – the 'spiritual' poverty of labouring for a money wage, going into debt to acquire and consume more objects offering the illusion of leisure and status. He enriched the language and sociology with the term 'conspicuous consumption' that increasingly drives our world. Second, patriotism and military discipline to maintain its aggressive imperialist expansion."

This might well have been written not in 1899, but the day before yesterday.

"Veblen provides a neat example of the 'double-think' of neo-classical economics when the factors of production are described in purely material terms. [He cites] John Bates Clark, an early American marginalist, dismissing the notion of capital as financial (money) value. In his view, it would be more accurate to regard capital as 'a fund of productive goods.' However, Veblen refers to Clark's own contradictory example of the transfer of capital from a whaling ship to a cotton mill. Plainly, 'capital *goods* are not purchase and sale.' Finance capital intervenese to change the nature of exchange' (Hutchinson, p. 113). Capitalism upsets all concepts of 'natural' returns to the factors of production."

Veblen emphasized the rigidities into which the concept of "class" led Marxists. "The complexities of class within capitalized money/market systems has been somewhat obscured by Marxist thinking that narrows the emphasis to capital-labour relations. This not only ignores the problems of unpaid work but cannot make connection with the position of debt-based, small-scale property ownership such as the peasant landholder. Veblen questioned Marx's prediction that agribusiness would absorb the small proprietor, converting them to landless labour. As early as 1906 Veblen suggested that socialists and small peasant farmers should have common cause in resisting finance capitalism. However, Veblen was a voice in the wilderness. Henceforth, the small farmer, classed as 'bourgeois' by 'socialists' sought to oppose the hated financial capitalism by adopting an ideology on the far right."

Broadening the Marxian Class Concept

More recently, under the impact of other cultures, this has begun changing with leftist politicians lending a sympathetic ear to land claims of indigenous peoples. In India Marxists are recognizing the links between the rural bourgeoisie with urban industrialists, that is influenced by the caste system. The authors of the book under review bring to centre-stage the exploitation that occurs within families where the women's unpaid labour is not recognized. "Social class is now just part of the set of resource factors and interrelated subjectivities such as gender and ethnicity that go into shaping social relations."

Obviously, the Social Credit people, no less than other reformers, will have to invest further effort in grasping how society is to move to the solution of the seemingly impossible problems that beset the world today. In an earlier issue of *ER*

(May 2004) we paid tribute to an earlier volume co-authored by Ms. Hutchinson in disclosing to us what had previously eluded us – what Douglas was saying with his A and B theorem. It was not capital budgeting, for capital budgeting which recognized the capital investment in equipment, buildings and much else that would come back to the producer only over a long period. During that time capital debt would have to be financed.

That was the entry through which exploitative financial capital took over. It had therefore to be bridged with a social dividend that could be justified by the heritage of all in previous generations who contributed in various ways to make possible the institutions, science, technology and social cohesion that made production possible in our day – slaves, martyrs, inventors, civic leaders, jurists. That social dividend would help make it possible to carry on production without being at the mercy of finance capital. Producers' banks would make its contribution to this end. That, however, does not mean that in addition to Douglas's A and B accountancy, we have no need of standard accrual accountancy (i.e., capital budgeting) that would keep us informed of when the total investment is to return and with what profits.

These two distinct gauges of the efficiency of a firm – or the economy as a whole – correspond to twin complementary concepts. One is liquidity that the Douglas A & B theorem addresses; and solvency which has to do with the existence of enough assets, liquid or otherwise, to cover the institution's debt.

One of the goals of the A & B Theorem is to avoid the need for external financing of the productive process. To close this monetary gap while production is being completed and the income from the sale has come in, Douglas depended upon the Social Dividend. This would help the producers organize their own financing.

Rethinking the "Inflation" Concept

There is another important detail that our Social Credit friends should look into. In recent election campaigns on all continents we have witnessed a fixation on balancing the national budget. That of course, conflicts with what we learned in the 1930s at a shattering cost. But so long as our central banks insist on identifying any rise of price indexes with inflation, we risk repeating that experience. Since World War II, the market economy has become a pluralistic one, in which more and more human and physical infrastructures are needed to serve ever more complicated technologies and intense urbanization. And these only the state can provide. The resulting taxation, however, inevitably becomes a deepening layer of price. Thirty-five years ago I identified this as "the social lien." This must be distinguished from inflation that properly refers to price rise resulting from an excess of demand over supply. Economics historians (notably the late Ferdinand Braudel) grasped the point. Economists have remained blind to it. Recognizing it would undermine the vested interests served by the self-balancing market construct, that dispatches all social and environmental concerns as "externalities." Economic policy has become increasingly identified with balancing the national budget that is increasingly in deficit because of governments' insistence on treating public investment as current spending.

Unless serious accountancy is introduced into our price theory, there will be no possibility of bringing in anything resembling the "social dividend."

William Krehm

1. The exponential function will repay a little attention. It is constructed to the specification that the rate of growth equals the value already attained by the function itself. That implies, of course, that the same is the case with the higher derivatives to infinity.

The formula is:

$$1 + x + \frac{x^2}{2 \times 1} + \frac{x^3}{3 \times 2 \times 1} \cdots$$

Differentiating the function for the rate of growth: 1 being a constant doesn't grow and hence becomes zero and x grows as the variable itself becomes 1 to replace the vanished first term on the left. The denominator of the next term is chosen so that its first derivative becomes x to replace the previous second term, and so on to infinity. Being an infinite series it doesn't matter that the first term disappears and the expression shifts to the right. There are an infinite number of terms available on the right to absorb the losses on the left. As they occur you pass on to the next higher derivative. In graph form this is a curve that starts almost horizontal but in no time at all stands vertical.

Our Tottering Fiscal Prudence

PICK THE MOST NONSENSICAL of nursery rhymes that starts a youngster chortling, take it as a key for understanding our world and you will still come closer than what passes for economic analysis these days.

Take the column "Until Debts Do Us Part" by John Ibbitson, in *The Globe and Mail* (14/07): "Congratulations to Alberta on retiring its debt. The rest of us should be so lucky. Debt inhibits a government's ability to stimulate the economy through investments or lower taxes, and siphons dollars that would otherwise be available for capital investment. All provinces suffer from the effects of one province's debt.

"Generally speaking, federal, provincial and municipal governments have been acting responsibly over the past decade to reduce the national debt which has fallen from the equivalent of 100% of the nation's GDP to about 80%."

The reference is clearly to the total of the federal, provincial, and municipal debt.

And the moon is a hunk of green cheese, and we must cut and package it and float an international cheese corporation to replace bankrupt Parmalat. For the only legal tender in the land *is* federal debt. Hence the only way our governments could meet Mr. Ibbitson's approval is for the federal government to issue more of its debt which is the only money of the nation. If our federal government repaid a major part of its debt, the provinces would be running up more debt, because there would be less money around, and greater need for provincial and municipal social programs. And the only way Ottawa could

pay off a big chunk of debt would be by slashing the tax base of the provinces, the municipalities and its own, As a result there would be an increased need for social programs.

The provinces and the municipalities and the private sector in a sense are seated on opposite sides of the great debt teeter-totter. The more Ottawa cuts its spending, the more the provinces must borrow. The more Ottawa borrows – providing that it uses the Bank of Canada for its borrowing so that the interest paid on those loans will come back to it substantially as dividends of the central bank. For the federal government since 1938 has been the sole shareholder of the Bank of Canada and with a reviving economy, the less the provinces and the municipalities would have to borrow.... There would also have to be enough unemployed, qualified workmen for the projects it finances with such loans, and enough materials within the country so that it does not have to borrow abroad. But unemployed and unsold goods we have in excellent supply. And above all the federal government's loans would not be wasted on paying interest to private banks, for borrowing that is available to it virtually interest-free from its own central bank.

It is shocking that so elementary a fact about money today has been made inaccessible to the media, parliament, and to our university students.

You can bring down this house of marked cards by asking politicians a simple question: "Since gold and silver – even in theory – have been demonetized, i.e., stripped of their role as legal tender, what would you have the federal government pay down its debt with? Federal debt bills of a different colour than those being retired? Or computer entries in a different shade of ink?"

And you could inform them of this suppressed cut of our history. In 1946, after 10 years of crippling depression and six of war, during which little was built or produced not for destruction, the ratio of federal debt to the GNP was 170%. Over the following 26 years, the country caught up with the neglect of the preceding 16 years, financing the introduction of new technologies, assimilated an unprecedented refugee influx to unheard of standards. Yet despite all this, by 1972 the above debt to GNP ration was reduced from 170% to under 20%. How was this done? By increasing the use of the Bank of Canada for holding federal debt equal to the mid-20 percentages. Today it hovers just over 5%.

In 1991 in the deepest stealth, to bail out our chartered banks from their gambles in the 1980s, they were bailed out, by an amendment of the *Bank Act* that did away with the statutory reserves of the need to redeposit with the Bank of Canada a portion of the deposits taken in by them from the public in their chequing accounts. These reserves earned them no interest, and thus made it possible for the government to borrow more credit from its own bank within the constraints established. The abolition of these reserves allowed the banks to increase their holdings of government debt by $60 billion without putting up a penny of their own money. (The Bank for International Settlements – a purely technical international agency that allowed no elected official of a government to attend its sessions – to help rescue banks in crisis throughout the world had already declared the debt of developed countries to be "risk-free" requiring no further capital for banks to acquire.) And that is where the nursery-rhyme nonsense comes in. The statutory reserves that were abolished by Ottawa had served as one of two tools for dealing with perceived inflation. In their haste to bail out the banks both Ottawa and the BIS overlooked that the end of the statutory reserves made the debt of any country anything but risk-free. Because whenever the central bank raises interest rates – its self-described "sole blunt tool to fight inflation" – those preexisting bond hoards of the banks would drop in market price. That oversight COMER picked up at once and warned the government about it. Reduplicated by every central bank in the Western world, it was the main cause of the international monetary crisis that began in Mexico and swept east Asia and passed on to Russia. It required Washington, the IMF and Canada to put up a standby fund of $51 billion to prevent a complete collapse of the world monetary system.

Deregulating Our Bailed-out Banks

But the scandal did not stop there. Having bailed out our banks in 1991, Ottawa proceeded to deregulate them to allow them to acquire stock brokerages, stock market underwriting establishments, and enter the credit card business in a big way. As a result three of our largest six banks featured along with the US biggest in some of the largest scams connected with Enron corporation. We learned of that involvement from the US government investigations, with settlements paid by our banks of as much as $80 million US.

All this is highly relevant, because the national elections both in the US and Canada were run largely on the basis of which of the major parties promised more loudly to balance the budget. Instead of useful economic theory that might help us understand society's needs, our government sets policy with nothing but a piggy-bank with a hole in its bottom.

These are details that we should have heard about in the recent election campaign. Hopefully we will in the next one. Without adequate information democracy risks becoming a nonsense rhyme.

William Krehm

Guantanamoing the Law Books

THE UNITED STATES did not join the Kyoto Treaty for the protection of the environment. That the world knows. What it doesn't know is that the Bush government has given similar treatment to legislation protective of the environment already on the books. That inconsistency perpetuates the pattern of the vote-counting in Florida that gave Bush the presidency despite the ballots cast. *The New York Times Magazine* (04/04/04, "Up in Smoke – The Bush Administration, the big power companies and the undoing of 30 years of clean-air policy" by Bruce Barcoli) tells a grisly tale.

"President Bush doesn't talk about new-source review (NSR) very often. Only once has he mentioned it in public, on Sept. 15, 2003, to a cheering crowd of power-plant workers and executives in Monroe, Mich., one of the nation's top polluters. Its coal-fired generators emit more mercury, a toxic chemical, than any other power plant in the state. Until recently, power plants like the one in Monroe operated by Detroit Edison were governed by NSR regulation, which required the plant's owners to install new pollution-control devices if they made any significant improvements to the plant. These regulations now exist in name only; they were effectively eliminated by a series of rule changes that the Bush administration made out of the public eye in 2002 and 2003. What the President was celebrating in Monroe was the effective end of new-source review.

"'The old regulations,' he said speaking in front of a huge American flag, 'undermined our goals for protecting the environment and growing the economy,' New-source review just didn't work, he said, It dissuaded power companies from updating old equipment. 'Now we've issued new rules that will allow utility companies to make routine upgrades without enormous costs and endless disputes. We trust the people in this plant to make the right decisions.'

"Of the many environmental changes brought about by the Bush White House, none illustrates the administration's modus operandi better than the overhaul of the New-Source Review. The president has had little success in the past three years at getting his environmental agenda through Congress. His energy bill remains unpassed. His Clear Skies package of clean-air laws is collecting dust on a committee shelf. The Arctic Wildlife Refuge remains closed to oil and gas exploration. Overturning new-source review represents the most sweeping change, and among the least noticed.

"The administration's real problem with NSR wasn't that it didn't work. The problem was that it was about to work too well – as it was designed to when it was passed by Congress more than 25 years ago."

A Costly Day of Reckoning

"Having long flouted the New-Source Review law, many of the nation's biggest power companies were facing in the last months of the 1990s, an expensive day of reckoning. The power companies were on the verge of signing agreements to clean up their plants. That would have delivered one of the greatest advances in clear air in the nation's history. Then George W. Bush took office, and everything changed.

"The *Clean Air Act*, adopted by Congress and signed by President Nixon in 1970 required polluters to clean up their operations. The law forced power plants and large factories to minimize their emissions of harmful pollutants, and it established national air-quality standards to be met by 1975. Seven years passed, and the national standards went unmet. Instead of building new, cleaner plants, many companies simply patched up and upgraded their old, dirty ones. So Congress updated the act in 1977, introducing a regulation called New-Source Review to bring older plants into compliance. A company could operate an old factory as long as it wasn't substantially modified. It was a way to let companies phase in cleaner factories over a number of years instead of all at once. During the 80s and 90s some power companies did replace coal plants with cleaner ones burning natural gas. But many other retooled plants to keep them running long past their expected life spans, and few were fitted with the scrubbers and other equipment required by NSR.

"The electric industry complained that NSR rules were so complicated that it was impossible for utilities to determine the difference between 'routine; maintenance, which wouldn't require an upgrade, and a significant 'physical change' that would. An examination of documents made public as a result of lawsuits, however, makes it difficult to credit these complaints. Beginning soon after NSR was implemented, the Environment Protection Agency (EPA) officials issued frequent letters and bulletins telling power companies exactly where the agency was drawing the line. Coal-fired power plants didn't move to the top of the agency's list until late 1996 when Bruce Buckheit, a former Justice Department lawyer who had recently joined the EPA as director of its air-enforcement division, noticed an article in *The Washington Post* about proposed changes to the ownership rules governing the power industry. 'The story predicted that deregulation would increase the use of coal-fired power generation in the Midwest. 'So we thought,' Buckheit recalled, 'If they're going to have all that expansion, they're going to have to pay attention to NSR rules.'

"Industry records indicated that many power plants had upgraded their facilities to burn more coal, which required new-source review permits, but [when] we started looking around for the permits, they weren't there." A lot of companies thought they could evade the law.

"At the same time a growing body of medical research indicated that industrial air pollution was making a lot of people sick. Power plants pump dozens of chemicals into the air; among the most harmful are nitrogen oxides, sulfur dioxide and mercury. Mercury, a highly toxic chemical emitted as a vapor when coal is burned, has been found to cause brain disorders in developing fetuses and young children, and unhealthy levels of it have been found recently in swordfish and tuna."

The Environmental Equivalent of Tobacco Litigation

"After two years of investigation, EPA had accumulated a daunting amount of evidence of wrongdoing by the coal-burning power industry. It was the environmental equivalent of the tobacco litigation. Former ERP officials noted that the agency might have enough legal leverage to force the industry to install up-to-date pollution controls.

"Attorney General Janet Reno announced the suits herself. 'When children can't breathe because of pollution from a utility plant hundreds of miles away,' she said, 'something has to be done.' The utility industry immediately turned to the Republican-controled Congress for relief from the lawsuits. But representative C.W. Bill Young, a Tampa-area Republican, unexpectedly turned a deaf ear to the overtures of his local utility, Tampa Electric.

"Faced with Congressional rejection and mounting fines – $27,500 per plant for each day a utility was in violation, some utilities struck bargains with the federal government. But others started writing checks to George W. Bush's presidential campaign fund."

The vote recount technique was broadly applied to the clean-up of pollution, and many other areas. It proved a pattern for holding at bay laws that were unwelcome to Bush's mega-campaign contributors. The decisions of such matters were simply moved beyond US legal jurisdiction.

"The coal-industry trade magazine Coal Age exulted in the industry's 'high-level access to policymakers in the new administration.'

"One key element of the strategy was putting the right people in under-the-radar positions – officials who came directly from industry to these lower rungs of power – deputy secretaries and assistant administrators. These appointees knew exactly which rules and regulations to change because they had been trying to change them on behalf of their industries for years.

"In January, 2002, the White House suffered a setback. The Justice Department delivered its report on the legality of the EPA's lawsuit against the Southern Company and other NSR violators. The department found that all of the lawsuits were legal and warranted.

"Shortly thereafter, White House officials decided it was time to try the Congressional track. On Feb. 14, 2002, President Bush unveiled his Clear Skies Initiative. The president declared that his proposed legislation 'sets tough new standards to dramatically reduce the three most significant forms of pollution from power plants – sulfur dioxide, nitrogen oxides and mercury.'

"Many Republicans and some moderate Democrats embrace the general concept of cap-and-trade, in which Washington sets pollution standards for the entire country, and then allowed companies that manage to reduce their emissions below the standard to sell their extra pollution 'allowance' to companies that haven't met the standard."

The oddity is that experts who worship marginal utility value theory as a biblical revelation, fly in the teeth of it when it suits their clients. An industry the reduces pollution beyond the national requirement trades that "extra" item at par for the same physical amount of pollution in an area where the cleansing is in short supply. If we translate the operation into the number of victims arising from such a deal, they are bound to increase since the lethal effect of pollution will increase with its intensity. Obviously anything goes when the self-interest of the empowered is concerned.

William Krehm

Reflections with a Sigh

AGE HAS ITS DISADVANTAGES: notably dimming vision, and the embarrassing elusiveness of familiar names. However, I suppose the vices of a lifetime do offer occasional consolation.... A stubborn curiosity about mathematics certainly has made such a contribution. It provided insight into the trained disability of distinguished economists to examine problems from new, revealing angles. Conventional economists too often miss important relationships by leaving it all to a "self-balancing market" that never existed and hence cannot

not be subjected to the Popper test of proving its *negative* version incorrect. Instead they simply declare the growing part of the economy outside that market – the environment, the family, the public sector – "externalities." The problems that this creates are then entrusted to "sufficient growth" that end up actually accentuating them. You will understand what I am saying if you consult the files under I for Iraq, and O for Oil. Because of the resulting dependence on growth, too often neither corporations nor the government even respect the elementary rules of accountancy. That leaves no standing room for the most elementary morality.

How Different the Record of Keynes

Note the contrary record of Keynes in this respect. Bred in the equilibrium school of economics – his father was an economics professor at Cambridge – a few years before the Depression he dismissed Marx as "unscientific." A decade later, however, he ate crow in an honest gesture that few of his colleagues have matched. He paid his tribute to Marx – whom he knew only through the intermediation of his brightest students like Joan Robinson and Sraffa – and acknowledged borrowing from him and from Major Douglas and Silvio Gesell, the elements for working out what came to be known as Keynesianism. That is what our government and orthodox economists are burying so deeply for their grave to qualify as upside-down skyscrapers in the ground. In doing so they are gambling away humanity's most precious talent: that it not only learns from its successes but from its defeats. Deprive it of that, and you debase human kind and make it a candidate for joining those species that geologists track down in primeval rock.

Nothing personal about being sent to Coventry by the right guys. It is not confined to COMER. Take the case of a distinguished economist at NorthWestern University much quoted in his day, Robert Eisner. Amongst much else, he did a careful study of the deficits of a celebrated alleged balancer of unbalanceable budgets, name of Ronald Reagan. In his attempt to "lick inflation," by slashing social services to fight inflation, and cutting taxes, Reagan actually stepped up the rate of inflation. Eisner did detailed statistical studies of how that inflation – when it got beyond a certain level – so reduced the real value of the national and private debt, that it actually revived the economy. That of course was related to the recent discovery of "good inflation," the first 2 to 3% that the Fed and the Bank for International Settlements fleetingly rediscovered, and apparently are in the process of being forgotten again.

Then the thought occurred to me: these scholars who believe in a self-balancing market that never existed are so locked in their faith that perhaps by sheer chance coincides with the interest of our financial institutions. Could they have simply and honestly just lost the ability of recognizing isolated self-balancing traits of the market price system even where they do exist?

And from the vantage point of ripe old age, certain perspectives are given us – for example, an increased interest in history, which is the memory of human kind seen through the warp of time. Orthodox economists who cannot even manage to remember what they swore by and were prepared to wreck the economy for, have no use for history. Nobody can mistake it for a self-balancing phenomenon. As though as a warning from heaven, all the great empires of the past – *with no exception* – have disappeared. The French *sou*, a negligible coin if it still existed when the euro came in, derived its name from the Latin *solidu*s. That was a gold coin used only by the upper class during the Roman Empire and in the Middle ages largely in transactions between states. Much of the less exalted transactions during the dark ages were transacted in kind, even taxes. Gold came largely from central Africa and ended up disproportionately in religious vessels and ornaments of the Church, i.e., the transactions between man and his Creator. Undoubtedly you know about Henry the Eighth and his wives. The reformation was supposed to have been a by-product of his divorce from Catherine of Aragon, so that he might marry Anne Boleyn, one of the wives he later beheaded. A more powerful motive, however, seems to have been to shake loose the gold hoards of the Church, so urgently needed by England, whose trading economy had come to depend upon an adequate supply of precious metals. The multiplier of banking that later made much money out of a little money base had not yet evolved. So the British monarch achieved that goal by hanging the odd abbot for hiding gold vessels – as in Glastonbury – and of course later by piracy on the seas.

Bumble-bees and Exposed Bottoms

That is the difference between number-crunching and economic analysis: recognizing the ever greater number of independent variables often identified by studying history. The methodology is otherwise known as systems theory, which the better economists are just starting to discover. May they persist and not be distracted by fellowships granted increasingly by central banks to distract them from their more honest investigations. Some of us have applied systems theory to economic matters for at least thirty years. That is part of the heritage that COMER is defending. The world has need of it. That is why it saddens us that the new leader of the NDP, Jack Layton, should apparently turn his back on the glorious traditions of the CCF in playing bumble bee to a Liberal minority government. There is no connection between the" bumble" in "bumble-bee" as in CCF headed for Mackenzie King's exposed bottom and "bumbling" as in Bob Rae. In his time as Premier of Ontario Mr. Rae was approached by COMER with a proposal to pressure the government to use the Bank of Canada to restore the funds that Ottawa had deprived the province of.

To that he replied – would you believe it? – he preferred having the federal government restore its grants to the province. That was considered "playing it safe and respectable" You just have to watch the performance of Paul Martin and his cloven-tongued promises to restore those grants to which Bob Rae was so attached. Were we all to become respectable by the standards of fiscal responsibility laid down by Brian Mulroney, society would be doomed. And for hedging against that, there is no derivative devised even by our banks.

William Krehm

Heroism or Foolhardiness?

THE FIFTEENTH ANNIVERSARY of the Tiananmen massacre has produced some poignant reflection from two of the principals on *The Wall Street Journal's* (3/06/04) oped page, of all places.

And these in turn lend themselves to some broader reflections on the fine line that separates heroism from foolhardiness – and on bills presented for settlement to the innocent, who cannot run as fast as the leaders, and whose survival rate may be smaller and still contribute to the survival of the tribe.

Wang Dan, one of the student leaders of the demonstration writes, "During the six years I spent in prison after the Tiananmen massacre, much of it in solitary confinement, I had ample time to reflect on whether we – the leaders of China's 1989 democracy movement made a mistake in encouraging the protests that culminated in the tragic events of June 4.

"Again and again I have asked myself if there was another path that could have avoided the bloodshed? Whether, by bringing students and ordinary citizens onto the streets to confront the Communist leadership, we frustrated the plans of reformist leaders, – such as former Communist Party General Secretary Zhao Ziyang – to engineer a peaceful transition to a democratic China. It's a question I've also often been asked during my public appearances in the US, since I was forced into exile in April 1998.

"Now, reflecting on the events of 15 years ago, it is clear to me as never before that the Tiananmen massacre was an unavoidable step in the long path to a free China, and that true political reform can never come from within the Communist Party. Indeed one of the real tragedies of 1989 was not that we jeopardized the efforts of so-called reformist leaders. Rather it is that they never had the vision or political will to lead China towards democracy.

"Encouraged by the brief relaxation in the political environment in Beijing in the months before the killings, which had even made it possible for me to hold workshops on democracy, we harbored false hopes that change could come from within the Communist Party.

"We petitioned the leadership in the hope of triggering a top-down reform. Yet the response of the 'reformists' in the leadership was disappointing. Had their hearts been with us, they would surely have seized this unique opportunity to publicly support our calls for democratization. Instead they continued to hide behind closed doors. Only after he had been outvoted in the Politburo Standing Committee did Mr. Zhao finally come and visit us in Tiananmen Square. And when our modest demands were answered with gunfire on the night of June 4, it shattered any remaining illusions.

"The experience of the 15 years since then has confirmed what we failed to understand in 1989. Namely the Communist leaders, be they conservative or reformist, are all wedded to retaining the current political system, complete with its corruption and lack of accountability. Instead the issue remains a taboo subject in Beijing. The new leadership now seems intent on extending their iron grip to Hong Kong.

"The Communist Party has reversed its official verdict on several other major political events in modern Chinese history. The Cultural Revolution, hailed by Mao Tse-Tung as a great proletarian movement, has long since been repudiated. Another popular protest that led to violent scenes in Tiananmen Square, the April 5, 1978, demonstration against the leftist leaders known as the 'Gang of Four,' was also initially suppressed. Within two years, that verdict has been reversed.

"Yet when it comes to June 4, there has been no change. That is because Messers. Wen and Hu realize that re-evaluating the official description of the 1989 movement as counterrevolutionary would shake the foundations of the Communists; grip on power."

"Only the cries for justice are getting ever louder. The Tiananmen Mothers have been gaining increasing domestic and international support in their fight to reverse the official version on the 1989 movement. They have been joined by Jiang Yanyong, the heroic doctor who blew the lid on China's initial cover-up of the outbreak of Severe Acute Respiratory Syndrome last year. In an open letter to the Chinese leadership, Dr. Jang recounted what he witnessed on the night of the killings and called on the government to review what he called the worst Communist crimes since the Cultural Revolution.

"This failure of the leadership to address the issue only increases the risk of further violent eruptions in the future, especially at a time of growing social discontent. With unemployed workers struggling to survive without welfare benefits, residents forced out of their homes without proper compensation and farmers living in extreme poverty, China is a tinder box that could be set on fire by the slightest spark.

"However, as more Chinese enter the private sector, the state is no longer able to control every aspect of life the way it used to. With the internet and modem telecommunications, it's become easier to break through the government's control of news and information and to organize campaigns for rights, be they the right to private property or freedom of speech.

"The 1989 democracy movement remains as much a part of my emotional present as my past. The fight for a reversal of the official verdict has become a goal which I can never abandon."

(Mr. Wang is today a doctoral candidate in history at Harvard.)

Two days later on its oped page, the *WSJ* carried an article "When Will Beijing Say Sorry?" by Wu'er Kaixi.

A Lot to Talk About All Night

"Shortly after he was released from prison in 1998, Wang Dan came to visit me in Taiwan. It was the first time two of

China's most-wanted student leaders of the 1989 Tiananmen protests had met in nearly a decade, and we had a lot to talk about.

"The June 4 massacre set our lives on different trajectories. Wang Dan had spent most of the intervening time as a political prisoner in China, before finally being forced into exile in 1998. I escaped shortly after the massacre and spent my time living the good life in France, the US, and finally in Taiwan. That didn't mean we didn't have a lot to talk about. Indeed, we were still talking the next day when the sun came up.

"We tried to work out whether we had done the right thing in encouraging the 1989 protests that culminated in the killings. Neither of us could be sure that we had, and the more we talked the more I realized that there was someone to whom an apology was long overdue. That person was Ding Zilin, who, as head of the Tiananmen Mothers' Campaign, has been relentless in her efforts to press China's government to accept responsibility for the bloodshed.

"On the night of the massacre, when I had already begun my flight to freedom (within a month I reached the safety of Hong Kong), her 17-year old son, Jiang Jielan, joined the protesters trying to stop the advancing troops – even though his mother had begged him to stay home. He was one of so many ordinary Beijing residents who took to the streets to protect us, and paid the ultimate price for doing so – shot dead three hours later, while Wang Dan and I survived.

"We don't know how many others were killed along with Ms. Ding's son. It could be hundreds, even thousands. But Ms. Ding, at least has spent the last 15 years reminding us there was a massacre. She still does, by persuading other families to stand up and count the ones they lost. She gets arrested on a regular basis, but she continues to remind us that 'the blood-spattered streets of Beijing have been paved over with a new concrete – brand-named 'economic progress.' She has been nominated for a Nobel Peace Prize, and in a braver, more honest world she would get it.

"When her name came up that night with Wang Dan, I felt guilty about having survived and made it to France and the US, when so many others had died. I felt guilty that I had not gone to jail like Wang Dan. I felt guilty of the death of Ms. Ding's son. I felt so guilty that we finally made a phone call that I've been putting off for far too long. 'Sorry,' I said to Ms. Ding. 'I can't even ask you for foreigveness.'

"'I'm just happy that you finally called,' she replied.

"All three of us began to cry, and I said: 'We can't replace the son you lost, but Wang Dan and I want you to think of us as your sons.'

"That telephone call, more than six years ago, was so painful that I have never publicly spoken or written about it until now. I will spend the rest of my life regretting the lives lost in 1989.

"Wang Dan and I were young men who thought we could change the world. Instead we inadvertently led a lot of people to their deaths. That caused a lot of pain to a lot of people. However, ours is not the most important apology, the apology that will allow my exiled generation to go home. That apology is still to come, from the men who ordered the killings.

"I have spent months thinking how today's 15th anniversary should be marked. The world has changed in so many ways. These are less idealistic times than those giddy days of the fall of the Berlin Wall – when anything briefly seemed possible.

"But if, for just one day, we could return to that idealism, I would ask the world to spend it looking hard at the China with which is has struck business deals, and remembering the mother in Beijing still waiting for that apology. Until it comes China will remain a dark place."

The Moral under Beijing's New Concrete

Or put in other words, those uncounted nameless martyrs, who have risked their existence and gone to their doom that future generations may live in a better world. Nothing was further from their minds than to patent the new society for which they were making such sacrifices. There were times when revolutions in military technology produced notable steps towards more democratic societies. Thus when the phalanx was introduced in ancient Greece and infantry formations with interlocking shields and overlapping spears stood up against war chariots, and upset social rankings. Or when the long bow drawn by sturdy peasant arms made its contribution to English democracy. But in general society's progress towards gentler regimes resulted over the ages from a vast input of "irrational" selfless sacrifice. A special breed of economic historian has arisen to track this down. Douglass C. North, who was awarded the Nobel Prize for Economics, is one of the most prominent of these.

Though of a Marxist background, for lack of anything better, he takes as his point of departure the standard neoclassical model to show how it misleads. This he achieves by extending that theory far beyond its traditional bounds. For example, he defines social capital as "human capital, natural resources, technology and knowledge." What a gust of fresh air! This breadth of definition of "capital" contrasts with the view of equilibrium theory where government capital is not recognized, and the destruction of non-marketed capital, is rarely reflected in government ledgers. To this he applies the maximising postulate [which] will result in investment in whatever part of the capital stock that has the highest rate of return. New types of physical and human capital will then be invented and types of natural resources discovered when the rate of return to be earned by investing forgone consumption in invention and natural resources exceeds the return in the existing machines and skills.

From the viewpoint of the economic historian this neoclassical formulation begs all the interesting questions. Its world is a frictionless one in which institutions do not exist and all changes occur through perfectly operating markets." It is a parody in short. "The costs of acquiring information, uncertainty, and transaction costs do not exist. However, throughout history, many resources are closer to common property than exclusively owned. As a result the necessary conditions for achieving the marginally efficient solution have never existed. He brings in, the 'national heritage' of Major Douglas without even intending to do so.

"Individuals may ignore an individual calculus of cost bene-fits. Mancur Olson in *The Logic of Collective Action* (1965) dem-onstrated when large groups were organized to create change but did not possess some exclusive benefit to members, they tended to be unstable and disappear. In essence, rational indi-viduals will not incur the costs of participating in large group action when the same benefits can be received as a *free rider*."

The reader may have been wondering where I was leading her by bringing in Douglass C. North, but we have arrived at its great relevance to the dilemma of the student leaders of the Ti-ananmen Square demonstrations. Why face the tanks and gun-fire in that slaughter, if you can let the others do so, and move in to share the benefits when they finally may come in for all?

North goes on: "The Marxist finesses the entire issue by ar-guing that it is classes that are the initiators of structural change. The best evidence that this is not standard behavior comes from Marxist activists themselves who devote enormous energies at-tempting to convince the proletariat to behave like a class."

Could it be that humanity up to now has survived as a spe-cies, because of a "rogue gene" that violates the "natural law" of the self-balancing market? That gene apparently occurs often enough to produce enough individuals ready to risk their lives that the tribe may survive. That will explain why a minority of people will put their careers as academics at risk, turn their backs on becoming big hitters in the world of high finance, or at least waver between the two dispositions. There are several items in this current issue of *ER* that echo this theme.

Our readers, we are sure, will have no difficulty in identify-ing them.

William Krehm

The Cambridge File

Cambridge Journal of Economics
Faculty of Economics and Politics
Cambridge, UK

2 March 2004
W. Krehm
COMER Publications
Toronto, Ontario

Dear [Mr.] Krehm,

Thank you for sending your paper "Homage to Newton – For a Proper Use of Mathematics in Economics" to the *Cam-bridge Journal of Economics*. Although your paper was well re-ceived at the Conference and made an important contribution to the debate, I am afraid that now the Editors have received and considered referees' reports it [sic],they have decided they cannot offer publication.

I enclose copies of extracts from the referee's comments for your information. I should add, however, that the Editors do not necessarily agree with all the points made by the referee and also that these comments do not necessarily give a com-prehensive account of the reasons for the Board judging your paper not suitable for publication in the *Cambridge Journal of Economics*.

With best wishes,
Yours sincerely,
Ann Newton, Managing Editor

Referee's Report

GENERAL POINTS

This paper raises an important question concerning the proper use of mathematics in economics, but doesn't begin to answer it properly. It makes no reference to the extensive literature on the topic by methodologists and others. Indeed, it makes no systematic use of the academic literature at all, and there is no list of references.

The paper rambles over a multiplicity of issues, from eco-nomic theory to trade policy. None is adequately treated. Much of the discussion is off the point. When the author comes to his own "Gaussian" (?) Solution it is entirely unclear what this means: there is no adequate attempt to explain what is involved to a general audience. Conclusions are drawn that seem totally unrelated to the mathematical concepts that are briefly and awkwardly presented.

Why Newton is singled out in the title is a mystery to me, especially as the paper attempts to put some weight on post-Newtonian developments in physics, such as thermodynamics. (But again there is no reference to the key figures on this topic, such as Georgescu-Roegen and Saviotti.)

Unfortunately, the paper is a failure. Its author should learn how to present and accredit and academic argument, before s/he claims to have answers to pressing questions.

PARTICULAR POINTS

P.1. The opening words are: 'A point has position but no direction. It is a scalar not a vector….' Wrong. A point is not a scalar. In n-dimensional space it can be represented by a n-dimensional vector. S/he continues, proposing that a point 'is useful only for number-crunching rather than analysis.' But mathematics is full of analysis of points in space and their meaning. These opening sentences set the tone for a paper that is mathematically ill-informed and weak in its own analysis.

P. 1 Systems theory does not assume that all subsystems have purposes.

P. 1. The author writes: "The goal of the market subsystem is to make a profit." This is open to objection on a number of counts. First, in what sense if any can the market have a "goal" especially as there is often no-one in charge and individual actors may disagree about objectives. Second, there is simply selling and buying (without new production) then some will make profits, others losses, and these will sum to zero. Third, the motives of some (if not all) may not be to make profits.

P.1 The author writes: "Under capitalism all subsystems speak the language of money." Dramatic, but what does it mean? Does it mean that money is used everywhere? We require precise language, not journalism.

P.1. The author describes money as a vector. In the context here s/he suggests that a vector necessarily involves movement. This is mathematically incorrect, and relates to the misunderstanding of mathematics in the very first paragraph, as noted above. A vector is simply a (Nx1 1xN) form of array.

P.1. The account and definition of entropy here is incorrect. Entropy is not energy, it refers to disorder. Conversely, negentropy is not "functional well-being" as claimed here: it refers to order and structure.

(Note that I have got only as far as the end of the first page. There are so many misunderstandings and mistakes here that the case for the paper is hopeless.)

P. 2 The author is right to point out that in much mainstream economics processes are often presented in a way that is time-reversible. But the problem here is not the lack of proof, as the author claims, but the assumption of models in which time-reversibility is inherent. The example that follows, concerning demand and supply, is trivial, and would be contested by no trained economist of any stripe.

P.3 "Tinbergen's counting rule: is not about equations as such, but policy objectives and policy instruments.

P.7 The brief discussion of the causes of inflation here is extremely and especially superficial. To blame it most on taxes is wrong-headed.

P.12. The example here from modular algebra is unclear, as the terms and rules are ill-defined.

The reader will ask why it is put in the paper as $(M+2)^2=M^2+2M+4$ and not $(M+2)^2=M^2+4M + 4$. And s/he doesn't need to be told that $2^2=4$?

P. 12. It is also entirely unclear how this mathematics leads to the proposition (attributed to Keynes) that countries should produce their own cookies rather than trade them.

Our Comment

COMER Publications
Toronto, Ontario

15/3/04
Ann Newton, Managing Director
Cambridge Journal of Economics
Cambridge, UK

Dear Professor Newton:

Thank you for making available extracts from the referee's comments on my paper read at your recent conference. That is a fair thing to have done, and should be helpful both to the Cambridge Journal of Economics and to me.

Let me draw your attention to a few key points of the referee's appraisal.

"'A point has position but no direction. It is a scalar not a vector.' Wrong. A point is not a scalar. In n-dimensional space it can be represented by a n-dimensional vector."

I quote from the *Principles of Mathematical Physics* by William V. Houston, Professor of Physics, California Institute of Technology, McGraw-Hill Book Company, Inc., New York, 1934, p. 74. "In the study of a physical problem it is usually necessary to establish a system of coordinates in which the various material bodies can be located. The position of the bodies, expressed in terms of these coordinates, are then the variables in the equations which state the laws of physics. Although these equations will contain explicit reference to the coordinates used, it is difficult to believe that the relationships expressed should depend upon the coordinates in any essential way. The laws of physics should be relationships between physical things, and these relationships should be true regardless of the language used to state them. In fact, it has long been taken as an axiom that the laws of physics must be expressible in a form which is the same for all systems of coordinates.

"The treatment of Hamilton's principle…has shown one method of expressing the Newtonian laws of motion in a form independent of any particular form of coordinates. The use of vectors is another way in which this object may be attained. A vector is independent of any particular coordinate system."

Obviously, price is amongst the most prominent coordinates used in just such a sense. You are undoubtedly aware that in the past year or so both the US Federal Reserve and the Bank for International Settlements, that had in the late 1990s militantly espoused "zero inflation," have now adopted the concept of "good inflation" (up to circa 2%) as well as "bad inflation." That would suggest a striving towards a concept that does not depend on the particular coordinate system chosen.

Your Referee: "The brief discussion of the causes of inflation here is extremely and especially superficial. To blame it mostly on taxes is wrong-headed."

There is nothing in my paper that blames it "mostly on taxes." I apply systems theory to show that the good functioning of the non-market subsystems of the economy are essential to prevent the breakdown of the system as a whole. These non-market subsystems – usually dismissed by equilibrium economists as "externalities" – depend on government for most of their funding, and that is why the population explosion, higher technology, [and] urbanization inevitably increased the layer of taxation in price. This effect on the price level is not to be confused with the result of an excess of demand over supply.

Oddly enough, my views of this and other items in my paper were actually covered approvingly by the *Economic Journal of Cambridge* in a review of my book, *Price in a Mixed Economy – Our Record of Disaster* (Toronto, 1975) by P.M. Deane in 1975 or 1976. A quotation from the review: "An unusual book. He is imaginative and well-read, over a wider range of past and present economic theory than the conventionally trained economist, and has some powerful arguments to deploy…. He is particularly persuasive about the need to base policy on what he calls 'a pluralistic notion of price….' This is not an easy book to read, but it has insights that make the effort worth while."

This book of mine was an extension of a 61-page paper that had appeared in *Revue Economique* in Paris in its May 1970 issue. I have misplaced the clipping from the *Economic Journal* and quote from a blurb from it from my second book, *Babel's Tower – The Dynamics of Economic Breakdown*, 1977. You should have no trouble in finding the full quotation on the Deane review.

I am sure that both Cambridge and COMER's own monthly publication, *Economic Reform* – now in its 16th year – will survive the non-acceptance of my paper by the *Journal*. But the referee's report reveals such a bottomless chasm that has developed between orthodox economic thinking and the issues that are pulling the world apart, that we should all be concerned.

I will just mention a few further items.

"Systems theory does not assume that all subsystems have purposes." The ecological subsystem, however, is defined by the need to look after the environment, the health [subsystem] to look after the physical well-being of society, etc. What is the objection of the referee about? An attempt to leave it all to the self-regulating market even in the non-market subsystems?

"The account and definition of entropy is incorrect. Entropy is not energy. It refers to disorder. Conversely, negentropy is not 'functional well-being' as claimed. It refers to order and structure."

The concept of entropy arose in the study of the flow of energy by the engineer Sadi Carnot and led to the science of thermodynamics. Its application to information theory was a much later derivative.

"Tinbergen's counting rule" is not about equations as such, but policy objectives and policy instruments." But in any mathematical procedure the solution of equations is involved. To solve them you must have as many independent equations as you have independent variables [to solve for].

"The example here from modular algebra is unclear, as the terms and rules are ill-defined. The reader will ask why it is put in the paper as $(M+2)^2=M^2+2M+4$ and not $(M+2)^2+M^2+4M+4$? And s/sh doesn't need to be told that $2^2=4$."

The explanation of the first question is that the writer is 90 years old and of failing eyesight, and does his own proof-reading for lack of budget. The important point, however, is the final 4 which is what modular congruence simplifies the operation to. It should not have puzzled our referee since it is all explained by the application of modular congruence technique by our remote ancestor in applying it to the names of days. Instead of giving every successive day a new name he adopted modular congruence and reverted to Sunday in cycles of module 7.

There has been a disturbing lack of communication between orthodox and really heterodox economic theory in the last four decades. Certainly the serious restrictions on public information on economic and monetary policy is a factor in this. As is the misuse of mathematics.

We should take to heart the comment by MIT professor Norbert Wiener in his final book addressed to the lay public, *God and Golem, Inc.* (1964): "The success of mathematical physics led the social scientist to be jealous of its power without quite understanding the intellectual attitudes that had contributed to this power. Just as primitive people adopt Western modes of denationalized clothing and of parliamentarism out of a vague feeling that these magic rites and vestments will at once put them abreast of modern culture and technique, so the economists have developed ideas in the language of the infinitesimal calculus."

With the twin heritage of Newton and Keynes, Cambridge should be in the van to straighten out this muddle. In that task I wish you godspeed.

Sincerely,
William Krehm

Cambridge Replies

Cambridge Journal of Economics
Faculty of Economics and Politics
Cambridge, UK

14 May 2004

Professor W. Krehm
COMER Publications
Toronto, Ontario

Dear Professor Krehm,

Thank you for your letter, which I have passed on to the Editorial Board. I hope to be in a position to respond in due course.

Yours sincerely,
Ann Newton, Managing Director

We Ripped the File Out of ER's June Issue

COMER Publications
Toronto, Ontario

21/05/04

Ann Newton
Cambridge Journal of Economics
Faculty of Economics and Politics
Cambridge, UK

Dear Ann Newton:

Yours of 14/05 arrived just in time for me to pull out of the June issue of *Economic Reform* our previous interchange.

I wish to assure you that I have no desire to embarrass your great university or anyone connected with it, and that I appreciate the many courtesies that came my way during my brief stay among you. However, I am convinced that in the present deepening world crisis the nexus between official economics and the reality around us still requires some effort. This past year my concern took me to conferences on heterodox economics as far as Tokyo, and my overall impression is that self-styled heterodox economists are prone to developing their own orthodoxy. Let us never forget that among the founding fathers and uncles of economic theory many – including Adam Smith, Ricardo, Stuart Mill, Karl Marx, Leon Walras – were without degree in economics, and that on one occasion President Ronald Reagan levied that charge against Keynes himself.

When I first contacted you, I made a point of emphasizing that though I have spent my life pursuing my studies in economics, I do not have a degree in that subject.

With best wishes,
William Krehm

Four Months Later

Since Ann Newton's letter of 14/05 over four months have passed, without further word as announced from the Economic Journal editorial board. What was urgent last May has become even more so in the interim. BIS and the Fed have apparently forgotten about the "good inflation" that they had announced, and higher interest rates are unlikely to make drilling for oil less costly. Major elections throughout the world are being contested with promises to balance budgets that lack meaningful accountancy. Hence our decision to make our Cambridge file public.

Hobson's Choice

I T ISN'T NECESSARILY the most pious that most frequently lay hand on the Holy Bible, for that would include those charged in our courts. Keynes's General Theory of Employment, Interest and Money, is in a somewhat similar position. Far, far more people swear by it, than actually read it. That is a shame, because Keynes has much to teach economists, not only about theory, but about the intellectual honesty that makes possible a theory that really counts. Perhaps his greatest achievement was in eating humble pie, when a whole series of economic theorists whom he had dismissed as "unscientific," were proved closer to being correct than seemed to him before the Depression. And then the great man, greater for doing so, didn't hesitate to say that he had been wrong in dismissing them. And by putting their varied contributions together he came up with a an understanding of what was necessary to pull the world out of depression and avoid getting into another one after the Second World War.

There is not only that monumental passage, never ever heard in our editorials or academic halls (*The General Theory*, p. 32): "The great puzzle of Effective Demand... vanished from economic literature.... It could only live on furtively, below the surface, in the underworlds of Karl Marx, Silvio Gesell or Major Douglas." Since Keynes himself was literally born into the academic tradition, and for most of his years delivered his heterodoxies from its pulpits, that sentence set a standard of selfless dedication that most of his colleagues did not understand or share. In the same great work whose opaque style bears witness to the urgency of its message, Keynes also pays tribute to J.A. Hobson, who anticipated by a half century an essential part Keynes's great contribution – the distinction between Saving and Investment. On page 365 of the *General Theory*, we are treated to this auto-biographical note of Hobson.

"Mr. Hobson has told how his book, *The Physiology of Industry* came to be written with A.F. Mummery. 'It was not until the middle eighties that my economic heterodoxy began to take shape. Though the Henry George campaign against land values and the early agitation of various socialist groups against the visible oppression of the working classes, coupled with the revelations of the two Booths regarding the poverty of London, made a deep impression on my feelings, they did not destroy my faith in Political Economy. That came from what may be called an accidental contact. While teaching at a school in Exeter I came into personal relations with a business man named Mummery, known then and afterwards as a great mountaineer who had discovered another way up the Matterhorn and who in 1895, was killed in an attempt to climb the famous Himalayan mountain Nanga Parbat.

"But he was a mental mountain climber as well, with a natural eye for a path of his own finding and a sublime disregard of intellectual authority. This man entangled me in a controversy about excessive saving, which he regarded as responsible for the under-employment of capital and labour in periods of bad trade. For a long time I sought to counter his arguments by the use of the orthodox economic weapons. But at length he convinced me and I went in with him to elaborate the over-saving argument in a book entitled *The Physiology of Industry* published in 1889. This was the first step in my heretical career, and I did not in the least realize its momentous consequences.

"For just at that time I had given up my scholastic post and was opening a new line of work as University Extension Lecturer in Economics and Literature. The first shock came in a refusal of the London Extension Board to allow me to offer courses of Political Economy. This was due, I learned, to the intervention of an Economic Professor who had read my book and considered it as equivalent in rationality to an attempt to prove the flatness of the earth. How could there be any limit to the amount of useful saving when every item of saving went to increase the capital structure and the fund for paying wages? Sound economists could not fail to view with horror an argument which sought to check the source of all industrial progress. Another interesting experience helped to bring home to me the sense of my iniquity. Though prevented from lecturing on economics in London, I had been allowed by the greatest liberality of the Oxford University Extension Movement to address audiences in the Provinces, confining myself to political issues relating to the working-class life. Now it happened at this time that the Charity Organisation Society was planning a lecture campaign upon economic subjects and invited me to prepare a course. I had expressed my willingness to undertake this new lecture work, when suddenly, without explanation, the invitation was withdrawn. Even then I hardly realized that in appearing to question the virtue of unlimited thrift I had committed the unpardonable sin."

Sound familiar? On two counts. "Unlimited thrift" these days has taken over all major parties throughout much of the world, and has cowed the minor ones to fear for their lives and even their careers as social reformers – to the point of not challenging the illusion of "paying off the national debt." Yet, since central government debt is the only legal tender in the world today, that would leave the world moneyless, and reduce us all to living on our credit cards. How long will it be before Visa and Citicorps issue a credit card to the government itself?

And the other bit of a too familiar landscape is what in polite academic parlance is known as "early retirement" for seditious views, or simple non-employment in the first place.

William Krehm

Thinking Out of the Box

W HY ARE MATTRESSES always sold with a box spring? The answer is, habit and good merchandising. When mattresses were just bags of straw – they were called ticks or pallets – having a spring under them gave you a little more, well, spring. When the manufacturers went to inner spring mattresses in the 1940s, springs were no longer necessary. But consumer habit made them a saleable product. So the box spring arrived to replace the old flat iron springs, even though a sheet of plywood is a lot cheaper. But that's habit and good merchandising.

We might ask also why most private houses have abominable windows which leak cold air and whose opening mechanisms always seem to be breaking. Large public buildings have airtight windows that do not open. Again, the answer lies in history: a long time ago, lighting and ventilation in a house were combined – in a hole in the wall. When window glass became affordable in the first half of the nineteenth century, ventilation suffered, and the openable window, with all its flaws, was invented. A vent that closes tightly when not in use, on the other hand is easy to devise. I have five of them in my lakeside cottage. My glass windows are sealed. In my city home…? Well, habit and good merchandising.

Speaking of household matters, can we ask why we require $230,000 to build ourselves a $100,000 house? Borrowing the first $100,000 from a chartered bank puts $100,000 of newly-created money into the economy. That could be inflationary. But taking it back, along with, give or take, $130,000 in interest payments over 25 years, must have the reverse effect. There are other ways to do it. For example, government holds the original right to create (interest-free) money. It can also hold mortgages. Why don't we insist that every citizen who wishes to build a house have access to such a loan? Habit and good merchandising, of course. That's why.

A recent report on executive compensation gave some interesting figures for the ratio of executive compensation to basic worker wages: Canada, 29:1; Switzerland, 12:1; Brazil, 110:1; US 349:1. We might ask, what explains the national differences? It would be thinking outside the box, however, to raise a wider, and fundamental, question: what determines how a society allots income to its people?

Conventional wisdom says:

1. Supply and demand. (If there are not enough computer techies, or brain surgeons to go around, competition drives up the remuneration.)

2. Personal gifts (brains, body type), education, "drive," and connections.

3. Collective bargaining (draws the line which divides the pie between workers and shareholders).

4. Government redistribution measures (disability pensions, graduated income tax, free public education).

In the case of corporate CEOs, supply and demand can't be the decisive factor; most CEOs have lots of people around them who would be glad to take on the job. CEOs don't bargain collectively. As for government redistribution, the figures are for pre-tax incomes. Graduated taxation, we might expect, would reduce the ratio between the CEO and the average worker. So the major factor must lie in the personal attributes: the typical Canadian CEO must be twenty-nine times smarter, taller, handsomer, better educated, more "driven" and better connected than the average worker. That seems reasonable enough. The only thing it leaves out is an attribute that was included in the evaluation of ancient Roman political appointees – luck.

Suppose we were to add still another criterion:

1. Value to the commonwealth (Now that's thinking outside the box!)

How about a national, or municipal, referendum in which each citizen was to arrange a list of occupations in an ideal order based on value to the community? For instance, how would you arrange this list: plastic surgeon, dentist, corporation lawyer, trash collector, high school teacher, plumber, auto mechanic, general of the forces, public school teacher, professional football player, president of a major bank, service station attendant, coffee shop waitress, test pilot, stock broker, autoworker. (In tabulating the results it might be justifiable to discount the top two occupations on each ballot, on the assumption that the respondent would put himself in first, or at worst, second place.) Seriously, how would the results of such a referendum compare with current remuneration arrangements?

Perhaps when a list had been developed in this democratic way, the tax system could be adapted to bring remunerations into agreement with it. Within the general brackets, supply and demand and personal attributes could still operate. Collective bargaining would be obsolete. And government could concentrate on the actual creating of useful work instead of on redistributing the income. Bears thinking on, even if only to point out the wide space available outside of the box.

Some Philosophy on Taxation

Still, that sounds like a pretty slippery tax system. What about that so-called "flat tax"? That sounds fair. Let everybody pay 20% of their annual income. Everybody treated equally; you can't get better than that.

So how much would my young cousin Sam pay with his $10,000 annual income? $2000. And my nephew, the lawyer, on his $100,000? $20,000. And what about my uncle, the financier, on his, let's say $1 million? $200,000.

Wow, Uncle Bill really gets hit hard! Wouldn't it be fairer if it were a real flat tax, not just a flat percentage tax? What if everybody paid exactly the same – say, just for the sake of argument, $50,000? No?

You could look at the 20% tax from another side. How much would Cousin Sam have left after taxes, to live on? $8,000. And Nephew Charles? $80,000. And Uncle Bill? $800,000. Doesn't sound quite fair. Uncle Bill, by his natural gifts, education, good health and application to his investments, gets out of the economy every year a hundred times as much as Cousin Sam.

Well, sure I said, "out of the economy." It doesn't come from his property on the moon. Not yet, anyway.

Funny the thoughts one has, lying on a mattress with no box spring.

Gordon Coggins

"Truth Will Out" — Too Often Only in Time for the Funeral

THE WHOLE INFRASTRUCTURE of economic relationships has been systematically distorted. The disciplines that were to watch over the soundness of society's reasoning have been hopelessly corrupted. When some of them eventually do get through, they are often too crippled and too late to deliver their message effectively.

Software and hardware have been tampered with. The language itself have become so mis-wired, that it is becoming easier for archeologists to reconstruct some relationships in ancient Troy that for our society to figure out whether it can afford survival.

The difficulty in reporting one of the cleanest breakthroughs of the facts of Ontario's only toll-road that was privatized by a Conservative provincial regime is a sample of the problem. In *The Globe and Mail* (12/08, "McGuinty's battle cry could set up roadblock's to investment" by Eric Reguly) illustrates the point:

Dalton McGuinty is the recently elected Liberal premier of Ontario, Canada's richest province. He succeeded a series of ultra-conservative governments who rode into power supposedly to clean up corruption, and straighten out provincial finances. Instead, this led to a series of suspect privatizations, details of which are only now coming to light.

"The Ontario government wants the world to know it won't tolerate the rape and pillage of its consumers. Governments are in business to protect the public interest and the public interest will not be served by giving the Spanish company that heads the consortium that owns Highway 407 the unfettered right to raise tolls for a century.

"That's why Premier McGuinty said the Liberal government 'won't back down in a fight with the owners of the province's only toll highway' to regulate the highway's fares, which are rising as fast as the Premier's ratings are falling. The vow came the same day the *G&M* reported the Spanish government might veto a proposed trade agreement between Canada and the European Union if Ontario blocks the highway owners' apparent right to charge what they want.

"Drivers rejoice. But will the public interest be served by stomping all over a business that is no longer a taxpayer-owned asset? If this happens, the message sent to the world won't be that Ontario protects its citizens; it would be that investing in Ontario [has] huge, and potentially profit-busting risks. And Ontario desperately needs private investors to finance tens of billions of dollars in new infrastructures, including a fresh fleet of electrically-generating plants.

"Construction of the highway among the northern and western fringes of Toronto was financed by the leftist New Democratic Party in the early 1990s. On the eve of the 1999 election, the Conservatives leased it for 99 years to an international consortium for about $3.1 billion. That was about $1 billion more than the development costs. It was a giveaway price. In 2002, one of the consortium partners sold a 6% interest for $178 million; it had paid $45 million."

Desperately Needing Private Investors to Run a Monopoly Highway Already Built

"The company's lead investor is Spain's Cintra Concesiones de Infrastructuras de Transporte." The heart of the business and the focus of the McGuinty government's ire, is the fee hikes. Some of the fees have climbed as much as 200% since 2000. The government claims the highway doesn't have the right to raise fees at will for the next 94 years.

"The basis of its argument is fairly simple. Two contractual documents exist. The first covers the main lease, the second, called the 'tolling agreement,' is a schedule to the main lease. The latter does not say the highway needs to grovel at the feet of Queen's Park [i.e., the government] before it raises tolls. But the government says the main lease specifically says tolling and other operational issues require government approval. The two contracts appear in conflict.

"So far the highway owners are winning. Last month, an arbitrator, retired judge Drew Hudson, said the highway owners don't need government approval to raise tolls. The Government went to Ontario Supreme Court to appeal the decision. Further appeals, lawsuits and legal stonewalling could drag this slugfest out for years. If the government wins, however, they risk building on the government's reputation as enthusiastic meddlers in private affairs.

"Reputation impairment among investors started with the Conservatives under Ernie Eves. The Tories announced the initial public offering of Hydro One; then cancelled it. They opened the Ontario electricity market to competitive forces, only to snap it shut, scaring away billions of dollars of investment in electricity generation. The Liberals' commitment to an artificially low fixed price for residential electricity only makes a bad situation worse. The result is an electrical energy shortage.

"It's not the Liberals' fault the Tories unloaded the 407 at a stupidly low price. But it will be their fault if the 407 wrangling provides another excuse for infrastructure investors to give Ontario a pass."

It is an evasion of the basic facts to label the former Conservative government's giving away the 407 at a ridiculously low price as a "stupidity." You will find the exact counterparts in Margaret Thatcher's privatization that rarely worked, but did put immense immediate profits into speculators' pockets. Like much under Thatcher, that was a carefully plotted redistribution of the national income.

COMER has for some years developed the view that a fundamental redistribution of the national income flow took place with the end of the statutory reserves that banks had had to put up with the central bank. This was justified by the declaration of central government bonds as "risk-free" requiring banks to put up no capital of their own to hoard, and with the deregulation of the banks to allow them to acquire mortgages, and every sort of stock market activities that had been since the mid-1930s separated from banking. All these measures led to the pyramiding of the powers of money-creation, the very essence of banking today, with the other important financial services that have their own pools of capital. Allow banks access to those, and the sky becomes the limit for the misappropriation of the national income. The rate of growth achieved in a single year, and the rate of growth of the rate of growth and so forth to higher powers are projected into the future and then capitalized for their present value. It is in fact the exponential series that is the mathematics of the atom bomb.

Two important points emerge from the nature of the 100-year-lease on Ontario's Highway 407 that gave the lessee vague competence to set rates for a century ahead.

1. It virtually embodies, or can at least be read to embody, this exponential pattern of stock market pricing.

2. But were all those "infrastructure investors" really needed? There was a simpler way out of the problem by making use of the Bank of Canada. Because the government of Canada is the sole shareholder of the central bank, practically the entire interest received by it on its loans reverts to the central government as dividends. Since the present hassle with Spain and possibly the European Union raises Highway 407 to a federal and not just a provincial problem, the two levels of government with a little foresight should have avoided privatization. It could have managed this with little sweat by restoring to Ontario the money already invested in building the toll road. For that no outside investors were needed. But the financiers at home and abroad fell over themselves for the opportunity to make a quick capital profit.

Surely that suggests the monopoly position of that highway, particularly because of the pace of urbanization of the whole Toronto area. That in itself should have alerted our governments to the fact that the price level would continue climbing. And once the monopoly character of that communication route had been established, our political leaders should have remembered that basic tenet of traditional economic theory, that in the case of monopolist services government control is essential, whether they are delivered by public or private corporations. Since the government had already built the highway, refinancing it through the central bank should have been a piece of cake. The alternative path was the one chosen: the reshaping of economic thinking to suit the interests of speculative finance does not merely open wide the gates to corruption. It imposes it.

Even a keen-eyed reporter like Reguly doesn't dare reach that obvious conclusion. When a common thief is caught with stolen goods, the court will not drop the case because the culprit produces a contract showing that he has already sold the hot goods. So long as the Bank of Canada was used for such long-term financing of vital capital projects by all three levels of government, the alleged obstacle that Reguly detects in the way of the Government defending its citizens simply did not exist. And treating such capital projects as current spending that is written off in the year of their completion and then carried on the government books at a token one dollar simply encourages the plundering of the public domain by the privateers. The nature of the bailout of our banks in 1991, followed incredibly by their further deregulation and the Bank for International Settlements' *Risk-Based Capital Requirements*, allowed them to load up with government debt entirely on the cuff. Rather than just 'stupidity' it all added up to a planned redistribution of the national income.

William Krehm

Never Underestimate Women, Banks or the After Life

MICKEY had worked all of his life, lived frugally, scrimped and saved. Before he died, he said to his wife, "Mary, When I die, I want you to take all my money and put it in the casket with me. I want to take my money to the afterlife with me, so I want a proper burial, not a cremation."

Mary promised him tearfully that when he died, she would put his savings in the casket with him.

When he was eventually stretched out in his casket, Mary was sitting nearby in black, with her friend Sarah. When the ceremony was finished, the undertakers got ready to close the casket and Mary said, "Wait just a minute, please!"

She had a small box with her. She put it in the casket. Then the undertakers locked the casket down, and rolled it away. Said Sarah. "Mary, I know you weren't fool enough to put all that money in there with your husband."

Mary replied, "Sarah dear, Mac and I had no secrets. I could not live with my conscience in the sight of God, if I broke my word to him. I promised to put all his savings in there with him. I wrote him a cheque for safety. Whatever he leaves in the account he knows I'll use sparingly."

With thanks to Economic Reform Australia Newsletter.

An Anatomical Morality Tale for Social Engineers

JOHN LOCKE'S *Essay Concerning Human Understanding* was a major step into the Age of Enlightenment and the systematic progress of knowledge. It was accepted rapidly because there was an important audience which had already demonstrated the principles there explained. For Locke knit together the consequences and implications of explorations undertaken by extraordinary intellects as they came together in founding the Royal Society for Promoting Natural Knowledge (1660). "[T]he virtuosi who emerged from the English Civil War pondered how they should go about gathering knowledge through experiments and observations, but only in an ad hoc way. It was Locke who transformed this kind of thinking into a full-blown philosophy, one that would become the heart of scientific method" (252).

One important focus of their research effort had been the human and other animal bodies, with a special interest in the systems that sustain life and constitute the rational soul. It entailed marathons of dissection, racing to keep ahead of decomposition amid the stench of rotting corpses, as well as surgical experiments on live animals. Participants included not only William Harvey but also such unexpected luminaries as Robert Boyle, William Petty and Christopher Wren, as well as Locke himself. The details are assembled in a new book by Carl Zimmer, *Soul Made Flesh: The Discovery of the Brain and*

How It Changed the World (New York: Free Press Division of Simon & Schuster, Inc., 2004, *xii* + 367 pp; illustrated; endnotes, bibliography, index). Zimmer's principal subject is Thomas Willis, whose anatomical explorations of the brain and nervous system inaugurated the modern study of *neurology*. Progress along these lines gradually identified physiological structures and processes as the demonstrably specific sites of faculties that had been attributed since ancient times to the ethereal *soul*. One consequence is that moral philosophers now study ethics using brain scans on living human subjects (with magnetic resonance imaging machines).

By the time of his death at 54, Willis was the wealthy physician of kings and lords, and had spent all of his adult life in collaboration with persons of restlessly ambitious genius. Zimmer affirms that Willis "did for the brain and nerves what Harvey had done for the heart and blood. His mixture of anatomy, experiment and medical observation set the agenda of neuroscience into the twenty-first century. [His] doctrines of the brain and soul became part of the bedrock of modern Western thought. And yet, despite his lasting impact, few people today know about Thomas Willis" (240). The lion's share of responsibility for his subsequent obscurity, says Zimmer, belongs to John Locke. The explanation of this assertion is the link to our subject of economic reform.

Shaking the Invisible Hand of the Creator

Soul Made Flesh provides illuminating parallels and instructive analogues between the medical arts and social engineering. Getting the anatomy right is an important step toward effective treatments. Willis and his collaborators were empiricists, seeking to understand the human being by dissecting it and examining its parts and systems. Along the way they encountered surprises, for what they found was not infrequently different from what they expected. Their expectations were based, of course, on the traditional explanations of their era.

Ever since Thomas Aquinas integrated the recently recovered works of Aristotle with Christian doctrines and affirmed that faith and reason cannot be in conflict since both have their source in God, this "natural philosophy" had dominated intellectual explorations. It became entrenched as universities sprang up across Europe in the 13th century. One part of the adaptation to ancient Greek texts was the concept that the soul is the *form* of the human body. It is also a spiritual substance that survives death and is the conscious self. Aquinas "made it clear that no *physical* organ could produce self-awareness or any other human thought" (18). Although dissection of corpses was a regular feature in those medieval halls of learning, the atmosphere of natural philosophy dictated that its purpose was always to demonstrate the handiwork of God. This meant exposing the liver, heart and head (open spaces in the brain called *ventricles*) while repeating the traditional explanation that these were the location of the soul's faculties, from whence they traveled around the body as invisible spirits to produce and maintain life. While that explanation sounds like nonsense today, the form of reasoning is still employed. It amounts to the assertion that "this is why the system works according to our

explanation" – begging the question of whether the explanation is in fact true. Among its contemporary practitioners are the professors of mainstream economics who employ a deductive apparatus to "demonstrate" that an invisible hand works to assure general equilibrium in that social handiwork of God, the self-regulating market system.

The ancient and medieval understanding of the soul was displaced from the heart to the brain and nervous system by dogged anatomical research – dissection, hypothesis and experiment. But it took a few centuries before anyone cared to use the dissection theatre for anything other than demonstration of the accepted doctrine. Eventually, however, one young surgeon was struck by inconsistencies between the ancient texts and what he saw in contemporary corpses. He came ultimately to the conclusion that the writers of those texts had not actually dissected and accurately described *human* bodies. This was Vesalius of Padua, whose empirical assault on the world *inside* was simultaneous with re-arrangement of the cosmos. In the same year (1543) that Vesalius "overturned the understanding of human anatomy", Copernicus "altered the anatomy of the world" (25).

Both understood that they were speaking sacrilege as well as nonsense, for they contradicted the authority of established knowledge and the recognized custodians of those beliefs. Caution is always in order when declaring that the emperor is naked, for even if the direct penalty is only social it can also be deadly.

Exploration of the world inside continued, but in a more tentative spirit given Vesalius' discovery (and the new spirit generally of looking directly at nature rather than relying on ancient texts). More than a century was to pass before Thomas Willis published *The Anatomy of the Brain and Nerves*, in 1664. (It was illustrated by Christopher Wren, who was working simultaneously on his first major triumph as an architect (182).) By that time explorers in the trail of Vesalius had made several strides, most important being those of William Harvey. As a young doctor, Harvey studied at Padua (1600) and became steeped in the empirical spirit by reading Aristotle and watching his professors apply it in the dissection theatre. In that context, he made the first observation (valves in the veins) that led him to discover the nature of the blood circulation system and the correct role of the heart. His focus on blood led him on to other observations that gradually developed into views that while obvious to his empiricist eye were nonetheless radical to his peers in the Royal College of Physicians. Once he had conceived the idea of the circulatory system, Harvey designed experiments to test it, and demonstrated them before the College of Physicians. Then, in 1628 he published the book which presented his argument "with terse, elegant precision". He dedicated it to the College in the hope of winning their endorsement, given that he had "first propounded it to you, confirmed it by ocular testimony, answered your doubts and objections, and gotten the President's verdict in my favour" (72).

Harvey's Professional Reputation Suffered

They dismissed his book, however, and Harvey's reputation as a physician suffered. Since he disagreed with the ancient authorities, he must be wrong. To many physicians, he "simply did not speak the language of medicine. They opened his book expecting a formal philosophical argument. Instead, they found something else entirely. To his contemporaries, Harvey seemed like the body's accountant, tallying up ounces and quarts when he ought to be thinking like a philosopher" (73). By that time Harvey was 50 years old, and hardly anyone in England accepted his idea for another 20 years. In the turmoil of civil war and revolution, however, he found a ready audience in the circle around Thomas Willis at Oxford. It was after learning from him about his discoveries – and most of all his methods – that this new generation began an intensive assault to understand the role and functions of the brain.

The year following publication of *The Anatomy of the Brain and Nerves* plague devastated London, and the next year it was destroyed by the Great Fire. On invitation of the Archbishop, Thomas Willis joined the rest of his Oxford circle colleagues in London to assist in the rebuilding. There Willis built the first major medical practice in England's history and became the most famous physician in the country, "perhaps in all Europe" (215-6). In the words of a contemporary, "never any physician before went beyond him, or got more money yearly than he." His theories were hugely popular, "yet his remedies remained, as ever, generally useless." He nonetheless became the first truly great neuroscientist in part because of his medical reputation. Because of it, he was permitted to dissect the bodies of aristocratic patients. "For the first time in the history of medicine, Willis could link the disorders that people experienced in life to the abnormalities he found in the brains after death. Because the brains belonged to England's ruling class, it became hard for his readers to dismiss his observations. The respectability of his success allowed Willis to expand his mechanical, chemical explanations of the brain to include the soul itself without being accused of heresy" (217).

Locke was an avid student of Willis, became a medical researcher and practitioner himself, and then veered away from the anatomical approach to one based on observation of symptoms and their response to different treatments. This search for patterns enables the identification and classification of disease syndromes – another kind of empiricism. Locke was following another transplanted Oxford doctor on this path. Thomas Sydenham's understanding was that "Nature by herself determines diseases, and is of herself sufficient in all things against all of them. The best a physician could do would be 'joining hands with nature.'" He and Locke did not believe that Willis's efforts to discover the mind by mapping the brain could ever succeed. Detailing the nature and structure of its parts could never explain its functioning (246). An analogue would be Keynes' impatience with the dogged focus on microeconomic analysis when it was the pattern of financial flows that was causing the symptoms of an acute social disease.

But for all Locke's skepticism about his teacher's project, Willis's neurology runs through *An Essay Concerning Human Understanding* like buried steel beams, invisibly bearing the weight of Locke's philosophy. Our understanding is limited by our anatomy – an anatomy which Locke quietly borrowed from Willis's dissections. Ideas, Locke wrote, come to the mind from the outside world through the nerves. None of the ordinary experience that Locke so treasured could have revealed this to him. Locke's isolated mind, its blank sheet of paper, and countless other details already existed in the lectures that Willis delivered to him in his student days. Locke was giving his old teacher a compliment that was at once backhanded and profound: Willis's brain had become an agreed-upon fact, one that didn't even need pointing out (256).

Dissecting Economic Dogma, an Inherently Political Belief

So ends the tale. Now, are there lessons for economic reformers? For one, structures are important and should be subject to examination, especially when the whole system is not working satisfactorily. A good example was provided by law professor Bakan's recent dissection of *The Corporation*. Similarly, we know that monetary and financial institutions have become a far different and more significant element in the economic system than they were at mid-century. Textbooks and core curricula in economics education, however, do not reflect this circumstance. Can this be because no one knows enough to look for structural and operational details? Doubtful, since such investigations used to be a regular activity for economists. Our problem seems not so much to exhume the structures, examine defects and prescribe cures as it is to resist a campaign for the Sydenham analogy that the mechanism is basically healthy and will self-correct. The difference for our domain is that cures from the past based on anatomical (structural) analysis are known to have worked. Our adversary is not ignorance of uncharted territory but rather the return to reverent contemplation of an elegant structure deduced from imaginary premises. Galbraith has called this an *Innocent Fraud*; others call it deliberate deception. Our problem is not one of knowing how to conduct effective research; it is rather one of resisting propaganda wielded by unconstrained power.

Economics is an inherently political discipline. It became the queen of the social sciences by providing the guiding logic for social reform from its emergence out of moral philosophy and political arithmetic in the 17th century. [Its practitioners] developed a rationale for freeing markets from the post-medieval privileges and power of Europe's landed aristocracies, bankers and monopolies. [Today], the vested interests are all for big government as long as they can control it. Real estate, minerals and finance have carved out niches to promote their interests while striving to paralyze the ability of government to regulate or tax them. The real aim of neoliberal ideology thus concerns who shall control government and the economy: elected officials or unelected financial managers. (*From Michael Hudson, in a forthcoming book.*)

Keith Wilde

Crazy Crossword Puzzle from Babel Tower

"GLOBALIZATION AND DEREGULATION" takes a beating as you browse through a single issue of *The Wall Street Journal* (8/07). The European Union is bringing in another 15 Eastern European nations, but Germany's road system is not up to the explosion of traffic that will ensue. The article "Roadblocks to EU Integration" by Matthew Karnitschnig informs us: "Germany's Autobahns Hit Bumps at Every Attempt to Expand: Dresden – As Europe struggles with political and economic integration of its new members, mostly in Eastern Europe, it has hit a very concrete problem: the sorry state of infrastructure linking the EU's old and new members. At its heart are Germany's once legendary autobahns, which over the years inspired other nations to build highway systems. Autobahns have become so contentious that building even the shortest link has become a near impossibility, leading to tie-ups at border crossings and traffic jams that snake across the countryside.

"Armin Beck, a senior official of the local autobahn office has spent years trying to persuade the local community to close the gap with a road that would allow seamless travel between Scandinavia and the Balkans. He peers across the Czech border and traces an index finger through the air along the contours of the hilly countryside to complete the missing link.

"'The opponents and interest groups range from residents to insects. At the moment bats are the big issue.' In Germany a spate of environmental laws – many adopted in the past 15 years – allow almost unlimited challenges to road construction. Despite the fall of the Iron Curtain over a decade ago, Germany hasn't been able to complete a single autobahn line along its 100-mile border with the Czech Republic. So in Dresden, an endless column of trucks snakes out of town [one of the architectural gems of the world beautifully restored] toward a narrow mountain pass and the Czech frontier. After German unification in 1990, the government made building the autobahn stretch a top priority. That is when Mr. Reck, a former political adviser and journalist, arrived to help sell local residents on the project. 'I had no idea what it would entail.'" Nor apparently did anybody else.

"It took seven years of meetings, environmental impact studies and public hearings to dig the first hole in 1998. Officials decided their best bet lay in accommodating the ever increasing list of demands. Stopping his truck on a deserted paved stretch near the beginning of the new autobahn, Mr. Reck hops out and points to a tunnel covered in fresh sod. 'This is the so-called green bridge, he says. The ¤5 million construction consists of two 1,100-foot long tunnels that wouldn't be necessary under normal circumstances. The hill it burrows under is made of soft soil, not rock. But preservationists demanded the tunnel to preserve a stand of trees on top of the hill.

"Further down the road, officials built a 600-foot bridge for deer and other wildlife. amphibians got 25 escape pipes and a 1,000-foot bridge. A rare species of bat known as 'small horseshoe nose' got a special tunnel that includes ultrasound technology to guide them through."

The point is not whether this is justified or not. Rather it is that such items – especially in a country where Greens are a political force – cannot be considered an "externality" to an all-wise "free market."

However, the absurdity of what passes as prudent budgeting only starts there.

How Germany Financed the World's Original Autobahns in the Depths of the Depression, But Can't Today

"Delays in improving and expanding the network in Germany have been compounded by new members' own transportation deficiencies. The EU transportation department says the region needs 12,500 miles of new roads, 18,700 miles of railroad track and numerous ports and airports, but such projects would cost $738.5 billion, money neither the EU nor individual countries can raise." Amazingly, it does not occur either to the EU, its component countries, or even the *WSJ* reporter to ask, if that is so, how did Germany manage to build the original Autobahns in the midst of the Depression, and how did the world manage to finance the reconstruction of Europe after a decade of depression and six years of war? And if the present impecuniousness were the case, why did they rush into the union and Globalization and Deregulation? Was it that they left such details to the eternal wisdom of a supposedly "self-balancing market"?

But immediately above this first article is another by Marcus Walker ("Germany Expected to Approve Deep Cut in Jobless Aid"): "Frankfurt – Officials expect a majority in Germany's upper house to approve – across party lines – a sharp reduction of generous state benefits for the long-term unemployed, a step aimed at pushing the jobless back to work. The measures go beyond the more modest abatements of other euro-zone economies, except for the Netherlands' changes in the 1990s. Until now, a German who hasn't worked for more than a year receives unemployment benefits at 53% of his most recent net wage, plus supplements for local and family circumstances, for an unlimited period. The new law would replace this with a flat rate of ¤345 (US $426) per month, plus rent and family supplements. Many economists say Germany's proposals will fall short of restoring economic dynamism.

"German employers have long advocated such measures, but labor unions strongly oppose the government's steps as socially unjust. Last weekend, former party members and labor unionists – who traditionally have backed the Social Democrats – launched preparations for a new left-wing political party to challenge the government in elections.

"The government also has sought to bring the present and long-term costs of state health and pension provisions under control. This year it has limited the number of prescription drugs covered by state health insurance and introduced a ¤10 fee per quarter for visiting a doctor or dentist."

Nor does that single issue of *WSJ* stop there in confounding the reader. Let's go back to the front page ("After Winning Jobs, European City Looks Over Its Shoulder – Timisoara, Romania, Struggles to Keep Outsourcing Boom" by Dan Bilefsky): "Timisoara – In this Transylvanian city, where the 1989 revolution that overthrew Romania's dictatorship began, dozens of young software engineers sit hunched over computers in a neighborhood still pocked with bullet holes inflicted by the Communist army. They are some of the beneficiaries of this city's decade-long drive to transform itself into a high-tech center.

"But Mirea Stoinescu, a 22-year-old in a Hugo Boss suit with the label left on the sleeve, says he would trade in Timisoara's war-scarred offices for the real Silicon Valley in an instant. 'Why would I want to wait around here 20 years for wages to rise when I can get what I want to-morrow? I want my Opel Astra and I want it now.'

"Timisoara spent years successfully promoting its pool of talented engineers and its prime location between East and West. The giant pig-processing plant that once dominated the local economy has been obscured with high-tech factories of Alcatel SA, Siemens AG, and Selectron Corp. Some 5,000 foreign companies have moved here, and still more are on the way.

"But Romania's push to join the European Union in 2007 will likely force the country to abandon many of the incentives drawing companies to invest here – including a zero percent income-tax rate for software engineers. City fathers worry that a brain drain could leave Timisoara little better off than it was in 1989, when 150,000 triumphant demonstrators unfurled a flag over the town's opera house proclaiming the city Romania's first democratic stronghold. Already wages are rising, and some multinationals warn they will move further east to Ukraine, Russia or China if the city can't retain its competitive advantage. Romanian technology specialists say about a third of the nation's information-tech professionals left last year, lured by pay increases as much as tenfold."

Romania's "Little Vienna" Faces a Trying Waltz

"The challenges Timisoara faces are part of the global chase to the bottom of the wage scale that is pitting Mexican manufacturing plants, which took jobs from places like Detroit and Raleigh, NC, against even cheaper producers like China.

"Timisoara, a city of winding canals and imposing squares, is known by Romanians as 'little Vienna' because of its baroque architecture. The first European city to install electric street lamps in 1881, it has always been more outward-looking than the rest of the country. During the Cold War, Romanians flocked here to buy black-market Levi jeans and banned copies of George Orwell's *1984* smuggled from nearby Yugoslavia. While state TV under the dictatorship consisted of two channels showing the late dictator Nicolae Ceausescu's speeches, Timisoara's technically-minded locals watched CNN, using makeshift satellite dishes hidden on their rooftops.

"Other eastern European countries such as Hungary and the Czech Republic that just joined the EU have been benefiting from a bigger flow of foreign investment. But Romanian costs are lower, and it has increasingly been stealing business from those countries as their wages advanced. While the average Hungarian monthly wage has jumped 20% in the past two years to about $720, the average in Romania is about a quarter of that. About 2,000 of Romania's 6,000 information technol-

ogy professionals emigrated last year, though the outflow has slowed with a tightening of the global job market. Romanian engineers are among the biggest group of foreign nationals working in Redmond, Wash.

"Others ask, 'Why should I want to leave?' He adds that his cost of living in Romania will buy him nearly five times as much as it would in Palo Alto."

To all of which, must be added a missing footnote. Every time, for any of multiple cut-throat reasons, a mass emigration takes place from one country to another, vast investments in plant, educational facilities, or in human capital become worthless, or lost to the jurisdiction that made them. What economist or accountant even tries to make that necessary adjustment to the "greater efficiencies" of Globalization and Deregulation that politicians prate about?

William Krehm

The Pressure Continues to Mount

Ms. Andrea Rivest
Town of Lakeshore
Office of the Clerk
Belle River, Ontario

Dear Ms. Rivest:

Mr. Andre Marentette has asked me to comment on the letter you have received from the Honourable Ralph Goodale, Minister of Finance of Canada dated 16/08, in reply to yours of June 11. In this I read this amazing passage:

"I have noted the suggestion that the Bank of Canada be instructed to hold a greater proportion of government debt by buying securities issued by municipalities and refunding interest charges. However, the problem with this action is that to acquire the government debt, the Bank of Canada would have to print new currency. The rapid growth in the money supply would eventually result in an increase in inflation and higher rates of interest."

Our Finance Minister misses the point. To bail out our banks from their speculative long-shots during the 1980s in financing gas and oil, real estate in New York and London, and the sudden urge of a well-connected Ottawa builder to collect entire US department store chains, the Mulroney government revised the *Bank Act* in 1991.[1] This discontinued the requirement that our banks redeposit with the Bank of Canada a modest part of the deposits received from the public in their chequing accounts. On these deposits the banks were paid no interest. These "statutory reserves" served several purposes:

A. They reimbursed the government for its surrender to the banks of much of the modern equivalent of the monarch's ancestral monopoly in coining precious metals – creating credit money. Since the early 1970s when the US went off the gold standard, the only legal tender has been central government debt. The statutory reserves provided the government with more elbow room for borrowing from the Bank of Canada within existing constraints. And since 1938, when a Liberal government nationalized the Bank of Canada, all interest paid on loans it holds – including those made to the government itself – finds its way back to the central government as its sole stockholder – less an overhead charge – as dividends. In essence loans made by the central bank to the federal government are a virtual interest-free loan to the government. By abolishing the statutory reserves, the Mulroney government increased the private banks' ability to take on more debt as a multiple of the cash it held, and decreased the amount of borrowing the federal government itself could do from its central bank. It therefore had to do far more borrowing from the commercial banks. On this it not only paid interest, but rates of interest that were being pushed into the sky by the wild policy of imposing a flat price level ("zero inflation") on a society that was providing costly infrastructures to accommodate new technologies, rapid urbanization, and a growing population. The Minister badly misstates the case in writing that "the bank would have to print new currency."

Shortly before the phasing out of the statutory reserves in Canada, The Bank for International Settlements' *Risk-Based Capital Requirements* introduced to deal with the crisis of banks throughout the Western World, declared the debt of the advanced countries to be "risk-free" and hence requiring no cash down payment.[2]

There is a ready answer to the Minister's concerns about inflation, one that worked spectacularly well in chapters of our history that have been suppressed. Our government's accountancy still makes no distinction between the federal government's investments in physical and human capital, between the purchase of soap for its lavatories and its outlay for the acquisition of a building, the building of a bridge, or its contribution to the education and health of the population. Though these assets will be used for decades, they are written off in a single year. Were that done in the private sector, there would be few solvent corporations in the land.

It is true that on the insistence of the previous Auditor General, Denis Desautels, Mr. Paul Martin as Finance Minister after weeks of bargaining agreed to phase in capital budgeting that would enter the value of the asset acquired to balance the cost of acquiring it. When the compromise finally reached between Mr. Martin as Finance Minister and the Auditor General was finally adopted in 1999, there was no parliamentary debate on the subject, no press release. Essentially it was accomplished in stealth. That is evidenced by the official position for paying down the debt to one half of its present amount. The fact is that, with proper accountancy brought into the federal books there would probably be little if any net debt. Be that as may, capital budgeting provides a strict disciplinary framework to avoid inflation. Only really necessary infrastructures – physical like water systems and sewers, or human like education and health – could be financed through the Bank of Canada over periods better reflecting their usefulness. And this could be done by an arrangement between Ottawa and the junior levels of government reducing the effective interest cost to the municipalities to a nominal amount.

In the last two years, the Federal Reserve System in the US and the Bank for International Settlements, came to make the distinction between "good inflation" (up to anywhere from 2% to 4%) and "bad inflation" beyond that. That was a less than forthcoming recognition of the fact that a high-tech, rapidly urbanizing society, such as ours, has need for far more elaborate infrastructures than the semi-rural Canada of a couple of generations ago, and such infrastructures are paid for through taxation. Our price level therefore must be seen as having two distinct components – one indicating real inflation and another portion of price rise that merely reflects that more infrastructure financed by taxation due to an excess of demand over supply throughout the economy.

No economist moving from a town of 10,000 to New York City expects his living costs to remain unchanged. Why then should they expect prices to stay flat when humanity as a whole is making just such a move? Such an agreement between the different levels of government would finally resolve the endless bickering amongst them that has made Canadian politics so ugly since the cost of bailing out our banks was passed on to the provinces and brought on the cutting of grants to our municipalities.

Please feel free to make whatever use of this letter that you see fit. I will make myself available to enlarge and further document its content wherever and whenever you feel that it might serve a useful purpose.

William Krehm, Editor, Economic Reform

1. Subsection (4) of Section 457 of Chapter 46 of the Statutes of Canada 1991.
2. This of course contradicted the policy of shifting the government's borrowing from an effective interest-free basis from the central bank to the private banks. For when banks load up with government debt 100% leveraged, and central banks push up interest rates to flatten out prices ("zero inflation") as happened at the same time, their previously acquired bond hoards with lower coupons than the current rate result in a massive loss of capital. That in fact almost brought down the world monetary financial system between 1994 and 1997.

Repetitive Fraud at Every Level of our Public Life Points to Something More Frightening

FRAUD IN OUR PUBLIC LIFE has echoed and spread on a scale suggestive of a deeper significance than is recognized by the guardians at our gates. Nortel, Canada's fourth most valuable company that a few years ago fell from $114 dollars a share into low single-digit territory in a matter of months, is once again stricken with dropsy. *The Globe and Mail* (16/03, "Nortel put money men on leave" by Dave Ebner) reports Nortel Networks Corp. rocked again as it put its chief financial officer and its controller on paid leave until a second review of the company's financial results is finished. This has driven its stock down nearly 20%. Nortel surprised investors last week when it said it would likely have to restate its financial results for the second time in several months. The second review, conducted independently by an external law firm and Nortel's audit committee, is continuing. Regulators in Canada and the US are now making enquiries as well. Such concerns slashed $6.5 billion from the market value of Nortel yesterday. The shares fell $1.60 or 18.7% – one of Nortel's worst percentage declines to date."

Portentously, Canada's foremost information technology corporation seems unable to transmit the most vital data on its internal affairs to its shareholders.

On the same front page of the *G&M* ("Banks to pay record fine in US mutual fund scandal" by Shawn McCarthy) relates "Bank of America and FleetBoston Financial have agreed to pay $675 million (US) over allegations of mutual fund industry abuses, the biggest settlement to date in continuing efforts to clean up the scandal-tinged industry. The deal was brokered by New York State Attorney General Eliot Spitzer and the US Securities and Exchange Commission and includes a reduction in fees at Mr. Spitzer's insistence. The settlement also requires eight members of the Bank of America's Nations Funds board of directors to resign their seats.

"The settlement is the fourth since investigations into trading abuses at mutual funds began last September. So far, these settlements have totalled $1.65 billion."

Canada, for its part, has still to even pretend reining in the massive irregularities on its stock markets. Possibly our Prime Minister will seize upon the US example to help his budget-balancing ambitions, and lay off victimizing the most vulnerable sectors of our society.

There are aspects of NY Attorney General Spitzer's activities that could serve as a model for Canada's authorities.

"Bank of America has agreed to pay and the significant reforms it has agreed to implement reflect the seriousness of the misconduct in this matter. The SEC's director of enforcement, Stephen Cutler, indicated that the investigation is not over and more actions against Bank of America employees could follow. Bank of America has agreed to pay $375 million, including $250 million in disgorgement of ill-gotten-profits and $125 million in penalties." These payments and the significant reforms it has agreed to reflect the seriousness of the misconduct in this matter,' Mr. Cutler said.

"FleetBoston will pay $149 million, including $70 million in disgorgement and $70 million in penalties Under a separate agreement with Mr. Spitzer's office, Bank of America and Fleet-Boston agreed to reduce the fees they charge to investors by $160 million over the next five years [all figures are in US dollars]." "Disgorgement" is an unlovely but apt word. Our banks, deregulated further after being bailed out in the early 1990s have likewise gorged themselves on the real economy.

"Last month the SEC and Mr. Spitzer alleged in a civil lawsuit that FleetBoston's two mutual fund subsidiaries engaged in massive trading abuses over a five-year period that harmed ordinary investors."

Here again, the abusive fees charged "ordinary investors" by Bank of America and FleetBoston were reduced by $160 mil-lion over the next five years. This might be a good example that Mr. Martin might take, since he has announced his intention to follow American leads more closely. It would also be a means of repairing his dented reputation amongst Canadians. Among the Canadian "ordinary investors" that we would particularly recommend to the attention of his government are the those with margin accounts who can only be described as fair game for bank-owned brokerages to recoup their losses and fines imposed on them by the US authorities.

In the US the SEC, spurred on by the prosecution successes of the Attorney General of New York, Spitzer, are moving towards investigating the prevalence of abuses throughout an entire industry, when detected in a few cases. Thus the *WSJ* (18/03, "SEC broadens problems" by Deborah Solomon): "SEC officials said they are trying to determine whether questionable behaviour in one or two companies signals problems throughout an industry.... The agency is now establishing an Office of Risk Assessment to help identify problems before they become widespread.... The enforcement division's broad inquiry into oil company reserves was based, in part on concerns raised by the corporation finance division. The SEC is investigating whether Shell overstated its energy reserve as well as El Paso Corp's reserve accounting.

Is Our Government Catching Bad Habits from Our Corporations?

"Another broad probe is examining whether some high-tech companies undervalued stock options for executives by issuing options just before valuing options to current stock price. If companies know positive information – such as good earnings – is coming that will raise the stock, they are obliged to value the options by factoring in the increased stock price."

Once such enquiry keeps on broadening to take in entire areas of the economy, it will not be able to stop before reaching the public sector. Because the games played by private corporations in treating liabilities as assets, and occasionally hiding this year's excessive earnings to create the impression of a steady escalation of earnings into the distant future, was never interrupted by a drop. That puffs up the stock price beyond reality. The case of Freddie Mac, the government-sponsored mortgage syndication corporation made the headlines for just such a scam. But is that not what our Mr. Martin has been doing salting away $4 billion dollars of "reserves," while exaggerating a deficit that was already rigged by treating government investments as current spending?

If you carry this further to take in broader ideological causes rather than just corporate crimes, you end up indicting an economic doctrine that identifies the economy with a highly idealized market that never existed. And attributing to it all the wisdom and treating all other non-market factors essential to social well-bring – health, education, environmental conservation of social well-being – as "externalities." Is that not exactly what rogue corporations do in their domains? And isn't the survival requirement of exponential growth imposed by the stock market a main source of the trouble? Does that leave any space for morality?

William Krehm

Why is the US Economy Still Slow?

NEW JOBS created in July came in at 32,000; well below the 150,000 new jobs the economy needs to create every month just to keep up with labor force growth. Since the expectation had been over 200,000, this was an unpleasant surprise. Obviously, the recovery is still in a painful phase seen from the point of wage earners.

Why isn't the economy returning to persistent job growth, when other key economic measures such as GDP and productivity growth are not looking too bad? Especially the strong growth of productivity – defined as value added of output per hour worked in the non-farm business sector – is puzzling. It reached a top of 9.5% in the third quarter of 2003 and 5% for the whole year, in an economy still with only sluggish job creation.

At the forefront of the debate about what caused this has been productivity measures' relation to offshoring. If offshoring widens the margin between a business's inputs and outputs, it can show in statistics as heightened productivity by the remaining domestic employees.

However, there are divergent views on the ramifications of cost and profit relations in offshoring. A view, critical of unbridled offshoring, maintains that it mostly is undertaken in search of lower labor costs to make room for higher profit margins. And in the next step, when the products from the offshore production reenter the domestic market, businesses depending on much higher labor costs cannot compete. Therefore, they either buckle under or themselves go offshore, causing further domestic job losses.

The defense for offshoring claims that many companies face competitive pressures, that make offshoring inevitable for survival. But, the claim is there is no need for worry for the process also weeds outs inefficient industries, freeing up resources to develop growth and jobs in more forward-looking sectors.

Certainly, but extending this happy scenario to a general rule is too optimistic. Among other things, it glosses over the fact that the production costs in developing countries are not just caused by lower wages attributable to lower living standards. Currency relations are also a major part of the picture.

Exchange rates are determined by a set of complex factors, among which traditional economics mentions trade balances, general level of economic development, expectations of future general growth. However, besides, the ability of such countries to attract and accumulate financial assets, also play an important role in today's currency relations.

These massively favour the economic developed nations, and creates a systemic overvaluation of their currencies compared to the levels that would prevail, if standards of living and derived local production costs were the main factor. Therefore, when companies from advanced economies invest in developing nations with the purpose of offshoring production (as distinguished from investments to enter the local market), their possible margin gains from the lower local production costs are amplified by the prevailing system of exchange rates.

The Marginal Productivity of Workers

Offshoring in manufacturing was already developing at a high rate in the mid-eighties. What is new is that it is now spreading to the services industries, causing jobs to be lost in market segments employing fairly high-skilled and high-paid workers, who used to think that job losses to offshoring only happened to other folks. This new reach of the phenomenon, and the perpetually growing trade deficit, has clearly sharpened the debate.

Neoclassical theory assumes that the marginal productivity of factors always will have a market price at which it becomes profitable for someone to employ them. This theory was formulated under the assumption of closed laissez-faire markets.

However, the current deregulated and open, globalized market conditions create large pools of liquid financial assets constantly sloshing around the globe seeking maximal returns. This is a very different picture than the one envisaged by the neoclassical economists. In their world, the role of financial markets was to passively connect demands for savings and investment. The reality is that modern financial markets, with highly asymmetric accumulations of liquid financial assets, instead of passively responding to trends in the real economy, often create the forces driving them.

Meanwhile, when outsourcing takes place within a nation state, or between nations having comparable level of economic development and asset accumulations, the marginal productivities of factors run along gliding scales. Thus, for example, if a company outsources a production to another company operating in a comparable cost environment, only relatively small shifts in the marginal relations will occur.

Most employees laid off as a result of such outsourcing will be able to find employment at similar wages, since their factor potential has not been significantly lowered. And since both the outsourcing company and the new producer reap comparative advantages by presumably focusing on what they are best at doing, the situation creates an aggregate productivity gain, much as predicted by neoclassical economics.

During the long economic expansion of the 1950s and 1960s, rising levels of trade took place between the developing nations. This was a result of increasing specialization along the above lines, connected to what Michael Porter has called the existence of differences in 'competitive clusters' between the developed nations. In other words, the growth in trade was caused by technological specialization in comparable cost environments, which meant that the gains primarily were caused by raising the marginal physical product.

Contrasting this, the growth in trade is today largely occurring between nations with very disparate levels of development and cost environments. Thus, the focus is no longer on technological specialization but on cost reduction. However, even though no enhancement of the marginal physical product have occurred, productivity – calculated as the money valued margin between businesses inputs and output per worked hour – will go up since the company's domestic operations will show a higher value-added generated by the remaining employees. If anything, marginal physical product is probably lower at the offshore location, but this is more than compensated for by the other, lower cost factors, including exchange rate differences.

When employees lose their jobs to offshoring under such conditions, it is often part of industry-wide trends, causing market demand for labour to fall precipitately. This makes it next to impossible for laid-off workers to find comparable work based on their current levels of skills.

This means that when offshoring and trade between nations with widely divergent development levels take place, marginal productivities of labor resources will no longer run along gliding scales but occur in downwards jump-shifts. Therefore, the process will not only lead to rising unemployment, but also cause the market price on the marginal productivity of workers to fall sharply, depressing the wages of workers still in employed in the sector.

As a result, if compared to outsourcing, offshoring is much more disruptive to employment. The connected sharp downwards shift in the market demand for workers with skills tailored to the affected industries means that many of them will never be able to find work at their previous income levels; and for those who will, it will take longer and involve retraining.

The Role of the Propensity to Consume

If productivity growth is high and wages stagnant, the productivity gains must turn up as income by other factors holders. Whether it is as executive pay, dividends, or retained earnings translating into capital gains, a reasonable assumption is that it mostly will accrue to individuals with higher incomes than wage-dependent workers.

Differences in propensities to consume between income groups play an important role in determining how offshoring influence domestic demand and consumption. Most wage-earners belong to middle-income households, which on a relative scale have higher propensities to consume than high incomes households. Therefore, if offshoring heightens productivity without generating a comparable growth in wages, it follows that it also affects the aggregate propensity to consume negatively. And since high incomes households also have a higher import ratio of their consumption, the propensity to consume domestic products, which stimulates the economy most strongly, falls even more.

Offshoring, a persistent trend since the mid-1980s, has created an accumulative effect as the growing trade imbalance bears witness. It has played a role in the stagnation of middle-class incomes, and the fall in the propensity to consume based on incomes.

What partly has kept consumption up and the economy going has been growth in debt levels. But as interest payments start to crowd out other expenditures, consumption will again show weakness. We appear to have reached such a point. Significantly, the tax cuts implemented by Bush missed their mark by failing to address this problem. In fact the tax cuts, by mainly benefiting high incomes households, added to the weakness of the aggregate propensity to consume.

Economic policies, which will restore wage growth and the share of disposable incomes for the middle class, as well as address the problem of the falling consumption of domestic produced goods and services, must return to center stage. Unless this happens, the US economy will not be likely to reenter a period of renewed stable growth,

Dix Sandbeck

Questions to The Globe and Mail

IN AN AMAZING EDITORIAL *The Globe and Mail* (16/10/04, "A few questions for Mr. Mulroney") poses queries to our former Prime Minister that bounce back to hit Canada's "national paper" squarely in the eye. It takes Mr. Mulroney to task for maintaining a suspect silence on dealings of his during and immediately after his tenure of office.

"By the time Brian Mulroney announced his retirement from politics in late February of 1993, he had become one of the most reviled prime ministers in Canadian history. One habitually heard jibes about his prominent chin, his mellifluous basso voice, his taste in footwear and his affection for Americana. On Feb. 25, 1993, this newspaper ran the headline, 'Mulroney resigns: Praise scant for PM's tenure, economic policy seen as main failing.'

"Perhaps partly because of Mr. Mulroney's unpopularity at the time, the investigative tomes that emerged soon after he stepped down – alleging rampant corruption and kickbacks during his tenure – found a ready audience. It was in this climate that the RCMP launched its now notorious corruption investigation in 1995. None of the RCMP's allegations against Mr. Mulroney were ever proven. He sued the government and won an apology and a $2 million settlement.

"Meanwhile the fruits of his 'failed' economic policies were just beginning to emerge, and his legacy was starting to crystallize. During his tenure, short-term interest rates had been pushed from the high teens to below 5 per cent. Inflation had dropped from 11 per cent to below 2 per cent. He had instituted the goods and service tax which became an enormous fiscal gusher, boosting federal revenues by $20 billion annually by the end of the 1990s. He had begun fighting the deficit, steadily reducing its size as a percentage of gross domestic product throughout his years in office, though the deficit grew in absolute terms to $42 billion in his final budget. More important, he had introduced free trade, which became an enormous growth generator. Between 1997 and 2001 exports grew by 37 per cent. Today, 85 per cent of Canada's exports go to the United States."

Short-Term Interest Rates had been Pushed into the Skies

"And yet, despite a policy record that bears up exceptionally well as the years pass, and despite the absolute discrediting of the RCMP's 1995 case against him, some of the more difficult questions about Mr. Mulroney refuse to go away entirely.

"Last year, *The Globe and Mail* revealed for the first time that Mr. Mulroney, within a short time of leaving office had accepted $300,000 in payment from German businessman Karlheinz Schreiber, reportedly in exchange for his help in launching a pasta business. In his new book *A Secret Trial,* author William Kaplan adds detail to those accounts. He chronicles how Mr. Mulroney, just months after leaving office, received $100,000 in cash from Mr. Schreiber. The money was stuffed into an envelope and handed over in a Montreal hotel. The rest of the $300,000 was paid the following year, always in cash, always in hotels.

"Mr. Mulroney has already tacitly acknowledged that he should never have met with Mr. Schreiber. In a *Globe* interview last November, he blamed the lapse on the people who introduced them, saying, 'If you accumulated all the sorrow over all of my life, it does not compare to the agony and anguish I have gone through since I met Schreiber. I should never have been introduced to him because the people who introduced me to him didn't know him.'

"Nevertheless, Mr. Mulroney refused to discuss the affair at length, instead relying on his official spokesman, Luc Lavoie, to repeat a simple mantra. The payments were legal. No rules were broken, all income taxes were paid. End of story.

"And yet there is a great deal that Mr. Mulroney could clarify. Why did he accept this much money, just months after leaving office, and with a businessman with a long history of lobbying the federal Tories? Why wasn't the payment made through a wire transfer or bank draft, as is common for large sums? What service, exactly, did Mr. Mulroney perform for the work? And what were the terms of the contract and why are the details about the pasta venture so imprecise?

"Nearly 12 years on, it's clear that Brian Mulroney made an exceptional mark on the economic life of this country. In service of that legacy, Mr. Mulroney should clear the air once and for all about his dealing with Karlheinz Schreiber."

Now let us have our former PM step out of the witness box, and let us ask the editor of *The Globe and Mail* to replace him there to shed light on the incredible assumptions in this editorial. For these suggest a cover-up even more fraught with consequence for this land than the Schreiber transaction.

There is the statement "Meantime, the fruits of his 'failed' economic policies were just beginning to emerge, and his legacy was starting to crystallize. During his tenure, short-term interest rates had been pushed from the high teens to below 5 per cent. Inflation had dropped from 11 per cent to below 2 per cent."

This was a time when Bill Clinton thrashed the elder Bush at the polls with the slogan "It's the economy stupid!." And even under a regime less servile than that of Mulroney, before the Canadian economy was opened widely to US domination as it is today, a prosperous Canada alongside a depressed United States was inconceivable The editorial cites 85% of our exports going to US as a strength rather than a vulnerability. The horrendous high-teen interest rates to which the editorialist refers did not drop from heaven, but were the "one blunt tool" that the Mulroney government imported from Washington.

That was imposed on this country to achieve "zero inflation." In the United States Paul Volcker, governor of the Federal

Reserves, was determined to "lick inflation," whatever the cost; and at the same time the Bank of Canada imported from the IMF John Crow, whose background had been in cracking the whip to keep near-bankrupt Latin American republics in line. Canada was not bankrupt, and in no way indebted to the International Monetary Fund, but the Mulroney government and the Bank of Canada acted as though it were.

Though the government has been the sole shareholder of the BoC since 1938, and Section 14 of the Act sets out the powers of the Minister of Finance to dismiss the Governor of the Bank in the case of a disagreement on basic Bank policy,[1] the Mulroney government conducted an elaborate campaign to introduce "zero inflation" and the independence of the Bank of Canada from the Government into the constitution. Only the opposition of the Finance Committee caucuses of the three major parties blocked the measure.

The Largest Bank Heist Ever

However, under Mulroney the government acted as though the proposed measures had become law of the land. University economic departments were purged through early retirement of any staff that did not conform to the new evangel. Economic texts were cleansed of any reference to the use of the Bank of Canada for which it had been founded – the low pegged interest rates that made it possible for the Bank of Canada to finance our Second World War at low rates, and catch up with ten years of neglect of our infrastructure and six years of war, while assimilating a vast penniless immigration from Europe.

And during this time our government managed to reduce a national debt that amounted to over 160% of the GNP at the end of the war to a mere 22% by the mid-seventies. It was under Mulroney, when bone-crunching interest rates were brought in to "lick inflation," that the debt soared once more. The great unspoken secret never even alluded to in *The Globe and Mail* or the other media, was the vast redistribution of the national income to permit the banks to recoup their stunning losses in financing speculative gas and oil, real estate and other ventures incompatible with responsible banking.

Prior to 1991, the Bank of Canada had two major weapons for combatting perceived inflation. It could raise the overnight bank rate that banks charged for making loans to one another to meet their overnight reserve shortfalls. This served as the benchmark for longer-term rates throughout the economy. Or, alternatively, it could raise the statutory reserves – at the time some 6% to 10% of the deposits it took in from the public in its chequing accounts. That decreased the amount of loans the banks were able to make, and thus cooled the economy without hitting everything in the economy with sky-high interest. But in 1991 Ottawa came to the rescue of our banks from their gambling losses by phasing out the statutory reserves over a two-year period. Those reserves had earned the banks no interest in recognition of the surrender to them of the modern version of its historic monopoly in coining precious metals.[2]

Even earlier the Bank for International Settlements, (BIS) a purely technical institution had come to serve as the bunker where central bankers plotted the undoing of the Roosevelt

banking legislation of 1935 that restricted the banks to banking. That had become the model for banking throughout the Western world. The BIS's effort to get the world's banks out of their losses in the 1980s was its *Risk-Based Capital Requirements*. This made a double contribution:

1. It shifted the assessment of their creditworthiness from their *cash* reserves to their *capital* reserves. Though banks do raise their capital in cash – by selling stock or through undistributed earnings, little of it is left in that form. Amongst bankers that is considered "lazy money" earning no interest. Most central banks paid no interest on the reserves they received from commercial banks because that cash simply replaced the gold or silver reserves that the banks once had to put up to back the paper money they were allowed to issue. or precious metals and paper bills that by their mere existence do not earn interest. In banking circles that is known as "seigniorage," originally resulting from the monopoly of the crown in coining precious metals at a cost well below their token value as money. That had been assigned to banks in issuing first paper money, and then credit to a multiple of the cash in their vaults.

2. The BIS *Risk-Based Capital Requirements* also declared the debt of OECD (the most developed countries) risk-free, requiring no money of their own for banks to accumulate. The immediate result of this measure and the ending of the statutory reserves was to allow the Canadian banks to quadruple their holdings of federal debt from approximately $20 billion to $80 billion dollars. When the Bank of Canada holds federal debt, the interest on that debt returns substantially to the federal government as dividends, since 1938 it has been the sole shareholder of the Bank of Canada. When the private banks hold such debt, such interest payments stay with them That restored to our badly distressed banks their lost capital. It also burdened our federal government with needless interest payments that go far to explain the explosion of federal debt under the Mulroney government. It was also the reason for the Goods and Service Task that simply shifted the burden for the bank bailout to the most vulnerable section of our population. Such is the "gusher" of revenue that the *G&M* editorial praises.

The increase of federal debt held by the banks amounted to an annual entitlement to the banks of $5 to $8 billion annually. The toll that high interest took on the economy amounted to many times the balance of the $20 billion "gusher" the *G&M* attributes to the GST. The phasing out of the reserves was slipped through parliament without explanation or debate. It was not reported by the media. The measure altered the distribution of the national income, surrendering to the banking sector the control of the economy. Nor has it rated a mention, let alone an explanation, in your publication to this date.

What the Gnomes of Basel and Ottawa Overlooked

These two measures for bailing out our gambolling banks, credited by your editorial as ushering in a golden age, had a sequel of disasters more numerous than one can recount.

In their haste to bail out our tottering banking system the experts of the BIS and our central bank overlooked a crucial detail. To save the banks they were allowed to load up with another $60 billion of federal debt, acquired entirely on the cuff. At the same time, as you mention, the Bank of Canada under John Crow drove up interest rates into the high teens to "lick inflation."

But when interest rates go up the market value of pre-existent bonds drop in market value. A similar cure for the banks' problems actually brought on a crisis that began in Mexico but soon spread to Eastern Asia, to Russia, and the world. It was well on the way to bringing down the world financial system, when President Clinton – without the support of his Congress – arranged a standby credit of $51 billion with the cooperation of the IMF and the Canadian government.

There is, moreover, an intriguing link between Mr. Mulroney's flawed behaviour, in and out of office, and the failure of our media to report so crucial a measure as the phasing out of the statutory reserves in 1991. In 1993 an American economic historian, Douglass North, was awarded the Nobel Prize for economics for a paper on the political consequences of a fundamental shift in the distribution of the national income. He showed that the latter can undermine the dominant political alliances based on the previous income distribution. The end of statutory reserves put our chartered banks in the direct line of succession of our ancestral monarchs in the creation of money. That spells power beyond anything decided at the ballot box. That was at once evident in the further deregulation of our banks shortly after their unpublicized bailout. This permitted them to acquire stock brokerages, enter merchant banking, underwriting, insurance, derivative boutiques – activities incompatible with banking. This has been expressly forbidden by the 1933 banking legislation of Roosevelt that threw up fire walls amongst the four pillars of the financial system – banks, the stock market, insurance and mortgages, and was echoed throughout the Western world.

Each of these financial specialties has its own pools of capital essential for the conduct of its particular business. Allow the banks with their multipliers of money creation access to these capital pools, particularly with the wild leverage that the end of reserves had allowed them, and the result was bound to be speculative inflation.

The Resulting Collapse of Political Structures

In the perspective of Douglass North's work, the break up of the reigning Progressive Conservative Party arising from Mulroney's surrender to the banks was inevitable. And, the surrender of most of our money creation to the banks was continued by the succeeding Liberal government with hardly a burp. *As a result the Liberal Party seems headed for a not dissimilar fate.*

Likewise, the decline of the Conservative Party after Margaret Thatcher had finished with it, and the Partido Revolucionario Institucional in Mexico after the ultra-corrupt Salinas regime that allowed the stock market to swallow the banks – a reversal of we might call the Brian Mulroney syndrome – where the banks gobbled up the stock market.

The Salinas episode resulted in 85% of the banking system of Mexico – a powerfully nationalist nation – ending up in foreign hands. Moreover, proclaiming interest rates "the one

blunt tool for licking inflation" was tantamount to waving a red flag to Islam for the Koran does condemn those persisting in taking interest to eternal hell-fire. Surprising that our big-time Washington terrorist-fighters should not have investigated that linkage!

William Krehm

1. *Bank of Canada Act* – Article 14(2).
2. Subsection (4) of Section 457 of Chapter 46 of the Statutes of Canada 1991.

BROMSGROVE PAPER 2004

In Celebration of Late Learners

IN SOME WAYS I am a late learner. It was only recently, that I grasped the important message Major Douglas was trying to convey in his cryptic language – his A and B theorem. I was nudged over that barrier by the previous writings of Frances Hutchinson. Almost as important was her recent essay in drawing on thinkers as diverse as Marx, Veblen, Schumpeter. If "late learner" refers to those who finally manage to climb over the fences that closed in their thinking, it can be a badge of honour. Keynes was a late learner who needed the Great Depression to shake him out of some inherited convictions. This last year I have spent much time and carfare attending conferences on heterodox economics from Kansas City to Cambridge, Amsterdam to Tokyo. And nowhere did I find such complete open-mindedness – with one possible exception – as in Bromsgrove. Let us then rejoice in our talents as late-learners. In a world of early-forgetters, late learning is a noble calling. The salvation of this troubled world could depend on it.

I will take as my point of departure an explanation of what Major Douglas's much-reviled A and B Theorem is about. It has nothing to do with the merits of capital accounting (a.k.a. accrual accountancy). That makes a clear distinction between the current and capital expenditure of government as well as in the private sector. But today almost all governments treat the cost of building a bridge or a school in exactly the same way as they do the soap for their wash-rooms. By now most of you will have heard COMER sing our song urging governments to recognize capital budgeting. Recently the party that Connie Fogal now heads in Canada, the Canadian Action Party, has joined us for the chorus. And the far greater reform party, the New Democratic Party, now lists Capital Budgeting as an option. Which is progress, but grossly understates the case. Without incorporating accrual accountancy into its national bookkeeping, any government is headed for disaster. We cannot go on treating crucial government investment in both human and physical capital as an extravagant current expenditure because it is not traded on the stock market. And most certainly we cannot bring in the national dividend of Major Douglas without it.

Our Governments' present accountancy mistakes the private sector for the entire economy. What is not marketed is taken to be an "externality." That is as though you calculated your personal net worth by mentioning only the mortgage on your home, but omitting the home that the mortgage financed. That is what has for years been fobbed off on the public as "prudent fiscal management." Nor is it an innocent error. It serves the interests of those who have for three or four decades been destroying the redistributive functions of the state.

If you carry capital assets on the government books at a token dollar, you can sell them for a tiny fraction of their real worth to deserving cronies or charming strangers. And then organize a public company, and earn a bouncing profit. And the taxpayers who have already paid once for those assets in taxes, will start paying for them again in user fees.

I can tell you stories out of Canada, and you can recount whoppers from the era of Maggie Thatcher.

Accrual accountancy will always be necessary with or without Douglas's A + B Theorem. The latter, is concerned with something quite different, and no less important. Together, they sing like two well-mated canaries.

What Douglas's A&B theorem is about is essentially *liquidity* – the length of time before new output can be marketed into *cash* to pay incoming bills. Until that happens the producers will depend on outside financing. And that's the fatal crack through which the Devil enters.

Sealing that opening is what the Douglas A&B Theorem is about. His way of doing so was to deliver a national dividend from the government to all citizens. The justification? It would represent the unrequited contribution of generations of slaves, martyrs, scientists, saints, engineers and other mortals who contributed to the cultural heritage that made possible our wealth-creating powers today.

Let us deal with these two very different concepts – capital budgeting and national dividend – and see how they overlap. Douglas's idea of a national dividend would serve more than a single purpose. It would help make possible alternate life styles less destructive of the environment and society than the compulsive accumulation of private wealth beyond all need or feasibility. It would liberate great talent to do what it was born to do, not compete on a balding wage market. But in the process of filling that important function, part of the national dividend would have to be kept in some cooperative form of banking controlled by small producers with government cooperation. For much of the soaring might of banks today has been based on their fairly recent engrossing of the farthings of the working population for their black arts. The very essence of banking is to lend out many times the money actually held by the bank. A long line of economists – including Karl Marx, Thorstein Veblen, Joseph Schumpeter – have described banking as a mixture of swindle and beneficent innovation. Increasingly, the deposits left with the banks by the public play hooky. Many times their total is lent out in the hope that there will always be enough money left in the kitty to honour any cheques written on it. However, should too many depositors ask for the return of their deposits at the same time, banks would close their doors, while desperate depositors lined up for blocks outside every bank in the land. Essentially, in the good and bad senses of the word banking is a *confidence* game.

That is why central banks were devised to act as a "lender of

the last resort." However, repeatedly the bankers pushed up the critical multiple of their credit creation beyond discretion Until the institution of the central bank and government-backed deposit insurance were introduced, runs on banks were neither infrequent nor pretty sights. Our trouble today is that the "lenders of the last resort" have mutated into "donors of the first resort," as finance capital corrupted our governments. And at the same time, the banks have been deregulated to gamble on an ever larger scale in every aspect of the economy. And those who produce our real wealth have been paying for the government's underwriting this sport.

Because of banking's sinister potential, in 1933, under President Roosevelt fire walls were thrown up between banks and other financial institutions. Brokerages, underwriters, insurance companies, merchant bankers, mortgage companies keep on hand pools of liquid capital essential for their businesses. Allowing the banks to get their hands on these and use them as base for their money creation is the surest way of guaranteeing that the economy will go up in smoke. And in being bailed out, the bankers will convert the experience into further ways of mulcting the rest of society – from wage-earners and industrialists to the sick and the dying. That contributed to the Great Depression and the Second World War. It is well on the way to similar results today.

Hence even if we should finally introduce a "national dividend," without obliging the banking system to stick strictly to banking, the national dividend would end up serving as just another pool for bankers to splash in.[1]

Retrieving the History of Economic Thought

The reform of the banking system is inconceivable without society retrieving the history of economic thought. Without the suppression of that record the financial community could never have highjacked power to the very hilt.

I am impressed by the way in which Frances Hutchinson and her co-authors have bridged the gulf separating Social Credit from other reform movements. However, there are a few details still needing attention from either side.

Let's begin with page 215 of Ms. Hutchinson's fine recent book *The Politics of Money* where a supposed document by Abraham Lincoln on monetary reform is reproduced. That document has long since been proved bogus. It dates from the period of the bimetallism debates that rocked the US. Monetary reformers felt free to put into words what Lincoln had enacted – his Greenback issue backed neither by gold or silver, but only by the nation's credit. While writing his fine works on money reform almost 20 years ago Bill Hixson, one of the founders of COMER, told me that he had considered using those supposed Lincoln quotes but decided they were not authentic. More recently one of our newer contributors, Keith Wilde, a federal civil servant who specializes in tracking down both neglected or fraudulent sources, arrived at the same conclusion. Lincoln did refuse to finance the North in the Civil War at the usurious rates that bankers demanded, and issued paper "greenbacks." And don't for a moment think that he had an easy ride with those Greenbacks. At no time did they rise to par and for stretches were under water. But they were redeemed at par. The bankers who bought them up saw to that. All that may have contributed to his assassination for putting an end to that other slavery. But I know of no evidence to prove or disprove that belief. What difference does it make if we stretch the facts in a good cause? An enormous one. Our opponents, having all the power at their command, have that privilege. We don't, nor do we need it. But if we are caught uttering a single remark that cannot be backed with hard evidence, it will be exploited to undermine decades of conscientious research.

On the following page Ms. Hutchinson quotes approvingly James Huber and James Robertson's *In Creating New Money* – not Robertson's fine recent collaboration with Bundzel – "calling on the UK and other governments to restore seigniorage, thereby ending the creation of money by the banks." That would in fact reduce the banks to the role of "intermediaries." Actually that is what they claim to be – at a time when their money-creation embraces nearly the entire money supply. However, most of our money is described by conventional economists themselves as *near-money* since almost all of it is interest-bearing, created by being lent out. Legal tender by definition should be interest-free – as was gold and silver, and as is paper currency. There is good reason for that, especially if the central bank has made overnight interest rates on interbank loans the benchmark interest rate the one blunt tool against inflation. For whenever the central bank raises its rate, the market value of preexisting loans with lower coupons takes a dive. That undermines the performance of such "near-money" as a store of value and much else.

The 100% money idea was widely espoused by many economists including Milton Friedman and Irving Fisher in the depth of the Great Depression of the 1930s. But that was a time when Henry Ford, Thomas Edison, and an amazing list of other mighty industrialists and even bankers were demoralized enough to listen to just about any scheme for getting the economy out of the ditch.100% money, however, excluded the socially useful banking function – supplementing the inadequate supply of precious metals when gold or silver was still legal tender. Properly controlled, the banking "miracle" could serve the world by supplementing our need for what we might call "complete-money," money not being loaned out, but by being spent into existence for essential "public capital," alongside a controlled amount of near-money loaned out for private profit. The private banks would have that field of providing banking services for the private sector, and creating near-money in the process. But a modest portion of the legal tender base on which this would be done would have to be re-deposited with the central bank on a non-interest earning basis. That is in return for the surrender of a part of the government's seigniorage rights – the ancestral monarch's monopoly in coining precious metals for a profit. That would provide the government with more room within the constraints in force to use the central bank to lend it money on a virtual interest-free basis. In countries like the UK and Canada where the governments are now the sole owners of their central banks that would take place in the form of dividends. But in the US and other countries where the central bank is owned by private banks, the dividends to those private shareholders are strictly limited, and the bulk of the profits also go to the government as consideration for part of the ancestral rights of seigniorage granted the banks.

Those statutory reserves have been abolished in Canada and New Zealand, or reduced to insignificance in the UK to 0.35 of one percent. In the US such statutory reserves are confined to working hours, like good trade unionists. When the banks close their doors their reservable deposits are shifted to non-reservable accounts and the reserves are no longer required.

The old statutory reserve system you will find described in minute detail in university economic texts published – in Canada – prior to 1991. In that year any reference to that chapter of our banking history suddenly vanished. That was the year when the statutory reserves were discontinued so that the banks could recoup their heavy losses in speculative investments during the previous decade in gas and oil and real estate. The Reichmann's building of Canary Wharf complex before proper transport connection with the City was remotely in place is but a sample of what brought on the revision of our *Bank Act* in 1991.

Does Bank-created Debt Live On?

But there is this about miracles: they tempt those who hold them in the palm of their hands to confuse themselves for the Lord Almighty. Vesting 100% of our money creation in our central bank would leave it to the government through the central bank to distribute the necessary credit to the private sector, and that prospect should make us wince. We are not short of public mega-scandals even today.

On the other hand, having the government borrow from its central bank at virtually zero interest rates would make possible essential investment in physical and human capital, including the national dividend.

And that brings me to another disagreement with something in the admirable Hutchinson book, *The Politics of Money*. I quote: "When loans are paid back they do not cancel out the debt and return to zero. Money created into existence by the repayment of debt remains tangible: the bank has got 'its' money back. As lenders to owners and investors, banks have become major owners and investors themselves in modern society."

This passage mixes up two very different things. If we keep them separate, we will gain not only in credibility but in understanding what must be done.

When the near-money created by banks out of thin air is repaid to the banks, that near-money is destroyed. But it is equally true that before their repayment those loans contribute to a higher profit for the bank in that year, and that *rate of increase* in their profit is automatically extrapolated on the stock market into the remotest future. And that increased stock price serves as collateral for further borrowing and investment.

The real problem is that the ghost of that loan after its destruction by repayment lives on in the fictitious growth rate of the banks' earnings and net worth. And the rate of that growth is automatically extrapolated into the remotest future. But you may ask what real difference there is between the two positions. In either isn't the end-product a huge speculative bubble bound to burst? The answer is: a crucial one. One answer to the question concentrates on a single number, i.e., a classic instance of *number-crunching;* Our approach is to *analyze the process.* And it is the process that we must grasp if we are to formulate suitable policies. Number-crunching concentrates on a single figure, often of dubious reliability. Analysis deals with the very different factors that may influence that figure in different ways. Very few phenomena in our ever more complex world can be really summed up in a single figure.

The mathematics of derivatives that dominates economic theory today deals not only with growth rates, but with the various powers of growth rates of increase in detached aspects of a security. Thus the growth rate of its yield, or of the currency in which it is denominated; complicated swaps and other combinations of two or more such derivatives are "customized" for their clients by our banks' "derivative boutiques." This opens an entire universe for the design of instruments for questionable deals. As in the Enron Corp.'s partnerships which were not even entered on Enron's balance sheet because derivatives are still unregulated and don't have to be reported. And once you start trading in the fragrance of roses rather than in the entire plant, you can skip the thorns and the sweat of planting and caring for the rose bushes. That permits you to control far larger quantities of such isolated aspects. That is how George Soros could outgun your Old Lady of Threadneedle Street to shoot down the pound. And then go on to do the same with the lira and other currencies.

Most economic reformists still talk about the voracity of compound interest, but we are in fact confronted with something infinitely more gluttonous. Alongside it compound interest is a mere Franciscan monk. Exponential mathematics deal with the indexes of infinite series of powers of growth rates rather than with the variables themselves. And here I used the word "infinitely" in a perfectly literal sense. Exponential infinite series were first explored by 18th century mathematicians and reached their pinnacle in the exponential curve. This is defined as follows: the rate of growth of the function always keeps up with the value already attained by the function itself. When you say that you imply that all higher derivatives to infinity do the same. The first derivative becomes the value of the function itself, the second derivative becomes the first which by definition is the value attained by the base function and so on into infinity. It is in fact the mathematics of the atom bomb.

Mention maths, and most people will head for the doors. But what is involved here is essentially taught in high schools today. It is both a sermon on and a diagnosis of our sick, sick world. I refer you to a footnote for some details.[2]

Road Blocks in our Derivative World

There are serious road-blocks in this derivative-run world to be cleared before the national dividend advocated by Social Credit and the rest of the reforms that we may be advocating can be brought in.

Balancing the budget, paying down the national debt and controlling inflation are seen as the main concern of governments. But is a balanced budget, based on what is essentially non-accountancy, possible? Even the suggestion of balancing a budget without capital budgeting is a scam.

Let the children starve, crime take over, our streams be poisoned, and our air polluted, while our governments use our surpluses to pay off the debt. But what are they going to pay off the debt with? Gold and Silver are no longer legal tender. Only the debt of central governments have that status. So the question arises: Will they then pay off the debt with government paper notes with a different colour? While trying to climb up this non-existent greased pole, the government would be reducing the money in circulation and driving up interest rates, and favouring the money-lenders once more.

There have been surreptitious introductions of partial accrual accountancy – in the US under Clinton at the beginning of 1996[3] and in Canada in 2002 relating entirely to physical capital, and with zero effort to explain to the public what is involved. Indeed, such information and the very introduction of accrual accountancy is kept a closely guarded secret. The growing layer of taxation in price reflects the need for increasing government investment in a society undergoing incessant technological revolutions, a population explosion, rapid urbanization. And all these factors are exerting increasing pressures on the environment. In distant periods when orthodox economists bothered trying to reply to such objections, the argument was that the growth of productivity would increase sufficiently to absorb this deepening layer of taxation in price without disturbing the price level. It is a long time since that argument – or any argument at all – has been employed to support the alleged need for "zero inflation." Figures on productivity, however, ignore the destruction of non-marketed resources essential for the preservation of human life. Into the 1990s the Bank for International Settlements (BIS) warned that the slightest amount of inflation, if not eradicated, would develop into the likes of the German hyperinflation of 1923, when it took a wheel-barrow of paper money to buy a glass of beer. But that German hyperinflation resulted from a lost world war, the occupation of the German industrial heartland by the French and Belgian armies to collect Germany's defaulted reparations in strong currencies that Germany could not earn. The BIS claim of the slightest "inflation," if not suppressed, would become a hyperinflation similar to Germany's in 1923 implied that if interest rates had been raised high enough in 1923, retrospectively there would have been no German defeat in World War I, no impossible reparations demanded, no occupation of the Ruhr by the French, no general strike across German in protest to it, no virtual resulting civil war.

Then suddenly – less than two year ago, we heard from the same BIS and the US Fed there is "good inflation" (up to 2% or even 3% or 4%) and "bad inflation" anything beyond that. Most alarming is the ease with which the group in command of official economic thinking reverse the dogma they impose on the world, without a word of serious explanation. The message is of irresponsible, brute power.

Meanwhile, governments are almost in unison attempting to balance budgets that do not distinguish between spending on capital account and for current account. In the US where

170 ∽

capital budgeting was brought in January 1996 for physical investments, and rolled back for several years, $1.3 trillion dollars of assets had been recognized for the first time.

French economic historians have caught up with the idea that urbanization has always led to higher price levels – an obvious point that still escapes our equilibrium-economists.[4]

Obviously a national dividend must add to the price level. The price level and balanced budgets however, have a very relative meaning when Wall Street's passions for balanced budgets come into play.

COMER was a pioneer in advancing the view that in a pluralistic society, price itself becomes pluralistic. It involves not only costs of marketed inputs, but increasingly of non-market areas of the economy, such as government-delivered services. Investments in human capital covered by taxation. must be treated as a public investment even though they are lodged in private heads and bodies. A better criterion whether they rate as a public investment is whether they serve to expand the tax-base.

We have made considerable progress in identifying the fatal factors that are leading towards to downfall of the prevailing system. We have also staked out some main traits of society – that should replace it. But how we will get from here to there is still unexplored. One thing is clear, the forces currently in control, are not going to give up easily. They organized their comeback from their disgrace during the last Great Depression with a brilliant thoroughness. They are determined not to let that happen again. Frances Hutchinson, (p. 206) has this to say on the subject, "Without a fundamental criticism of capitalist theory and practice many innovations are doomed in the long run by the underlying social structure and its political-economic inequalities. The danger is that they will tend to reproduce underlying social inequalities rather than overcoming them. In this sense they may offer false hope. At the same time, people involved in developing new strategies may gain substantial empowerment or heightened awareness, and the value of these achievements must not be neglected. Every attempt to transform lives within capitalism is potentially an attempt to transform capitalism itself."

The present free-for-all that has taken over in the world economy is bound to lead to confrontations of a degree of violence overshadowing even what we are currently experiencing. All the diverse reformers, each concentrating on a neglected aspect of social relationships can and must make their contribution in addressing the whole of this staggering problem. But that requires careful consultation and the pooling of ideas. A clear line must be drawn between what we can compromise on, and on which compromise would be surrender. We must persist in listening critically to what other reformist streams have to offer, and learn to regard the variety of views as an important asset. For a knowledge of supplementary policies may serve to protect the flanks of a common cause.

Discussion in itself is an invaluable resource, whether it leads to agreement or not. The suppression not only of alternate views but of our history threatens society's survival. By repeating our disastrous errors on an ever more monumental scale,

humanity risks self-destruction. And then some wiser species succeeding man in control of this planet may speculate who it was that left it so cluttered with poisonous debris.

William Krehm

1. In Canada in 1946 the ratio of assets to cash held by banks had amounted to 11 to one. Currently it is close to 400 to 1.

2. Financial derivatives derive conceptually from the rates of growth of a function with respect to its independent variables in differential calculus. The first derivative is the velocity of their growth rate, the second is the acceleration of that growth rate, the third the increase in the rate of growth of the acceleration and so on to infinite order. It is one of the marvels of the human mind that a few decades after John Law built his financial castles the most prolific mathematician of all time, Leonard Euler not only developed the full potential of derivatives to infinite degree, but also pioneered the exploration in the realm of imaginary numbers (based on the non-existent square root of-1) – a virtual mathematical parallel of Law's far frailer innovations in high finance. These had to do with paper money wholly without backing of precious metals. Likewise he stretched the concept of the corporation and anticipated the Physiocratic School of proto-economists in France who saw in land the ultimate sources of all economic value. These three components Law mixed into a powerful witch's brew to become the virtual economic dictator of France financing the luxuries and wars of Louis XIV by issuing paper currency backed by the future development to half of the wilderness of North America to which France laid claim.

Marx, Thorsten Veblen, and Jospeh Schumpeter paid tribute to John Law as half genius, half swindler.

In financial circles today an abstracted aspect of a given security is taken as the variable, and various derivatives to any order are calculated. Operating in this fairyland allows a far greater command of crucial abstracted aspects of a given security – say the value increase of the security on the stock market, or of the exchange value in which it is denominated, or endlessly ingenious swaps of such derivatives. With this new technology in blowing financial soap-bubbles, it becomes possible to incorporate in the present price of a security or the derivative of its future price. But essentially this is a deal with the Devil. Once such artificial valuations have been attained, its promoters are committed to maintaining them including their growth rates into the indefinite future. Any shortfall leads to the collapse of the house of cards. This is the root of the seemingly endless financial scandals that are clogging the American courts. There is in fact no room left for morality. That explains the endless resistance in the financial community to the oft-heard recommendations for the control of derivatives in even exalted circles.

3. In Canada the situation is far worse. Over three years after the US government smuggled in the essence of accrual accountancy in its handling of physical assets, the then Finance Minister Paul Martin was still slugging it out in private with the then Auditor General Denis Desautels resisting the latter's ultimatum that he would not approve the government's balance sheet unless accrual accountancy had been brought in. The result: a compromise whereby it would be brought in initially only with respect to fulfilling the treaty obligations with the aboriginal peoples of the country and the environment. This meant that until the obligations under the treaties with

the aboriginals and the Kyoto agreement respecting the environment were fulfilled, the unfulfilled obligations would be treated as budgetary liabilities. However, the settlement of the dispute included demeaning a statement from the Auditor General, that the assets recognized under the agreement would represent no new money coming in to the treasury and hence would not justify further expenditure. A decade ago the increased budgetary deficit arising from the shift of federal debt from the Bank of Canada to the banks had created an annual entitlement of between five and $8 billion. To fill the hole in the federal budget created by that, Ottawa slashed the grants to the provinces who passed the treatment onto the municipalities. This has contributed to a severe crisis in municipal finances across the land.

4. I made the point in *Revue Économique*, Paris, May 1970. "La stabilité des prix et le secteur publique." Significantly, the publication has since disappeared.

OBITUARY

Walter Stewart, 1931–2004

THEY DID NOT BREAK the mould when they made him. He was not cast, and there never was a mould. For forthrightness, honesty, courage, and resourcefulness, he never had his match. The outpouring of tributes from the media bears witness to this but his full import is in most instances hidden by references to his eccentricities. The truth is that his record and lasting contribution makes most others in the sorely tried profession of journalism in no small degree ashamed of themselves.

Roy MacGregor in *The Globe and Mail* (17/09) wrote: "You can understand what former *Maclean's* editor Peter Newman was getting at yesterday when he said 'he may have been the engine driver – but Walter Stewart was the magazine's conscience.' Peter Newman should know.

"The secret of his success as a journalist, Walter Stewart said, when he was regularly tilting at the privileged establishment, lay in his battered briefcase. The leather was frayed; the handle broken. 'It's got me past more office doors than any phone call or business card or fancy title.' The battered briefcase, he claimed instantly convinced clerks and secretaries that he was a lawyer, and all he had to do was swagger into any office, plunk it down on a desk and they would immediately begin answering questions as if he had just held out a Bible and sworn them in to the truth, the whole truth, and nothing but the truth, so help you Walter Stewart.'"

The second bit of advice that he gave his colleagues was to write each article as though you had just arrived in town that morning and were going to leave town that evening.

It tells you much of the state of affairs in the banking world that as enquiring a mind as Walter's should have had to learn from me that the statutory reserves that banks had to leave with the central bank were phased out over a two-year period beginning with a bill sneaked through parliament in 1991. It had not been reported in the media or debated in Parliament.

We had learned of it from a sympathizer who had the bad habit of sitting in libraries reading *Hansard*. One of these days *Hansard* will be kept under lock and key. At our next meeting he told me that he had mentioned it to a friend who had been a former cabinet minister, whose name he was not free to divulge. "Couldn't be!" the friend exclaimed. "Why that would leave them nothing but to push up interest rates to fight inflation!" By the time he spoke at a public meeting on the subject he had obtained permission to reveal the identity of the shocked friend – Eric Kierans, minister in the Trudeau cabinet, and a former head of the Montreal Stock Exchange!

Eventually Walter devoted himself entirely to writing books that combined scholarly research with a social conscience. His biography of Trudeau set a high bar for political biography in the land. I was flattered to be one of those to whom his final work on Canadian banks was dedicated – his *Bank Heist – How Our Financial Giants re Costing You Money* (1997). It will remain an essential reference book on Canadian banking. Walter Stewart will be long remembered for good cause.

Bill Krehm

REVIEW OF A BOOK BY NICOLA PARISE, DONZELLI EDITORE, ROME, 2000

"La Nascita Della Moneta — Segni Premonetari e forme arcaiche dello scambio" ("The Birth of Money — Pre-monetary tokens and archaic forms of exchange")

UNDER OUR VERY EYES, the essence of money is undergoing change. Time was when money, in the form of gold or silver or notes issued by a government, earned no interest by the mere fact of its existence. Giving off interest was a function of *debt* denominated in one currency or another, but not of the currency itself. That contributed to the relative stability of currencies for it made them less dependent on current interest rates. Today, since all currency is lent into existence and thus bears interest, the value of existing debt is doubly interest-sensitive: once since a rise in interest rates depresses the value of previously issued debt, and again due to the higher exchange value of the domestic currency due to increased foreign demand for it.

The time has come for rethinking the very nature of money. An interesting contribution to this is being made by studies in the literature of ancient Greece, particularly of the Homeric poems. One overriding conclusion: rather than a natural phenomenon, money is a social product, and like society itself, its nature is constantly undergoing change. And this was often determined by factors quite other than trade. More remarkable still, some of these researches help us understand aspects of the changing role of money today.

"Louis Gernet[1] sees in the difference between symbol and token that the first is imbued with direct emotional power, whereas the latter has to do with broader social usages. If so, the origins of money would largely evolve from symbol to token. The research of Gernet on the pre-monetary attempts in ancient Greece to find a measure of universal value remind us of M. Mauss's Essay on Gifting amongst 'primitive' peoples."[2] He held that it was not likely that the notion of money arose all at once. It makes more sense to seek the potential qualities of money in the properties of the materials exchanged in archaic and primitive societies. One thing is certain: pre-money was associated with magic powers. And objects used as money had to be suitable as a measure of value: they could not be physically consumed when used, but had to last for further circulation as a means of acquiring perishable consumption items. That was soon transformed into power that compelled subjects to perform services for those possessing such magic items.

"Bronislaw Malinowski, in a polemic with Charles G. Seligman (1910), protested against the abuse of the designation 'money,' and refused to include bracelets, sheets of green stone and other symbols of wealth in the category of money.

"In all archaic and 'primitive' societies, that did not have money or monetize either gold, silver, or bronze, sea-shells, precious stones and precious metals performed the function of 'means of exchange,' but not in the modern manner. Such objects rather had the character of talismans. Their powers were essentially subjective, whether associated with individuals or groups, and basically unstable, depending on the number of transactions for which they were utilized.

"Circulation combined economic and non-economic considerations. It was an archaic form of exchange that related to marriage, military and juridical services, divinity, and wealth" – with no lack of mystique that in fact still occurs in our day.

"Only later did the magic and precious objects that the community had earlier associated with purchasing power become permanent instruments for the universal measurement of value."

Money — A Social Phenomenon

"Economic theory, however, views the economy as something wholly autonomous and isolated from the rest of social life. It represents the beginnings of economic activity as a period of pure "natural economy" practising forms of barter. In fact no archaic or 'primitive' society appears to have practised barter among individuals. Instead, as Mauss observed, exchange seems to have been an affair of groups or of their leaders, or of both. What was involved was not only institutions of economic utility, but banquets, rites, courtesies, women, games and military display.

"And though the manner in which the successive ceremonies of gifting – the original gift, its acceptance, and the requital – appeared voluntary, they were in fact obligatory. No one had the right to refuse a gift offered, or not to reciprocate. That would be equivalent to a declaration of hostility. The prestige of the groups concerned and the authority of their leaders depended on respecting this etiquette.

"The role of pre-money was assured by magic and the value attributed to precious objects due to the prestige of the chain of its earlier owners, and how long it had remained in circulation.

"Indeed, all social groups involved in such gifting seem to have been based on blood ties. Once that was left behind, economic factors emerged as determinants of other social relationships. The structure of the community was no longer that of a family tree. Gifting and economic exchange thus appear in two distinct stages of development. But traces of the old rules lived on long after in juridical, political and religious practices. To the 'wanax' [king] in Mycenian Greece were attributed certain cosmic powers like rain-making, and he presided over the religious, economic and political life of the community. His palace was seen as a repository of precious things: talismans. The memory of these lived on through the disturbances and invasions which led to the destruction of the old order by invasions and internal turmoil towards the end of the second millennium BC. Administrative control of society and the use of writing were lost by the time the cities of Greece described by Homer appeared on a more modest scale. The custom of gifting lived on within families (the oikos), but not grandly organized by a central bureaucracy out of palaces. More modest rivalries amongst equals took over. And the gifts now given and received symbolized the wealth under the dimly remembered ancient regime were now replaced by prized objects that served as wedding gifts, to guests, and blood relationships."

Once the blood-relationship is left behind as a basis for exchange, the family tree is replaced by the relationships of production in the structuring of the community. That becomes the arch-type of all groupings founded on reciprocity. On the other hand, when the implications of mutual gifting were largely religious, they symbolized the wealth and power of the donor. These contrasted with another item of gifting-the heads of cattle, more often serving the more utilitarian function as a unit for counting, than to set out the grandeur of the donor.

Gernet emphasizes the notion of social power originally vested in many of these precious objects. They may, for example, have served as wedding gifts in the family. They thus carried a cluster of personal merits and expressed other values than strictly economic ones. In Homer it was above all the heirlooms kept in the bedroom that the master of the house had received as gift and was restoring to circulation. They symbolized a social accumulation of the qualities of previous donors.

"The division of booty, votive offerings and wedding presents were all occasions for rising above the concrete individual form of value to a more general aspect of equivalent values."

The importance of cattle in Homer for valuating other assets suggested to Bernhard Laum the religious origin of money.[3] In turn the value of pottery, bronze armour, a girl, bars of metal, or the sumptuous fare the guests had eaten in Odysseus's house were valued in terms of oxen.

Laum concluded that it was not the object exchanged that acquired value because it was employed for a religious purpose, but rather that it could be employed for ritual purposes because it already had something sacral about it.

Laum and other scholars have ransacked the great Homeric poems for evidence on this dawning period of money. "He was struck by the progression of the various numbers of cattle by which Homer expressed the value of other items: 1, 4, 9, 20, 100. Likewise the number of cattle that were mentioned in sacrifices were 100, 20, 12, 9, 1. There is no mention of a sacrifice of four oxen, for example. From the identity of the number of cows used to evaluate other assets and for religious sacrifice, Laum concluded that the measurement of value had a religious rather than a commercial connotation.

Of course, you are free to conclude that it might be as a sort of throw-back that so many wealthy folk make it their purpose to collect money today as a sort of religious mission.

Any "circulating value" could do as value equivalent. However, the role of general measure of value came to be filled not by some "circulating value," but by oxen. Although oxen did not offer durability or the possibility of hoarding, or easy transport, they were ideal sacrificial victims. And that determined their choice as a value measure. By their part in the religious rites were ideally suited for the early expression of abstract value. Sacrifice led directly to instruments connected with such rites. Thus the spit, originally a tool of sacrifice, gradually became metal money, as did the tripod and the double-axe.

In this way the process began in which circulating objects of wealth, became pre-monetary tokens, filling the functions as autonomous media of exchange, in no way dependent on the prestige and connections of their previous owners Since the contribution of the recipient was much to the fore, the choicest part of the animal sacrifice went to the greatest heroes according to merit. What finally remained was divided amongst the rank-and-file, the small pence of the occasion. This was an essential link in the chain of development that led to the introduction of money in Asia Minor in the last decades of the 7th century BC.

Light Shed on Contemporary Money Mutations

This little book of which we have covered less than a half because of space limitations, sheds light on the more recent transformations in the role and nature of money. There is a powerful suggestion of symmetry in the traits of pre-monetary exchange media, and the most recent degenerative trends in money. Of necessity it had to be cut loose from identification with precious metals by the sheer volume attained by world trade, and above all by the explosion of speculative activities. But the process has been very one-sided favouring those with control over credit money creation. The notion of abstract valuation was retained only when it suited those in charge, while on the contrary when it suited those in the saddle monetary policy seemed to work on the assumption that money remained something concrete that we would run out of unless it reduced its spending for social purpose. On the other hand when the very valuation extrapolated the rate of growth of profit rates already attained into the indefinite future and then incorporated them into current price, its availability is deemed unlimited. Booms take on the headiness of religious orgies. In general the trend was to deal with growth rates of perceived values rather than with the value

themselves. And the real production is guided by the interest rate (again a rate) as the one blunt tool. The values placed on various gifts in pre-monetary society reflected in part the value real or fictitious of goods and people in long extinct societies.

Our current governments are driven by an unrestricted pursuit of monetary accumulation that can never be sated. From a medium of exchange money is becoming primarily a means for gambling leading to the accumulation of personal fortunes that bear no relationship to the real human needs. Distribution between countries and between classes within even the richest lands is unsustainable since credit requires a certain balance of revenue between debtor and creditor.

The pre-monetary periods of the Greeks were motivated by gifting that looked back to a richer, more cultured age, that may have been idealized, but actually had existed. The present goal is inspired by a vision that at no time existed or could exist: a self balancing society where all agents and the power distribution is assured by the infinitesimal size of all actors of production. There is a systemic evasion of a basic constraint of credit money – there must be a substantial access to credit on terms repayable by the borrowers.

Meanwhile, these researches in the Homeric poems and other great ancient literature allows us to grasp the pre-monetary traits that never quite gave up the ghost and that are becoming ever more evident.

Though they may be found falling short of the epics in the Iliad and the Odyssey, there are some striking parallels with them in the following extracts from a front-page story in *The Wall Street Journal* (27/9, "Lord Black's Board: A-List Cast Played Acquiescent Role" by Robert Frank and Elena Cherney): "On a winter afternoon four years ago, Hollinger International Inc.'s directors met with the company's chief executive, Conrad Black, for an especially busy board meeting.

"Gathered around a mahogany table in a boardroom high above Manhattan's Park Avenue, eight directors of the newspaper publisher, owner of the *Chicago Sun Times* and *Jerusalem Post*, nibbled on grilled tuna and chicken served on royal-blue Bernardaud china, according to two attendees, Marie-Josee Kravis, wife of financier Henry Kravis, chatted about world affairs with Lord Black and A. Alfred Taubman, then chairman of Sotheby's [tip-top auctioneers who have handled more celebrated magic trophies than Homer sang of].

"Turning to business, the board rapidly approved a series of transactions, according to the minutes and a report later commissioned by Hollinger. The board awarded a private company, controlled by Lord Black, $38 million in 'management fees' as part of a move by Lord Black's team to essentially outsource [not to China, however] the company's management to itself. It agreed to sell two profitable community newspapers to another private company controlled by Lord Black and Hollinger executives for $1 a piece. [That dollar was replete with the Lord's charisma.] The board also gave Lord Black and his colleagues a cut of profits from a Hollinger Internet unit.

"Finally the directors gave themselves a raise. The meeting lasted about an hour and a half, according to the minutes. The board of Hollinger – a star-studded club with whom Lord

Black had long-standing social, political and business ties – is emerging as a particularly passive watchdog. Hollinger directors openly approved more than half the of the transactions that allowed Lord Black and his colleagues to improperly siphon more than $400 million from the publisher, according to a company investigation overseen by former Securities and Exchange Commission Chairman Richard Breeden.

"The board rarely asked basic questions to get the facts it needed, despite warning signs. In addition to the management fees and other payments, the report says the board approved retroactively use of $8 million to buy Franklin D. Roosevelt memorabilia. A company jet, a platoon of servants, four homes, and a constant round of parties – all partly funded by Hollinger – were left largely unscrutinized by the board, according to the Braden report."

Those who explained as vanity Lord Black's determination to become a British lord even at the cost of losing his Canadian citizenship misread him. As a scholar of self-advertised depth, he was undoubtedly aware of the role of the previous owners' charisma in the valuation of whatever they touched, and he was simply applying it in keeping with the tenor of our times. Surely branding and the whole cult of advertising have their affinities with the of the valuations of pre-monetary times.

William Krehm

1. Gernet, Louis (1983). *Anthropologie de la Grece Antique*. Paris. Italian translation by A. Rocchini, Milan, 1968.
2. Mauss, Marcel (1965). *General Theory of Magic and Other Essays (1950)*. Translated into Italian.
3. Laum, Bernhard (1924). *Heiliges Geld. Eine Historische Untersuchung ueber den sakralen Ursprung des Geldes*. Tuebingen.

Putting our Government on Credit Cards to Pay Its Rent

A FEW YEARS AGO when I was still regularly invited to appear before the House of Commons Finance Committee, a charming, young Conservative member from the Maritimes often managed to sit beside me. In that way we had many interesting, light conversations. From these it emerged that Scott Brison was not only highly intelligent but extremely well-informed. There seemed nothing I could tell him about Canadian banking and its tortured history that he didn't already know. Naturally I wondered what a bright young man like that was doing in the Conservative Party.

Now I am equally puzzled why he would have crossed the floor into the Liberal Party. Currently, of course, he is the Public Works Minister in the Martin Government in charge of "a massive sell-off of federally owned buildings toward finding billions of dollars that can be diverted to health care, urban infrastructure and other core programs" (*The Globe and Mail*, 21/09).

This program promises to end up as a massive grab of public property that may even match the bail-out of our chartered banks by ending their statutory reserve requirements in 1991; and their subsequent further deregulation to take over brokerages, underwriting establishments, derivatives boutiques, and just about every other activity incompatible with banking. It could, indeed, become the Mother Hubbard of Canadian political scandals, leaving the Quebec sponsorship an epic at the starters' gate. I could cite a half-dozen reasons for this conviction, and partly because I admire Mr. Brison as one of the most interesting fauna in the Canadian political jungle, I shall proceed with my first instalment of the task.

It is one of the picturesque oddities of our politics that we still do not list the real estate holdings of our government at more than a token value on the asset side of its balance sheet. It is true that in 1999, the then Finance Minister, Paul Martin, conducted a many-week-long wrangle with the then Auditor General Denis Desautels, who declined to give unconditional approval of two successive annual balance-sheets of Ottawa unless this elementary requirement of double-entry bookkeeping were introduced. It ended up in an unlovely compromise whereby Mr. Martin agreed to phase accrual accountancy (a.k.a. capital budgeting) into the governments books; and Mr. Desautels issued a humiliating statement to the effect that the introduction of accrual accountancy, while recognizing the physical assets of the government currently disregarded, would bring no new money into the game, and hence must not be taken as making possible increased spending. That statement alone vitiated the long-postponed benefit of bringing serious accountancy into Ottawa's books. It was like a person calculating his personal worth by listing the mortgage on his house as a liability, but forgetting the value of the house itself as an offsetting asset. Accordingly, the citizen in question couldn't afford to fill the doctor's prescription for his heart complaint and a spot of cancer. When the error was brought to our citizen's attention, he made the entry into his books, but reasoned that no new clinking coin had entered into the situation he could still not afford survival.

During his brief term as Finance Minister John Manley actually used the term "accrual accountancy" in the hallowed House of Commons, where some unidentified unofficial speaker keeps such obscenities unmentioned. Yet no harm done: the puzzled members, most of whom in 1999 had actually voted for its introduction, unless my boob-tube was lying, seemed not to know what he was talking about. In any case Mr. Manley soon gave up even using the term and in the debate – before, during, and since the election – the term accrual accountancy, alias capital budgeting, was never mentioned again – even though it had, to a limited extent, become the law of the land. Of course, since Mulroney much that is still in our law books – e.g., the vital passages of the *Bank of Canada Act* – are never referred to and have long been sent to Coventry.

Instead, elections are being focused on reducing and even paying off the national debt. I myself, though not a drinking man, with my own ears heard the campaigning Prime Minister at a CBC town hall, declare with a straight face that the government should and will reduce the federal debt by one half.

Our PM, however, omitted to mention what he will use to pay down the 250.5 billion smackers needed for that. Gold won't do, silver won't do. They were demonetized over 30 years ago. This high state secret should be divulged without delay. For until it is, the voters will continue being hoodwinked with promises that are simple nonsense.

Whereas the former Auditor General – one of a long line who had tried before him – obtained a messy compromise with Finance Minister Martin, it really didn't begin to deal seriously with the issue. In the early 1960s, pondering the unexpectedly rapid recovery of Japan and Germany from the physical destruction of World War II, Western economists had recognized that the reason that they had failed to foresee how soon these two defeated countries would become formidable competitors again on the world market. The reason, it was agreed, is that the numerous young US economists, who had been sent to those lands to study the problem, had concentrated on the physical destruction of the war, but overlooked that their human capital in education, health, had been left substantially intact. From that they recognized that human capital, rather than machines, buildings and other physical capital was the most productive investment a country could make. Theodore Schultz of the University of Chicago was awarded a Nobel Prize for Economics on the strength of that discovery. That being so, should health, education, and social welfare not be listed as assets in calculating a country's net worth to show how much financing it can do to acquire more of this most productive investment? Why then are we selling the government buildings to be able to invest more in health, when our most productive of investments already made has not been entered in the federal books – even at a token dollar. Isn't this madhouse masquerading as fiscal prudence?

Is Henry George in the House?

And now a word about government buildings. For the most part they tend to be located in downtown areas of large cities. Given the rapid urbanization underway in recent centuries, urban building sites in strategic centres have always soared in value. Henry George, 19th century reformer who narrowly failed becoming mayor of New York City, even proposed that only land be taxed. Certainly a stretch, but it is a fact that much of the great aristocratic fortunes of Britain can be traced to the ownership of much of downtown London. For the most part most of that land is merely leased to developers, who inherit the land plus improvements. Once speculators get their mitts on such land in a significant city, they rarely let it go. It makes them landlords with a capital L, a guaranteed free ride to the moon. The sensational rise in value of such urban sites is entirely due to the vast investment of government in culture, health, education, in short in public capital investment that stokes the dynamism of a large city.

By putting federal office buildings up for sale, the government is almost literally throwing away the crown jewels without even a historic record of their costs, let alone their present and future value. Poor Henry George is left standing on his head.

Directly or indirectly, it will be the banks who will finance the acquisition. But why should anybody believe that the banks are in a better position to finance this irreplaceable real estate than the government, whose credit is the only legal tender in the land? Along this path we will end up paying tolls to get into our bedrooms.

Almost thirty years ago, I proposed that before a new subway line is built, the government (municipal, provincial, or federal or *tutti quanti* in collaboration) use their own inside information to quietly buy up key sites along its routes and lease them to private builders for putting up buildings on them That would keep much of the rise in the value of such sites out of the price of rents, residential and commercial.[1]

In 1991 it was these same banks who had gambled themselves to the brink of illiquidity and even insolvency financing massively real estate ventures in Toronto, Calgary, New York, and London. To bail them out the Mulroney government slipped through Parliament without debate, or press release, the phasing-out of the statutory reserve requirements that a modest part of the deposits they received from the public in chequing accounts be redeposited with the Bank of Canada. Those reserves earned them no interest, but gave the federal government more elbow room in borrowing from its central bank within the existing constraints. When the government borrowed from the BoC, of which since 1938, it has been the sole shareholder. The resulting loan was almost interest-free, since apart from overhead expenses, all the interest it pays its own bank on those loans comes back to it as dividends.

When the government borrows from the private banks, the interest, of course, stays with them. That was part of the bail-out rationale. And then these banks, having again been bailed out, were deregulated further, so that they could gamble themselves into the gutter once more.

They have to go on gobbling and growing, since their already attained growth rate extrapolated to doomsday has already been incorporated into their stock market price. So now Mr. Brison, who understands the vulnerabilities of this madhouse economy so well, has been entrusted with managing this grand sequel to the privatization of the CNR and Ontario Hydro scandals.

But isn't real estate a risky, speculative operation, given to tremendous booms and busts that have brought many mighty corporations low. And isn't that too risky for governments to engage in? Must it not be left to private corporations that have the savvy to manage to get bailed out by the government, whereas the government is too simple-minded to bail itself out, even though it does own the central bank?

But real estate is a gamble only for private speculators. When owned by the government – and, of course, serving a real purpose for government functions – government-owned real estate has a unique feature. When the economy swoons, more government services are required, and there is a greater demand for floor-space to deliver them, at the very time that private lessees go bankrupt in droves and leave their landlords in straits. What the project that Mr. Brison has been charged with will guarantee is that the private owners will up rents drastically as the government needs ever more space, and are functioning in rented space. I know that Mr. Brison – a dazzling gem in Ottawa's drabness – will already be informed about the present hassle on the toll rates on Ontario's 407 bypass of Greater Toronto that was built by the Ontario government and then sold to an international consortium. Tolls have risen by 200% in five years, and have nowhere to go but to hit the heavens. Imagine a similar effect on Ottawa's support of education, health, and social services programs when the rents housing them in buildings the government itself once built and owned join that witches' sabbath.

We leave it to Mr. Brison to take it up from there.

His well-wisher,

William Krehm

1. Appendix "Vanishing Shelter" by Sam Madras, Faculty of Science, York University in Krehm, W. (1997). *Babel's Tower: The Dynamics of Economic Breakdown*. Toronto. The late Sam Madras, who first taught me the elements of systems theory, fleshed out the idea in this appendix.

When the Guardians of Morality Survival Take to Crime

BANKS AND BROKERAGES are about making money, in both literal and metaphoric senses. There are, however, other institutions that are formally dedicated to protecting and healing society. When these lapse into social banditry the time has come for some serious questions. In turn some huge American private hospitals, pharmaceutical companies, and now insurance companies are being investigated by regulatory authorities in the United States for what would be more readily expected from gangsters. The techniques for bringing these to light were indeed perfected by the experts who devised and whetted their weapons in dealing with the latter category. These include deadly subpoenas widely cast that the recipients dare not answer untruthfully, since the example of Martha Stewart has been singed into their brains. Hence the scurry of the guilty squealers to get there first so that their penalty will be less. Accordingly the software for handling white-collared crime bids fair to outstrip that for handling convictions of darker hue. What is still missing is a way of handling corruption well connected politically.

In *The Wall Street Journal* (18/10/04, "Insurers Reel from Bust of a 'Cartel'" by Monica Langley and Theo Francis): "Inevitably the search was directed toward catching up with insurance where everything gets expressed in dollars. On a Friday afternoon last month, the nation's largest insurance companies were served with subpoenas from the New York Attorney General asking an explosive question: Had they ever engaged in bid-rigging?

"By the next week, several of the biggest insurers told the Attorney General's office that they had paid kickbacks for having business steered to them and had submitted sham bids to mislead customers. Their panicked responses revealed evidence of a broad scheme of collusion and price-fixing within the $1.1 trillion insurance industry.

"It's [about] the same kind of cartel-like behaviour carried out by organized crime that Attorney General Eliot Spitzer pri-

vately told his top officials. 'It's like the Mafia's "Cement Club,"' added Peter Pope, his chief criminal investigator, referring to construction projects when a corrupt contractor rotated cement companies into jobs based on kickbacks. The bid-rigging allegations raise the possibility that the scandal could engulf other major players and lead to the overhaul of the insurance businesses. Marsh, AIG and Ace have suspended the practice of 'contingent commission' in which an insurer pays a broker in exchange for steering business its way. The practice has been standard for decades.

"Next on the hot seat: Aon Corp., the second-largest insurance broker with more than $6.7 billion in brokerage revenues world-wide last year. Investigators are examining whether the Chicago-based firm improperly steered its customers based on fees from insurers and whether it engaged in bid-rigging. Mr. Spitzer is also probing whether Aon directed business for its services to insurers ready to use its services when buying 'reinsurance,' or insurance coverage for insurance companies This practice is known as 'tying' or 'leveraging.'

"Aon, which was first subpoenaed when Mr. Spitzer opened an investigation into the industry's pricing practices, said in a statement last week that soliciting fictitious quotes, bid-rigging and accepting payments from insurers in exchange for not shopping around 'would violate Aon policies.' Aon said 'to the best of our knowledge, our employees have not engaged in those practices.' It also said it is cooperating with Mr. Spitzer's office. However, the head of the investment protection unit in Mr. Spitzer's office, David D. Brown IV, said 'Aon is dragging its feet as much as it can.'

"Already there are signs that the scandal could spread. Mr. Spitzer plans to examine whether life and health insurers engaged in bid-rigging. On Friday two companies reported receiving fresh subpoenas from the Attorney General: life insurer MetLife Inc. and National Financial Partners Corp., a broker of wealthy individuals and smaller companies. Both companies had received subpoenas earlier in the probe. National Financial Partners said the new subpoena asked whether the company 1requested any insurance companies to provide fictitious or inflated quotes to clients.' It said it 'it is not aware of such activity.'

"Insurance stocks have plummeted by tens of billions of dollars collectively. Marsh stock has fallen by more than one third. For now the hottest seat in the industry is occupied by Jeffery W. Greenberg, Marsh's chairman and chief executive. At last Thursday's news announcement in the case against Marsh, Mr. Spitzer said, 'The leadership of that company is not a leadership I will talk to.'

"Mr. Greenberg is part of an insurance dynasty that has been shaken by Mr. Spitzer's charges. His brother runs Ace and his father runs AIG – and both insurers were among the first to finger Jeffery Greenberg's company as a possible wrongdoer.

"Twice in the past year, the Attorney General has found problems at Marsh units. Last fall its Putnam Investments became the first mutual fund company charged in that industry's trading scandal for allowing favored customers to buy and sell shares in ways that cheated other investors. And earlier this year, the firm's Mercer Human Resource Consulting unit admitted to giving the New York Stock Exchange's board inaccurate or incomplete information about the pay of former stock exchange chief Dick Grasso.

"At the heart of the insurance scandal are allegations of bid-rigging and 'pay to play' deals. Businesses seeking insurance often hire a broker such as Marsh, which in turn solicits bids from several insurers. Marsh is alleged to have sought artificially high bids from some insurance companies so it could guarantee that the bid of a preferred insurer would appear cheaper and would win the business at hand. According to Mr. Spitzer's complaint insurers were willing to put themselves out of contention for these bids because they expected Marsh to protect their bids on other occasions. Such machinations violate New York state anti-trust laws and the broker's fiduciary duty to act in the best interests of its clients, Mr. Spitzer charges.

"The lawsuit also charges contingent commissions, the widespread practice among insurers of paying brokers commissions based on the volume or profitability of the business the broker directs to them. These commissions, which have been disclosed poorly if at all, gave Marsh an incentive to direct business to insurers paying the best price or terms, Mr. Spitzer alleges.

"It was the industry's use of contingent commissions that initially triggered Mr. Spitzer's investigation. Within a few months hundreds of boxes of documents littered the 23rd floor of the Manhattan high-rise where the Attorney General's investment protection bureau is located. The interns and students enlisted to plow through them found many instances of Marsh brokers steering business to insurers paying the most in contingency commissions. By mid-September evidence had begun appearing of the Marsh firm bid-rigging. On Septemberp 17, a wave of subpoenas went out under the state law prohibiting fraud and under the *Donnelly Act*, New York's antitrust law. Insurance companies had two weeks to respond.

"Among the first calls to the Attorney General was one from AIG, headed by Maurice R. 'Hank' Greenberg, whose eldest son is Jeffery Greenberg, Marsh's chief executive. Another early call came from yet another insurance firm headed by a Greenberg – Ace, whose president is Evan Greenberg, Jeffery's younger brother. Ace and AIG jockeyed to be the first to meet with the Attorney General. 'They were racing to be the first to acknowledge the bid-rigging,' says one official. They wanted to appear most cooperative to get the best treatment.'

W.K.

On Our Jobless Recovery

IN *The New York Times* (5/10, "A Missing Statistic: US Jobs that have Moved Overseas"), Louis Uchitelle boldly attacks a many-storeyed problem without a ladder.

"The job market finally showed some life in September, but not enough to sidetrack a growing debate over why employment has failed to rebound nearly two years after the last recession ended. The debate intrudes increasingly on election politics, but in all the heated back and forth, an essential statistic is missing: the number of jobs that would exist in the US today if so many had not escaped abroad.

"The Labor Department, in its numerous surveys of employers and employees, has never tried to calculate this trade-off. But the 'offshoring' of work has become so noticeable lately that experts in the private sector are trying to quantify it.

"By these initial estimates, at least 15% of the 2.81 million jobs lost in America since the decline began have reappeared overseas. Productivity improvements at home – sustaining output with fewer workers – account for the great bulk of the job loss. But the estimates made suggest that the work sent overseas has been enough to raise the unemployment rate by four-tenths of a percentage point or more, to the present 6.1%."

That, however, is just the ground floor of our leaning edifice. But there is, too, a vast educational and training structure developed in the early postwar decades to educate and train the skilled workers and engineers in the developed countries. If we are outsourcing more and more of our semi-skilled and even skilled work, is it not inevitable that we should have less use for much of this infrastructure? And is this not a neglected factor in its notorious deterioration – from sheer crowded classes, ever higher fees, increasing inroads of the influence of corporations who are expected to provide more of its funding? Surely there is an important interrelationship there. But economic theory has been castrated to the point that it does not even recognize the role of human capital, though four decades ago it was recognized as the most productive of all investments.[1] That leaves statisticians blind without the assistance of seeing-eye dogs.

The relationship becomes still more complicated when we recognize that we depend for ever more of our engineers, medical staff on the emerging world. This represents a depletion of their scarce human capital while we are ever more niggardly in developing our own. The flow is thus a two-way affair, and should have a place in the world's capital flow statistics.

But back to the Uchitelle article. "That [job-] leakage fuels the political debate. The Bush administration is pushing the Chinese to allow their currency to rise in value, thus increasing the dollar value of wages in that country, a deterrent to [the US] locating jobs abroad. The Democrats agree, but some also call for trade restrictions, and they attack the Republicans for cutting from the budget funds to retrain and support laid-off workers in the US." That in fact should be considered as demanding a recognition of the capital loss suffered by the very outsourcing process. It thus represents a shift in capital losses to the public sector and to society to increase the bottom line of private corporations.

"While most of the lost jobs are in manufacturing or in telephone call centers, lately the work sent abroad has climbed way up the skills ladder to include workers like aeronautical engineers, software designers and stock analysts in China, Russia and India."

When the outsourcing was of low-skilled manufacturing jobs to overpopulated, emerging or Third World lands like Mexico, Central America and the Caribbean, one country was played off against the other – for tax exemptions that ruled out the physical and human infrastructures required to support the new urbanization arising from the outsourcing. The result can be seen in the *maquiladora* slums on Mexico's northern border. Today, however, the outsourcing is to countries better able to defend themselves, by independent currency policies, and by utilizing the levers of international policy – above all China. It is visibly becoming an ever-more complicated game. And as such, it requires a far more complicated accountancy to keep track of its real net significance. Above all the distinction between current spending and capital investment must be made.

Outsourcing then comes in a variety of forms and with a whole gamut of consequences.

"'All of a sudden you have a huge influx of skilled people; that is a very disruptive process,' said Craig R. Barrett, CEO of Intel, the computer chip manufacturer.

"Intel itself has maintained a fairly steady 60% of its employees in the US. But in the past year or so, it has added 1,000 software engineers in China and India, doing work that might have been done by people hired in the US. To be competitive, we have to move up the skill chain overseas." Or otherwise expressed, move down the chain of environmental and living standards.

"The trade-off in jobs is not one for one. The work done here by one person often requires two or three less efficient workers overseas. Even so, the total saving for an American company can be as much as 50%, even allowing for the extra cost of transportation, communication."

What is not included in this estimate is the cost to the general public in taxation, inconvenience, and security risk from congested airways, roads, and seaports.

The Job Costs of Outsourcing

"The estimates of job loss from offshoring are all over the lot. Among professional economists the high-end estimate comes from Mark Zandl, chief economist at economy.com, who calculates that 905,000 jobs have been lost overseas since the last recession began in March 2001. That is 35% of the total decline in employment since then. While most of the loss is in manufacturing about 15% is among college-trained professionals.

"Morgan Stanley, the investment firm, is adding jobs in Mumbai, India, but not in New York – employing Indian engineers as well as analysts who collect corporate data and scrutinize balance sheets for stock market specialists in New York. Lehman Brothers, Citigroup and J.P. Morgan are also setting up shop in India.

"Near the low end of the job-loss estimates sit John McCarthy, research analyst at Forrester Research Inc., and Nariman Behravesh, chief economist at Global Insights. For them the loss is 5,000,000 to 800,000 jobs over the past 30 months, again almost wholly in manufacturing. Starting in January 2000 and running through 2015, globalization of American production will have eliminated 3.3 million jobs at home, he estimates.

"Some are trying what amounts to niche estimates. Roshi Sood, a government analyst at the Gartner Group, for example, estimates very roughly that state government cutbacks have pushed overseas the work of 3,400 people once employed in the US, either on public payrolls or on the payrolls of companies that contract with state government.

"In Indiana, for example, the Department of Workforce Development recently chose an Indian company, TCS America, to maintain and update its computer programs, utilizing high-speed telecommunications to carry out the contract. The TCS bid was $8 million below those submitted by two American competitors."

Trying to balance state budgets does little for bringing down the US's worrisome international trade deficit. At every level there is a simple-minded approach to problems of ever more tangled complexity.

William Krehm

1. See Krehm, William, *Price in a Mixed Economy – Our Record of Disaster*, Chapter 13.

Letter from Barcelona

October 14, 2004

Dear *ER*,

I took a bus-man's holiday recently, when an intended sight-seeing visit to the Pyrenees turned into attendance at a conference on economic policy in Barcelona. The Basic Income European Network was holding its 10th conference (after twenty years of existence) as part of a larger event called *Dialogue on Human Rights, Emerging Needs and New Commitments* organized by the Catalonian Institute of Human Rights, with a heavy involvement by UNESCO. I had been alerted to the existence of this movement six or seven years ago by Sally Lerner (University of Waterloo), and since UNESCO events always treat important subjects with high quality presentations, I stopped in to find out more of what Basic Income is about.

The plenary sessions were interesting and vital, but tended to treat the issue only in its moral and sociological aspects. I selected from the program two of the parallel sessions that seemed to be the only ones to address economic feasibility and financial techniques for achieving the BI goal, which is stated as a payment made by the state, as a right of citizenship to every full member or resident of a society, even if he or she does not work, or is unwilling to accept a job if offered, and irrespective of whether he or she is rich or poor, in other words, irrespective of other possible sources of income and domestic arrangements.

On the way to the session breakout rooms I stopped to look over the BI literature table to get a better idea of scope and focus. There was not a lot, but the quality seemed good and I purchased one monograph and a compendium of past papers prepared by members of the Network. I will pass along my evaluations when I have had time to read them more carefully. My cursory examination reinforced the view obtained from printed program and plenaries that economics and finance have not been well represented in BI discussion. After having sat through two sessions titled "Innovative and Sustainable Financing for

Basic Income," I asked why, after twenty years, did this topic have such a tentative feel, as if it were only now getting underway? The moderator passed my question to one of the speakers who he said had been present from the beginning. Yoland Bresson answered by observing that those who came together in the founding of BIEN were mainly sociologists, political scientists and moral philosophers, and that they had never sparked much interest among economists.

I think that Bresson's confirmation of my superficial observation is still surprising to the man-in-the-street, as it most definitely would have been to adults of 30-plus years ago, but given that BIEN is only twenty years old, maybe it isn't. It is consistent with my discovery exactly one year ago that the professional literature of public policy and administration does not touch the subject matter of monetary and financial policy. (I had this observation confirmed by a political science professor with a strong personal interest in economic policy and a sociologist who has spent a career surveying all the literature that bears on public policy as it is affected by technological, environmental and social change. Monetary and financial policy are in the domain of economics, and other social science specialties leave it alone.)

And it bears on your opening question in the September *ER* of "why so many unanswered, and indeed unasked, questions are leading the world where it does not choose to go." I wonder if you saw the essay by Lewis Lapham, "Tentacles of Rage: The Republican Propaganda Mill, A Brief History" in the September *Harper's* magazine? It goes a long way toward the explanation, providing the background to an emergent effort to influence the thinking of academic economists that I observed as a graduate student in the US almost forty years ago, and which apparently succeeded. In brief, money power bought the academy and converted it to a propaganda machine. Since observing those early efforts in the sixties, I have watched from the inside as government authority, will and muscle to regulate money and financial power in the public interest have been progressively stripped away. Today, it is rare to find an economist who makes empirical investigation of the institutional structures that check and shape the behavior of individuals and groups (corporations) as they express their private drive for more money and power.

One of them who does showed up at the BIEN conference and provided one of the most useful presentations. Myron Frankman of McGill University argued that there is plenty of money at the top of the world's income distribution to provide $1,000 per year to everyone on the planet, and that this abundance is even more striking when wealth distribution is brought into the picture.

Much of his paper is devoted to problems of measuring and comparing incomes, within and among countries, a difficulty that is only compounded w.r.t. wealth. Available data nonetheless justify his figure of $1,000 per person/year and more accurate measurement could only make it higher, in his considered opinion. He notes with regret that most of the effort expended on this kind of measurement is focused on the poor, in spite of Susan George's warning of 30 years ago that in order to help the poor, one should study the rich. This is especially impor-

tant and difficult because the rich are so successful in keeping their wealth and incomes hidden from view. Frankman's paper can be viewed at http://icesuite.com/myron.frankman/files/mjfbien10.pdf.

I enjoyed a few conversations with Myron over lunch and dinner, and he affirmed the observations above about the decline among economists of interest in empirical study of market structures and related institutional frameworks from a regulatory, public policy perspective. He said that when he himself and colleagues of his generation retire, there will be virtually none left. Content of the mainstream economics literature today, and hence of university instruction, is so focused on modeling the behavior of "free" markets (do they portend equilibrium or chaos?) that economics departments are driven to hiring new professors straight from graduate programs in mathematics. The implied emphasis on deductive reasoning at the expense of empirical research can only reinforce economist jokes like the men in a lifeboat with only canned provisions and no can opener–the economist's solution is "assume a can opener."

Some BI Authors

From the literature table and the sessions I attended, I observe that when Basic Income authors do get into the domain of economics and finance they lean toward the traditions initiated by the likes of Henry George, Veblen, and C.H. Douglas. I heard two presentations in this vein, both focused on the unearned income associated with site values (land) and other essentially public or collective resources that have been seized as private property by robber barons of the past or present. As do several other BI authors, these speakers poured scorn on the slogan popularized by economists of the past 35 years that "there's no such thing as a free lunch." The essence of *rent* as explained in the textbooks of neoclassical price theory that I studied and taught from is that it is unearned income – a payment for which the owner has done nothing but collect it.

Jeffrey Smith of the Geonomy Society of Portland, OR gave a cautiously positive answer to the question "Can Rents Fund an Extra Income for Everyone," and Charles Bazlinton, a British surveyor and author of *The Free Lunch* (the monograph I purchased and will review) cautioned against implementing a Basic Income without a deliberate system for taxing land values along with it.

Coincidentally, while attending the conference I was corresponding frequently by e-mail with another author who is a prolific contributor to this line of thinking – empiricist and institutional. Michael Hudson is Distinguished Research Professor of Economics, University of Missouri at Kansas City, and he says it is one of the few departments that has not been completely taken over by the post-Keynesian, Chicago-led fad of monetarism in the neoclassical resurgence. (See the Lapham article mentioned above for added flavor.) Hudson has a book in preparation which addresses your observation about "so many unanswered, and indeed unasked, questions leading the world where it does not choose to go." In reviewing drafts of his Introduction I can see the struggle entailed in assembling information that is publicly available (if one chooses to look) and then to present it in a way that gives a fundamentally different concept of the world than the one that is driven by the doctrinal fixation of the age–in this case the neoclassical, monetarist resurgence that is assisting finance and property power to reverse 800 years of progressively democratic policies. (A generous sample of his writings is available at www.michael-hudson.com.)

The situation of contemporary economic thought seems to be reflected in an appreciation of Jacques Derrida that appeared in *The New York Times* on October 14. A close professional friend wrote that The guiding insight of deconstruction is that every structure – be it literary, psychological, social, economic, political or religious – that organizes our experience is constituted and maintained through acts of exclusion. In the process of creating something, something else inevitably gets left out. These exclusive structures can become repressive – and that repression comes with consequences.[W]hat is repressed does not disappear but always returns to unsettle every construction, no matter how secure it seems…. Mr. Derrida understood all too well the danger of beliefs and ideologies that divide the world into diametrical opposites: good or evil, for us or against us. He showed how these repressive structures, which grew directly out of the Western intellectual and cultural tradition, threatened to return with devastating consequences. Mr. Derrida does argue that transparent truth and absolute values elude our grasp. [I]t is necessary to recognize the unavoidable limitations and inherent contradictions in the ideas and norms that guide our actions, and do so in a way that keeps them open to constant questioning and continual revision. There can be no ethical action without critical reflection.

A distinctly novel approach to financing Basic Income was provided by a youthful Australian engineer who pointed out that all the non-human energy that is currently used to do the world's work could be generated in a space one-quarter the size of South Australia using available solar collection technology. The value of this opportunity would go a long way toward providing a universal income supplement. Further exposition of this idea (adapted from the late Buckminster Fuller) and some of its limitations is provided in the an upcoming review of *Cosmic Accounting* that I wrote as a letter to the author.

Keith Wilde

Hi Keith:

Gratifying to learn that you were attending the Barcelona conference while I was away at the fruitful Bromsgrove annual gathering. I met Steve Zarlenga there and I will be reviewing his book hopefully in the December issue. Meanwhile note my review of an Italian study by Nicola Peresi, the premonetary chapters of which covers much of the ground that Zarlenga does in his early section. In view of this your reference to the deconstructionalists is extremely timely. Your point is well taken – you cannot ignore millennial achievement in separating the proto-commodity concept from the proto-exchange medium. (Marx's concept of abstract labour brushes on this in a way.)

In any case, our point that salvation of the thinking process on economics may be salvaged abroad by fresh conceptual contacts to make up for the suppression of anything resembling a serious discussion at home. And the vehicles for that are the internet and the better of the spate of congresses abroad. Eventually we will organize one of our own right here.

All best, *Bill Krehm*

Mail Box

Encouragement from our subscribers helps keep us in fighting trim.

Guelph, ON
I have learned a lot from your wonderful articles.
Vi Morgan

Edmonton, AB
Hopefully there may still be a few dollars left [from the enclosure] to help fill the financial hole your so worthy endeavour no doubt digs.
Roger Swan

Formosa, ON
Please send me a copy of each video. I will show them to as many as I can. Keep up the good work! It is better to die trying than to lose hope. Your efforts are an inspiration.
Josh Benninger

The Dead Rat Under our Floor Boards

NO PRIVATE FIRM could survive if its books made no distinction between current spending – floor wax, fuel and such things – and investment. It is high time that our governments heeded the advice of their auditors and started doing just that. President Clinton as of January 1996[1] actually moved in that direction, under strange circumstances. A previous government had bailed the banks out from their speculative losses during the 1980s in gas and oil, real estate and much else incompatible with banking. This was achieved by reducing to insignificance the statutory reserves that they had to leave with the Federal Reserve. These were redeposits with the central bank of a modest portion of the deposits that they had received from the public in chequing and other short-term accounts. Such redeposits earned them no interest. Previously they had served several purposes:

1. They were a payment to the government for having assigned to the banks much of its powers of money creation – originally the monopoly of the ancestral monarch in coining precious metals. Today gold and silver are no longer legal tender. The only legal tender for the past thirty years has been the credit of the central government. And like currency this bears no interest. That in fact is an important feature of legal tender. Were legal tender to throw off interest like a bond by virtue of its very existence – the value of our money supply would drop whenever interest rates went up. And that is hardly what the central bank, supposedly above all else devoted to preserving the value of our money supply, should be advocating. However, that is precisely what all central banks did in the early 1990s when they were bailing out our improvident banks.

Such reserves left more elbow room within existing constraints for the government to borrow from its central bank at virtual zero-interest rates. In countries like Canada or the UK, where the government is sole shareholder of the central bank that takes the form of dividends, which return to the government whatever interest it may have paid on its debt held by the central bank less a modest handling charge. But even in the US, where private banks own the central bank, a fairly similar portion of its earnings reverts to the government, because the dividends to its private shareholders are severely capped.

2. The statutory reserves allowed the central bank to control the price level without moving interest rates. Raising or lowering the percentage of the deposits the banks received in chequing accounts that had to be redeposited as reserves with the central bank did the trick. If it were lowered, the banks had more base money on which they could raise a superstructure of say ten times that amount in the loans they made. When you raise interest rates, you hit everything in the economy that

moves or stands still. If the central bank lowered the amount of lending the banks could do by raising the reserve rate, they were better able to focus on what really had to be done in cooling or stimulating the economy.

Exit the Bank Reserves

However, to restore the banks' massive capital losses the statutory reserves in Canada were phased out over a two-year period starting in 1991. In the United States they were substantially reduced, and by various devices further downgraded to practical insignificance. At the close of business hours such redeposits are automatically swept into non-reservable accounts, and at the opening hour of the next business day returned to a reservable account.

That left the benchmark rate of the Federal Reserve – its fund rate at which one bank can borrow from another overnight to meet its cheque clearances – the "one blunt tool" for "fighting inflation" and otherwise controlling the economy.

But in their haste to cast a life-line to the floundering banks, the high international rescue team overlooked an important detail. The Bank for International Settlements (BIS), a sort of club of central bankers that made a point of being beyond control of governments, had in 1988 brought in its *Risk-Based Capital Requirements* declaring the debt of developed countries risk-free and thus requiring no additional capital for banks to acquire. However, during this period BIS itself was urging central bankers to fight inflation with higher interest rates right until "zero inflation" were attained. Anything less, thundered Alexandre Lamfalussy, General Manager of BIS, in his 1991 annual report, would lead to the runaway inflation as in Germany of 1923.

However, the BIS and the central bankers overlooked an important detail. When interest rates are pushed up to achieve "zero inflation" the huge bond hoards of the banks – totally leveraged – drop in value like stones. And that risked bringing down the world banking system.[2] I and other members of COMER tried sending warning of what would happen to Ottawa via the retiring head of the Office for the Superintendence of Financial Institutions (OSFI), Michael Mackenzie. A complementary copy of Economic Reform that repeated the warning has been sent to every member of parliament for years. But it has been to no avail.

The day of reckoning blew out of Mexico in 1994. There the peso, under a burden of corruption and dollar-denominated debt, collapsed, as money fled the land. President Clinton, without the backing of his congress, patched together a $51 billion standby fund with the help of the IMF and Canada. The losses sustained in Mexico, nonetheless, were an important indirect factor in the East Asian crises of 1977, and that in Russia of 1978.

A more durable solution was designed by Clinton's Secretary of the Treasury, Robert Rubin, an alumnus of a top Wall St.

firm. As of January 1966, he smuggled capital budgeting (a.k.a. "accrual accountancy") into the Department of Commerce figures for "savings." For the first time physical investments of the federal government were treated as "savings" which they most definitely were not, since that implies cash reserves, and the assets retrieved for the government books were in bricks and mortar and equipment, highways, bridges, and so forth. Carried backwards for several years they restored to the asset side of the government's balance sheet some $1.3 trillion. That provided the solitary statistic that Clinton needed to convince the bond-rating agencies that the government merited a better rating. The resulting lower interest rates at which the government could borrow from the banks produced a budget surplus, assured Clinton's re-election, and brought on the great boom of the latter 1990s, and the subsequent bust – all without disturbing the sleeping dogs of the right. All this was in accord with Clinton's guiding principle: keeping the political center.

And note well, that had still not recognized the vast federal investment in human capital – education, health, social welfare. In the 1960s economists, studying the surprisingly quick recovery of bomb-devastated Japan and Germany, had concluded that investment in human capital was the most productive of all investments. But that great discovery was simply buried almost as soon as it was made, because it contradicted Wall St.'s marching plans.

The Wall Street Journal (18/11, "Fed Chief's Style: Devour the Data, Beware of Dogma" by Greg Ip) discusses the management style of Alan Greenspan as Chairman of the Fed, and makes much of his hunting instincts for data. In fact much of the article is focussed the very year of 1996 when accrual accountancy was brought in by Clinton for physical investments. But in an entire page there was no mention of that key event. Instead Mr. Greenspan assigned the drop in interest rates to the delayed effects of private investments on productivity. But how could you possibly measure productivity, without noting how much government spending was for physical infrastructures vital for every aspect of life and the economy? And what would the effect be on the appraisal of the government's "fiscal prudence" if the vast investments in health, education and social services were recognized for what they are?

In the United States and Canada, as throughout the world, there is a growing concern about what is happening to our democratic system. But there can be no democracy unless there is a serious flow of information. Why then would a bungled half measure like the partial introduction of serious accounting be kept a state secret?

Canada's Even More Sordid Record

Canada's experience with politicians and serious accountancy has been even more sordid. At least three royal commissions and an uncounted line of Auditors General recommended it to the governments of their day. To no effect. However, in 1999 a very determined one in the line refused to give unconditional approval to the governments balance sheet unless he complied. What ensued was weeks of rancorous bargaining between the auditor Denis Dessautels and the Finance Minister of the day,

Paul Martin, in which harsh words like "cooking the books" filled the air. Finally Martin agreed to start recognizing government investments as such, but extracting from the Auditor General a demeaning statement to the effect that since the switch to accrual accountancy would bring no new money into the treasury, it would not justify additional spending. However, when the banks were bailed out, it was the misrepresentation of essential investments as current spending that justified Mr. Martin not only in slashing grants to the provinces, but in downloading programs to lower levels of government without adequate funds to take care of them. Instead of accountancy, Mr. Martin favoured stashing away not only capital investments, but unassigned funds, so that when the results for the year were reported he could bring forward funds that he denied the existence of, let alone assigned to necessary capital programs, and take his bow as "fiscally responsible."

Accountancy should not be a game of hide-and-go-seek amongst politicians, but a means of tracking the needs, the failures and achievements in our ever more complex world.

William Krehm

1. First reported in the *Survey of Current Business* for January and February 1998, p. 13, and *Economic Indicators*, p. 34, and the *Federal Reserve Bulletin*, Table A-40.
2. In the 02/1994 issue of *Economic Reform* ("Supplementals to the Finance Minister"), I wrote: "Our banks are well on the way to becoming government pensioners. According to Bank of Canada figures, bonds issued or guaranteed by the federal government and held by the Bank of Canada dropped by 37% between 1987 and the same month in 1993. But over the same period similar securities in the portfolios of our chartered banks had risen by 768%."

The Coming Depression in China

LATELY the business press has been salivating over the Chinese economic miracle – double digit growth for a decade, a huge trade surplus, booming real estate and manufacturing, etc. *The Globe and Mail* recently devoted an entire edition to China.

Most of the coverage is of the cheerleading sort. Here's the next super tiger economy. Don't miss this opportunity! There is the occasional nod to problems and divisions in Chinese society such as the lack of democracy and human rights, but the general tone is strongly positive.

For a different (and more realistic) assessment of China we have Russian economist Krassimiv Petrov (www.gloomdoomboom.com). He sees an economic bubble building in China, similar to the one in Japan in the 1980s. As always, the Chinese bubble is derived from a huge credit expansion. The Chinese money supply, according to the Chinese central bank, rose from 11.89 trillion yuan in January 2001 to 22.51 trillion yuan in January 2004 – almost a 100% increase. This is greater than the credit expansions that preceded the Great Depression in the

US, and the Japanese depression of the 90s. Lately the Chinese central bank has attempted to dampen the boom by raising interest rates and restricting credit to certain sectors, but these measures appear to be having little effect (*The Globe and Mail*, Oct. 30). Petrov predicts that the bubble will inevitably burst by 2008, and the great Chinese depression will ensue.

The effects will be felt here. The credit expansion has helped maintain a low exchange rate for the Chinese currency, which in turn has fueled a huge trade surplus. The US has a vast trade deficit with China, but that is covered in part by the Chinese purchases of US debt. A Chinese depression will, of course, end this symbiotic relationship and the US economy will plunge into depression as well as China is forced to repatriate its US assets.

Petrov postulates an exact parallel between the current US – Chinese relationship and that which existed between the US and Britain/Europe in the 1920s. At that time Britain was an overstretched imperial power (as the US is today) trying to maintain a strong currency but heavily dependent on borrowing abroad. The US extended loans to Europe in order to maintain demand for US exports (like China today) but most of the loans were unsound, and could not be repaid. So the bubble inevitably burst and the Great Depression followed.

Of course the root of the problem then as now is a monetary system that facilitates such a credit expansion and its subsequent collapse. The Chinese banks, like their Japanese counterparts in the 80's, have been pouring money into real estate and the other expanding sectors. These loans are predicated on continual high rates of growth. When the growth slows or stops, many of the loans become "non-performing." The banks are forced to retrench and the money supply falls. It is a pattern that repeats endlessly with disastrous consequences yet, when the crash comes, you can be sure that the media will advance any number of explanations that have nothing to do with the root cause.

David Gracey

America's Foes Prepare for Monetary Jihad

From "The New Statesman," Monday, October 4, 2004

"THE US DOLLAR has long been the currency of the oil industry. But members of OPEC are contemplating ditching greenbacks. The results could be catastrophic for the American economy, reports Janet Bush. However darkly terrifying America's Iraqi horror story, a small voice of comfort has broken through US night sweats. You are still the most powerful and richest nation on earth. You will get through this, it murmurs. But that reassuring whisper comes from a small devil on America's shoulder, speaking mischief that will land the listener in deep trouble.

"A great many people – if not in the White House – have grasped the reality that America's huge, all-conquering economy is genuinely vulnerable for the first time since the 1930s, and that its fragility coincides with a period of expanding and expensive military exposure around the world. US bestseller lists are stuffed with books agonizing about whether the American empire is finally coming to a close; uncanny parallels are drawn between the military and financial overstretch of imperial Rome and imperial Washington. George W Bush's pre-emptive doctrine in foreign policy is enormously costly; on top of billions of dollars' worth of tax cuts, largely for the rich, it is prohibitive. It is predicted that the federal budget deficit will reach $2.4 trillion over the next ten years. To finance that deficit, the US needs to persuade investors – more often than not from overseas – to lend it up to $4B net every day.

"Even without America's apparently infinite capacity for foreign military adventurism (how much would tackling Iran or North Korea cost?), its fiscal outlook seems dire. Two experts on the US budget position, Niall Ferguson and Laurence Kotlikoff, estimate that the country faces a $45 trillion gap between the money it has and the money it needs to finance existing social security, Medicare and pensions commitments ahead.

"It is not just the federal government that is in trouble. When adjusted for inflation, the wage for the average American male working full-time has fallen over the past 30 years; and, because of that, five times as many mothers – even those with young children – must now work to make a decent living wage. Not since the Depression have Americans saved so little and, at the same time as running down their rainy-day money, been so neck-deep in debt. By 2003, total debt had soared to $37 trillion; that's $128,560 for every man, woman and child in the country. Some of that debt has been racked up on mass retail therapy (Americans love to say 'when the going gets tough, the tough go shopping'), but a lot of it has been the inevitable result of the Average American Joe struggling to make ends meet."

The Deeper the Deficit, the More Reckless the Administration

"The richest nation on earth is living way beyond its means, and yet the Bush administration blithely continues to spend. It takes no steps to rein in the deficit – sometimes, indeed, it seems that the deeper the deficit, the more reckless the administration becomes. No other nation on earth can behave this way – in every other case, governments know that if their deficits run out of control, they will be 'punished' by the market. Investors will lose confidence, interest rates will have to be raised to attract capital, financing the deficit will become more expensive, and a vicious spiral will be in place. Why, then, can the US run a deficit of more than 5 per cent of its gross domestic product and still manage to attract $4B a day at interest rates of only 1.75 per cent?

"The US has been running a bubble economy for decades; the recent dotcom boom and bust was a minor episode in a history of deficit-financing since the 1960s. Then, as now, the US borrowed with impunity, whereas other countries have always had to choose between guns and butter – foreign policy expansionism or domestic prosperity – the United States has spent profligately on both. President Kennedy spent freely on New Deal social programs and the Vietnam war; George W. Bush has emptied the coffers on tax cuts and Afghanistan and Iraq.

"There has never been a shortage of people willing to lend to the US; after all, as the richest nation on earth, it has to be good for the money, doesn't it? Even when investors have become nervous about its profligacy, there has been plenty of credit because the US economy is a crucial market for the world's producers. In living memory, the United States has been the sole engine powering the world economy; there has been no alternative to continually injecting it with fuel.

"But the US has a stick to add to the carrot since the end of the Second World War, it has had the unique privilege of 'owning' the world's reserve currency – the notes and coins used for trade and investment more than any other currency for 60 years. This confers unimaginable advantages. America is able to ignore the discipline of having to balance its books because, if it runs out of money and can't find anyone to bail it out, it can simply print dollars, inflating away the value of its debt and destroying the value of the assets held by its creditors. In other words, it can threaten financial blackmail."

"In the 1970s, European and Asian governments started complaining about lending America the money to finance the Vietnam war; the US simply responded by engineering a catastrophic fall in the dollar, which erased its deficit over time but also crucified the economies of its trading partners in the process. Now, with the deficit soaring again to finance foreign wars, the US is repeating the trick. It has encouraged the dollar to fall; exporters to the US such as China and Japan have had no choice but to try to arrest that decline to protect their trade. How? By buying dollars, which they invest in US treasury bonds, thus financing the deficit. How very neat. But the United States cannot count in perpetuity on winning this game of financial chicken, based on the pre-eminence of the dollar. Its angriest political enemies have worked out the game and have been mulling over their counter-moves. Al-Qaeda has already targeted the soaring symbols of US economic power, from the twin towers to the New York Stock Exchange; now Muslim fundamentalists are trying to topple the dollar. A plan being pushed in particular by Mahathir Mohamed, former prime minister of Malaysia, for a new gold-backed Islamic currency – the dinar – is a rallying point. 'Stealth Bomb to Dollar Islamic gold dinar!' one website proclaims, describing the currency as 'the second prong to planned Muslim terrorist attacks on the United States, intended to annihilate US economic power in a world of rising gold prices and a persistently declining dollar.' The dinar, it says, is the tool of 'monetary jihad.'

"Rejection of the dollar is increasingly being used as an act of political aggression, and nowhere more acutely than in oil-producing countries. The trailblazer was none other than Saddam Hussein who, in 2000, announced that Iraq would henceforth make all its oil trades in euros, a decision that conspiracy theorists – and not a few eminent Middle Eastern experts – say triggered the US invasion. The United States derives substantial benefits from the dollar being the established currency of the oil industry. Because most countries import oil, they must maintain reserves in dollars to pay for it – two-thirds of the world's currency reserves are kept in dollars. This is a major factor upholding the dollar's position as the world's reserve currency; a switch out of dollars in the oil industry would be a major assault on the currency's pre-eminence.

"In April 2003, Indonesia's state oil company, Pertamina, said it was considering using the euro for its oil and gas trades. Even more significantly, in October last year President Vladimir Putin hinted that Russia, the world's second-largest oil exporter, might switch to euros. A Russian move would be enough to tip the balance for other major oil producers. As Arab disapproval of the US war in Iraq has mounted, so a consensus for switching out of dollars has been building; OPEC has openly discussed the option and even Saudi Arabia, once America's staunchest Middle Eastern ally, is reported to be considering rejecting the dollar. For now, the euro is the most viable alternative; in future, it could be the Islamic dinar or, far more likely, a new Asian currency. Western storytellers would relate the tale of the emperor, his new clothes and the little boy who saw his nakedness; perhaps Arab fablers might talk about desert mirages. America's economic dominance was once real; it is now a receding reality, a confidence trick. Washington might ponder that before scattering its dollars and daisy-cutters next time around."

Janet Bush

Editorial Comment

The situation is indeed grave, not only for the US, but for the rest of the world. So, grave, indeed, that before panicking over all that gold that we have been led to believe that society as such owes, we must realize that what it owes is credit essentially owed to itself. And to meet that challenge the first step is to introduce some serious accountancy to replace the hysteria that bankers and conventional politicians whip up to hide the facts. The first step in that direction is to make a clear distinction, as all accountants in the private sector do, between spending on current items like floor-wax or fuel, and long-term investments, like buildings, or in the case of governments, roads, buildings, schools, jails, hospitals that will last for years. The latter should not be treated as a current debt, but depreciated over their useful lives. Few governments, if any, do that. Until they do, all the hand-wringing about the debt that we are handing down to our children and grand children is honest ignorance, or a cunning decoy. Your next step for your mental detoxification on such matters is to turn to "The Dead Rat Under the Floor Boards" on page one of this issue.[1]

Another point of importance: the article mentions the US attracting foreign money at 1.75%. That is a common error. The then 1.75% benchmark "fund rate" was strictly for overnight loans between American banks under the Federal Reserve to help them meet their cheque clearances. Though longer term rates – as for example credit card rates at 18% and higher – were affected by that benchmark rate in their movements up or down, they were at nowhere near 1.75%. To pretend they were is to misread the whole record of debt slavery.

The Editor

1. In its February 1994 issue, for example (reproduced in *Meltdown* on page 123) you can read: "Our banks are well on the way to becoming government pensioners. According to Bank of Canada figures, the amount of bonds issued or guaranteed by the federal government and held by the BoC have dropped by 37% between 1987 and the

same month in 1993 (when the reserves had finally been phased out). But over the same period similar securities in the portfolios of the chartered banks had risen by 768%.

"The fly in this balm is that when the economy starts recovering and prices point up, the BoC will raise interest rates 'to lick inflation.' That will collapse the value of the banks' fully leveraged bond holdings and their capital will go up the chimney. We have tried alerting the government and the media to this. To no avail.

"Now *The Wall Street Journal* ('The Fed Can't Control Interest Rates' by Martin Mayer of the Brookings Institute) offers a similar warning."

A Well-hidden Blessing in the US Election?

THE US ELECTIONS may have bestowed a well-hidden blessing on Americans and the world. For many recent decades could be summed up as a reversal of the earlier democratization which not only had brought us greater literacy, but a freer flow of information to give our improved minds more to chew on. The great depression of the thirties and the war that it led to had eventually ushered in a new freedom in asserting moral issues in deeds rather than only in quotes from the Holy Scriptures. Let us face it: the depression and the war had frightened hell out of human kind, and they made as though to turn over a nobler leaf in the relations of classes at home and amongst nations.

But the devil is never idle. The very prosperity of the postwar heaped new temptations before our leaders. And step by step they have succumbed. Little remains of the moral rebirth that seemed so fully paid for by the Depression and WWII.

It was soon to become largely a balancing of superpowers and super-wealth. As riches became ever more plentiful, they became more ill-distributed – at home and abroad. Chicanery and secrecy increasingly took over as the Soviet super power – far from an incarnation of virtue itself – succumbed, and the United States was confronted with the fleshy lures of sole superpower status. Enrichment and military muscle became ends in themselves. This was marked by the furtive undoing of legislation that impeded the pursuit of these irresistible goals. Even the virtuous legislation ever more rarely passed has been adopted in stealth because it belied what had been proclaimed laws of nature. Programs of aid to the impoverished world were converted from grants to loans, at times on usurious terms. (See the review of the Wood book in this issue.) A chasm came to yawn deep and wide between Islam for which any interest taken is a mortal sin, and the West that has elevated raising interest rates to the sole blunt tool for running the economy. Our universities and their textbooks have been purged to distort rather than to study our history. Morality has been relegated to orphan status.

What more natural then that the more underprivileged, less educated sections of the United States should be repelled to the point of turning their backs on New York and the areas that are home to the best educated, and wealthiest Americans? And with the decay of the American social institutions, and the decline of the job situation, it is the undereducated and underprivileged areas of the United States that are expanding in territory rather than the privileged ones. You can see that in the distribution of incomes. There should then have been no surprise in the election results. The less opulent, less educated, less prosperous part of the world's mightiest nation, themselves either victims of outsourcing in lost industries or the recipients of outsourcing themselves on degrading terms, have responded in the most obvious way open to them. They have sought morality in the arms of a militant version of old-time religion. Much of our crucial history has been suppressed, and the media gagged in the reporting of crucial legislative U-turns. Yet the stench of the Dead Rat under the Floorboards can't be hidden. It has simply engulfed the American electoral process, as it has our own.

Wall St.'s gambols that helped bring on the Great Depression of the 1930s in many respects anticipated those that are clogging the US criminal courts today. It was a period of mammoth loans to Latin American dictators with blood on their hands. The age of financial mergers flourished – power companies as today were a favorite field. The stock market spread its lures to the most humble – shoe-shine boys took to giving their clients tips on what stocks to buy. Of course, in no time they lost their shoe-shine stands, as brokers jumped out of their skyscraper windows. Breadlines three or four abreast inched around city blocks. Financiers with patrician names were sent to jail.

When the clean-up of the mess was begun under Roosevelt, bankers landed in the doghouse under the *Bank Act* of 1935 that soon came to serve as a model throughout the non-Communist world. It established firewalls between the four segments of the financial sector – banks, insurance, real estate mortgages, and the stock market. For good enough reason. Each of these needs a pool of liquid capital to conduct its business, but the banks are unique in having the power to lend out many times their cash reserves through the cheque-clearance mechanism. Give the banks access to these liquid capital pools of the other financial segments, and they will compound their credit creation and expose themselves to hazards incompatible with banking. This happened on a huge scale in the real estate and gas and oil bubble of the 1980s, with disastrous results for the banks' solvency. At that point both the US and the Canadian governments stepped in to bail them out in the shadows. We describe the process in an article, "The Dead Rat Under our Floor Boards," the leading article in this issue and we will try not to repeat ourselves. In Canada this took the form of phasing out the statutory reserves – a percentage of the public deposits that the banks took into their chequing accounts This increased the multiple of their cash holdings that the banks could lend out.

The American Fed through the Bank for International Settlements had been the main inspirer of this policy, but to itself applied it on a more discrete scale. It did not abolish outright its own statutory reserves – that treatment was for emerging or third world countries in difficulties with the IMF like New Zealand or Latin American countries. Canada owed nothing to the IMF, but its Conservative Prime Minister of the time had as his first principle of statesmanship to anticipate Washington's wishes. Washington for its own use reduced its statutory reserves drastically and shifted deposits requiring reserves at the close of business hours to non-reservable accounts and back again at the opening of the next business day.

Canada's University Texts are Revised

The end of the reserves in Canada was kept a closely guarded secret – and only a minimum of publicity was given to their steep downgrading in the US. The giveaway was so huge and so raw that not surprisingly the textbooks were revised to eliminate any reference to it. It took almost a year before COMER tracked down the bill in Canada that did the job. For our reader's convenience we pass on its reference number: Subsection 4 of Section 457 of Chapter 46 of the Statutes of Canada 1991.

So big and raw was that bailout that it changed the power structure of Canadian politics. It left the road clear to deregulate further the banks that had just been made whole from their losses in previous gambles. Practically all of what remained of the Roosevelt banking legislation was done away with. The banks were able to acquire brokerages, insurance operations (in Canada they still can't sell insurance from their bank branches), and mortgages, establish derivative boutiques. A derivative deals not with the whole security but with an abstracted aspect of it. For example, the rate of growth of its stock quotation, the acceleration of that rate of growth, the foreign exchange in which it is denominated, and so forth. The banks' derivative boutiques not only sell such items, but customize complex combinations of them – e.g., "swapping" the rate of increase in its yield with that of an unrelated stock. This allows those who use them to command a far greater leverage – control over the value of such shares – than if they bought the entire underlying securities or currencies. They are also unregulated despite countless recommendations of experts over the years that they be brought under government control. Unregulated, they are not subject to being reported. That has allowed our banks while seeming to retain their interest in the underlying securities that they may have just sold to trusting clients, to short their future revenue. For derivatives, being unregulated, do not have to appear on their books.

Compared to this state of affairs, the Depression of the 1930s was an age of innocence.

The Roosevelt Government didn't really know what it was doing, but it did keep an open mind. When Keynes visited Washington and met the President, Roosevelt found it hard grasping what he was talking about. "Some sort of mathematician," he commented. But that didn't stop his enquiring mind. And that made possible hope and considerable redemption. Every proposal to get out of the mess was considered. Young academics who could not get tenure at their universities because of their unorthodox views were brought to Washington and given a hearing. That is how John Kenneth Galbraith, a graduate from what was an obscure agricultural college in Canada – now the University of Guelph – recounts in his latest book that when he applied for a job in Washington he was hired so fast, that they forgot to ask whether he was a US citizen. He wasn't. But

he soon set up the price department of the US government. A couple of agricultural economists who were gold bugs convinced Roosevelt and his Secretary of the Treasury that raising the price of gold was the solution. Every morning soon after his Treasury Secretary, name of Morgenthau, breakfasted with Roosevelt in his bedroom while they studied the movement of the gold market the day before and decided how high it would be allowed to go that day.

US Open-mindedness during the Great Depression

Despair produced an open-mindedness unknown in public affairs before or since. Long lines of once conservative heads of large corporations, Henry Ford, Thomas Edison, the heads of General Motors, even banks, espoused views of Social Credit, and even 100 percent banking, out of a deeply felt need to lift the economy out of the gutter.

Government capital programs like the Tennessee Valley Administration were brought in with heavy central bank financing. Post offices were built at a small fraction of the cost had they been postponed a decade or two later. when folks could actually afford the price of postage stamps again. The lack of jobs and economic activity was recognized as the key problem. The essence of Keynesianism – that savings and investment must not be confused for they pull the economy in opposite directions and cannot be kept equal in times of depression – prevailed. A Utah banker, Marriner Eccles, who had never even heard of John Maynard Keynes, let alone read him, developed that conclusion from his observations of his own business, and was appointed Roosevelt's Secretary of the Treasury. Once the Depression and the War were behind, he became something like the Judas of the New Deal.

That is our first important bit of evidence in situating the Dead Rat Under the Floor Boards. In 1951, when the Americans had removed price controls – on the very eve of the Korean War! – as prices started climbing it became necessary to move the peg that had put a ceiling over interest rates during the war. In his memoirs President Harry Truman recounts that he was given to understand that the Treasury on behalf of the executive was negotiating with the Fed towards that end. When the Treasury-Fed Accord was closed, however, it turned out that his Treasurer – under the influence of Marriner Eccles – had betrayed him, and the peg instead of being raised, had been abolished. That underhanded act in high office launched a dreadful chapter in the history of the world that we have still not seen the end of.

Then came the evangel of the supposed independence of central banks from their governments so that they might better pursue the goal of "zero inflation."

The introduction of accrual accountancy to end the writing off of physical investments of the government in a single year and amortizing it over its useful existence was a most virtuous deed.

But when it appeared for the first time in federal statistics in January 1996 it was in the greatest secrecy – under the heading of "savings." That it most certainly was not since the $1.3 trillion dollars that brought to light for this first time in the public domain was not in cash, but already invested in bricks and mortar and equipment. In the private sector keeping assets or liabilities off balance sheet is an offense that has sent more than one high executive to jail. However, hiding the significance of that introduction of serious accountancy into the government's books was not mentioned in the press or in parliament.

Nor was the public instructed in the consequences of writing off capital assets of the government in a single year – a virtual home-run in economic book-cooking. Such a writeoff exaggerates the deficit monstrously in year one of the investment, since it is treated as a current expense that should be paid off when incurred. That results in more taxation being raised than necessary. A deeper layer of taxes in price is mistaken for "inflation," which allegedly can only be cured by high interest rates. Then since the capital asset – a building or a highway, appears on the government's book at a token value of one dollar, it can be privatized at a small portion of its real value to produce an apparent surplus that can be patriotically applied to reducing the deficit.

The citizens whose taxes have already paid for the facility once with its privatization have to begin paying for it in users' fees a second time.

And on top of it all, the most productive of all government investments – investment in human capital – education, health, and social services – is still ignored and not even treated as capital but as current spending.

William Krehm

REVIEW OF A BOOK BY MALCOLM J. GREENSTUART. PIGTALE PUBLISHING, YANAKIE, VICTORIA, AUSTRALIA, 2001

"Cosmic Accounting"

THIS IS AN UPDATE and modest extension of Buckminster Fuller's vision of potential abundance by means of a global electric energy grid, an idea for which there was a boomlet of enthusiasm in the early eighties. It emerged out of the energy crunch of the early seventies and the concomitant notion that since usable energy is the most critical element in any economic system; it ought to be the standard of value. Some thinkers extended this reasoning to propose that money should represent a measured quantity of free or usable energy (a Joule standard in place of the gold standard). Fuller's grid brought this notion closer to feasibility, for it would permit thousands of mini-generating facilities of great variety to feed into it, especially from solar collecting devices. Since the sun is shining somewhere all the time and energy can be transmitted speedily around the grid, every continent can be using solar power 24 hours a day. Part of the enthusiasm for the Fuller vision was its democratizing potential. If everyone had a device for collecting and transforming free energy from wind, sun, or falling water and a connection to the global grid, then consumption from the grid when one's own generator was idle could be likened to withdrawals from a savings account. Once wired up in this way an individual would never again have to pay to get his or her work done. That would be a very substantial contribution to equalizing incomes around the world. It is therefore a highly appropriate item for consideration by campaigners for social justice, and so it was that I encountered Greenstuart's presentation to the Basic Income European Network (BIEN) at Barcelona in September of 2004. He appeared on a panel with others who argue that opportunities for "free lunch" are abundant and in fact enjoyed by the most wealthy members of our species.

The main departure of *Cosmic Accounting* from what I remember of Fulleresque ideas in the eighties is the focus on concentrated energy farms as contrasted to the great variety and number of independent generators feeding into the grid from the user's own location. The author would give a jump start to energy money by giving it away to everyone, in equal shares, from more centralized power stations. He imagines that recipients would start using their endowments of free energy as a replacement for money and that the attractions of this system would encourage its spread over all the planet. The metaphorical equivalent of Net National (Global) Income would be collected and tallied each day and divided equally among all individuals on earth. Each would have his/her allocation recorded in a central computer and their usage would be constantly monitored, by meter and the equivalent of a debit card. The central computer keeps track of distribution and consumption, and the individual accounts and debit cards enable participants to spend and to keep track of their credit balances. (Unconsumed daily budgets could be converted into an energy savings bank, such as a seawater desalinization plant; technological progress will overcome the objection that we are heavily reliant on petroleum fuels for transportation.) This system permits the transfer of energy credits to whomever is interested in receiving them, at the discretion of the owner.

Greenstuart is an Australian engineer, and he reports that with a solar collecting device (parabolic dish) recently perfected at Australian National University it is now possible to generate all of the energy consumed annually on earth, from every source ($6 \infty 10^{14}$ Kwh), on a collector farm equivalent in area to one-quarter that of South Australia. He proposes a pilot project in that region, to serve a community of about 20,000. He estimates the cost of the parabolic dish energy farm and the necessary gridwork to cost $70 million (AUD). This amount should all be raised by donations from about 10,000 people, none of whom would expect any return on their contributions other than the resulting endowment of a perpetual energy income– plus the satisfaction that they are taking a critical step toward transforming the world to a sustainable basis. "All we need is the money to build the generation and distribution facilities in the first place so we can start giving energy away at no charge." While we are still wide-eyed, he goes on to affirm that "a first thing it will take for this initiative to start moving is to discard the disbelief that 10,000 people won't sponsor a scheme that does not produce a financial return. [I]t will take believing that it is possible to get over all the other potential hurdles." This can be accomplished, he believes, by spreading the good news about "the very attractive possibility and wonderful outcomes that are associated and naturally delivered with this system" (i.e., the negation of all the environmental and humanitarian horrors lamented by doomsday prophets of the past half century).

A Free World Power Dividend?

The notion of free electrical power strikes one as preposterous in 21st century Ontario, but the context of the Barcelona conference lends some plausibility. The energy grid by itself (as illustrated in Fuller's "dymaxion" projection of the globe as a flat map) is doubtless feasible from the technological standpoint, and this possibility is an endowment of "free lunch" from collective human ingenuity and effort over thousands of years. It is owed to no one of this generation.

There is a clear affinity with the Social Credit principle of cultural inheritance. And the arguments for Basic Income offered by the author's co-panelists in Barcelona make a persuasive case for the availability of unearned rents that could be taxed away from their privileged recipients at no cost to overall economic performance. It is therefore supportable on the financing front from a principle that is regularly developed in textbooks of economics–or at least used to be. Greenstuart's arguments for a donated investment and free distribution of energy credits are unnecessarily convoluted because he has apparently not become aware of the daunting social impediments to Fuller's vision of a sustainable system.

Fuller is quoted as having said that "wealth is the accomplished technological power to [provide for human needs and wants]. Money is only an expediency-adopted means of interexchanging items of real wealth." It is further noted that Fuller was encouraged, near the end of his life (in 1983), to observe that the idea of energy-money had become a topic of conversation (115). That gave him hope that humanity might survive. (For he recognized the non-sustainability of the existing monetary and financial system with its requirement of economic growth to distribute income.) Energy as money did indeed become a topic of conversation as the environmental movement gathered strength in the sixties and seventies. *Cosmic Accounting* gives us no information about the momentum or lack thereof that followed that awakening, and it seems to have fallen below the horizon since about the early nineties. The author mentions his contacts with Global Energy Network International and the Buckminster Fuller Institute without implicating them directly in his enthusiasm for *cosmic accounting*. Only one paper in his list of references addresses the topic of energy accounting as a monetary system, and it was published in the first volume of *Ecological Economics* in 1989.

The notion that energy be used as money stems from the observation that energy is the principal or critical component to any production and the only truly scarce or limiting element to fulfilling human needs or wants. All inorganic materials can be recycled, and biospheric management and interpersonal services will be provided by willing volunteers once people do not have to worry about where their most basic income (embodied energy) is coming from. Energy is therefore the true *cost* of everything. The next step in this line of reasoning is to infer that the *price* of everything should be the same as its cost. Cosmic accounting presupposes that all (legitimate) costs are energy costs, and that it is the sum of these costs built into any item that should determine its price. This is a near equivalent of saying that the price of an item ought to be the same as the value of the labor that went into it, with an implicit judgment that everyone's labor should be counted equally. Part of the appeal of energy accounting as replacement for the monetary system is its anticipated contribution to the elimination of non-productive and wasteful activities. (For example, energy conservation would be a paramount consideration in resource allocation, and most of the existing financial system could disappear.) Those services that are useful, even though not directly productive of physical output, would be voluntary (teachers, physicians, artists, entertainers, etc.). Handicrafts and other activities that do require a large share of human physical input relative to inanimate energy would be exceptional in having prices that exceed their (electrical) energy cost. Instead of recognizing this as a payment for labor, however, Greenstuart calls it "profit."

His solution therefore depends on the good will of people who may have expended considerable effort to accumulate skills that are in demand. It also would have to win over the agreement of the owners of inorganic (recyclable) materials out of which machines, grids, buildings, etc. are made. For example, the energy cost of a parabolic collector disk is said to be six months, but the money cost is so high that it takes 20 years to repay. The premium in money terms is a social obligation to people with unique skills and rare property resources. Whether it is a mine, junk yard or patent, these people have claims against others that are protected as legal rights to property. Property values (claims of ownership) regularly reflect an element of rarity.

Air is supremely valuable to humans, but it usually is not sufficiently rare to command a price. At the level of interpersonal services, rarity is also a factor and regularly entails the social element of obligation. The idea of *value* is deeply linked to interpersonal obligation. Diamonds are a favored illustration. Now that they can be manufactured, diamonds are less rare, but they have maintained high value due to their accumulated symbolism of interpersonal obligation.

The link of values like these to energy costs of production is tenuous at best. Conventional accounting keeps track of them in terms of money. Balances accumulate, which gives a *storage* aspect to money. Storage is much less convenient for electrical energy. Greenstuart counters (private communication) that the storage defect can be mitigated by technological development. This is doubtless true, but if it were removed completely then cosmic accounting seems likely to suffer from the same defects that give rise to the phenomenon of unearned income in the existing system.

Part of the appeal of energy-as-money probably stems from the notion that money should have intrinsic value–real value that can be stored up and consumed on a rainy day. Just as old, however, is the understanding that no kind of money can really perform this function, as Midas learned when he tried to eat or embrace gold. Clarity in thinking about money is enhanced by thinking of it as *claim* on value as contrasted to value in itself or a *store* of value.[1] Greenstuart's scheme for transition to cosmic accounting requires that *some* people voluntarily give up part of their claim on other members of society. It therefore entails issues of social justice that are as old as humanity. And although modern technology is introduced, it does not seem to have the capacity to make those old issues go away.

Inanimate energy slaves do make more production possible with less human labor, but the social issue remains and is inextricably linked to the observation of economists that human input is the ultimate source of all value. It was always possible to reduce toil, pain and social injustice if one could attribute different motivations to members of our species. Many visionaries have devised schemes for social organizations that would overcome human nature. Thomas More anticipated Fuller's vision, 500 years ago in a fantasy-land he called *Utopia*. He made an estimate of how much work per day from every individual it would take to do all the work necessary to feed, clothe and house the population.

It was only a few hours. The rest of the time they could spend in creative and socially uplifting activities of every kind–just as Greenstuart has suggested is possible in the world of abundant energy slaves (inanimate). That amount of work per person would cover all real costs, and there need be no accounting at all, since everyone would be paying full price for everything, every week of his or her working life. Everything necessary (and jewelry was not on the list) would be available in abundance, so nothing would have a price. Costs were already paid, so there was no need for money. His requirement of a few hours of work per day from everyone is the equivalent under different technological circumstances of the proposal to share the annual solar energy endowment equally. Greenstuart stops at that point, in the belief that he has completed the theoretical work. Thomas More, however, did not stop there. Having laid out an energy distribution system as initial conditions, he then carried those assumptions forward to examine every implication he could conceive for what social life would be like if the system worked according to plan. When he was finished, he surmised that no group or nation had ever, nor probably would ever, put it into practice. Fuller's vision did not get beyond the human barriers perceived by More.

Keith Wilde

Editorial Comment

The concept of using energy flows as a measure of value enjoyed a flare under the sponsorship of the Club of Rome in the 1970s, as is reflected in my book *Babel's Tower: The Dynamics of Economic Breakdown* (1977). In it I have the following criticism of the book of Howard T. Odum and Elizabeth C. Odum, *Energy Basis for Man and Nature*, McGraw Hill Book Company, New York, 1976:

"The attempts of ecologists to integrate price into their models have not been more successful than the efforts of economists to work non-renewable fossil-energy factors into theirs. On either side the tendency has been to ignore the different subsystems contributing each its specific input into price.

"The Odums set up a direct equivalence of monetary and fossil-energy units. 'The following explanation suggests that energy flows are a measure of value and are ultimately responsible for the values humans attribute to money…. The town isolated in an agrarian region in a steady state…helps us understand how energy flow represents value for survival and why circulating money helps keep track of their values…. Money circulates from rural forms to the town and back. The money flows as a counter-current to energy flow. It starts as low-quality energy in the country and then is transformed and concentrated by production process and the transport of product to the town. In the town, the energy is concentrated further in high-quality-goods and services that are returned to the country. For a regional system to compete well and thus survive, it must use its energies in the least wasteful way while generating the most energy flow…. When such an energy arrangement exists, it is an equal-value loop. The circulation of money around that loop is the way human beings recognized that the flows are of equal value. The fossil-fuel equivalents of the energy flow around the loops are also equal, since both were generated from the same energy sources…. In steady-state conditions fossil-fuel equivalence can be used as a measure of contribution to survival and thus to value.'

"The excursions of the Odums into social theory suffer from improvisation. The circulation of money can hardly be described as 'the way human beings recognize that the energy flows are of equal value.' There are societies in which money plays a quite marginal role, but energy flows effectively enough for survival. The 'steady-state' which serves as king-pin in the proof of the equivalence of energy and money is a monistic abstraction – very much the counterpart of the equilibrium points of marginalist theory in economics.

"It is out of the question that our society should revert to a steady state – even if such actually existed in a remote past. We must balance our consumption and supply of energy. But to do so we shall have to introduce some highly dynamic changes in the structures, ethic, and motivations of our society. That implies that it will be anything but stationary, though its energy consumption may become static or even decline. A society that has attained our level of technology and pluralism is inescapably subject to a high momentum of change. That change must be patterned so that we do not destroy our ecology and ourselves, but that will call for 'organic growth' rather than a stationary state.

"Far more than physical energy enters into the production of high-quality goods and services. It is impossible to reduce the work involved in the writing of James Joyce's *Ulysses* to their equivalence in fossil-fuel units of energy. If such an equivalence existed, we would be helpless to explain the phenomena of classical Athens, Elizabethan England, or Renaissance Italy. The entire consumption of physical energy in such societies was negligible by our standards.

"The fallacy of the Odums is that they treat our economic-ecological complex as though it were a homogeneous system, when it is in fact composed of several subsystems, each with its specific logic. The Odums attempt to assimilate everything into the ecological-resources subsystem, just as conventional economists try imposing the logic of the 'pure and perfect market' on the other subsystems."

William Krehm

1. A distinction made by Gunnar Tomasson recently on the "Gang8" Internet forum that may be viewed at http://finance.groups.yahoo.com/group/gang8. Tomasson is a Washington-based economist in private practice with special interest in monetary and financial reform. He spent a 23-year career in the IMF.

Mail Box

Hon. Ralph Goodale, Minister of Finance
House of Commons, Ottawa, ON

November 5, 2004
7 Grant Street, Stratford, ON N5A 1L5

Dear Minister:

In the October issue of *Economic Reform*, Mr. William Krehm, editor of the monthly publication, responded to a statement made by you in a letter to Mr. André Martenette re: governments, federal, provincial and municipal, borrowing from the Bank of Canada instead of Canada's commercial banks. In your letter you wrote that:

"To acquire the government debt, the Bank of Canada would have to print new currency. The rapid growth of the money supply would eventually result in an increase in inflation and higher interest rates."

But even I know that statement to be incorrect – for two basic reasons:

1. There is in existence a total of Canadian coins and paper money worth approximately $35 billion. Yet at any moment there is business being conducted using Canadian currency involving the exchange of goods and services worth approximately $135 billion. That means that there is approximately $100 billion dollars that exists as nothing more than a temporary blip on a computer screen, a blip that will be relocated as that bit of business is concluded and another entered into.

2. If, when governments borrow from commercial banks, the commercial banks do not print more bills or strike additional coins, why would the Bank of Canada be forced to do this? Yes, I realize that only the Bank of Canada has the right to create and add to the money supply, but why would it be necessary to do so when commercial banks temporarily create additional money based on loans they make to facilitate business?

The sole difference between borrowing from the Bank of Canada and borrowing from Canadian (or foreign or international) commercial banks is how much it costs the borrower to service a particular debt.

Canadian commercial banks charge interest at a rate which adds tens of millions of dollars per quarter to their profits. The amount garnered from loans to government is listed in the quarterly reports and sometimes shows up in newspapers. That profit goes straight into the pockets of shareholders and is lost to taxpayers and their government representatives, especially if it goes offshore.

The Bank of Canada's sole shareholder is the Government of Canada. Any profits accrued by this shareholder are available for ongoing and new government programs, and to pay down the debt. Borrow from the Bank of Canada and save twice: get back all the interest paid on the loan except what it takes to actually operate the Bank, and borrow less the next time because you've got that interest to spend.

The commercial banks would miss their quarterly subsidies, but then I don't think their bottom lines should take precedence over the welfare of all Canadians who would certainly benefit if the Government of Canada took advantage of this savings that is available.

Sincerely,
D. Rhea East

EDITORIAL NOTE: Ms. East is a retired geography high school teacher who taught her students to think and write lucidly about vital matter concerning society and its planet. It would seem that our Finance Minister or the hacks who churn out the replies to taxpayers' correspondence have flunked this test.

Economics and the Corporatist Culture

MOST PEOPLE participate in activities creating economic value in the hope that it can lead to a better quality of life for them. But in the real world, all activities occur in a social context. Therefore, enhancing the quality of life entails both a quantitative and a qualitative aspect.

The quantitative aspect is closely connected to the direct economic activity, which earns the money income allowing people to buy goods and services. The qualitative aspect, while also partly a function of the level of goods and services we can buy, are however mostly decided by how the surrounding social context provide us with a responsive background for social and creative activities. The latter is the type of activities that the American psychologist, A.H. Maslow (1908-1970), called self-actualization, which constituted the highest needs driving human activities in his hierarchical system.

In a normal human environment, quantitative inputs arising from the economic system have thus to be integrated in the general social context in a way that creates qualitative enhancements of social expression.

The Corporate High-jack

Unfortunately, the social context of society has been high-jacked by a corporatist culture, which has harnessed our current high-tech industrial society to serve a narrow set of goals. The key aim is to maximize the economic surplus available for distribution among a small elite at the pinnacle of the corporate system.

As the corporate system has transmogrified into its present all-compassing form, it has effectively waged a slash and burn war against all other forms of social expression. As a result, people in modern societies no longer have a varied palette of cultural, educational and leisure options for a socially meaningful lifestyle. At all crossroads they are met by a few highly commercialized choices, with little difference in substance.

The result is a culture transfixed on material objects and their possession. Questions as to whether they actually fill any positive role are pushed into the shadows. When Maslowian self-actualization becomes replaced by a drive for fulfillment through possession of material objects, it often leads to a pathologic state of self-centeredness, where ability to communicate or empathize with others is lost. And not only ordinary people fall victim to this pathology. In most cases the corporate elite succumb to a personality-deforming sub-culture where self-actualization is substituted by role-plays advertising unrestrained ability to disregard the money-cost of their lifestyles. This, of course, is the very opposite – the enthronement of money as the only valid measure of social worth.

The Strip-down of Economic Theory

The new corporate culture has also pervaded academic environments. A symptom of this is the naming of almost all new campus buildings and research centres across North America after corporate sponsors, rather than after historical figures or famous scientists which had been the tradition.

A more serious question is how scientists and university teachers have adapted to the new corporatist culture. In no discipline has this been more evident than in economics, which has allowed itself to be reduced to a theory without much validity outside the narrow scope of portfolio management for the wealthy, or determining which conditions best ensure unrestrained corporate growth.

The Illusionary World of Equilibria

At the center of corporatist economics is an illusionary world, in which economic forces move up and down curves, depicting imaginary points of equilibria at their intersections. Government interference in "free" markets is decried as creating local inefficiencies. The whole exercise is made to look plausible by a few crude observations that everyone can recognize as their own: e.g., such as we will buy more ice cream if it is cheaper, and paying taxes reduces our potential for buying all the CDs we would like.

In this environment, theories such as the Keynesian derived IS-LM model has been turned upside down. The IS-LM model, in its original form, was part of a theory that advocated a strong government role in supporting the economy under downturns by among other things raising governments' discretionary demand. The key methods advocated was expanding the money supply, which would drive interest rates down.

In the interpretation of modern corporatist-inspired economics, the IS-LM model is used as a defense for the policies of central bankers when they use interest rates as the all-important weapon against inflation.

For most people with ordinary incomes the marginal propensity to consume is almost static, being very close to 100 percent. The influence of interest rates thus has very little influence on the reciprocal, the marginal propensity to save. In these incomes ranges, the main consequence of higher interest rates therefore means higher costs of already existing loads of consumer debt. And since debt repayment is non-discretionary spending, when its cost rises, it will either crowd out real spending, or alternatively force debt to higher levels.

The Great Upcoming Fire-sale

Interest payments made by ordinary households do not disappear. They are simply paid to someone else. At first, they are paid to banks or credit card companies. But these are only intermediaries. The final owners of debt are the portfolio – holding wealthy households belonging to the corporatist elite at the other end of the economic spectrum.

These high-income households have a low marginal propensity to consume, and since a lot of their consumption consists of luxury imports, an even lower marginal propensity to consume *domestic* products. Current economics only focusses on the standard effect of higher interest rates that temporarily reduces interest-sensitive demand. It ignores the important side-effect that further lowers spending by shifting income from households with high marginal propensities to consume to those with low propensities to consume. Furthermore, this shift lowering the propensity to consume real goods and services is lasting.

If governments carry large debt loads, higher interest rates will also crowd out their discretionary spending or force them to add to debt. But unrestrained growth of government debt has traditionally been seen as unacceptable since it can crowd out real investments of firms. This might not only lead to reduced future economic potential, but also put further pressure on interest rates.

Under the old banking system demanding reserves as a fixed proportion of banks' portfolios of debt instruments, this consequence was more or less assured.

The great trick that governments and their central bankers came up with in 1988 was the Basle Accord. It eliminated the requirements for reserves in exchange for risk-weighted capital requirements. In this scheme of things, the government debt of the developed countries was assigned a zero-risk weight, making it possible for government to expand debt almost without limits. In particular, the effect of crowding out private investments was eliminated, since accumulating government debt no longer affected banks ability to expand their credit to private borrowers.

But there are still no free lunches. As the whole process pushes a rising number of the economic chips over to the side of the table where the wealthy sit, they will eventually demand that some of their chips be cashed in. The only means available will then be fire sales of public assets at fire sale prices.

And that of course is where we are at the moment – at a climactic point of disequilibrium rather than of equilibrium.

Dix Sandbeck

Review of a Book and a Social Conscience

In Retrospect: The Tragedy and Lessons of Vietnam by Robert McNamara with Brian VanDe Mark, Random House, New York, 1995.

MCNAMARA opens with an explanation why he should retell his story once more, an ancient mariner who with each retelling reveals a bit more of what weighs heavily on his conscience. "My associates in the Kennedy and Johnson administrations were an exceptional group: young, vigorous, intelligent, well-meaning, patriotic servants of the United States. How did this group – 'the best and the brightest,' as we eventually came to be known in an ironically pejorative phrase – get it so wrong on Vietnam?

"The story has not yet been told.

"But why now? Why after all these years of silence am I convinced I should speak? The main [reason] is that I have grown sick at heart witnessing the cynicism with which many people view our political institutions and leaders.

"Many factors helped lead to this. Vietnam, Watergate, scandals, corruption. But I do not believe, on balance that America's political leaders have been incompetent or insensitive to the welfare of the people who elected them. Nor do I believe they have been any worse than their foreign counterparts or their colleagues in the private sector."

Such comparison standards, of course, in this day of manipulated memory suppression, severely limits McNamara's soul-searching. For in this era of Globalization and Deregulation foreign governments and above all the private sector, are no acceptable yardstick for decency or responsibility. On matters that count our history is the main tool in humanity's survival kit. Not only for what did work, but from the evidence, what can't. It is from society's disasters quite as much as from its successes, that humanity can learn what makes survival possible or rules it out. History, a key resource, has, however, been twisted and even – as in economic theory – completely ruled out.

"The US commanders in Vietnam – as did I – viewed the conflict as primarily a military operation, when in fact it was a highly complex nationalistic and internecine struggle."

Yet all those other key aspects, had simply been declared "externalities" an atrocious habit that spread to government from the degenerate discipline that passes for economic theory. In an ever more complex world, the concerns of a privileged class was mistaken for a guide, and other problems were declared self-balancing – i.e., automatically balancing themselves so that they can safely be ignored.

What has Happened to the Absent South East Asian Experts of the US Government

Since the writing of this book – and more recently a film done based largely on this book – the age of Globalization and Deregulation has made devastating progress. The outpouring of scandals involving the largest corporations of the private sec-

tor, and the number of big and little Vietnams across the globe have multiplied. Our review of what is still the latest Vietnam soul-searchings of the Secretary of War when US intervention in Vietnam was initiated is still incomplete. What is still unaddressed is almost as revealing as what is brought forward.

"Many political leaders and scholars in the US and abroad argue that the Vietnam war actually helped contain the spread of Communism in South and East Asia. Some argue that it hastened the end of the Cold War. But I know that the war caused terrible damage to America."

Much of the book – in contrast to the far better edited film produced in the light of the Iraqi experience during the subsequent decade, is confined to judgments based largely on criteria within the US hierarchy. Yet there are telling passages.

Example: "Our government lacked experts to consult to compensate for our ignorance. When the Berlin crisis occurred in 1961, President Kennedy was able to turn to senior people... who knew the Soviets intimately. There were no senior officials in the Pentagon or the State Department with comparable knowledge of South East Asia. The irony of this gap was that it existed largely because the top East Asian and China experts in the State Department had been purged during the McCarthy hysteria of the 1950s. Without men like these to provide sophisticated, nuanced insights, we – certainly I – badly misread China's objectives and mistook its bellicose rhetoric to imply a drive towards regional hegemony. We also totally underestimated the nationalist aspect of Ho Chi Minh's movement. We saw him only as a Communist and only secondly as a Vietnamese nationalist." Why did we fail to consider China and Vietnam in the same light as we did Yugoslavia – a Communist nation independent of Moscow: Tito seemed unique, because he and Stalin had openly fallen out. And Cuba's recent tilt toward the Soviet Union seemed illustrative of how ostensibly independent Third World movements placed themselves within the Communist orbit. Thus, we equated Ho Chi Minh not with Tito but with Fidel Castro."

The "domino theory" that had already dunked a good part of Latin America in blood, was in a sense a premonition of "Globalization and Deregulation." It held that the world was an indivisible prize contested between the Soviet Union and the US, and signified that any challenge to American overlordship wherever, unless checked with full military might would inexorably work its way to American home territory. No room was left for other interpretations, or alternatives to scotching any movement that didn't conform to the "Washington Consensus." The US at its most aggressive, was always cast as being concerned only with the defence of its homeland and the all the nobler virtues that reigned there. Amongst the more bizarre consequences of such a doctrine was the complete disregard of the alienation of the rest of the world's respect for the country that invented modern advertising and public relations.

William Krehm

REVIEW OF A BOOK BY ROBERT E. WOOD,
UNIVERSITY OF CALIFORNIA PRESS, BERKELEY,
1986

"From Marshall Plan to Debt Crisis — Foreign Aid and Development Choices in the World Economy"

AN APOLOGY for our habit of reviewing books long in the tooth and falling short of best-seller status. The Nazis burned books. Allowing them to languish virginally on library shelves is a more efficient way of sending them to Coventry.

"In 1955, at the close of his account of the origins of the Marshall Plan, ex-US State Department official Joseph Jones [remarked], 'The Marshall Plan's creation suggested 'not the limits but the infinite possibilities of influencing the politics, attitudes and actions of other countries by statesmanship in Washington.'"

As a sociologist, Wood begins with an apology for "his boldness in tackling a subject generally the preserve of economists, and to a lesser extent of political scientists. I have not felt that I have left my sociologist's craft behind. It has become increasingly apparent to me that foreign aid plays a significant role in shaping those aspects of the social world that sociologists commonly look at: social equality, class structure, politics, gender relations, rural-urban relations, and so forth." It is high time that economists availed themselves of help from other disciplines to tidy up the mess in their workshop.

"The central focus is on how this structure of access to aid has changed over time and shaped development options in the Third World. From this perspective, the emergence of the debt crisis is closely connected to the role of aid in the world economy. The debt crisis has profoundly altered the international environment that Third World countries face; and the legacy of debt will continue a central focus of international relations and development choices for years to come."

A far cry from the self-congratulation of official scribes on the success of the Marshall Plan that put the show on the road!. "For one thing, the activity financed by aid may not be the true measure of aid's impact because the recipient government might have carried out such activity in the absence of aid. The real impact of aid in such cases may be to finance some alternative government activity or simply to underwrite higher domestic (often luxury) consumption.

"The Marshall Plan has come to symbolize boldness and success, and virtually whenever new directions in US foreign aid programs have been proposed, the theme of 'a new Marshall Plan' has been pressed into service. Officially known as the European Recovery Program (ERP), the Marshall Plan dispensed over $13 billion between 1948 and 1952 to Western European countries. Over 90% of this aid was in the form of grants.

"By the end of 1951, indeed, the Marshall Plan was in a deep crisis that was resolved only through rearmament and the expanded aid of its successor, the Mutual Security Agency. The real success of the Marshall Plan lay in its contribution to the construction of a new international order, not in the quantity of capital and raw material it provided Western Europe.

"Five sets of changes in the world economy created the dollar shortage that was the basis of the worldwide postwar economic crisis.

The Breakdown of Trade between Eastern and Western Europe

"First, the breakdown of trade between Eastern and Western Europe. In 1948 Western European exports to Eastern Europe were less than half of the prewar level, and imports from Eastern Europe were only one third. Instead of recovering, this trade declined over the next five years. This meant that European countries had to rely on dollar imports from the US to fulfill needs formerly met by trade with Eastern Europe.

"Second there was the loss of important colonial sources of dollars. Vietnam was in rebellion. So was the Netherlands' major dollar earner, Indonesia. Guerrilla insurgency was increasing in Britain's most profitable colony, Malaysia. France had 110,000 troops in Indochina, and the Netherlands had 130,000 in Indonesia. Britain had 1.4 million troops around the world. South Africa took its gold sales out of the sterling area dollar pool.

"Third, there was Europe's loss of earnings on foreign investments. Continued sales of these investments was a condition of lend-lease aid during the war. For both France and Britain, overseas investment earnings had long helped offset trade deficits. In addition, Britain had run up $13.7 billion in debts, known as sterling balances, to other sterling area countries, particularly India. These countries now clamored for the balances to finance their development plans.

"Fourth, many of the European countries and their overseas territories were hit with declining terms of trade. 'Had the price of gold and rubber gone up as those of other items traded, the same exports to the US during the five years following the war would have earned an additional $3.5 billion for the sterling area. Total Marshall Plan aid to Great Britain came to $2.7 billion.

"This left them susceptible to small fluctuations in the US currency at the same time that no new mechanisms had yet been approved to provide the kind of international liquidity that sterling had once provided. Britain's need for aid after the war was partly rooted in US aid policies during the war. It was official US policy to administer lend-lease in such a way that the UK's gold and dollar balances would not fall below $600 million or rise above $1 billion. This was secured by altering what the British were expected to pay for in dollars and what would be included in lend-lease. The US reasoning was that reserves less than $600 million would force Britain to resort to the kind of economic controls the US was dedicated to preventing, whereas over $1 billion would leave Britain too independent of postwar US influence." That fell short of "leaving it all to a free, competitive market."

However, largely domestic concerns prompted Washington to begin preparing the Marshall Plan long before the Cold War cast its shadow over the landscape and was fully exploited to get the Marshall through Congress. "A 1941 survey of the American Economic Association found 80% of its members predicting a postwar depression."

It early became evident that Europe's dollar-earning capacity would not solve the US's problem in exporting enough to keep their economy from relapsing into depression. "US imports from Europe constituted only 0.33% of US GNP. Politically untouchable tariff walls made increasing most European imports impossible. US policymakers looked instead to the overseas territories of European countries to bail out their colonial masters. This description does not accurately portray the way the colonial powers acquired the dollars their colonies earned. The basic idea of triangular trade was reiterated again and again throughout the Marshall Plan.

"Its most fateful error was that it overlooked the powerful movements arose throughout the colonial territories to cut their ties with the wounded imperial powers. It imparted an incoherence to Washington's policies *vis à vis* the colonial insurgencies – encouraging them at times and supporting the colonial powers' efforts to suppress them at others. Arms sales were not an unimportant overarching factor in this ambiguity. Military Keynesianism, of all versions of the doctrines of the Wizard of Bloomsbury, was most acceptable to the US Congress. Europe's quality troops were never where Washington wanted them.

"Secretary of State Marshall reported in 1949: 'When we reached the problem of increasing the security of Europe, I found the French troops of any quality were all out in Indochina, and the Dutch troops of any quality were all out in Indochina, and the one place where they were not was in Western Europe.'" In one way or another the colonial wars had to be resolved (p. 43).

"The brutality with which the message to was imparted to Latin America that the Marshall plans they expected were not in the cards contributed to the riots [the *"Bogotazo"*] that marred the Bogota Conference of 1948. For Latin America reliance would be entirely on private investment. *The unspoken footnote was that the CIA and the American military, were already mobilized to guarantee that the economy of the region would be wide open to American corporate investment on its terms.* [Our italics.]

"But bridging the dollar gap with the rest of the world – the initial goal of the Marshall Plan – was not doing well. In 1951 the dollar gap was the worst since 1945. However, the [Marshall Plan] came to be popularly defined as a success partly through a redefinition of goals. At the end of the Marshall Plan, conservative social forces had greatly strengthened their political control in all Western European countries. European resistance to rearmament had been overcome. In the popular mind, the Marshall Plan had prevented Europe from 'going communist.'

"In this context of deep pessimism about an economic solution to the dollar gap by 1952, a massive military buildup emerged as the only practical solution of the Truman administration months before the Korean war broke out. One State Department document, for example, justified a military approach by observing that Congress was more favorably disposed to military aid than to aid for economic recovery." There was the added advantage to military Keynesianism abroad, that it ensured a sustainable relationship with Europe by tying it to American military hardware, whereas purely economic aid might prepare the recipient nations for uniting to assert their autonomy from the US.

"The Marshall Plan created a body of operating principles and procedures that remain an integral part of the aid regime. Although aid's use to block socialism has been well understood, its role in limiting national capitalism extends beyond the Marshall Plan period. The hammer to achieve this has been debt.

"Over one-fifth of US aid between 1948 and 1952 went directly to the underdeveloped areas. In both Europe and the underdeveloped world, specific procedures and techniques were devised in the aid regime. The use of counterpart funds (money to be advanced, but held back as security for the fulfilling of specified conditions), became a widely emulated method of expanding the leverage of aid."

The Proliferation of the Aid Regime

"By the 1980s, however, the aid picture had become enormously complex. Separate aid programs were now administered by all sixteen countries of the Development Assistance Committee (DAS); by at least eight communist and ten OPEC countries, by approximately twenty multilateral organizations in addition to various components of the United Nations system, by hundreds of private organizations. Aid programs had even been initiated by Third World countries.

"The 1950s were a period of the dominance and diversification of bilateral aid programs of the advanced capitalist countries – a state of affairs, ironically, assured by the advent of smaller Soviet and Chinese aid programs. The 1960s were marked by the emergence of new forms of multilateralism, largely either under the auspices of, or modeled after, the World Bank. The 1970s witnessed the sudden emergence of Middle Eastern oil-producing countries as major aid donors, as well as an expansion of World Bank that consolidated its position as leading aid institution. In the mid-to-late 1970s, the expansion of non-concessional private bank lending in lieu of official financing came to constitute a fundamental challenge to the aid regime, culminating in the debt crisis.

"The specter of communist aid led the US to press the OEEC countries (constituted in 1961 as the Organization for Economic Cooperation and Development [OECD], with an expanded membership including Canada and Japan) to initiate or expand their own aid programs.

"New multilateral institutions accounted for 40% of multilateral aid in 1970, and 50% by 1980.

"The institutions emerged largely in response to Third World pressure, but they represented a defeat of the effort of Third World countries to establish a UN institution providing capital assistance over which they would have control.

"The most unexpected institutional development during the 1970s was the explosion of aid flows from the major oil-producing countries of the Middle East, members of the Organization of Petroleum-Exporting Countries (OPEC). By far the greatest proportion of their enormous dollar reserves was placed on deposit with commercial banks in the advanced capitalist countries, but some was lent directly to Third World countries at concessional rates.

"Marshall Plan aid was overwhelmingly in the form of grants, but aid to Third World countries in the later 1950s and 1960s was increasingly on a loan basis.

"The most striking innovations in external financing in the mid to late 1970s occurred not in the aid regime but in the practices of private commercial banks. But whereas in the 1950s they consisted almost entirely of direct private investment, in the later 1970s lending by private commercial banks far surpassed direct private investment.

"This had to do with the growth of the Eurodollar market. This refers to the offshore markets for loans in any strong currency. The offshore venue of such loans not only kept them free of taxation and other restrictions. Those who lent on the eurodollar market, in effect created their own notional money supply, effectively off their balance sheet so long as contractual obligations were honoured. Not only did it by-pass home-based restrictions and controls, but circumvented invasions of privacy in other respects. Unless repatriated, it has a tenuous connection with the real economy.

"The Third World thus became entangled with the wrong end of the credit spectrum. Its finances, at best vulnerable enough, became exposed to every wiggle in short-term funds. That tended to repel productive investors.

"The oil price increases in 1973-4, resulted in OPEC countries placing $22 billion in Eurocurrency deposits in 1974. But the expansion of the banks' financing of the Third World began earlier. Between 1965 and 1976, the number of US banks with foreign branches rose from 13 to 125 and the number of branches from 211 to 731. Faced with stagflation at home, the banks of the First World turned to the Third World for expansion. It was seen as an "economy of scale" making multimillion dollar loans to a single minister or dictator, rather than having to deal with thousands of small borrowers at home. Besides, the buzzword of the day was the risklessness of 'sovereign debt,' i.e., loans to governments. Corruption took care of any doubts that surrounded that concept. Much of the money lent to Third World lands stayed in special accounts in the US as undeclared commissions.

"External financing for underdeveloped countries has become highly differentiated. The number of bilateral donors has increased, and multilateral institutions have proliferated. No formal mechanism of systemwide coordination exists. The United Nations has virtually no influence over bilateral aid programs and practically none over the multilateral institutions officially affiliated with it, such as the IMF and the World Bank."

The jungle that dominates the international aid field flies in the face of proposed sets of principles.

William Krehm

How the Debt-based Monetary System Functions in Canada

(Presented by Connie Fogal, leader of the Canadian Action Party, at the Bromsgrove Conference in the UK in October)

RECENT FIGURES from Statistics Canada and the Bank of Canada show that the total debt of all levels of Canadian government, individuals, and corporations is $2.27 trillion. Canada has a total money and near-money supply of 800 billion dollars. Therefore, the debt owing is three times the amount of money around with which to pay it off.

Of the $800 billion money supply, only $38 billion is legal tender (currency in circulation) created by the Bank of Canada interest free. The remainder is credit created by the major chartered banks as loans (mortgages, credit card loans, home equity loans, business loans, etc.) on which interest must be paid.

Thus the Canadian economy is run on a debt-based monetary system, where legal tender amounts to 5% of the money supply and credit amounts to 95%.

We must ask ourselves:

1. How do we pay off a $2.27 trillion debt with a total money supply of $800 billion of which only $38 billion is legal tender?

2. What would happen to the Canadian economy if all Canadians stopped borrowing and started saving instead at the same time?

Canada is part of a world debt-based monetary system controlled and managed by bankers rather than sovereign governments. It was that world debt-based monetary system that was responsible for the Great Depression of 1929.

In recent years, millions of the world's people have lost all, or nearly all, of their retirement savings. Corporations and individuals have gone bankrupt. Millions have lost their jobs and homes. Governments have cut spending. Several nations around the world are trying to stave off banking and economic collapse. Over 4 billion people live on $3.00 a day or less.

By 1929, bankers, brokers, and corporate leadership ran the economic systems into collapse. In Canada, part of the solution was the nationalization of our Bank of Canada. The nationalized Bank of Canada did not materialize without work, struggle and deep political debate.

In Canada one such political person was Gerry G. McGeer. During 30 years of political life, he was a BC Liberal, a member of the BC Provincial Legislative Assembly, a Member of Parliament, a Senator. He was Mayor of Vancouver City in 1935 and 1936. In 1936 McGeer published a book called *Conquest of Poverty, or Money, Humanity and Christianity*.

Gerry McGeer — Trailblazer

In the preface of his book he wrote:

"Ever since the passage of the English *Bank Act* of 1844, the creation, issuance, and the regulation of the circulation of the current medium of exchange, though being duties that constitute the most conspicuous and sacred responsibilities of government, have been in large measure delegated in blind faith and absolute confidence to bankers and financiers.

"Necessity now compels all to recognize that the creation and issuance of the medium of exchange, the monetization of public credit, the circulation of the medium of exchange, and the general supervision of the monetary system must be restored to government."

McGeer's insight into the debt-based monetary system of the 20s and 30s and his persistent fight to change it was rewarded when the government of MacKenzie King in 1938 nationalized the Bank of Canada, returning to government the control of the creation of the nations' currency and credit.[1]

The legislated mandate of the nationalized Bank of Canada states:

"It is desirable to establish a central bank in Canada to regulate credit and currency in the best interest of the economic life of the nation to control and protect the external value of the national monetary unit, and to mitigate by its influence fluctuations in the general level of production, trade, prices, and employment, so far as may be possible within the scope of monetary action, and generally to promote the economic and financial welfare of Canada."

This mandate was followed from 1938 until the mid 1970s, Canada's best financial years in the interest of the citizens in financing our infrastructure, housing, and all our proud social programs. In the mid 70s, a change of policy took place which gradually gave back the control and creation of credit to the private banks.

It was the Conservative governments of Brian Mulroney that initiated the erosion of the legislative mandate of our Bank of Canada in a number of ways, and successive Liberal governments continued the abuse. The powerful mandate still remains, but government practice refuses to honour it. To wit by the following:

1. Since 1975, our governments have decreased the use of our Bank of Canada to hold Canada's debt. Result? A dramatic increase of unnecessary interest paid. In 1975 the total federal debt was $37 billion. By the year 2000 it was $585 billion. This dramatic increase was due to borrowing money from foreign and domestic banks at market rates of interest, rather than borrowing from our own Bank of Canada at nominal rates of interest, the payment of which come back into government coffers as dividends.

The Erosion of our Legislation

In 1975 our own Bank of Canada held about 22% of Canada's debt. By 1991 it held only 8% of our debt. By 2000, only 5%. Borrowing at market rates ranging from 6% to 18% (in the 80s) rather than at about 1% from our Bank of Canada.

When the Liberals replaced the Conservatives in government in 1993, the debt was $408 billion. By the year 2000, the debt was $585 billion. By year 2004, the Liberals reduced the debt to $510 billion. To effect this reduction, the Liberals viciously slashed social program spending, and created surpluses which they applied against the debt. They starved the people to feed the banks.

2. In the mid 80s the Mulroney government initiated a policy of "Price Stability" through the increase or decrease of interest rates rather than requiring the banks to increase or decrease their cash reserves (statutory reserves) with the Bank of Canada.

3. During the Mulroney years, the government further deregulated the banks. That is, government removed the firewalls between banking, stock markets, real estate mortgages, and insurance. The regulations had been there since the mid-1930s to protect the public interest.

Deregulation allowed the banks to gamble in derivatives (an aspect of securities, instead of the securities themselves), merchant banking (trading and warehousing in entire non-banking companies), underwriting (guaranteeing the distribution of a new issue of stocks), stock brokering, and insurance.

With deregulation, banks could now access pools of capital previously unavailable to them. This process gave the banks inside information as a result of their now wearing many hats. Small business and farmers experienced increased difficulties in accessing loans, and local branches disappeared as banks chose to gamble in the great casino of international finance (except when they got burned and came back to peddle more credit cards at home).

4. It was to restore the capital that the banks had lost in their gambles that the Mulroney government eliminated the statutory reserves.

By law (statute) our chartered banks were required to deposit with our Bank of Canada a modest part of the short term deposits they received from the public. This "reserve" was the price that banks had to pay for the right to create most of our money supply as "near-money" (i.e., money bearing interest by its mere existence).

The reserves that were deposited with our Bank of Canada earned the banks no interest. Those reserves put at the disposal of our government over $120 billion of interest-free money that would grow from year to year with the economy (William Krehm, *Economic Reform*, Vol. 16, No. 1, January 04). The quantum was even more when the amount of reserves, i.e., percentage of deposits, was higher. Prior to 1980 there had been "secondary reserves," income-earning securities required to support the deposits in chequing accounts.

To make matters worse, then Mulroney's government, having lost the use of that reserve money, turned around and borrowed from those same banks, either directly or indirectly, the money it needed to make up for the loss of the statutory reserves. It began paying those same banks $5 to $8 billion per year on that money that previously had been interest free (William Krehm, *ibid.*). Naturally these figures go up as the economy expands.

After depriving itself of the use of the statutory reserves, interest free, the Federal government cut grants to provinces who then cut grants to the municipalities.

Deregulation Leads to a Larger Bank Casino

5. Bank deregulation and bank gambling resulted in the bankruptcy of a number of small Canadian banks. In the early 80s a number of minor banks went belly up in a cloud of scandal: Canadian Commercial Bank, Northland, Unity Bank and

others (Walter Stewart, *Bank Heist*, Chapter 9). Depositors were caught. Business loans were caught. The government bailed out the banks paying off the protected deposits by underwriting deposit insurance, and negotiated settlements with the depositors and other creditors (called workouts).

"Cooking the Books" — Thereby Undervaluing Canada's Worth

6. "Cooking the Books" – thereby undervaluing Canada's worth. Until 2004, the Canadian government was "cooking its books" – an accusation made by Canada's own Auditor General in 1999. They used cash flow accounting when they should have been using accrual accounting (capital budgeting). They pretended that assets did not exist which did exist. For years, except for Crown corporations, governments did not show the full asset side of their balance sheet, thus exaggerating the net debt. Government was writing off assets like a bridge or a building in one year, and then showing them on their books at a token $1.00 value. It was by this method that government has sold off buildings, land, railways, to private parties at bargain basement prices.

In 1999 after a fight with the auditor general of Canada who refused to sign off unconditionally on two years' balance sheets Martin agreed eventually to using proper accounting procedures in two areas, environment and aboriginal matters. In the year 2004, our government has finally committed itself to eventually reporting all its physical assets as such Canada's accounts. But this was not explained to the public or to Parliament. Nor was there a mention of the government investment in human capital – education, health and social services – which economists in the 1960s had recognized to be the most productive investments a nation can make.

Why have our governments been acting so contrary to the interest of its own citizens? It is because we have had leaders and parties in control who are part of and agree completely with the New World Order, i.e., globalization. They are willing participants and major players in the international financial regime being imposed on the world by the International Monetary Fund (IMF) and the World Bank They are submitting Canada to the regime of "structural adjustments" – the process of removing government from its role in the economy – and "privatization" – the process of wholesale sellout of public assets and government responsibilities.

In 1995 Paul Martin slashed federal health care transfers to the provinces by $28 billion. Sheila Copps, a former MP in the Chrétien government cabinet, recently revealed that in 1995 Paul Martin was lobbying the Chrétien government hard to scrap the medical care program. In the June 2004 election campaign, Martin promised to return a mere $9 billion to health care. Martin's years of starving our once proud health care system are still ricocheting as provincial governments dismantle and privatize such services.

Between 1999 and 2003, in addition to slashing funding for health care, our Canadian government slashed funding for education, unemployment insurance and various other social programs. The results for people have been deaths, debts, drop-outs, poverty, homelessness, marriage breakdown.

The result for government has been massive surpluses. Between 1999 and 2003, the Canadian government accumulated a surplus of $46.7 billion (Alternative Budget of the Canadian Centre for Policy Alternatives).

Canada is in the process of being "structurally adjusted." It is just that the process cannot be accomplished so easily here as in underdeveloped countries. The phrase "structural adjustment" is a euphemistic one created by the IMF (International Monetary Fund). When countries need financial assistance they go to the IMF who in turn demand "structural adjustment" (the process of removing government from its role in the economy) and "privatization" (the process of wholesale sellout of public assets) in return for the money. This impoverishes the people as their resources are stolen out from under them. One structural demand is that national central banks be removed so that there is no national power to create and control their own money supply. Herein lies the explanation of why our governments refuse to use the power of our own Bank of Canada. They are complicit participants in the IMF regime and are moving Canada by stealth into the regime.

So what is to be done?

We have to inform people that they have a choice about money. Money can be their master, or money can be their servant. This will not change until we have politicians, i.e., true representatives of the interest of the people, who understand the issue of monetary sovereignty vs. monetary slavery; and more importantly, who have the will to say NO to monetary slavery.

Connie Fogal

1. The following interchange took place between McGreer and Graham Towers, the first governor of the Bank of Canada in 1938 when Towers, a former vice-president of the Royal Bank of Canada, testified before the Subcommittee of Banking and Commerce in 1939:

    McGreer: But there is no question about it that banks do create the medium of exchange?

    Mr. Towers: That is right. That is banking business in the same sense that a steel plant makes steel (p. 287).

    Reproduced in Vol. 5, No. 10 of *Economic Reform*. Carried in *Meltdown: Money, Debt and the Wealth of Nations*, COMER Publications, 1999, selections from the first decade of *Economic Reform*, p. 117.

The Municipalities Fight Back

IN OUR OCTOBER ISSUE we reproduced the crucial portions of the letter sent by the Honourable Ralph Goodale, minister of Finance of Canada, dated 16/08. This was in reply to a letter from Ms. Andrea Rivest, of the office of the Clerk, Belle River, Ontario, with copy to Mr. André Martenette, resident of that municipality and member of COMER, on loans from the Bank of Canada to municipalities for the construction and renewal of infrastructure. We publish below extracts from the submission of two members of Comer supporting Mr. Martenette, Gordon Coggins and George Crowell, both retired university professors, on the Minister's reply to the municipality's correspondence:

"If the Minister's letter aims to confuse the issue raised by the Town Council – a request that he exercise his statutory authority under the *Bank of Canada Act* to instruct the Bank to make low-interest loans to municipalities for major infrastructure projects – it is eminently successful in its aim. Another interpretation of this letter is that the Minister himself is confused."

Getting the Minister to Stick to the Problem

"Addressing the second possibility, we respectfully note the following:

1. The Minister says (paragraph 2): "the problem with this action is that to acquire government debt, the Bank of Canada would have to print new currency. The rapid growth in the money supply would eventually result in an increase in inflation and higher rates of interest."

"There are two points here:

(a) "The Bank of Canada would have to print currency." This is not correct; as paragraph 5 of his letter indicates, the Bank is totally empowered to create credit – that is, loans – as credit not cash.

(b) The "rapid growth of the money supply" is mostly rhetoric. First, the rate of growth of the money supply would be only as rapid as the Bank decided, in its wisdom and according to its mandate 'to regulate credit and currency in the best interests of the economic life of the nation, to control and protect the external value of the national monetary unit...and generally to promote the economic and financial welfare of Canada." (*Bank of Canada Act*, Preamble). The Bank would presumably be wise enough to set a reasonable cap on the amount at any given time. Further the municipalities making such a request are not asking for a government *expenditure*; they are asking for a Bank loan, which in due course would be repaid. As participating municipalities repaid their loans, new loans could be made to them or other municipalities for other useful projects, without an increase in the money supply beyond the initial cap.

Since the request is not for the creation of currency, but for the creation of credit, the references to the possible evils of currency creation – greatly exaggerated in any case – in paragraphs 3, 5, and 6, are irrelevant.

The "What if" case in paragraph 4 is a red herring. First, the municipalities are not asking for loans to the "Government of Canada," but to the councils of municipalities. Secondly, it would be dumb indeed for the Bank to borrow money (perhaps from private banks, which already create more than 95% of the Canadian money supply) when it is empowered to create credit, and did so extensively during and after World War II. The war expenses ran up a national debt that was successfully paid down without inflation.

Paragraph 6 is essentially correct. Some nations have overdone the creation of money to meet government expenses. Others, Canada included as noted above, have made controlled use of credit creation without inflationary disaster. This is like saying, "if you eat too much you will make yourself sick, therefore you should not eat." A further point compromising this comparison-based argument is the fact that not only does

Canada own its own central bank, as the Minister acknowledges, but Canada is one of only three countries in the developed world which does. That should limit the comparison with other countries to Switzerland and England.

Paragraph 7 argues from a hypothetical supposition – "that the Bank of Canada did not want to change the total amount of loans it had outstanding." We can suppose it, but we cannot imagine a reason for such a policy under the Bank's mandate "to promote the economic welfare of Canada."

Getting the Issues Straight

First, note once again that the municipalities are not asking for loans to the provincial government, but to municipal governments, for useful public infrastructure investment. Secondly, "federal taxpayers subsidizing provincial governments" is a curious and false distinction. There is only one taxpayer. Whether he or she pays to the municipal government, the provincial government or the federal government, is a matter of convention; and the redistribution of tax moneys is and has been since the founding of the nation, a major policy function of federal and provincial governments.

Incidentally, since the founding of the nation, municipalities have grown to be the predominant centres of population. It is a far different country from the Canada of 1867. The new political and economic reality needs to be faced: the now huge responsibilities of municipalities give them a respectable claim on a larger share of the tax pie than they had 175 years ago. But, note once again, the municipalities' specific request is not for tax expenditure, but for loans that will be repaid.

The only negative effect of a moderate application of such a policy would accrue neither to the governments nor to the municipalities. Where a municipality, in its need for a particular project, was able to avoid borrowing money created by the chartered banks, but instead could access a well-managed Bank of Canada low-cost loan policy, the banks, of course, would be the losers. Obviously, the minister must expect some protest from their spokespeople when he instructs the Bank of Canada, either under his existing statutory authority or through legislation, to make such loans available to municipalities. A precedent for such legislation, incidentally, was part of the initial establishment of the government-owned Bank of Canada in 1938 – Bill 143, the *Municipal Assistance Act*.

Respectfully,

Gordon Coggins, PhD, and George Crowell, PhD

Notice of Council Decision

Windsor City Council adopted the following resolution at its meeting held November 15, 2004:

CR1014/2004

1. THAT the report of the General Manager of Corporate Services and City Treasurer dated October 14, 2004, regarding Ontario's Municipal Taxation System and Loans from the Bank of Canada BE RECEIVED for information.

2. THAT the City of Windsor support initiatives such as interest free loans as part of a comprehensive "new deal" for Municipalities.

3. The City of Windsor requests THAT the Provincial Government consult with Ontario Municipalities and Municipal organizations, such as the Municipal Finance Officers' Association of Ontario (MFOA), regarding future changes and improvements to Ontario's Municipal Taxation System.

4. That copies of this resolution BE FORWARDED to the Association of Municipalities of Ontario (AMO), and to the Federation of Canadian Municipalities (FCM).

Carried, Councillor Jones was absent from the meeting when the vote was taken.

BASIS report Number 10928 AFT2004 12

Steve Vlachodimos
Manager of Council/Committee Services/Deputy Clerk
November 16, 2004

Face Lift for our Stock Markets?

THERE ARE TWO WAYS of appraising our stock markets. One is crunching figures. Another is taking a hard look at the figures themselves, what they include and what they omit. The trouble is that the figures you have for that exercise may have been dressed up by the corporation officers, not infrequently in cahoots with their auditors. The media have been overflowing with tidings of the investigations of this in the US. Those investigations have even led to some mammoth fines levied on three of our six large Canadian banks because of their part in connection with Enron, one of the least fragrant of Wall St.'s scandals.

Quite understandable then that sections of Wall St. should feel the need for a bit of cosmetic surgery, to help it back to a youthful innocent glow.

Thus *The Wall Street Journal* (27/07, "Hedge Funds Stake a Claim in Acquisitions" by Henry Sender) "Even as their traditional trading strategies are drying up, hedge funds' coffers are creaking with cash. So some of the biggest funds have decided to take a page from the playbook of buyout funds – well, most of the book, actually – and get into the business of buying companies.

"Just how serious these funds are about their new business line was underscored last week when a group of about a dozen hedge funds made it to the final round of bidding for the Texas Genco Holdings Inc. unit of CenterPoint Energy Inc.

"In early spring, invitations to participate in the auction of the merchant energy company went out to about 100 potential buyers, including other power companies and the usual megabillion investment funds, including Kohlberg Kravis Roberts & Co. LLC and Blackstone Group. But in May, as the list of potential acquirers for Genco was being winnowed, a group of hedge funds unexpectedly got in touch with Citigroup Inc., which was orchestrating the auction, and notified them of the funds' interest in acquiring Genco.

"Last week, a group made up of Blackstone, KKR and two other big-name private equity funds won the prize, agreeing to buy Genco in a deal valued at $3.85 billion.

"But the hedge funds in the running were powerful contenders, lasting to the final round of three bidders. Some of these hedge funds, or private investment pools, had war chests of $10 billion and more. Traditionally the funds haven't been involved in takeovers. Indeed, most hedge funds haven't been known beyond their own clubby world consisting of other funds run by tight-lipped managers on behalf of wealthy investors and institutions.

"Their presence and persistence at the Genco auction is one more indication of their growing clout across all financial markets and activities. Though they are new to acquisitions, as the Genco auction showed, they are expected to get up to speed soon and become formidable competitors.

"Such activity goes against type for hedge funds. These have always eschewed both the limelight and a long-term investment horizon. But as the funds accumulate ever-more massive pools of capital, they can no longer just deploy their money in short-term trading of everything from Australian dollars to the shares and bonds of merger candidates."

As the stock market becomes iffier, the bigger, more successful operators not only have outgrown it, but are looking for a safer place to park their winnings.

The Search for Safer Places to Park Super-profits

"And as they look for other homes for their money, hedge funds are increasingly competing with private-equity funds, endowments and wealthy families. These private-equity funds buy private companies and aim to sell them later at a profit, and are looking enviously at the ability of hedge funds to trade in and out of public companies. At the same time, hedge funds – which generally allow investors to withdraw their money as often as every month – hope that the acquisitions business will allow them to hold onto customers for longer stretches.

"As they venture into acquisitions hedge-fund managers may end up being better, or at least more frequently compensated than private-equity managers. The latter pocket performance fees only after they sell out the companies they have bought, a process that may take several years. Hedge funds, however, estimate the value of their positions at year end and managers pay themselves performance fees accordingly."

Like so much in the financial world value can be a not entirely objective affair.

"Take Perry Capital. That hedge fund isn't a household name, but it has about $8 billion under management. It has provided capital to some troubled energy companies, including a $100 million revolving credit to Xcel Energy Inc. Perry was also the dominant investor in a $300 million convertible trust of preferred security for Allegheny Energy Inc.

"'Hedge funds are the most flexible, the fastest, and in many cases the cheapest source of money,' said George Brokaw, partner of Lazard Frères & Co. 'Indeed, hedge funds can look past governance issues, or other matters, like a lack of audited financial reports, whereas these matters would put off banks, insurance companies and other tenders.' In a healthy market that might appear an efficiency, something even to be monetized. If the market becomes problematical this can become the stuff of future newspaper captions.

"Some hedge funds already have a history of investing in distressed companies, including the energy sector, where they cannot easily trade out of their positions. 'Now the first question my clients among energy companies ask is whether hedge funds would be interested in providing money,' said Marco Masotti, a lawyer with Paul, Weiss, Rifkind, Whatton & Garrison LLP in charge of the firm's hedge-fund and private-equity practice.

"Genco, of course, isn't troubled. But it did have a feature that made it particularly attractive to hedge funds as they migrate from trading positions to longer-term control positions: 19% of Genco's shares trade publicly. That meant the hedge funds could easily obtain information about the company while considering a deal and still buy and sell the shares."

The Wall Street Journal (27/07, "Independent Research Hits Wall Street" by Ruth Simon and Louise Story) reports of "a whole new world when it comes to stock research for individual investors. Beginning today, 10 of the nation's biggest brokerage firms – among them Credit Suisse First Boston, Morgan Stanley and Citigroup Inc.'s Smith Barney unit – must provide clients with a second, independent source of research in addition to reports by the firms' own analysts. The move was part of last year's $1.4 billion settlement with the Security and Exchange Commission and state regulators. The agreement resolved charges that the brokerages issued research tainted by investment banking conflicts of interest."

The more logical remedy would have been to undo the deregulation that united the incompatible activities of underwriting stock and then peddling it to the public. That separation was imposed by the Roosevelt government because of a mishap known as the Depression of the 1930s introduced by the Great Wall St. Bust.

"Each of the ten firms was required to hire an outside consultant who would then select at least three outside firms to provide independent research to its clients. The firms must spend anywhere from $7.5 million to $75 million each on independent research over the next five years."

Unfortunately, the same money can be used to buy supervision or to bribe. In a pinch of temptation such things are known to happen on Wall St. as in the recent Enron case of "auditors" who are supposed to be the supreme cops on the corporation-book beat.

But then how long are facelifts supposed to last before they sag again?

"The newly available research, however, will present a fresh set of challenges for investors. People will now have to negotiate different methodologies and standards for rating a stock as a buy, sell or hold. Another problem: what to do when the recommendations conflict as they do in a surprising number of instances."

SEC Goes Solomonic and Cuts Baby in Two

Surely, that frequency must tell us something: that the urge of the financial conglomerates as underwriter of the stock to profit from a sale may outweigh its loyalty to the client that it is selling to while wearing its broker hat. The only way around

that is to license banker types as one-stop financial servers only after checking their qualification for canonization as saints. And besides if you found and hired the future saint, he would be fired in no time flat for not meeting the prescribed quota of profit for his clients.

"The Bear Stearns Co. analyst and the independent research firm disagree nearly 55% of the time, says Michel J. Downey, the independent consultant who selected the outside research firms used by Bear Stearns. Bear Stearns says it has not instructed its brokers to 'prioritize' one research report over another." But isn't that precisely where we came in?

"Starting today, investors can obtain the reports via their brokerage firm's web site or by calling its toll-free number. The firms are required to provide one independent report per stock but some are giving their customers as many as four reports for the same security.

"Investors might have been able to pare their losses had outside research been more widely available in the past. Consider the case of WorldCom, which filed for bankruptcy in 2002 after a massive accounting scandal. Kevin Calabrese, an analyst with Argus Research, downgraded WorldCom to a sell on Jan24, 2002, when its shares were trading at $10.40. Jack Grubman, Citigroup analyst, maintained a buy or hold rating, on the other hand, until late June when the shares had sunk to $1.22."

It is impossible injecting morality into a set up constrained to show ever-mounting returns by ordering that more money be spent for independent research. In the universe of "bigger is better" what cannot show ever mounting returns – be it consultant bankers or an auditing firm – is eliminated as inefficient. In this way the economy races on to the precipice and beyond.

W.K.

Portrait of a Virtuoso in Sleight of Tongue

IN THE SECOND of a two-part series in *The Wall Street Journal* (19/11, "A Less Visible Role For the Fed Chief: Freeing Up the Markets") Greg Ip examines the less public side of Alan Greenspan's lengthy record as chairman of the Federal Reserve Board in the US. What emerges is a masterful portrait of a past master in the art of not saying what he means or not meaning what he says.

"Consider what happened in 2002, when Democratic Senator Dianne Feinstein proposed new rules to govern how traders buy and sell contracts through financial instruments known as derivatives. Her move came after Enron Corp. and others sent electricity prices soaring in California by manipulating the market. When she telephoned Mr. Greenspan for support, he declined, telling her the proposal threatened the multi-trillion dollar derivative industry, which he considers an important stabilizing force that diffuses financial risk."

The operative words in that mouthful are "diffusing financial risk." The meaning of "risk" should be clear – the Enron boys by dealing with isolated aspects of energy deals, e.g., the rate of their price increase down the line – were able to control a far greater multiple of future energy production than if they had to acquire future deliveries of energy as such.

Because such derivatives were unregulated, there was no obligation for them to report what derivatives they or others in these deals might buy or sell. In that way three large Canadian banks who had a hand in designing the notorious arrangements under which those banks were able to acquire shares in partnerships in which Enron high executives played a key role, not only in selling their exposure to the risk but more than their exposure – i.e., sell their interest short through derivatives, without any outsider being aware of their betting against the position that they had marketed to their customers. The magic word is "diffuse" which my dictionary defines as meaning "spreading widely." Translating Greenspanese into ordinary prose it means applied to markets: "non-transparency."

Obviously, spreading resulting loss to countless smaller investors in Enron and the energy-consuming public, the risk may have been spread from the point of view of the gamblers in derivatives, but it is painfully concentrated for the humbler folk who lost their investment or were stuck with the exorbitant electricity prices.

But let us resume Ip's tale. "Mr. Greenspan persuaded other Bush-appointed regulators to join him in a critical letter that Sen. Feinstein's opponents wielded as a weapon on the Senate floor. The bill was narrowly defeated on a procedural motion. Sen. Feinstein reintroduced the proposal a number of times and at least twice Mr. Greenspan rallied fellow regulators to oppose. 'I believe it would have passed without his opposition,' Sen. Feinstein says.

"In addition to thwarting the post-Enron impulse to regulate derivatives, Mr. Greenspan helped remove Depression – era barriers between banking and securities industries and has blessed mergers creating banking behemoths. He has implored regulators to keep their hands off hedge funds and other markets that are replacing banks as financiers of American businesses. Although the Fed is a major bank regulator, it has become a less intrusive one under Mr. Greenspan."

The Secret of Mr. Greenspan's Popularity

This, it would appear, is at least a great part of the secret of the blind trust that Mr. Greenspan commands. It is a vote in support of the logical acrobatics that Mr. Greenspan performs on behalf of those in power.

"Critics say his hands-off regulatory philosophy has made the Fed a less effective watchdog, citing complicity by Fed-regulated banks in recent corporate scandals.

"Behind the advocacy is a passionate belief that freely functioning financial markets are better than government regulators – and even central bankers – at protecting the economy from booms and busts. The result is a paradoxical position for one of the world's most influential civil servants. His ideal is the pre-Civil War period when the federal government was so invisible that it didn't even issue a national currency."

And yet that was hardly a time when banks did not disappear

with their depositors' savings.

The sphinx – combining the head of a man with the body of a lion, and the wings of a great bird – defied the laws of biology and much else. That indeed seems the essence of the Greenspan miracle. Imagine a police chief who believed in leaving the field open for lawbreakers.

"Mr. Greenspan first articulated many of his views in the 1960s when he was part of the intellectual circle surrounding libertarian philosopher Ayn Rand. If businesses were solely responsible for their own reputation, he said at the time, they would do whatever necessary to maintain it or ultimately fail."

Would that "ultimate failure" not be a simply synonym for the "boom and bust" that we all of us – not excluding Mr. Greenspan – say they want to put behind us?

"'It is in the self-interest of every businessman to have a reputation for honest dealings and a quality product,' he wrote in Ms. Rand's *Objectivist* newsletter in 1963. Regulation, he said, undermines this 'superlatively moral system' by replacing competition for reputation with force. At the bottom of the endless pile of paper work which characterizes all regulations lies a gun."

As though there is a lack of firearms around today, at home and abroad!

"His language has moderated but he still admires the laissez-faire capitalism of the mid-19th century. Banks, for example, issued their own currency whose value fluctuated with the issuer's reputation." It certainly did, and entire rooms were papered with worthless bank currency.

"In 1913, the very organization in which he made his name, the Federal Reserve, was created. As lender of the last resort, the Fed could prop up failing banks, reducing the incentive for bankers and businessmen to act prudently.

"Market discipline weakened further when the government created federal deposit insurance in 1933, making depositors less concerned about the reputation of the bank to which they entrusted their money. That was compounded when the US went off the gold standard in 1933. 'A kind of vicious circle of government replacement of market oversight [was] clearly set in motion,' he said in a May 2001 speech."

If you replaced all the learned apologies for our current financial system with a single man, that man would be Alan Greenspan. For those in the saddle, he is worth a library of treatises that no one else would quite dare write, and a clutch of votes in the electoral college.

William Krehm

Translating the Upside-down Official Economic Model into Architectural Terms

IT IS BECOMING increasingly apparent that our world, mis-motivated and misinformed, is headed for a major disaster. Past defeats are reclassified as victories suffering only from a shortfall of "growth." That excludes society learning from its previous missteps.

Above all, there is a studied lack of clarity of just what is supposed to be "growing." That is why the comedians in the US have been having such a field day. But we can't leave it all to the comedians. Not only are the necessary questions not asked, but the necessary information for framing them is being buried ever deeper by our governments, universities, and our media.

And that is why we are going to adopt a *reductio ad absurdum* method to a tragically absurd situation: we will translate the economic problem to its equivalent in a more accessible field, where the ridiculous and the disastrous hit you in the eye.

We have chosen architecture, and specifically its great American enrichment – the skyscraper, but adapted to the alleged need for growth. Our model is thus a special sort of skyscraper that will add new storeys each year and a growing rate of growth; i.e., a derivative of the growth already attained. And since the very idea is fantastic, this skyscraper will be topped surrealistically with a Castle in Spain. Needless to say its moats and parapets will also go on expanding in all directions.

Now comes the crucial feature that relates the model to the reigning model of our world economy: defeats are reclassified as victories, up becoming down, and down up. Accordingly our expanding skyscraper grows upside down burying itself ever deeper in the ground. For greater efficiency, the ever more numerous underground storeys are used as parking space available only to the latest, biggest models of gas-guzzling SUVs.

The Editor

Our Banks are Coming Back Home with their Tails between their Legs

BY THE LATE 1980s our banks had been deregulated to allow them to gamble bigger and better. The statutory reserves – the proportion of the deposits taken into their chequing accounts that had to be redeposited with the central bank – had been decreased progressively from the 10% that it had

been. That decrease in the statutory reserves allowed the banks greater leverage of the credit banks could create on the cash base they receive from the public as deposits. These primary statutory reserves deposited with the Bank of Canada earned them no interest.

In addition there had been secondary reserves which were interest-bearing government securities that had to be left with the BoC, but these had been abolished in 1980. Thus in Canada all statutory reserves were abolished outright. In the US, they were reduced to insignificance. In addition in 1988 the Bank for International Settlements, an appointed body in Basel, Switzerland, issued its *Risk-Based Capital Requirements* guidelines, proclaiming the debt of developed countries "risk-free" needing no additional capital for banks to acquire. The rationale of such a bailout was to allow the banks to load up with government bonds without putting up any money of their own, because of the supposed risk-free nature of government credit in developed countries. In Canada by 1993 our banks had quadrupled their holdings of such government debt to $80 billion entirely on the cuff. Those in charge of the bank bailout went on to the next step in repairing the banks' capital losses and providing them with an annual entitlement to fund their future market plays: the BIS declared even the slightest rise in the price level unacceptable, that had to be repressed by raising interest rates. That was a perfect bondholders' reaction: they are always jumpy about the currency in which their bonds are denominated losing its purchasing power. Obviously, with their hoard of government debt, banks would stand to gain immensely by higher interest rates. Or so they thought.

But they and their advisers in Ottawa and the BIS had overlooked a crucial detail: when interest rates climb, already existing bonds with lower interest rates drop in market value because you can do better buying new bonds at par yielding a higher rate. Repeatedly COMER warned the government that the combination of bailing out the banks by allowing them to take on huge bond holdings wholly leveraged, and high interest rates would bring the banks into crisis. To no effect.[1] The truth blew initially out of Mexico that under a crushing burden of its traditional corruption and a load of dollar-denominated government debt threatened to collapse and bring the whole international monetary system down with it. On the advice of his Secretary of the Treasury, Robert Rubin, a bright alumnus of Wall St., President Clinton at the last moment saved the day by patching together a standby fund of over $51 billion US, with the help of the International Monetary Fund and the Canadian Government. This incredible blunder of our governments in bailing out the banks damaged their ability to think straight. And since the details of the banks' previous bailout had been kept a secret from the media and parliament itself, there was no possibility of their being corrected by a public review of what they proposed doing. That irresponsibility of our government led to further deregulation of the banks so that they might gamble in still further areas incompatible with banking.

Razing the Financial Fire Walls

President Roosevelt in the US had in 1935 set up "fire walls" between banking and other financial activities insurance, the stock market, mortgage financing. For good cause. Each of these industries keeps a pool of capital essential for running its own business. Give the banks' access to those pools of capital through deregulation, and they will gamble themselves under the table in no time flat. And indeed that brought about the East Asian meltdown of 1998, the out-gunning of the Bank of England by speculators operating with derivatives – a new highly leveraged option play of conceptually isolated features of securities.

Derivatives are notable for being completely unregulated so that any bank selling its customers stock of questionable worth through its banking arm, can short the same stock on a highly leveraged basis by selling derivatives, without even reporting that on its balance sheet. Such scams in sports are much in the headlines. The power of muscles honestly earned through exercise and talent can be increased by shots of steroid. Because for athletes steroids are prohibited, that has separated more than one cheating sport star from his gold or silver.

Oddly enough in the banking world the financial equivalent of steroids in athletics is not frowned on. Governments in fact rewarded the cheaters with new shots of steroids. That enabled the mega-financier George Soros a few years back to outgun the Bank of England and shoot down the British pound to earn his group a reported profit of a cool billion.

Then he went on to do a similar job on the Italian lira. COMER in good time warned the government of the danger of giving our banks further shots of steroids. But to no avail. There were only five or six biggies left, but many mergers with trust companies helped keep the mergers going. The argument was that to survive and go out there and beat the really big international banks on their home turf, they need to become bigger. I remember appearing before the committee that was touring the country to hear evidence with the chair providing an eloquent defence of further bank deregulation by citing the size of the Japanese banks they had to stand up against. I tried pointing out that the big-time Japanese banks that our banks had to be beefed up to compete against were already in trouble with their euro dollar loans and had in fact had already stopped lending. You might question my mixed metaphor in shifting from skyscrapers standing on their heads to steroids. But in that I was just copying our government in their attitude to the banks. Instead of being held to concentrate on banking to provide useful services to those in Canada who needed them, the banks were suddenly viewed as a sort of national hockey team whom we were obliged to applaud and cheer as they pushed on to a world championship.

Now the verdict is in, though its true significance is buried. Increasingly the talk is of further bank mergers, Not a word about using the Bank of Canada for the purposes for which it was intended: to finance the infrastructures of Canadian soci-ety. Instead all those bonds that the banks hold and on which the government pays interest stays with the banks. Most of our government's deficit has been the result of this, and of course the lack of accrual accounting that distinguishes between current spending and investment. Ottawa's much-cited deficits of the past were the excuse for the wholesale downloading of social programs onto the provinces, who have passed on the treatment to the municipalities. Our education system is in tatters. Our roads are potholed. Our health system is at risk. Valuable public assets – the CNR, Ontario Hydro have been sold off for songs. And the banks? How have they fared in their conquest of the bigger challenges of the world market? Dismally, if we are to take the most recent reports of the auditors of the largest of our banks the Royal Bank of Canada. *The Globe and Mail* (23/11, "RB Set to slash hundreds of jobs" by Sinclair Stewart): "Royal Bank of Canada is expected to cut 'several hundred' more jobs at its Toronto head office in the next two weeks as part of a continuing effort to slash costs and streamline a bloated corporate structure. The country's largest bank has already chopped 150 positions, largely in dribs and drabs, since earlier this fall. Sources say RBC will make its next round of Canadian cuts on Dec. 9th, with further reductions slated for January to be focussed mostly on the global technology and operations unit. David Moorcroft, a spokesman for RBC, said the banks has yet to determine how many of its roughly 7,000 head office jobs will be slashed. However, if the bank does get rid of hundreds of additional positions, it will have downsized its head office by between 5 and 10 percent. RBC has stressed that it is shifting resources more toward areas of the bank responsible for generating revenue, and does not plan to slash the front-line work force at its branch network."

In short it is not resuming its shutting down of local branches that service personal and small business loans to play the big game on the US and world stage. Instead it is back to pushing credit cards to humble individuals at home to make up for its mammoth losses and moral black eyes suffered in the company of the big banks abroad. Side-shows in the Enron super-scandal have been amongst their costliest disappointments.

"Scott Custer, the recently appointed CEO of RBC's US retail bank, RBC Centura, said this month that RBC would ease the pace of new branch openings in the south-eastern US, and would also reduce its head office roster.

"RBC's expenses grew by 8% percent in the first three quarters of 2003, four times as fast as its revenue growth. This, coupled with anemic returns from its US retail banking operations, prompted CEO Mr. Nixon to overhaul his senior management team in September and embark on a reorganization of the company's business lines. Several of the bank's top executives, including three vice-chairmen, retired as part of the make-over, as did the former head of RBC Centura."

Canadians Learn of our Banks' Quixotic Fortunes from US Investigations

"Analysts have predicted RBC could take charges of between $500 million and $1 billion in the near future to write down goodwill on its faltering US businesses, and to bolster its legal reserves to cover any potential damages from its involvement with Enron Corp. RBC, TD Bank and CIBC are each defendants in a massive $25 billion (US) class action suit launched by shareholders of the disgraced energy trader. TD took a $300-million (Canadian) charge last spring, but RBC and CIBC have so far not taken any specific provisions.

"Speculation about an Enron-related charge for these Canadian banks has heated up after J.P. Morgan & Co. set aside $2.3 billion (US) to cover possible legal fallout from its entanglement with Enron, and another US financial institution, Bank of America Corp., struck a settlement with the company's investors. A few days later the *G&M* (11/12, "Hunkin is de-risking the place" by Sinclair Stewart and Andrew Willis) reported that the CBIC chieftain, John Hunkin, launched a personal campaign disavowing just about everything that it claimed to be on the verge of achieving a decade ago when Ottawa had put it on steroids and sent it out to conquer the financial world. And Andrew Willis: "John Hunkin has met with investors about 50 times in the past several weeks, and each one has pressed him with the question: How in the world does the CBIC intend to grow?"

Unexpressed is the rest of the sentence: "Now that you guys are off steroids?" This is unfamiliar territory for the 59-year-old CEO who for the past five years has presided over a bank known as much for its aggressive deal-making as for its willingness to expand into the US and go toe-to-toe with some of the biggest names on Wall St. After myriad gaffes during the past two years – the failure of its US electronic banking unit, a costly settlement with the regulators over Enron Corp., entanglement in the US mutual fund scandal, and even the recent embarrassment over faxing confidential information to a West Virginia junkyard for months on end, even when the honest junkyard owner warned them of what they were doing – CBIC has largely retreated to Canada, and is the only one of the Big Five [banks] without a significant growth strategy.

"'One of the biggest compliments I've heard about us now is that we may be the most conservative bank in Canada,' he told the *G&M*. 'I think that's a major swing. I feel great about that. I actually have the hope that some day you guys in the media will find us uninteresting.' CIBC has been so conservative with its cash, in fact, that many on Bay St are referring to it as the income trust of the banking sector. Last year it paid out $781 million in common stock dividends and bought back 8.4 common shares at a cost of about $1.24 billion. 'John Hunkin is de-risking the place, and that's not a bad idea,' says Gavin Graham, a portfolio manager of the Guardian Group of funds. 'Ed Clark is doing the same at Toronto-Dominion Bank.'"

There is in short a retreat of the entire Canadian banking community with their tails between their legs from their grand international careers for which the government ran up its deficits to equip them to move Wall St. to the banks of the Ottawa River.

Isn't it time that we heard from Mr. Martin, our PM, who presided as Finance Minister during this period and exerted himself to ensure that the handiwork of the Mulroney Conservative Government lived on?

Since the promised conquest of foreign markets has fallen on its face, isn't it time that we withdrew the pensioning and deregulation of our banks so that we can return the funding that was diverted to them from key social programs?

In short if Ottawa refunded the banks from their vast losses in the round of speculative losses in the 1980s by shifting money creation powers from the government-owned central bank to the commercial banks revamped as something like a national hockey team. For the talk is of bank mergers once more, and that means positioning the banks to elbowing out the most needy portion of our populations – our aging, our unwell, and our students – from essential government assistance.

William Krehm

1. See *Meltdown: Money, Debt and the Wealth of Nations*, COMER Publications, 1999, p. 89, reproducing an early warning on this point that appeared in *Economic Reform* in December 1992.

The Political Economy of No Tomorrow

Distributing the Cost of Externalities

In the economically advanced nations, manufacturing, transportation, and an ever-increasing number of household functions are dependent on large energy inputs generated by fossil fuels, predominantly oil. This gives rise to a number of so-called externalities – costs that one person's (or economic agent's) activities causes others to bear. In the case of burning fossil fuels, the main externalities are air pollution, which can have serious health effects; and emission of green-house gases, which trap the sun's rays and raise the Earth's surface temperature with a major climate change as a possible outcome.

In an economic system where cost distribution is closely tied to private ownership and market exchanges, distributing the costs of externalities creates problems since they typically pass through a medium that nobody owns before their effects arise. Neoclassical market fundamentalists, unwilling to assign the public sector a role in any economic matters, have tried to solve the conundrum of distributing these costs with Coase's Theorem.

According to this theorem, activities which harm other economic interests should be litigated away. This, the theorem claims, is possible even though no property rights exist for the intermediate medium, just as long a clear cause – effect can be proven. As usual in neoclassical contexts an assumption of perfect conditions is necessary, in this case that litigation costs are zero (or fully recoverable) and that all parties are in possession of the same full information.

Coase's Theorem might look good in the university auditoriums, where fantasies are known to flourish. In the real world of modern business enterprise dominated by secretive corporations, well staffed with highly paid in-house counsel that know how to proactively knock unfriendly litigation off the board before it reaches serious stages, Coase's Theorem has little practical merit. For Coase's Theorem to work, market power must be symmetrically aligned and no market agents able to bend legal conditions to favour their interests.

But even if these unlikely conditions were fulfilled, Coase's Theorem still has problems. It becomes ineffective if (A) the externality loss is created and/or borne by a large number of agents (as is the case with air pollution); and (B) if the time lag between cause and effect is protracted (as is the case with a potential climate change).

Continuity of Self-interests

The problem that arises when cause and effect are separated by a substantial time lag is not restricted to externalities, but common to economic activities in general. All projections about future outcomes are given probability weights by market participants, both with regards to whether or not the forecasts' assumptions are realistic, and as to whether or not new technologies or other changes are likely to change a given market's supply and demand.

Assigning probability weights lie fully within the scope of rational expectations theory. But there are other aspect of economic projections that neoclassical theory gives little weight to because they do not conform to its assumption of rationality and continuity. Economic continuity is the expectation that within firms, executing agents act in full continuity with the owners' interests.

Continuity, as all other economic principles, is dependent upon a set of conditions specific to a given situation. One important aspect is the fact that an executing agent has what can be defined as an activity horizon. Within the activity horizon, value projection and estimations are connected to the agents' direct self-interest and will therefore, by and large, follow patterns according to the neoclassical prescription. The threat of being fired or losing economic incentives ensures that executing agents will follow owners' interests.

However, if the value formation that firm generates as a result of an agent's executive activities falls outside of the agents activity horizon, it will not be connected to direct self-interest, and therefore will be assigned a much lower value. For example, if an employee's actions are detrimental to the value formation of his firm, if that first becomes visible after he or she has left the firm, the employee might be relatively unconcerned about it.

The tendency of self-interested individuals and executing agents of firms to assign different value to outcomes of market events according to whether or not the value manifestation occur within their activity horizon multiply exponentially in the case of externalities, which, per definition, are not governed by individually assignable property rights. In most cases there is a continuity between owners and executing agents interests in disregarding externalities and not deal with them, because the costs they thereby dump on society has little chance of getting back to the firm.

In cases when an executing agent of a firm knows that activities he directs cause externalities that are sure to lead to a Coase litigation, the continuity principle should direct him to avoid causing externalities. However, if the externalities first become visible after he plans to leave the firm, it becomes his economic self-interest to disregard the externalities and maximize short-term profit. This strategy will enhance his remuneration while still at the firm and thus becomes the dominant self-interest, even when it is a certainty that the Coase litigation later on will re-impose the cost of not combating the externality on the firm.

A Public Role

With regards to externalities, when they arise from the actions of individuals as private citizens and not as agents of firms, neoclassical general market principles, including Coase litigation, is even more helpless. This is a function of the very large number of individuals both causing and being affected by such externalities.

In recognition of this, many governments in the economically advanced nations have recognized that only measures with a strong public role have any hope of dealing with these problems on the scale and commitment that is called for. A result of this realization is the Kyoto treaty – designed to reduce emissions of green house gasses on an international basis – which the majority of developed nations, including Canada, have signed on to.

At first, the American government under Clinton appeared to be on board. But the treaty had problems getting through Congress where it still was pending when Bush took office. Of course, it didn't take Bush long to dump it.

The Bush administration basically is an alliance between the oil industry (directly represented by the Bush family and Cheney) and a powerful group of neoconservatives centered around the think-tank with the interesting name "The Project for the New American Century" (Cheney, Rumsfeld and Wolfowitz, all belong to this think-tank). In their view, environmental and energy policies should be left to the markets, which as we saw, inherently means short-term interests. And public bodies should stay out of such matters avoiding impeding these interests.

A problem for governments in the advanced nations is that the environmental file has become something of a wild card in elections that can move swing voters unpredictably, dependent upon what context they connect to it. On one side, people are concerned by the rising levels of pollution and congestion where they live. But on the other hand, many people fear that implementation of effective pollution controls, including international treaties such as the Kyoto, might restrain their ability to freely indulge in their high energy-consuming lifestyles. This creates a split-personality attitude toward these problems for many people.

A Day at the Races

"Gentlemen, start your engines." Clad in a black Nascar Jacket to fit the occasion, Bush in February 2004 was the starter of the Daytona 500 race, the highlight of the Nascar circuit.

But the president of the United States doesn't pop up at such events just because he thinks it is fun. They are carefully selected events designed to send important political messages. At Daytona, the goal was to ensure that the environmental questions played to his advantage in the upcoming election by having the fear of restraints on the American life-style dominate in the voters' minds.

Essentially, at Daytona, when Bush mingled with the players of this fuel-smelling macho world, he sent the message that on his watch, nobody would be allowed to mess with Americans God-given right to their energy-guzzling life style.

It has been said that America has become more conservative and many in this respect points to the surge in conservative Christian fundamentalism. However, this surge can be seen as a result of the fact that more and more people know that America's way of life can not be sustained if it were the global norm. Therefore, its continuance demands a policy of political and economic dominance that, increasingly, embraces a readiness to take control of global resources by military means.

To justify the exploitative attitude the battered Christian faith is once again pulled out. On the individual level, it creates an escapist unreality. In this unreality, the unpleasant truth, that one's political choices have become part of an exploitative system that enables one to live a materially comfortable life denied to the majority of people in the world, is shrouded in hymns and prayers to God. This leads to a fixation on political questions connected to religion, but which, in the big picture of the current worlds' state, are of very little relevance.

On the other side, backward-looking Islamist fundamentalists use the anger of the denied peoples to launch their own power play, having successfully replaced formerly more secular oriented progressive political movements in the Islamic world. Since the world's main oil reserves are located in the predominantly Islamic Middle East, this region of course has a crucial strategic importance.

As a result we seem headed for a new Thirty Years War over power and resource control centred in this region, the justification for which, like many past wars, is couched in religious terms on both sides.

In this scheme of things, the real global problems, such as climate change, global social justice, and developing meaningful and sustainable life quality patterns are lost in the smoke of the bombs.

Dix Sandbeck

Mail Box

A Letter to Finance Minister, the Honourable Ralph Goodale

As was recommended to you in an open letter dated August 16, 2004, by William Krehm, I recommend that the Government of Canada (GoC) immediately start to do more of its borrowing from its own public central Bank of Canada (BoC). If the GoC were to instantly borrow all of its $510.6 billion debt from the BoC how much profit do you think it would make? Well! – I'll answer for you. It would make $35.2 billion because that is exactly how much the BoC would give back to the GoC

of the $35.4 billion in interest that it would charge it. Don't you think that that would be a good deal? So why don't you do it? Let all of us Canadians know! – and don't give that old worn-out incorrect answer that this would create inflation, because it would do the opposite! – it would create no inflation in comparison to the GoC's present practice of doing most of its borrowing from private-for-profit banks.

Albert Opstad, Edmonton

The New York Times Makes Amend for being Scooped in the Twin 11/9 Atrocities by Peterborough High School Student

T HE NEW YORK TIMES appears to have been scooped by Liam Rees-Spear, a Peterborough, Ontario, high school student on the identical anniversary of the Twin Tower atrocity in New York and the US-sponsored overthrow of the democratically elected Allende presidency in Chile. That identical anniversary was almost as though Someone on High wanted to nudge us to important comparisons. In any case, as though to make amends, *The New York Times* has come in with a one-and-a-half-page story on the mounting evidence not only of the murderous record of the Pinochet regime, but of its corruption to the very marrow of its bones. In assessing the preemptive military program of the Bush regime, the congressional evidence on which the *NY Times* story is based is crucial. Anything less would be a continued whitewash of one of the bloodiest stretches of military intervention to suppress democratically elected regimes throughout Latin America. That undermines Washington's credentials for teaching the Iraqis or anyone else very much about democracy.

We quote from the *Times* piece (12/12, "The Pinochet Money Trail" by Timothy L. O'Brien and Larry Rohter): "Santiago, Chile – Gen. Manuel Contreras is a religious man. A bas-relief of the Last Supper hangs on his dining room wall, not far from a thick, leather-bound Bible that rests on a table. As the former head of Gen. Augusto Pinochet's secret police in Chile, General Contreras is also a controversial man. A large silver plate given to him by Argentina's intelligence services sits on a shelf, a few feet from the Bible. The inscription on the plate reads June 1976, the same month and year that General Contreras and other South American intelligence chiefs authorized assassinations of exiled political dissidents in a wide-ranging conspiracy known as Operation Condor. Although General Contreras denied the existence of such a plan in a recent interview, the plot has been amply documented in US intelligence records.

"According to a declassified 1979 State Department memorial, Gen. Contreras opened a 'secret bank account' at Riggs Bank in Washington, when he was a young soldier based in the US. The State Department report noted that General Contreras's balance at Riggs was as high as $26,000 in the mid-1970s. But Gen. Contreras was less certain about funds Riggs held for his former boss, Gen. Pinochet, whose accounts are among those at the center of a sweeping money-laundering investigation of the bank. The sums involved – as much as $8 million according to an assessment by the US Senate – have left even Pinochet's staunchest allies wondering about their origin."

Pinochet as Financial Genius

"'The problem with Pinochet is that he got quite a lot,' Gen. Contreras said. 'Army wages were very low, even for someone as senior as Gen. Pinochet.' As Chile's strongman from 1973, when he overthrew Salvador Allende to 1999, Gen. Pinochet presided over a purge of political opponents. But he also laid the foundations for what has become Latin America's most stable and promising economy.

"In the US, however, Senate investigators published a lengthy report in July that detailed multimillion-dollar accounts that Gen. Pinochet and his wife, Lucia, held at Riggs. The funds were disguised and moved around the globe for years with the cooperation of Riggs officials, said Senate investigators, even after he was detained in London in 1998 and held under house arrest on Spanish court accusations of human rights abuses and genocide.

"Regulators fined Riggs $25 million earlier this year for failing to comply with bank secrecy laws and an investigation of the bank and its executives for possible money laundering is under way at the Justice department.

"In Chile, the fact that Gen. Pinochet secreted large sums of money in other countries has forced a reassessment of his legacy. The Chilean Congress has established a commission to determine if the Riggs accounts contain stolen government funds, an investigation that is moving apace with a separate judicial inquiry and a tax evasion investigation.

"'Let's not kid ourselves,' said Juan Pablo Letelier, chairman of the Chilean congressional commission and son of Orlando Letelier, a former Chilean foreign minister assassinated in Washington as part of Operation Condor. 'Obviously no public servant, even one who is head of state and commander in chief of the army, amasses that sort of wealth in this country, based on public income alone.

"Exactly how the general supplemented his modest salary – never more than about $40,000 a year as president – with bank accounts holding millions of dollars remains unknown. His financial adviser has told the Chilean press the general's fortune could be as much as $15 million and that all of it was accumulated legally, through shrewd financing.

"Chilean officials have openly ridiculed that explanation. The general's own sworn financial statements, released in recent weeks by US Senate investigators and approved by a Riggs executive, indicate that he received large 'commissions from service and travel abroad" during his nearly 25 years as Chile's ruler and military chief.

"Based on the examination of other documents, Chilean of-

ficials said Gen. Pinochet, now 89, participated in lucrative real estate deals and may have received some of his biggest riches as a result of industrial privatizations engineered by his administration. Those transactions benefited numerous members of his government, the Chilean military, a core group of businessmen who were his avid supporters and his former son-in-law.

"Chilean authorities are examining whether the general received kickbacks from insiders in the privatizations.

"[Certain] sometime supporters have had their faith in the former dictator shaken. Gen. Contreras's wife complained in the interview that she and her friends sold their jewelry to raise money for Gen. Pinochet's legal defense in the late 1990s, only to learn through the Riggs investigation that he had much more money than they ever suspected.

"Gen. Contreras, who said the secret police kept its own funds at the Bank of New York during the 1970s because the CIA told us that was a 'good bank,' and that the entire Chilean military should not be suspected of financial improprieties simply because Gen. Pinochet was now on the hot seat.

"According to the 1979 State Department memo, American authorities initially examined General Contreras's account at Riggs Bank as part of their investigation into the murder of Mr. Letelier and his assistant, Ronni Karpen Moffitt, whose car was blows up by a bomb as it approached the Chilean Embassy in Washington. But the memo said it was impossible to determine the source of Gen. Contreras's funds because officials at Riggs had destroyed all relevant records. Riggs declined to comment. Funds that Riggs maintained for Gen. Pinochet are proving equally murky and difficult to trace. As Gen. Contreras himself said, his former boss's wealth appears quite large for a man who spent his entire professional life as a soldier and public official. Gen. Pinochet's financial adviser, Oskar Aitken, said that he believes his client's $15 million fortune is the result of an unusual amount of high level hand-holding. The general's accounts were personally managed by Joseph Allbritton, who remains the single largest shareholder of Riggs, as 'Pinochet's biggest admirer in the banking world.' Mr. Allbritton, Mr. Aitken said, 'promised and delivered rates of return that doubled the General's capital every three years.'"

Pinochet's Booming but Elusive Accounts

"A Riggs spokesman said that Mr. Allbritton didn't personally manage the general's accounts and that the two men had met in person only on two occasions. Riggs' own records indicate that most of the general's accounts were earning interest of only 2% or 3%. Riggs, according to American investigators, did not inform regulators, as required, about the existence of the accounts when asked about them four years ago. Moreover, the bank, in a maneuver that it conceded was improper, changed the names on the accounts from 'Augusto Pinochet Ugarte and Lucia Hirtart de Pinochet' to 'L. Hirtart and/or A. Ugarte.' While banking at Riggs, the general also went by the names Ramon Ugarte and Daniel Lopez, two of the financial aliases that Gen. Pinochet's financial and legal advisers say he used.

"When the Riggs bank reviewed the propriety of maintaining the general's accounts after his arrest in Chile in 2001, a memo prepared by Steven B. Pfeiffer, a Riggs board member observed that the general's indictment 'describes with excruciating detail in over 270 pages the facts and lists thousands of people assassinated, tortured, or disappeared during Mr. Pinochet's tenure.' Still Riggs kept the accounts open.

"The mailing address for one of the Riggs accounts, it turns out, is a park in downtown Santiago, across the street from military headquarters.

"The Chilean authorities are focusing special attention on privatizations of former state-owned companies in sectors like steel, electricity, mining and telecommunications and financial gains the general might have secured through these transactions. The most lucrative privatizations were from 1985 to 1999 when it was clear the Pinochet government's days were numbered. Privatizations were largely controlled and overseen by a small group of senior Chilean military and civilian cabinet members and economic advisers, a number of whom later got shares and high-paying positions at the very companies they helped privatize.

"When Gen. Pinochet seized power on September 11, 1973, Julio Cesar Ponce Lerou was just one of many ambitious young Chileans, just graduated from forestry school. Today he is one of Chile's richest people and president of a mining company that controls some of the world's largest deposits of nitrates, iodine, and other minerals and chemicals. At the time of the coup he was married to Gen. Pinochet's daughter, Veronica, and at various times not long after, he was both president of the agency that supervised the privatization of all state-owned companies and the military dictatorship's representative on the board of the company he now heads, called Soquimich.

"Mr. Ponce Lerou led a group of investors who acquired parts of Soquimich, according to an investigation conducted by the Comptroller General's office after the dictator's fall in 1990, at less than a third of their market value. Despite Mr. Ponce Lerou's youth and inexperience in 1978 he was named president of a state-owned cellulose company that the dictatorship planned to sell to private investors. He secured the presidency of two other major state-owned enterprises, and by 1983 was the general director of the agency in charge of supervising the privatization program.

"Today, Soquimich's shareholders include foreign investors like the Bank of New York and Citigroup. But the largest block of stock remains in the hands of a holding companies called Pampa Calichera which Mr. Lerou controls."

The philosophy and practice of privatization underpinned the celebrated friendship between Margaret Thatcher and Gen. Pinochet.

Many forms of torture employed by the dictatorial regimes in Chile, the Argentine and Brazil, had been taught those who used them at a special school set up in Panama by the US army shortly after the end of WWII for just that purpose.

W.K.

An Instructive Double Anniversary — 9/11

REMEMBER 9/11/73: the year that a democratically elected government was toppled by a fascist military junta, a country was thrown into darkness and bloodshed. A heroic leader was murdered in the presidential palace after delivering a speech of defiance to his attackers, and a message of hope and solidarity to his fellow countrymen.

I am referring to the military coup that took place in Chile on September 11th 1973, that some of you may not even have heard of, though it affected the lives of many millions. The coup was supported by the United States, indirectly through the funds of massive multinationals like the ITT (International Telephone and Telegraph Company) and directly through the CIA. Together these organizations brought about the regime of Augusto Pinochet, the infamous dictator whose regime of violent oppression and murder was smiled on by successive US administrations and policy makers. The coup ousted the democratically elected president Salvador Allende. President Allende had favored the people and the well being of his country over the interests of the US multinationals and the wishes of the State Department. This was a deadly sin for a South American leader.

Allende's leftist Popular Unity Party implemented agrarian reforms. They redistributed the land, bringing an end to a medieval system of property ownership that the large landowners and corporations had imposed on the Chilean peasants. The government nationalized the copper mines (which were owned primarily by two massive US companies) so that they could be an asset to Chile as opposed to some CEO in Dallas.

On September 11, 1973, the coup began. General Pinochet, and two other generals of the Air Force and Navy, quickly took power. Allende was assassinated after making his speech of hope to the Chilean people ending with "these are my last words." Yet the deaths continued: students, artists, union members, members of the Popular Unity Party and anyone who opposed the coup were rounded into a sports stadium in the capital where they were tortured and executed. Their deaths were reported as "disappearances" and even seven Americans "disappeared" in the course of the first few weeks of the coup. To all of this the United States turned a blind eye, deliberately hindering the efforts of the American victims' families as they tried to discover what had happened to their loved ones. To this day, bodies turn up in mass graves all over Chile as more of the "disappeared" are found. Still powerful interests have managed to protect Pinochet from standing trial for human rights abuses. [After this piece was written a Chilean court ruled that he is fit to stand trial.]

Perhaps if the US had never taken such an attitude to Chile, or Guatemala or Nicaragua or Iraq or Afghanistan where they imposed leaders and regimes that created such pain and suffering, then we would not have to remember the more recent September 11th in Lower Manhattan. But when people in Canada and all over the world line up on September 11th to mourn beside the American flag. they also should remember the other 9/11, because regardless of belief all human life is equal.

Liam Rees-Spear
Grade 11, PCVS, Peterborough, Ontario

PART 1: REVIEW OF A BOOK BY STEPHEN ZARLENGA, AMERICAN MONETARY INSTITUTE, NY

"The Lost Science of Money: The Mythology of Money — The Story of Power"

THIS IS A REMARKABLE BOOK on two counts: the author has staked out a subject in so all-embracing a way that, to my best knowledge, has no precedent. The "hidden science of money," in its misty origins and seductive ambiguities, has always been a happy hunting ground for the devil's minions. Zarlenga draws a bead on the entire process from its sacral beginnings to the latest financial scandals. With careful documentation he explodes the myth of the founding fathers of economic theory, who, peeping beneath Adam and Eve's fig-leaves, saw in them destined traders frustrated by barter.

That is to misread what money is about. Considered just as another commodity – gold, silver, or whatever – has little to do with what it is or how it is measured, once it is enlisted as a monetary device. The Greeks called its latter role "nomisma." Its value as such is set not by its worth as a commodity but by the fiat of a political or quasi-political authority that launched its circulation. Thus the value of a paper dollar bill may be five cents if we consider the costs of its physical production. However, as a token claim (or ticket) for the purchase of any commodity backed by the credit of the government, it is worth a whole dollar. And note well, this is not a *debt* of the government to be paid, but a medium to facilitate the exchange of commodities or other values.

Obviously this gap between the "commodity value" of the material substance of the monetary unit and its token worth is a bottomless well of temptation, and must be protected by a strict limit on its issue. Exceed the social need of it and the value of the nomisma will shrivel "*Nomisma* comes from the Greek *Nomos* meaning *law*. And earlier meaning of the root is pastureland (the Greeks were originally a pastoral people) with strong hints of a shepherd guiding his flock, but not necessarily to the slaughterhouse.

In that derivation is embedded the forbidden secret of money. Mistake the two valuations of the nomisma with the value of its material content and you have 95 cents of play room for scams. As little-known chapters of history, it has accounted for the purloining of the wealth of empires. Unless a public body retains the power of creating money and keeps alive the distinction between the legal tender that can take the form of paper bills and the worth of the material, inked paper or whatever, society is flying blind, and inviting robbery.

Money was not Just the Result of the Inconvenience of Barter

No single work on so vast a theme can cover all bases. I missed reference to the Homeric poems that bear witness to gifting rather than individual barter as the remote source from which the money concept developed. This aspect was explored by M. Maus and others of the French Durkheim school of sociology. Or the use of cattle as a measure of the piety of religious sacrifice, and then shifting to the bronze, iron or whatever the material of the tools of the sacrificial rites to the nomisma role for the metal itself. There seems to be a greater variety of evidence of the origin of proto-money in religion rather than in trade. While economists sucked out of their thumbs the frustration of barter as the source of the money concept, more serious investigators tested that view and found it wanting. What led them to this conclusion were ancient poems like those of Homer and the customs of primitive peoples today. They concluded that barter when it occurred was rarely between individuals but between tribes or their leaders, and was largely ceremonial. Particularly in ancient Greece, the cow was a measure of value, obviously stemming from the its role in ritual sacrifice. The precious metals rather than a means of circulation of goods and services, were originally accumulated for burial in the foundations of temples and shrines. Temple prostitutes were a common means of attracting precious metals for such pious hoarding rather than trade. Money arose then as a much broader social phenomenon than merely man's alleged instincts as an irrepressible trader. The sacred roots of money, moreover, have a way of resurfacing even today in darker, demanding ways.

The take-over of the economy by bankers has thus required the suppression of much of our history and literature, beginning with Aristotle and Plato who were explicit on the distinction between the two aspects of money. There were always two distinct and incompatible ways of appraising the precious metals – as plain commodities, and as money or proto-money where the value was what the monarch stamped on a sample of the metal. Treating money as a simple commodity thus requires a high degree of obfuscation.

The introduction of smaller silver coins into ancient Greece introduced money to the small farmers. Previously if they borrowed commodities such as grain before harvest was in, they repaid it in kind. But with the introduction of small silver coins they might borrow the grain when its market value was low and then by the time repayment was due, find the value of the currency in terms of grain had risen ruinously. Or they may have received the loan in money at the Athens rate but were required to pay interest at the Corinthian or Aeginaian rate which could be 50% higher. Where you have several different coining authorities – there were three in ancient Greece – the repertory of possible tricks multiplies. That is why in Sparta Lycurgus outlawed the use of gold and silver as money and introduced iron "cakes," whose usefulness as a commodity was deliberately destroyed by being dipped in vinegar while still hot. Thereby it became unambiguously a nomisma, worthless *except* as a medium for trading.

When Copper and Bronze were more Useful than Gold

The Romans made a point of keeping the commonly used money strictly nomismata – coins of bronze – a mixture of copper, tin, with a little lead. This was introduced by Rome's second king, suggestively called Numa (718-672 BC). In this way they were insulated from the influence of the Middle Eastern powers who coined gold and silver as their money.... Gold and silver could be traded in Rome as merchandise, but the ability of the eastern temples or merchants to control and disrupt Rome's money was greatly reduced by the Numa innovation. The fate of Greece was partly determined by the orientation of its money. Greece faced east; Rome faced West.

It was only during the Punic Wars that the powerful defence thrown up by its bronze currency against foreign monetary intervention was sapped.

J.W. Frazer's *Golden Bough* tells how in 204 BC, after enduring 16 years of Hannibal's rampage and 70 to 100 thousand dead, the war-weary and desperate Romans were seduced by a prophecy concocted from the Sibylline books: 'The foreign invader would be driven from Italy if the Oriental Goddess, the Phrygian "Mother of the Gods" were brought to Rome. The small black stone which embodied that mighty divinity (Kybele) was conveyed to Rome. In the very next year Hannibal embarked for Africa. The Phrygian Goddess' sanctuary was established on Palatine Hill. Some have argued that the cultic success in ridding Italy of Hannibal threw open the gates of Rome to a variety of Eastern cults. But the warfare had already helped bring down the money system and Roman justice with it.

"The 'commodization' of Rome's money system dramatically accelerated the emergence of a plutocracy – a ruling order based on wealth. 'By the time of the 2nd Punic War there were already significant accumulations of capital in the hands not only of the Roman Establishment, but of a non-Senatorial business class. This capital may have been the fruits of the profits made during the 1st Punic War. Contractors commanded sufficient reserves to make deliveries to the Government on credit from 215 BC onwards.

"Our hypothesis that silver was provided to the mint at a six-fold overvaluation can help explain where the money came from. And the timing also works (p. 65).

"For the loans were being repaid even before the war was over. Then immediately upon defeating Hannibal, there was a political thrust to start a new war with Macedon. Apparently those benefiting from warfare didn't want any interruption to their profiteering."

This eventually brought on a revolt on behalf of the small farmers led in turn by two aristocratic brothers, the Gracchi, inspired by Stoic philosophy. Both were martyred, and the era of Julius Caesar and his dictatorial successors took over. Each of these, while still striving for power, minted his own gold coins. This had a double purpose – financing their attempt to seize supreme power and advertising the extent of power already attained. Under Augustus the ratio of gold to silver was raised to 12:1, and an end was put to coining by patrician families. Julius Caesar had directed his conquest to gold sources, that amongst

much else would allow him to handle his huge personal debt. With every new colony founded, a new coining was launched under the Roman stamp to take care of its monetary needs. Despite Rome's Eastern conquests gold and silver drained off to the east, largely because of the luxury imports by the high-living new rich of Rome. Slaves replaced free labourers on the vast latifundia that took over as usury ruined the small farmers.

All this echoes strangely familiar in the claim of central banks to be independent of their government, no matter what their charters may say. That is notably the case even in Canada and the United Kingdom, where the central governments are in fact the sole shareholder of its central bank with the explicit ultimate responsibility for its basic policy. Moreover, the official goal of "zero inflation" is unrealizable in a pluralistic urbanized high-tech society, in which ever more indispensable infrastructures are provided by the state. The coining of gold was considered the ultimate sign of sovereignty. Strip government of that prerogative, and what is left is no longer a truly sovereign power.

For a later period, after the Roman Empire had declined, it worked like this: the gold/silver ratio in the West was kept high, ranging over millennia, from 9 to 16 to 1. However, the ratio in India and Asia was kept low – usually around 6 or 7 to 1. This meant that silver taken from Europe to India was exchanged for nearly twice as much gold in India as in Europe. The nexus of this trade was the land bridge above the Middle East. Whoever controlled that area usually controlled the trade.

"If it was controlled from the West, they got 100% more gold for their silver than the local value. It worked just as well from the East. If they controlled the trade they received 100% more silver for their gold. If control was shared, trade would probably have been at a 9 to 1 ratio, giving each establishment a profit on exchange.

"The existence of this dichotomy and its significance is almost unknown (Jacobs, William, *The Precious Metals*, 1831, reprinted NY, A.M. Kelley, 1968). Alexander Del Mar also discovered it. While the mechanism is still [generally] unrecognized, we can identify its traces in the work of modern historians such as M. Rostovtzef's *Social and Economic History of the Hellenistic World:* 'The Ptolemies [Macedonian successors to Alexander the Great in Egypt] 'for reasons unknown to us but probably dictated by economics...separated themselves and their Kingdom from the rest of the Hellenized world. It seems to have been an accepted fact that they derived an enormous reserve of gold from the Arabian caravan trade.

"Pliny [the Elder] wrote that 100 million Sesterces of silver, equivalent to one million gold Aurei, was annually exported to India and China from Rome. He had been appointed Procurator in Spain and entrusted with managing the Revenue. But the secrecy of the mechanism is underscored by the fact that its workings were not known to him, for he couldn't understand why his countrymen always demanded silver and not gold from conquered races."

It should be made clear that what Zarlenga has to say about the handling of money creation in the contemporary world in no way stands or falls with his espousal of the price ratio of gold and silver in remote and more recent times.

This is how Zarlenga sums up his views on the reasons for the decline of the Roman Empire. "The combined evidence on wealth concentration, the absence of mining, the normal erosion of the coinage through usage and the tendency of the precious metals – especially silver – to flow eastwards, present a powerful argument that an inadequate supply of circulating medium of money – was a (the?) major factor in the continued decline of the Roman Empire.

"Behind that scarcity, ultimately, was a huge error in monetary theory that some ideologues still make today – the false belief that money should be a commodity or economic good, that is, wealth, rather than a legally based abstract power."

On the High Social Cost of Commodity Money

Then in his Chapter 4, "Re-Instituting Money in the West," Zarlenga takes an entirely different approach to the question of fiat money – money whose worth does not depend on the intrinsic value of the material enlisted for the money role, but on the credit (a.k.a. these days as the "productivity") of the nation.

"'The advantage to society of having enough rule of law to create fiat money is enormous and not just a matter of degree.' The breakdown of law and of money continued to operate negatively, the one upon the other for centuries, in a slow downward spiral of societal decay. Re-building them would take centuries more. In that process we observe several attempts to resurrect commodity-based money, which in many respects are more of an advanced form of barter than a true money system." For if you consider money just another commodity, three not just two commodities are involved in any exchange.

"Creating such commodity moneys requires expending a great deal of work in prospecting, mining, refining and minting. Maintaining that money against the attacks of coin clippers, metal exporters and normal wear and tear over the decades also requires great energy.

"These heavy burdens tend to neutralize the benefits eventually derived from such money systems, leaving mankind trapped on an economic treadmill. This is especially true considering the low state of resources that societies had available to deploy in those darkest ages of Europe. At first the precious metals systems continued well into the 17th, 18th, and 19th centuries. Modern 19th and 20th century money systems, which claimed to be precious metals systems, generally depended on an element of fraud rather than force, as we shall see.

"Thus the advantage to society of having enough rule of law to create that money system is enormous. It is just not a matter of degree, but produces a different kind of result altogether. It would take until the 13th and 14th centuries to reach that critical threshold in Europe.

"An early attempt to rebuild the money system was made by Charlemagne (742-814), often credited with establishing a new monetary standard and with re-instituting weights and measures in the West, from which the pound, shilling and pence notations evolved. More accurately, Charlemagne's system was a revival of some Roman coining traditions. Charlemagne's

system of Livres, Sols and Deniers had existed from at least 418 AD as seen in the Roman Code of Theodosius. This 'money of account' system had served to unify different Roman Coinages issued over time. The alternative would have been an expensive re-minting and the loss to the melting pot of the numerous historical commemorations in the old coins.

"The basis of Charlemagne's Empire was military conquest and the enslavement of subjugated people, mostly Saxons. Using this extensive slave labor he re-started or intensified precious metal mining at Chemnitz, Kremnitz, and Rauthenberg, mostly of silver, working the slaves to death in the mines. Those slaves not needed for mining were sold to the Moslems through Jewish and Venetian intermediaries. To mint Charlemagne's silver into pennies, many new mints were opened at Dorestad, Aachen, Bonn, Cologne, Maastricht and Namur. At one point he considered producing all the coinages at his Palace mint at Aachen." That, of course, indicates how much wealth and effort was dedicated to provide the semblance of a commodity currency.

"However, the coinage was still scarce as indicated by taxes being collected mainly in services and produce, rather than coinage." And in the well-known fact that for centuries later, royal courts moved around from royal domain to domain as they consumed the resources grown locally. All this indicated the crushing cost of trying to maintain a commodity money system when there was neither the precious metals nor skills and institutions available for that or the alternate fiat currency."

Zarlenga traces the different ways in which successive regimes exploited the discrepancy between the gold-silver ratio in India and Europe. The Venetians learned to live with the Muslim conquest of the Eastern Mediterranean, by adapting their trading to the Muslim injunctions against the taking of interest. The Venetians replaced it with profits by the Venetian financiers who shared with the active entrepreneurs the actual risks. But those profits included the huge discrepancy in the gold-silver ratio between Europe and Asia. The basis for this collaboration was in Egypt which was kept isolated from the rest of the Muslim world, undoubtedly for this purpose. The Portuguese by discovering the route around the Cape of Good Hope cut into Venice's monopoly which had brought Italy the Renaissance, and the European basis for the collection of the ratio bonus shifted from Pavia to Antwerp. The Jews came to play an increasing part in communications across the ratio frontier. From Portugal it shifted to Holland, largely because of its prowess in shipbuilding. And from there to England. Then with the discovery of America, far cheaper sources of gold became available.

Zarlenga aims some well-directed irony at Marx's labour theory of value that joins with an equality signs the value of gold to the hours of average labour needed for its production. The average hours of labour needed for the production of gold might seem irrelevant, given the fact that the gold that flooded Europe after the Spanish conquest of America was not mined by the Spaniards but stolen – once by the Spaniards from the Amerindian civilizations that they destroyed for the purpose, and then much of it by English pirates from the Spaniards. Two radically different social systems reigned on either side of the equality symbols. Moreover the same scenario had been reenacted three hundred years earlier fuelled by the same famine for an exchange medium in Europe that had been bleeding its scant silver into Asia.

"In 1095 Pope Urban II passionately called for an expedition to take Jerusalem from the Muslims. 'It is the will of God' chanted the multitude, and every village in Europe was affected by this greatest undertaking of any kind since the time of Imperial Rome.

"But after all Moslems had ruled Palestine for over 400 years. The Emperor asked for help in retrieving the holy lands to remove the military pressure the Seljuk Turks placed on Byzantium. At the time the larger part of the Jewish population had moved from Asia to Europe. The occupation of Spain by Islam had brought a wave of Jews with it. Much of the East-West trade was in their hands through Spain. The massacre of Jews in Europe by Crusaders as they left on the first Crusade may indicate that constricting the Jews was a motivation on more than one level.

"But the Papacy also wanted to end the dominance of the Basileus in Constantinople which was apparently still recognized as the supreme religious authority by most of the Western leadership. Or if a large Western force could be moved near Constantinople without raising alarm over the many years it would take to assemble, that force could ultimately be used to topple the Emperor."

The Hidden Monetary Drive behind the Crusades

"All these high level objectives and more were in fact achieved during the Crusades. The Basileus succeeded in dislodging the Moslems from Jerusalem for almost 100 years and forever from Spain. The Mediterranean was reopened to general Christian traffic. The significance of the Jews in international trade was 'drastically reduced' after the Crusades broke the Moslem-Christian barrier, breaking the trading links of the Jews in Europe with the Radanites of Egypt, who held long-standing trade relations with India. Many poor Crusaders were responsible for the massacres of the Jews. The attacks were said to be religiously motivated in that anyone who accepted baptism was not harmed – for example all the Jews of Trier. However, many massacres occurred elsewhere: in the Church at Rouen; at Speyer 800 Jews killed each other to avoid baptism In Mainz, 1014 Jews similarly died together, and massacres occurred at Altenauhr, Xanten, Mors, Kerpen, Gelden and Cologne (James Parkes, *The Jew in the Medieval Community,* Hermon Press, New York, 1976). 'Unless the reader can seize some of the horror of those fatal weeks it is not possible to understand the hatred of Jews of the Middle Ages for Christianity and for those Jews who accepted it.'

"When the Crusaders reached Constantinople they were awe-struck by the sight of the great walled city. Nothing like it existed in the West. The various leaders took oaths of loyalty to the Emperor and agreed to give him all conquered territories. The Army went on to Jerusalem, remaining orderly in spite of poorly planned logistics. There was no fodder for the animals. Sheep, dogs, and even pigs were used as pack animals. Desertions were heavy. The Emperor had been advancing behind them to take possession of his new lands, but heard of their problems and turned back to Constantinople. Somehow on July 15, 1099, they took Jerusalem, and an ecclesiastical Kingdom was set up there with Godfred de Bouillon as king. They then took one city after another, perpetrating many horrors in the name of Christianity.

"Christian behaviour contrasted poorly with that of the Muslims, especially Saladin the Great. A Kurd born at Takrit, Saladin had united the Muslims to fight the Crusaders. In 1183 he retook Jerusalem, granting merciful terms. Saladin's guards kept such order that no Christian suffered any ill usage.

"Over time the Crusaders, always a small minority in the cities they conquered, became orientalized. They inter-married with the 'infidels,' and didn't think much of home. Both Christian crusaders and Moslem defenders eventually sought alliances in battles against co-religionists. Christians came to boast of Moslem descent. The Moslems had preserved elements of Greek learning and Roman law in a better form than the West. Despite the Clergy's falsified reports on conditions in the Holy Land, the fame of Saladin the Great spread throughout the West and members of the educated classes desired to convert to Islam.

"The Crusaders also came into closer contact with the origins of Judaism and Christianity and some found reason to question their faith. This led to a new freedom of mind in some individuals. One important result of the 1st Crusade was the formation of the Knights Templar, originally called the Poor Knights of the Temple of Solomon. They were formed in 1114-18 to protect pilgrims in the Holy Land. Questions have arisen as to their humble origin and goal.

"'The evidence suggests that this avowed goal was a facade and that the Knights were engaged in a much more ambitious, grandiose geopolitical enterprise (*The Temple and the Lodge*, Arcade, Little Brown, 1989). The Templars' original membership simply appears too high-powered and their growth too rapid. They were involved with the Cistercian order, which became a primary promoter of the 4th Crusade. The nine Knight members in 1128 included Fulk, Comte d'Anjou (father of Geoffrey Plantagenet and grandfather of Henry II, King of England), Comte de Champagne; and Hughes de Payens, who became the order's first Grand Master. Within one year they owned lands in France, England, Scotland, Spain and Portugal. Within a decade their possessions would extend to Italy, Austria, Germany, Hungary and Constantinople. By 1150 the Temple had begun to establish itself as the single most wealthy and powerful institution in Christendom, with the sole exception of the Papacy (Dana Carlton Monroe, *The Kingdom of the Crusades*, Port Washington, Kennikat, 1966).

The Father of a Thousand Forgotten Novels

And here the plot thickens to father a thousand forgotten novels. "Byzantium had obstructed the 3rd Crusade and formed an alliance with Saladin, who held Jerusalem. Elements in the

West, including the leadership of Cluny, France's greatest religious house, and especially members of the Cistercian Order, plotted Byzantium's downfall. The plan was to divert the 4th Crusade into an attack on Constantinople under the pretext of re-instating Emperor Isaac and his son Alexis, who had been deposed in a palace coup. Venice's fleet would be crucial. 95-year-old Enrico Dandolo readily agreed to lead the expedition. He had been partly blinded by Byzantine officials, a favorite method of torture. The appearance of the Venetian fleet in the harbour of Constantinople was enough to make the acting emperor flee and have the deposed Emperor Isaac reinstated, but when his son told him of the agreement made to cede religious sovereignty to Rome, he objected. When the Byzantines learned of the agreement in January 1204, they murdered both father and son and installed Canabus as Emperor." With sovereignty Rome and countless principalities in Europe would revert to do their own coining of gold and silver.

"On April 9th, the Crusaders attacked and defeated the Byzantines. From April 13 to 15 the Christian invaders were turned loose on the greatest Christian city in the world. They went wild. They preserved the foolish relics – the bones of the Saints, pieces of the Cross, milk from the Mother of God, and destroyed the great artworks: the bronze charioteers of the Hippodrome; the She Wolf suckling Romus and Romulus; Paris presenting the apple to Venus; an exquisite statue of Helen of Troy; statues commissioned by Augustus; all the great works taken by Constantinople over nine centuries from the ancient temples. All were melted down into bullion or coin. Thousands of manuscripts and parchments from many personal libraries were now burned and from that time on the works of many ancient authors disappeared altogether.

"Baldwin of Flanders was elected Emperor and Venice took control of the Patriarchy and Churches. The loot was gathered up and divided. The Pope ratified these decisions. The schisms between the Latin and Orthodox churches became irrevocable. Michael 8th recovered Constantinople from the Latins in 1261. It fell to the Ottoman Turks in 1453.

"The fall of Constantinople in 1204 formally ended the Empire's monetary powers, which had held sway in Europe from the time of the Caesars.

"The 'secret' dynamic behind this 'sacred' monetary system was that the Basileus would be ready to exchange centrally minted gold Bezants for locally minted silver coinage at a 12 to 1 ratio, when it could exchange that same silver for up to twice as much gold bullion in India and points east. When Byzantium fell, control of money slipped from sacred hands into secular hands. While the Lateran Council would soon (1211) declare the Papacy's supremacy over all earthly sovereigns, they couldn't make it stick. Frederick 2nd assumed the sacred prerogative of the Basileus and minted gold coins at Naples in 1225. Local rulers all over Europe began minting gold coinage.

"Vast amounts of spoil were brought back to Europe from Constantinople, more than the official figures, because the marauders cheated their fellow Christians and did not put all their loot into the official pool, which totaled about 400,000 marks weight worth of silver. Forty barrels of gold were found beneath the altar of St. Sophia alone. The plunder of Constantinople by the Venetians and other of the Crusaders probably transferred more metallic wealth to Western Europe than all the commerce of the centuries that preceded it (William Jacobs, *The Precious Metals*). The return of this metallic plunder to Europe gave a crucial monetary boost to European life and was probably the main factor in Europe finally reaching the magic threshold, the critical monetary mass where a truer, more advanced monetary system could function. Nomisma could be introduced. The hoarded coinage and bullion had been less than useless in Constantinople, where it required heavy storage expenses and served as a magnet attracting conquest. In Europe it would be put to much better use: by Venice in her commercial activities, by the Princes in their realms, by the Church in helping to finance construction of the great cathedrals of Europe by individual crusaders and by the Knights Templar in their growing financial activities."

William Krehm

G.G. McGeer on Monetary Policy

MCGEER has been mentioned in these pages at least twice before in the past year (May and December). He made important contributions to the argument that private banking companies have too much latitude in expanding and contracting the supply of money and that governments should have a monetary policy and exercise control over it. His expository power is familiar among money reformers and conspiracy theorists although his name is not, for he drafted what they revere as "Lincoln's Monetary Policy." To be compared with Lincoln as a writer, and especially to be mistaken for him, is a high compliment to McGeer's skill with words. His 359-page book containing that Lincolnesque statement was published under the title *The Conquest of Poverty* in 1935. (See my article in the May *ER* for details.) I know of at least two other works by him on the same subject matter. One of them is the primary subject of this essay and was issued in 1933 as a pamphlet of 36 pages that you can read and download at www.yamaguchy.netfirms.com/mcgeer_r/mcgeer.html.

You will notice that it has the same *Conquest of Poverty* title. The third work is a clothbound book titled *The Need for Monetary Reform*. I know of it only through a publisher's advertisement in the back of another book. From contextual circumstances I am confident in inferring that it was published prior to 1935, and I am guessing that it post-dated the document you can get electronically.

Gerald Grattan McGeer ("Gerry") was a colorful presence on the Canadian scene in from the early 1920s through the '40s, as a successful promoter of local development, an MLA, Mayor of Vancouver and Senator. He was celebrated by Clyde Gilmour in an entertaining biography that appeared in *Maclean's* magazine just a couple of months before McGeer's untimely death at age 59 ("The Great McGeer," April 15, 1947). To really appreciate the flavor of *The Conquest of Poverty* I do recommend Gilmour's "album." A book-length biography was published much later (in the mid-1980s as I recall), in BC, written by an author with the interesting name of David Ricardo Williams. I have seen this book, in the National Library, but had spent very little time in it before it was spirited away from my locker by the request of another user. My notes say that the Foreword is by Bruce Hutchison, with other comments by him salted around in the book. Hutchison is cited for the observation that McGeer was neither a socialist nor a Social Crediter. Instead, he says that McGeer's ideas most closely resembled those of Hitler's finance minister/monetary czar, Hjalmar Schacht, and that after the War, admirers and detractors alike began to realize that those ideas "presupposed a very tight brand of government control over most aspects of life and commerce." (Note that comment, for it is the key issue on which evaluation of McGeer's contribution will depend.) McGeer was in fact a vehement Liberal and ally of MacKenzie King. He campaigned for King in his successful return as Prime Minister in 1935, and was appointed by King to the Senate in 1945. See the Gilmour article for an account of the impact he made in Parliament when he came to Ottawa to present the contents of the 1933 document. Subsequent passage of the Bank of Canada Act did not achieve McGeer's ideal, of course, but the new central bank was brought closer to it a few years later when it was nationalized by MacKenzie King's government.

The pamphlet version of *The Conquest of Poverty* at the Yamaguchy site is further identified on the cover as a "Report to the Vancouver Trades and Labour Council." ("Gerry" had by that time established a solid reputation for himself as a successful crusading lawyer.) He opens with a stinging criticism of the Macmillan Banking Commission which had recently made recommendations for Bank of England policy and, then turns on the government of R.B. Bennett with contempt for having hired Lord Macmillan to repeat his performance here – a gesture of impotent complacence in the face of the Depression crisis enveloping working-class Canadians. There were some members of the Macmillan Commission whose views he respected, however (naming J. Maynard Keynes, Reginald McKenna and Ernest Bevin among others). In this document he therefore singles out portions that he likes of the Commission's report for British policy and attributes them collectively to those individuals, assembling the favored ideas as a "minority report." (He may have been fully justified in making this interpretation of their intent, but it is nonetheless a rhetorical trick that one could miss in the vehement flow of his prose. He then did much the same thing with some rather thin documentation when giving credit to Abraham Lincoln for his own monetary and banking prescription in the 1935 book.) His biographers note that McGeer did carry on a correspondence with Keynes. At the end of this pamphlet he acknowledges other monetary reformers such as C.H. Douglas and Silvio Gesell for having contributed ideas and techniques that might be added as important refinements once the immediate crisis of the Depression had been countered by an expansion of government spending. For the mo-

ment, however, his prescription was to simply have government finance important public works, using fundamentally the same techniques that had fueled the war effort of 1914-1916 and that paralleled Lincoln's in financing the Civil War. The current argument for financing municipal infrastructure by direct Bank of Canada loans is an obvious extension.

Verbal Choreography Around a Solid Centre

Following is a sample of Gerry's head-twisting prose:

"Surely, no one can justify as sound the practice of governmental borrowing at interest of credit from a private monopoly when the government has the power to set up a national banking system through which can be issued paper currency and bank credit more valuable as purchasing power medium of exchange than that which is issued by private bankers. Our department of finance, exercising one of the powers enjoyed by Central Banks patterned after the Bank of England, issues Dominion legal tender notes redeemable in gold, which are loaned to the private banks at interest in the vicinity of 3 per cent. This the banker calls cash and treats as the reserve basis for the issue of bank credit. Varying with the conditions of the times, the banker then issues bank credit from 5 to 15 times the value of his legal tender cash on hand with which he finances loans and buys and finances government interest-bearing bonds and any other form of liquid assets producing interest or profit.

"The idea that a government should issue national legal tender cash to a private banker at 3 per cent and then permit the bankers to issue on that reserve bank credit on the average of ten times its value, and compel the taxpayers of national, provincial and municipal governments to pay from 3 to 6 per cent for bank credit to finance all governmental activity reduces our world to the topsy-turvy level of the 'Land of the Mad Hatter.' Such an absurdity is beyond the comprehension of intelligence, but its acceptance as sane and sound economy is nevertheless a fact."

That is what he prepared for his labor union clients and delivered for them in hearings of the House Banking and Finance Committee. It is said of that event that his Ottawa auditors were virtually speechless in the face of this vehement clarity, reduced to asking polite but essentially innocuous questions. It is highly pertinent to ask whether and by whom that argument has been cogently refuted? The founding of COMER half a century later and its stream of arguments and publications pressing much the same theme suggest that the challenge has not been answered. The context of our times is doubtless more complex, but the core issue seems to be with us still. McGeer's arguments do seem to have some presence in favorable aspects of the Bank's legislative mandate, as described by Krehm in *The Bank of Canada: A Power Unto Itself*. The clarity of McGeer's prose and the simplicity in which he perceived the circumstance can be a lever for understanding more complex times and institutions. It illuminates, for me, the pages of *Babel's Tower: The Dynamics of Economic Breakdown*, and the issues discussed in this publication. It might be useful for COMER members to read it critically and to collectively annotate it with sufficient detail to bring it up to date and to then re-publish it as a primer for monetary and banking discussion and education. I should add that McGeer's prescription for avoiding the inflation bogey is just as limpid and persuasive as his argument for expansion of the money supply – but read it for yourself.

One further selection from the pamphlet report is especially significant in these days of "privatizing" established government functions, including social security and medical care. The "new" direction for government-directed social policy is to have poor people take care of themselves by investing their meagre savings in the stock market lottery. It is called an "asset-based approach to poverty." McGeer again:

"Now people do say that bank dividends to bank shareholders do not disclose any such lucrative activity as the possible manipulation of credit I have outlined indicates. But they have never had the opportunity of examining...the private profits of our banking leaders and their associates, gained largely through credit manipulation. But investigations in the United States of recent date give some indication of what they are. The great profits of the credit system do not go to the bank shareholders, but to men like the Morgans, Mellons, Holts and Wood Gundys, who enjoy the power of rule by credit control. The information disclosing their activities, profits and possession of wealth would be forthcoming only under a most careful and efficient investigation. The reputed wealth of certain bankers and well-known groups indicates that the profits of our credit barons are not to be considered as being in the same class as bank shareholders' dividends."

In other words, don't believe everything you read in audited financial reports of banking corporations. That may be a redundant warning in these post-Enron days, but McGeer stands as a witness that we are naive not to think about who is paying the auditors and why.

One source of the power in McGeer's prose is his appeal to a populist, democratic instinct that money ought to be something that is provided and controlled by governments – especially democratic ones. This idea appeals to our sense of justice; it seems right and hence strikes us as "natural." If there is any activity that qualifies under the economists' definition of a public good, provision of a sound and stable money supply ought to be it. And if it is not operated solely as a function of government, then it ought to be closely regulated by government as a public utility. But that is old-fashioned political economy; in these days the "economists of innocent fraud" have taught us that we live in the best of all possible worlds where markets are completely self-regulating. Indeed, money is a special case because it is so commonplace. We handle it every day as something that is simply "there" like the sun in the morning and the moon at night. Money is so familiar as the price of everything that it takes a conscious effort to conceive of money itself as produced by an industry and having a price. McGeer tried to give us an idea of that price (in the passages excised from the quotation just above) by calling attention to the enormous value (social cost) that we transfer to private bankers via the absurdity of letting governments borrow from banks when they should be themselves the ultimate and inevitable monetary authority.

But while the idea of government monetary management

may sound "natural" it has rarely if ever been an established fact. Even the old Soviet Union was forced to cope with international money changers and financiers. Monetary management and policy are the subject of a perennial contest between democratic governments and private bankers. These days it is the big players in the "private" sector that appear to be winning most of the time, which calls forth effort from groups like COMER to regain balance. The bankers' side wins when they can convince folks that government is bad for them and that "free markets" or "the market system" is the real state of nature to which we must always be striving to return. Thus we get the comment attributed to Bruce Hutchison above. And even though the host of the "Yamaguchy" site generously provides this McGeer text for us, he is wary of Gerry's fulsome attribution of honest and intelligent professionalism to public servants as managers of a government monetary system. That is his reason for not posting the 359-page book version of *The Conquest of Poverty* to his very valuable website (even though he has done the work of scanning it).

The Underground Longevity and Continuity of Monetary Reform

It is rare to see references to McGeer in economic or financial histories. This does not necessarily mean that he didn't have some impact at the time. (It has been found more effective to marginalize the bearers of bad news than to make martyrs of them.) But a reader of this document cannot help but wonder how Gerry developed such a mastery of his theme. And that raises a question about the longevity and continuity of a "money reform" underground. It seems unlikely that he came by these ideas in isolation and as a consequence of only a few months as counsel to the Vancouver labor group. He doubtless had some contacts with the populist tradition in America, for it is said that he was frequently invited to give Lincoln Day speeches. We do know that he had an admirer in the person of Robert L. Owen, drafter of the Senate version of legislation that created the Federal Reserve System (*ER*, May 2004). Perhaps his eloquence on this subject stems partly from the fact that he didn't have the crutch of "unconstitutional" that his American counterparts could appeal to. He had to develop another approach, and so chose Jesus for the principle of controlling the money changers and the probity of professional public servants for assurance that it could be done. (Noteworthy here is the comment of Milton Friedman to Joel Bakan. See my review in September *ER*.)

Keith Wilde

China's Resourcefulness in Deflecting the Pressures to Push up its Currency

GLOBALIZATION AND DEREGULATION has led to some difficult confrontations between national economies. Many of the traditional arrangements for the defence of national living standards and cultures, tariffs, labour and health standards have been scrapped, and that leaves the national currencies – where they continue to exist – overloaded with the responsibility of protecting national standards. Not only has the European Union added to this discrepancy, especially with the imminent entry of new Eastern European candidates to the EU. A North American currency union was a highly promoted goal before the Iraqi adventure has put that issue to rest. Yet, it should not be assumed that we have heard the last of that initiative.

Against this background, intriguing strategies have been devised by countries under pressure to increase the value of their currencies.

In the 1970s the abandonment of even the pretence of a gold standard, much of that pressure was directed against Japan by the United States. Involvement in Vietnam and the oil crunches of that time were playing havoc with the US dollar, which was increasingly exploiting its privileged status as reserve currency of the world. The Americans countered with the demand that the Japanese allow their currency to rise. The Second World War and the Cold War were still vivid memories, with Japan still in a Madam Butterfly role, she could hardly counter with an outright refusal to strengthen the yen. Instead, she had recourse to artful evasions, drawing on the rich courtesy resources of her culture towards that end.

However, the low yen was vital to the continued export successes of Japan in making good its war losses, and its lack of natural resources. For a while the Japanese thought they had improvised a practical rather than just a diplomatic strategy. It was to load up with American securities, and even real estate. They had the bad luck, however, to hit the near top of both the US real estate and the stock markets, and in addition to some sizeable losses, they also garnered some unpopularity for having picked up some of the cherished icons of US real estate.

We cannot help admiring the superiority of the current Chinese response to the American pressure to raise the yuan to rein in the sweeping powers of the Chinese export drives. Rather than targeting over-priced US real estate icons, they have drawn a bead directly on the exports and domestic markets of just about every industry, garnering much technology and marketing know-how in the process. For that their own rich cultural past was immensely useful, as was their recent familiarity with variant social systems, and of course, their almost endless supply of dirt-cheap and highly motivated labour. Plus the sheer massive allures of a 1.3 billion eventual market that serves them far beyond anything that the Japanese had to fall back on.

The Wall Street Journal (26/11, "Shopping for China – A scourge of the Rust Belt Offers Some hope There too" by Peter Wonacott") tells a fascinating tale:

"When Lu Guanqiu, his wife and five others pooled $500 to start a tractor repair shop in rural China in the late 1960s, local officials laughed off their efforts. 'You're a farmer. You should be in the fields,' he remembered them saying.

"Today Mr. Lu is one of China's wealthiest men, founder and chairman of Wanxiang Group Co., that country's biggest autoparts supplier with $1.5 billion in sales last year and $3 billion this year. Now he is setting out to compete with the world's biggest parts suppliers on their home turf in the US.

"Mr. Lu has assembled interest in more than 30 ventures around the world that make most of the components in the underside of a car. Wanxiang's US sales are expected to grow 60% to about $400 million in 2004, company executives say. Its smaller European division is on pace for a 30% revenue rise this year.

"Mr. Lu is helping write a new chapter in the story of China's surging economic growth. He is swooping into the American rust belt and scooping up investments on hard-hit auto suppliers. Some of them are finding that the remedy for Chinese competition is an infusion of Chinese money, and a timely means to cut costs.

"Last year China was the largest recipient of foreign direct investments; now the funds are starting to flow the other way, too.

"This month, Shanghai Automotive Industry Corp. announced it was planning a merger with Britain's MG Rover Group. In September it acquired a controlling stake in Korean car maker Sangyong Motor Co. China Minmetals Corp. is pursuing a $5.5 billion bid to buy Noranda Inc., Toronto's zinc and nickel miner. Meanwhile, telecommunications giant Huawei Technologies Co. has acquired two US equipment makers and set up research centers in Dallas and Silicon Valley.

"Though still a trickle compared with Japanese investment in the US in the 1990s. Chinese investment is starting to grow. Chinese companies invested $2.9 billion overseas last year, a 5.5% increase from 2002 but still less than 1% of the world's total, according to China's National Bureau of Statistics.

"In joint ventures in Illinois, Minnesota and Ohio, Wanxiang has sought alliances where it can move into more sophisticated products and pick up big new customers. It has looked for ways to cut costs, including shifting some production of low-end parts to China.

"Mr. Lu's rise began in 1962, when he was tossed out of his job as a blacksmith's apprentice. The small steel plant he was working in closed down amid the tumult of China's Great Leap Forward, a campaign to rapidly industrialize the nation. Instead of heading back to the farm, he started repairing bicycles, and went on to service tractors as well.

"He built a small village commune into something rare for the era: a market-driven family enterprise. Mr. Lu's wife, Zhang Jinmei, became an expert welder and worked through four pregnancies. In 1972, she gave birth to her only son, now Wanxiang's chief executive, Lu Weiding, literally on the factory floor. Three of Mr. Lu's daughters work at Wanxiang.

"When private companies were still illegal in China, the nation's political spasms worked to Wanxiang's advantage. With managers of state-owned companies often tied up in political struggles, Mr. Lu attended to their neglected customers. In 1973, his factory bought 300 tons of cannon barrels from the Chinese army because local authorities kept steel for state enterprises. His wife cut open the barrels with an electric saw and transformed them into brisk-selling tractor blades.

"Mr. Lious later used a precious steel quota from the government to begin producing universal joints, a palm-size component that transmits power from the engine and drive shaft to the wheels. Wanxian, Chinese for universal joint, began to supply tractors, trucks and – in the early 1980s – an exploding number of cars.

"As more multinationals arrived in China, executives from General Motors, Ford Motor and Volkswagen sought out Wanxiang as a supplier; Wanxiang racked up global orders, many coming from other parts makers such as Visteon which bought the Chinese company's chassis auto parts. His single workshop spawned more than 30 factories and 31,000 employees in China. From its whitewashed headquarters in Xiaoshan city, Wanxian has diversified into securities, banking, property – and even toothpaste, crawfish and US oil wells.

"Wanxian's US operations, headed by Mr. Lu's son-in-law Pin Ni, grew by offering bargain prices on auto parts. By 1995, it was posting $3.5 million in revenue and had moved into a small warehouse to store the auto parts coming from China. In the late 1990s, Mr. Ni began gobbling up American companies. Some needed cash because Chinese companies like Wanxiang were eroding their business. It bought five companies making bearings, drive shafts, and other auto parts. In 2001, it spent $2.8 million for a 21% stake in Universal Automotive Industries Inc., a Nasdaq-listed brakes maker. All told, Wanxian's investments brought close to 1000 new employees under its umbrella." As Mr. Ni sees it, Wanxiang is helping the rust belt stay alive. Just west on Interstate 90, on the border of Wisconsin, those efforts are getting a test in Rockford. Since the mid-19th century this city has churned out much of the country's power tools and lots of auto parts. But lately small factories that form Rockford's industrial backbone have fallen on hard times.

"Wanxiang, one of its suppliers, came to the rescue. It invested an undisclosed sum to form a joint venture and has reaped the returns of reducing the axle-maker's costs. Executives of both companies say the Driveline is profitable and expects a 30% sales increase.

"Across the street, Driveline Rockford Powertrain is also trying to carve out a global niche with Wanxiang. In October, 2003, Wanxiang took a substantial a stake in the private company which supplies drive shafts and other equipment to heavy equipment makers such as Caterpillar Inc. Powertrain shifted its universal joint production and other manufacturing to Wanxiang in China.

"'We couldn't reduce our costs without Wanxiang,' says Thomas Corcoran, Powertrain's chief executive. They're an outstanding partner.'

"Those on the factory floor aren't so upbeat about the relationship. Powertrain workers, who average 50 years in age and $16 an hour, complain they can't hope to compete with low-cost Chinese labor. In the last three years, about one-third of the company's jobs have disappeared. Some components Powertrain gets from China deviate in size and are made with poor quality steel, according to Randy Whelchel, the Powertrain representative to the United Auto Workers union. 'Basically junk,' he says.

"Powertrain's Mr. Corcoran acknowledges 'some major quality issues' with Wanxiang products. But he says the Chinese company responded quickly by dispatching engineers and ironed out the problems."

In short, rather like the contents of a wan ton in a Chinese Dim Sum meal, the contents, though succulent, are not always familiar to Westerners.

W.K.

Pollution, Too, Grows and Gets Globalized

WE HAVE LONG QUESTIONED the consoling way of governments handling the growing problems of pollution. You simply squeeze the problem into a market format, organize a system of credits for firms who have cut their pollution of a given sort beyond the legal requirement, and presto you have a market solution! And when you have a market trading such credits, and enough profits made, that by definition *is* success. No further questions are asked. When you land in heaven I am sure you will not criticize the cooking, and likewise on earth when a fat enough profit is made, the supposedly perfect system is working. It is that simple. At once a whole corps of professional pollution traders springs up, dealing not only in actual pollution but in options on future pollution credits. Nobel prizes for economics are issued for those who set up the best model loaded with bogus mathematics, and nothing is left to do but to market the model.

Globalization — A Conveyor Belt of Blessings?

Frequently we expressed our doubts that you could find a useful measure for such exchange of polluting rights. For one thing a certain added unit of a given pollution could have a far more deadly effect on the population in an already heavily polluting area. But the latest news – a by-product of China's sensational wild and wooly industrial expansion paints a picture of the problem in far more disastrous terms. Rather than being cut up into tidy markets, the earth is a single biosphere. And it is already groaning under the stresses imposed on it. Evidence is at present flowing in of the disastrous results for the Western World of China's astonishing capitalist growth, on which we have come to depend for avoiding a deep economic recession.

The Wall Street Journal (17/12, "A Hidden Cost of China's Growth: Mercury Migration" by Matt Pottinger and Steve Steklow in Beijing and John J. Fialka in Washington):

"Conveyor Belt of Bad Air. On a recent hazy morning in eastern China, the Wuhu Shaoda power company revved up its production of electricity, burning a ton and a half of coal per minute to satisfy more than half the demand of Wuhu, an industrial city of two million people. AES Corp., an American energy company, owns 25% of the 250-megawatt facility, which local officials call an 'economically advanced enterprise.'

"The plant is outfitted with devices that prevent soot from billowing into the sky. But other pollutants, such as nitrogen oxides, sulfur dioxide and a gaseous form of mercury, swirl freely from the smokestacks. Rather than install more sophisticated and costly anti-pollution equipment, the plant, majority-owned by state-controlled entities, has chosen to pay an annual fee, which it estimates will be about $500,000 this year. That option meets Chinese standards, but wouldn't be allowed in the US. The airborne output of Chinese power plants like Wuhu Shaoda was once considered the price of China's economic growth, and a mostly local problem. But just as China's industrial might is integrating the country into the global economy, its pollution is also becoming a global concern. Among the biggest worries: the impact of China's vast and growing power industry, mostly fueled by coal, on the buildup of mercury in the world's water and food supply.

"Scientists long assumed mercury settled into the ground or water soon after it spewed forth as a gas from smoke stacks. But using satellites, airplanes and supercomputers, scientists are now tracking air pollution with unprecedented precision, discovering plumes of soot, ozone, sulfates and mercury that drift eastward across oceans and continents. Mercury and other pollutants from China's more than 2000 coal-fired power plants soar high in the atmosphere and around the globe on what has become a transcontinental conveyor belt of bad air. North America and Europe add their dirty loads. But Asia, pulsating with the economic growth of China and India, is the largest contributor.

"'We're all breathing each other's air,' says Daniel J. Jacob, a Harvard professor of atmospheric chemistry and one of the chief researchers in a recent multinational study of transcontinental air pollution. He traced a plume of dirty air from Asia to a point over New England, where samples revealed that chemicals in it had come from China.

"One reason China's power industry spews out so much pollution is that under the nation's rules, many plants have the option of paying the government annual fees rather than installing anti-pollution equipment."

That is a formula that calls for some contemplation. Given what passes for economic reasoning, it would seem a winner: it improves the budgetary performance of the country at the seemingly trifling cost of what official economists call an "externality." But, of course, that logic which confuses an idealized market with the economy cooks the books by such soothing nomenclature in many areas.

Poisons We Breathe and Eat

In the US the consequences are being detected not only in the air people breathe, but in the food they eat. The US Environmental Protection Agency recently reported that a third of the country's lakes and nearly a quarter of its rivers are now so polluted with mercury that children and pregnant women are ad-

vised to limit eating fish caught there. Warnings about mercury, a highly toxic metal used in things ranging from dental fillings to watch batteries, have been issued by 45 states and cover four of the five Great Lakes. Some scientists now say 30% or more of the mercury settling into the soil and waterways come from other countries – in particular, China.

"Officials in some countries are using the presence of pollution from abroad as an argument to do nothing at home,' says Klaus Toepfer, executive director of the United Nations Environment Program in Nairobi, Kenya.

"Yet global remedies – primarily treaties – are even harder to achieve. The last such initiative, the Kyoto Protocol, limiting emissions related to global warming, was rejected by the US, the largest contributor of such emissions – and doesn't apply to China, the second largest emitter. The best shot at a treaty for transcontinental pollution, Mr. Toepfer believes, would be to regulate a single pollutant that everyone agrees is hazardous. He recommends starting with mercury.

"China is already believed to be the world's largest source of non-natural emissions of mercury. Jozef Pacyna, director of the Center for Ecological Economics at the Norwegian Institute for Air Research, calculates that China, largely because of its coal combustion, spews 600 tons of mercury into the air each year, accounting for nearly a quarter of the world's non-natural emissions. And the volume is rising when American and European mercury pollution is dropping. Chinese power plants currently under construction – the majority fueled by coal – will alone have the capacity of more than twice the electricity-generating capacity of the UK."

Natural Sources

"EPA scientists estimate that a third of the mercury in the atmosphere gets there naturally. Traces of the silvery liquid in the earth's crust make their way into the sky through volcanic eruptions and evaporation from the earth's surface. It took the industrial age to turn mercury into a health concern. Mining, waste, incineration and coal combustion emit the metal in the form of an invisible gas. After it rains down and seeps into wetlands, rivers and lakes, microbes convert it into methylmercury, a compound that works its way up the food chain into fish and eventually people.

"The dangers of significant methylmercury exposure to the nervous system are well documented, particularly in fetuses and children. Permanent harm to children can range from subtle deficits in memory and attention span to mental retardation. In January, EPA scientists released research indicating that 630,000 US babies born during a 12-month period in 1999-2000 had potentially unsafe levels of mercury in their blood – about twice as many babies as previously estimated.

"China is phasing several measures to tackle air pollution. But soot plus sulfur dioxide and nitrogen oxides – often referred to as Sox and Nox – are understandably taking priority over mercury. Even with the existence of entire [mercury-]poisoned villages, other pollutants affect even more Chinese people. Airborne particulates are a suspected leading cause of respiration disease around the country. Acid rain from sulfur dioxide now pelts a third of China's territory, a ratio that is 'expanding not shrinking,' says Pan Yue, the deputy director of China's Environmental Protection Administration, or SEPA.

"Mr. Pan, an outspoken champion of stricter environmental standards, says there currently aren't any rules being drafted to address mercury. 'As for China's impact on surrounding countries,' he says, 'I'm first to admit the problem. But let's talk about this in the context of international fairness,' he says,' before firing rhetorical questions at Washington: 'Whose development model are we emulating? Who has been shifting all of its pollution-heavy factories to China? And who bears an even greater international responsibility than China – but has yet to shoulder it – on matters like greenhouse gas emissions?'"

W.K.

Municipalities to the Fore on the Internet

MUNICIPALITIES across the world have been getting the wrong end of the big stick. In a rapidly urbanizing, high-tech world much of the responsibility of running our society is being downloaded onto them, without the funds to pay for it. Thus *The Wall Street Journal* (7/12, "Economic Time Bomb: US Teens Are Among the Worst at Math" by June Kronholz) brings the shocking tidings that "the US ranks near the bottom of industrialized countries in [student] maths skills, ahead of only Portugal, Mexico and three other nations, according to a new international comparison. Economists say this is bad news for long-term economic growth.

"Two of the study's most unsettling findings: the percentage of top-achieving maths students in the nation is about half that of other industrialized countries, and the gap between scores of whites and minority groups – who will make up an increasing share of the labor force in coming decades – is enormous. The US ranked 24th among 29 countries that are members of the Organization for Economic Cooperation and Development, which sponsored the study. Using the OECD's adjusted average score of 500 points, the US scored 483 – 61 points behind top-scoring Finland and 51 points behind Japan. In a wider group that also included 10 non-members, many of them developing nations, the US tied Latvia for 27th place. The OECD study, called Program for International Student Assessment or PISA, also looked at reading and science skills, where US students scored slightly higher than in maths, and at general problem solving skills, where they scored close to the bottom. In science, US youngsters scored 491 points, in reading they scored 477, all using a 500 point average."

Neglected Contributing Factors

The important detail is that not only application, talent, and the standard of teaching enter as determinants of these results. Hardly less important will be the presence of the mother in the home or absent helping to earn the family's living, the cultural level and the quality of family relations, and access to cultural influences outside the schools.

Squeeze municipal budgets like a lemon to provide geopolitical statistics to keep Wall St. in a perky mood, and education and other social services take a beating. In the long run, of course, that does the finance markets no great good. A swarm of parasites too gluttonous of their victim's blood, may have a merry future, but hardly a lengthy one. That is the message carried by these indecent statistics: a country whose elite has taken upon itself to set the world aright by futuristic military means is not able to educate its young generation better than the tiny ex-Soviet republic of Latvia.

A complementary message from another angle comes from the *WSJ* (23/11, "Telecom Giants Oppose Cities On Web Access" by Jesse Drucker): "Dozens of cities and towns across the country are rushing to offer low-or no-cost wireless internet access to their residents, but the large phone and cable companies, fearful of losing a lucrative market, are fighting back by pushing states to pass legislation that could make it illegal for municipalities to offer the service."

When Corporations Block Increased Productivity

"Over the past few months, several big cities – including Philadelphia and San Francisco – have announced plans to cover every square block with wireless internet access via the popular technology known as Wi-Fi, short for wireless fidelity. Cities say these plans will spur economic development and help bridge the digital divide, making Web access nearly ubiquitous."

Ponder that expression "the digital divide" – it decides who may have access to vital skills for earning more than a pariah's living, or have enough information to know whom he is voting for, and who remains completely out of the loop. The importance of this for raising educational levels should be evident to the most obtuse free-market fanatic.

"But that is bad news for the large Bell telephone companies and cable operators, who are looking to their digital-subscriber-line (DSL) and cable-modem businesses for growth. Wi-Fi, technically known as 802.11, takes existing high-speed internet connections and wirelessly extends them by several hundred feet, allowing dozens or even hundreds of people to share one subscription."

That sounds to my ears like increased productivity that is supposed to keep the creaky market system "growing."

"Philadelphia announced during the summer that it would hook up the entire city with Wi-Fi. Its current Wi-Fi service is free, but it hasn't decided whether that would continue with wider deployment. 'There are some very specific goals that the city has that are not met by the private sector: affordable, universal access and the digital divide,' says Dianah Neff, the city's chief information officer. She says that less than 60% of the city's neighborhoods have broadband access.

"However, last week, after intensive lobbying by Verizon Communications Inc., the Pennsylvania General Assembly passed a bill that would make it illegal for any 'political subdivision' to provide to the public 'for compensation any telecommunications services, including advanced and broadband services within the service territory of a local exchange intercommunications company operating under a network modernization plan.' Verizon is the local exchange telecommunications company for most of Pennsylvania, and it is planning to modernize the region using high-speed fiber-optic cable. The bill has 10 days for the governor to sign or veto.

"The Pennsylvania bill follows similar legislative efforts earlier this year by telephone companies in Utah, Louisiana and Florida to prevent municipalities from offering telecommunications services which would include fiber and Wi-Fi.

"Critics denounce this legislative tactic, arguing that the US lags behind other countries in broadband internet access because the phone and cable companies have been able to roll out the service in some areas."

"'We should be encouraging our municipalities to take a major role in broadband, the way other countries are doing,' says James Baller, who represents local governments on telecommunications issues."

Are the Competing Services Really Equal?

"The telecom companies argue that it is unfair for them to have to compete against the government. They say that the legislation enables them to improve service to their customers by investing in their networks. If we put that money at risk and here comes the government to compete against us, with advantages that government has – not paying taxes, access to capital at good rates."

But are they really providing the same services? We assume that municipalities would provide internet services affordable to most families that would be less soaked with advertising, sex, violence.

Besides was it not a basic principle of anti-trust doctrine of the late last century that where a monopoly service is being provided, there should be a measure of government control to keep the private sector straight?

William Krehm

Use of Public Credit for Public Works Proposed in UK

"THAT THIS HOUSE is concerned by the conclusion of the report by the Association of Chartered Certified Accountants (ACCA) that private finance initiative is an expensive way of financing and delivering public services; urges the Treasury to commission an independent review of the benefits of using public credit and increasing the proportion of publicly created money as alternative means of financing public works; notes that the case for using public credit in this way is strengthened by the fact that, as measured by the proportion of publicly created money in circulation, public credit fell from 20 per cent of the money supply in 1964 to 3 per cent today; suggests, therefore, that an increase in the proportion of publicly created

money should be used to cut the costs of public investment and to boost the total amount of public spending without borrowing or taxation; considers that this can be done without any impact on inflation; and therefore urges the Chancellor to develop and use public credit rather than accumulating even more debt or enriching the private finance initiative and public private partnership contractors who are making vast profits from the Government's desire to provide alternatives to borrowing, even though this one is more expensive in the end."

To me this is VERY encouraging and I plan to organize a Forum event in the New Year to celebrate our "progress through persistency."

Meanwhile, do think about asking your MP to sign this important EDM 327 which you can find on edm.ais.co.uk/weblink/html/motion.html/ref=327. For real progress we need more than 29 signatures this year!

This most convenient way is via www.faxyourmp.com; i.e., you compose your text on-line which gets faxed to your MP.

With best wishes until 2005,
Sabine McNeill
Organizer, Forum for Stable Currencies
www.monies.cc
This is an initiative that our parliamentarians should be encouraged to imitate in Ottawa.

An Internal Flight from the Besieged US Dollar?

THERE WAS A TIME in the early 1990s when the message beamed out from most central banks and their private club, the Bank for International Settlements (BIS) in Switzerland, was clear and simple: there is no compromising with inflation. Instead of allowing even 1% or 2% of price increase as acceptable, that little shortfall from an utterly flat price level, if neglected, must end up in as runaway an inflation as the one that collapsed the German Reichsmark in 1923. To reach that "scientific conclusion" BIS brushed away a whole set of historical circumstances that led to a situation where Germans had to bring wheelbarrows of paper marks to the beer hall to buy a mug of tepid beer. They drank their beer tepid during that crisis, because if they waited for it to be cooled, the price might double or triple. There was a whole mess of history that had to be put out of sight to reach this conclusion. Germany had lost the First World War. The French had insisted on heavy reparations being imposed on her, and on receiving them in a strong currency which Germany was not allowed to earn by high tariffs. When the payments weren't made, the French and Belgian armies occupied Germany's industrial heartland, the Ruhr. A general strike supported by the whole German political spectrum broke out in response. Virtual civil war took over.

To claim that such runaway inflation would happen in any country that accepted a 1-2% rise in its price index is to imply that if interest rates had been pushed up to the dizzy levels that were being applied in the early 1990s to attain "zero inflation," there would, by retroactive miracle, have been no lost war, no reparations, no occupation of the Ruhr basin, no general strike and no civil war. All that is implied in flapping around propositions like pancakes.

But who would have imagined that within fifteen years many of the symptoms of an internal flight from the powerful US currency would be taking place in its homeland? Yet to get rid of history, it is not enough to ignore it. Do that, and that sharp-toothed beast is certain to exact a bloody revenge.

Listen to *The Wall Street Journal* (24/11, "In Tug-of-War on Stocks, Some Pull Away from US Market – Foreign Shares, Commodities Appeal to Skeptical Pros; A Bet on Illinois Farmland" by E.S. Browning): "Steven Leuthold has snapped up warehouses full of lead, copper and aluminum for the mutual fund he manages in Minneapolis.

"In Cleveland, investment adviser Tim Swanson is putting his wealthy clients' money into stocks in Indonesia, Poland and the Philippines.

"Ray Dalio in Westport, Conn., has been buying the Australian dollar, Swedish krona, Chinese yuan, gold and European bonds for his investment firm."

Some Prefer Farmland to the Once Almighty Dollar

"Most mainstream investors still believe that US stocks are the right place to put a big chunk of the American public's assets. These investors generally think stock prices will continue to post modest gains next year even if they can't match the big double-digit increases of the late 1990s.

"But in contrast to much of the 1990s, when US stocks were often perceived as the only game in town, a small but growing segment of professional investors is now weighing a wider range of choices. Some of the skeptics are betting against the US dollar by investing abroad. Others are buying gold, copper, lumber, even farmland." [In Germany in the doleful time mentioned above there was even an attempt to float a new currency with a real estate backing for no other possibility was in sight. It didn't work.]

Some are going into US bonds, despite tiny yields. "All these investments are putting pressure on stocks and creating a tug-of-war over the market's direction.

"It could be that these investors are outsmarting themselves. If the Bush administration's proposals for shifting Social Security money into stocks were adopted, that could spark a lasting stock-market rally. And some analysts may overestimate the average American investor's appetite for Hungarian stocks, aluminum and the like."

On the other hand, if climbing interest rates play havoc with the stock market, oops there could go another big chunk of US pension money leaving still further millions of Americans facing a beggarly old age.

"If stocks are going to resume the rally that sent the Dow Jones Industrial Average up more than 25% last year, they are going to have to overcome forces they didn't have to face in the 1990s – among them worries about the dollar, bullish feeling about oil and other commodities, and growing interest in developing countries.

"'In the next 10 or 15 years, I expect it to be like the 1970s in market dynamics,' says Edgar Peters, chief investment strategist at Pan Agora Asset Management, which manages $13 billion in Boston. 'We are going to have strong run-ups and then strong bear markets.' Stocks had trouble making lasting progress throughout the 1970s, and frustrated investors swung towards money funds, commodities and real estate. That's somewhat similar to what is happening today, although inflation, a big problem in the 1970s, remains quiescent.

"In less than three years the dollar has sagged 15% against the currencies of America's major trading partners. A lot of traders are betting that the trend will continue. A country with a mounting trade deficit such as the US is often tempted to weaken its currency to make its products more competitive in overseas markets. US Treasury Secretary John Snow has suggested he won't step in to try reversing the dollar's recent weakening.

"'The big collapse in the dollar is likely close, and speculators are starting to see the blood in the water,' warns Mr. Dalio's investment firm, Bridgewater Associates, which manages $92 billion for pension funds, endowments, foundations, and governments. Mr. Dalio who is 55 years old and founded Bridgewater in 1975, has a small position in US but is more active buying futures in the currencies of Japan, Australia, Canada, New Zealand, Switzerland, Sweden, Korea, Taiwan and even China. His hunch is that Japan and China will have to let their currencies rise against the dollar, although they are reluctant to do so for fear of damaging their own manufacturers. And as the dollar falls, he adds, he expects China to shift some of its foreign currency away from dollars and towards gold and European bonds – both areas in which he is investing more money.

"Andy Engel couldn't believe his ears. He and his colleagues at Leuthold Weeden Capital Management were sitting in a Minneapolis conference room, planning 2004 investments for their mutual fund, and his boss, Mr. Leuthold was suggesting industrial metals. Not stocks of companies that make metals, not futures, but millions of dollars worth of crates containing the lumpy products themselves. Mr. Leuthold had personally invested in commodities in the past, but his $600 million Leuthold Core Fund hadn't."

This signified a distrust of the complicated superstructure of financial ownership of production that in recent years had become the dominant force in the American world empire. To the point that a trust fund – an important arm of the financial empire – was making a decision to bypass it and load up with the actual material products that had been downgraded to the mere dice in the great game. And as though to make the point in a still more embarrassing way, the prospects of those crates of metals depended basically on how America's main emerging rival may overcome its own jungle of uncertainties and keep up its economic ascent.

"Chinese demand would help send metals' prices soaring, Mr. Leuthold explained. They could hold the crates for a few years and sell them as a big profit."

Providing of course, that the Chinese government could deal with its job-seeking displaced peasants flocking into the coastal cities. And it is a touch-and-go matter whether China's troubled banks can maintain the appearance of solvency. And supposing that they cannot, where does that leave Mr. Leuthold, and indeed the United States of America in its wilting grandeur?

Especially if it cannot shake itself loose from its commitment to military adventure across the globe.

"Mr. Engel, 45, recalled his early days in the business 20 years ago, when he was a Dean Witter stockbroker and the commodities brokers were kind of off in a back corner. They were viewed as a variety of crackpots.

"Not any more. His mutual fund wound up putting 7% of its money into the metals and cutting back its stock exposure. Aside from a fire in one of the aluminum warehouses, which necessitated sending cleaners in to wipe down the crates, the investment has been a lifesaver. The commodities are up 14% this year and without them the fund would probably show a loss for the year.

"'We do pay a custodial fee, and an insurance fee, but even with that it is attractive,' Mr. Engel says."

And yet the financial, abstract end of things remains the driver's seat, even though a leg or two of the chair may be wobbling: "Other investors are making bets on oil, which helps explain why its price has gone up sharply. In a world where big US stocks are trading at an above average 20 times corporate profits for the past year some think it better to bet on raw materials whose prices have long stagnated than on expensive stocks of the companies that use them. Mr. Dalio, who also is betting on commodities, has calculated that oil would have to go up to $120 a barrel before America's annual oil bill got back to the same share of economic activity as in the 1970s."

Just weeks ago that sort of reckoning had been left to the Saudis, Venezuelans and the Iraqis to worry about, while Wall St. indignantly protested about oil prices (unadjusted for inflation) had surpassed the record prices of the oil crunches during the 1970 decade. But now with all those barrels of oil they have in storage, Walls St. is coming to factor inflation into its musings.

All in all, it doesn't seem an ideal time for Washington to undertake imposing its version of free elections on the rest of the world by military adventures.

Other Alternatives

Nor do the surprises end there.

"Until this year, Cleveland banking group National City Corp. was pretty conventional with clients' money. It invested it in stocks and bonds.

"That has changed. Concerned that standard investments weren't going to generate enough gains, Mr. Swanson, who oversees investments at the bank's wealth-management division began looking for something with more pop. He didn't want commodities like copper or gold, because the insurance and upkeep fees could drain clients' holdings. He settled on developing countries. Bit by bit, he moved about 5% of client's money out of the US and other developed country stocks and into mutual funds that invested in the markets of developing countries in Asia, Eastern Europe and Latin America.

"Using mutual funds reduces the risk of a blowing up in any one country or stock." It also adds to the number of administrators who have to be looked after whatever the result of their ministrations. Note, too, that Asia and Latin America and Eastern Europe have been considered up to now the walking wounded, victimized by American banks and the IMF. And now they are seen as a refuge from the mighty US economy!

"Brett Gallagher, who helps manage $17 billion in New York for the Zurich financial group Julius Baer Holdings, has been fleeing US stocks and put 15% of his investments in developing country stocks. 'Our number one play would be Turkey,' he says. Other countries he likes include the Czech Republic, Hungary and Russia. He has more money in developed Europe and Japan together than in the US.

"Jim Brorson, who invests in stocks for a living for New York money manager Neuberger Berman from his office in Chicago, is keeping his money closer to home, Looking for ways to hedge stock holdings in his personal portfolio he bought farmland in Illinois. He happens to know an Illinois farmer willing to find the land and grow crops on it. The money manager figures the land has appreciated 7% a year in value, plus income off of it, and I get to go down there and kick dirt around which is better than sitting in front of a computer."

So every body is happy. But not quite.

"Perhaps the single biggest sign of skepticism about US stocks has been the surprising strength of the US bond market.

"Since the Federal Reserve began raising its target short-term interest rates at the end of June, US Treasury bonds actually have risen in price – an anomaly that few investors predicted. The Fed is expected to keep raising rates for months to come, gradually moving them up from 45-year lows. Rising rates are usually bad for bonds, because new bonds, with the higher rates, return more money than existing bonds. That causes the price of the older bonds to fall.

"So why have Treasury bond prices been so resilient? One answer is that Japan and China have been buying dollar-denominated bonds in an effort to keep the dollar from falling against Asian currencies." It was just such an agenda – allowing our stressed banks to load up with bonds without putting up money of their own with ever higher rates, that almost brought down the international financial system in 1994. It folded the Mexican banking system and moved on to produce financial havoc in East Asia and Russia. And now the world is risking a similar disaster on an even greater scale in pursuit of another such agenda – the reluctance of Japan and China to reduce their currencies so that they can continue to compete the pants off the United States. Buying US bonds has the effect of supporting the US dollar and retaining low competitive prices for the yuan and the yen, despite the pressures from Washington to push them higher.

The article continues: "And some American investors are leaning towards bonds because they remain nervous about US stocks after the post-bubble bear market, although buying bonds won't protect the investors against any future fall in the dollar."

On this tangled skein of conflicting agendas depends the future of a planet where the talk is of increased transparency.

William Krehm

What the Tsunami Teaches Us

AS WE RIP UP the 2004 calendar we face the world in a state of confusion and dilemma. We are locked in a blind faith in those in power and in the pap they feed us.

Listen to *The Wall Street Journal* (3/01, "For 2005, Rising expectations" by E.S. Browning): "As the 2005 trading year opens, the anomaly of rising rates and rising stocks has begun to spark concern and debate in the investment community. Either the rules have changed, people are saying, or stocks are overdue to decline.

"Seasoned investors tend to wince whenever someone tells them that things are different this time. But at least as far as the recent Fed rate increases go, a surprising number of old hands think this is a special case: inflation simply isn't serious enough, they say, to force the kind of sharp Fed rate increases that markets fear.

"In a typical business cycle, the Fed steps in because the economy is accelerating and inflation is beginning to rear its head. The Fed sends rates sharply upward in an effort to force the economy to slow by boosting borrowing costs. As businesses pay more for their money, profits suffer. Consumers get hit with higher costs, too; mortgage rates rise and people stop buying new houses and cars. The stock market tanks."

Let us stop right there to note that the analysts – though a breed obsessed with number – have lost the power to distinguish between the singular and the plural, certainly the very root of the number concept.

Our Teeter-tottering Economies

For there is no longer – even to the extent that there ever was – a single economy. Today in many ways, at home and abroad, it is sliced into contrasting fragments, seated on opposite sides of giant teeter-totters. One side rises not only *as* but *because* the other drops. The same *Wall Street Journal* has kept us well informed about the outsourcing of an increasing portion of the actual production of the West to countries of abysmally lower wage and living standards. This began in relatively unskilled manufacturing processes to backward countries in Latin America and then rapidly began scaling the technological ladder in China and India. In many industries there it is moving from actual physical production to call-centers, engineering, planning, and even working out business strategies for American corporations. This results not only in deflationary price trends in many economic lines in the countries of the first world, but at the same time in a patchy financial boom reflecting the incorporation into the growth rate of current stock prices growth rates already attained and more particularly of such growth rates into today's *financial* prices. Securities and detached aspects of security prices – say the current growth rate, real or contrived, serve as collateral for more credit creation. What results is a growing inflation of the financial sector at the same time as there is a considerable deflation in many lines of physical production. There is no way of accommodating these two clashing dichotomies under a single diagnostic term. Indeed, it is deflation of the real economy that feeds the illusion that the economy is inflation-free and permits the over-confident to treat the future itself as a bankable asset.

Obviously this ultimately involves a dangerous flirtation with infinity – the very mathematics of the atom bomb. All the constraints of society and the environment that interfere with this game are simply declared "externalities," a fancy word for putting them out of mind. These barriers to unlimited growth incorporated in current prices and valuation of collateral have to do with forces that are within human power to deal with by imposing social controls. The recent tsunamis with their incredible destruction of human lives ought to serve as a reminder, that beyond forces within human power to control, there are those almost wholly beyond such regulation. At best human societies could limit their exposure to such natural disasters, and devise what limited means of foretelling them may be possible. Place limitations on globalization, on pushing urbanization to its ultimate limits. Leave areas of ready refuge to which humans may retreat in the event of natural catastrophes. But that almost certainly would require limits to the blind expansion of human societies' rates of profit within their economies as narrowly defined at present.

At the moment the public's attention is almost wholly absorbed by coping with the victims of the disaster, dead and living. But already a trickle of information on what might have been done throughout the Pacific and the Indian Oceans to establish early warnings systems, and preserving natural defences. Thus *The Globe and Mail* (06/01, "Did deforestation add to tragedy?" by John Vidal, London) informs us: "As the full damage is assessed, there is growing consensus among scientists, environmentalists and Asian communities that the impact of last week's tsunamis was considerably worsened by tourist, shrimp farm and other industrial development that destroyed or degraded mangrove forest and other defences against the sea.

"Reports from India, Sri Lanka, Indonesia and Malaysia suggest the worst damage is in places with no natural protection from the sea, and that communities living behind intact mangrove forests, in particularly, were largely spared. According to leading Indian agricultural scientist M.S. Swaminathan, chairman of a government inquiry into cultural developments, 'the mangrove forests in Tamil Nadu's Pitchavaram and Muthupet regions acted as a shield and bore the brunt of the tsunamis. But in other areas, such as Alappuzha and Kollam, where forest had been cut down and there is sand mining and developments, the devastation is more widespread. The dense mangrove forests stood like a wall to save coastal communities living behind them,' he said.

"While most Asian countries have strong environmental protection laws governing coastal development and coastal forests, these were widely ignored by the powerful tourist and aquacultural industries, which rapidly encroached onto beaches and cleared inter-tidal areas to provide better views, wider beaches or the brackish water in which shrimp and prawns thrive."

As with Fossil Fuel so with Beaches

"'The full fury and wrath of the waves were felt in areas where nature's green belts of coral reefs and mangroves no longer exist or were never present in the first place,' said a spokesman for Walhi, Indonesia's leading environmental group.

"'The US-based Mangrove Action Project, a network of 400 non-governmental agencies and more than 250 scientists and academics in 60 countries, said such areas may be disappearing even faster than rain forests. Vast tracts have been cleared in the past 20 years in India, Thailand, Bangladesh and Indonesia,' a spokesman for the project said. Mangroves once covered as much as 75% of the coastlines of tropical and sub-tropical countries, but less than 50% remain today. And of this remaining forest, more than half is degraded." (Guardian Service News.)

There are in fact no externalities – neither within and beyond human control. The very idea of a self-balancing market must be expunged. The obscene notion of using interest rates of any sort as the "sole blunt tool" for regulating the allegedly self-balancing market has helped excavate bloody trenches between the Islamic and Western societies. It is a needless provocation to a religion that holds that the very institution of risk-free interest – other than the bankruptcy of the debtor – is a sin calling for eternal hell fire. The recent tsunamis with their incredible loss of human life show that we cannot afford to indulge in such deadly games of blocking human foresight to further the scope of human greed. It is time for checking the credentials of *a priori* certainties.

William Krehm

A Disturbing Parallel between Nortel's Accountancy and That of our Government

T HE GHOST of the once great Nortel, for decades the high-tech flagship of Canada, seems ever with us. At one time that company accounted for fully a third of the value listed on the Toronto Stock Exchange. Accountants, most incredibly, seem to have contributed to rather than prevented Nortel's epic disasters. So great was their complicity in Nortel's that it added up to a corporative culture rather than an occasional lapse into white-collar delinquency. It was as though Canada, in our view a demurely decent land, had chosen a pirate vessel for its flagship. And considering the losses inflicted on so

many of its shareholders, the number of hopeful loyalists the stock still commands is amazing. From a price of $124.50 at the peak of the high-tech boom it dropped to less than a dollar. Currently it sells at the $4 level, to ready takers. The headline in the stock market section of *FP Investing* (12/01, "Nortel Gains Help Cushion Falling Index") bears out the dictum of the great Barnum: "One is born every minute."

The Peril of Dating

By now Nortel has parted with two thirds of its staff, and has been the subject of a further board shakeup as a result of a review by a Washington law firm Cutler Wilmer Pickering and Dorr LLP. But that review stopped notably short of implicating the corporation's auditors, Deloitte Touche LLP. Yet former executives are quoted stating that the questionable accounting practices, were not only a major ingredient of the puffery of its stock prices, but made possible bonuses delivered by virtue of fictitious improved earnings. Accountancy as practised in this world-rank corporation under successive CEOs seems less an attempt to understand its inner workings than a conveyor belt to delay essential bookkeeping corrections to make possible the vesting and cashing-in of options by the commanding brass.

A key feature of such bookkeeping has to do with the handling of capital losses in the valuation of the corporation's equipment. Frequent excessive provisions for such losses were taken. That excess was corrected, but not transferred to the company balance sheet until the alleged improvement in operational results would become useful in vesting options already issued to high executives so that they could be sold at a profit.

Yet *The Globe and Mail* (13/01, "This Stock Still Holds Power Over Investors" by Simon Tuck) informs us that Marilyn Schaffer-Francis, who had worked at Nortel almost fifteen years ago and is now an independent communications consultant confesses to a "tough-to-define attachment to the communications equipment maker that goes far beyond any analysis of the company's financial prospects. Not only has she invested another ten thousand dollars [despite her previous losses on the stock] but says her confidence in the Brampton, Ontario-based company is rooted not in patriotism but in a belief that Canadian companies tend to be better governed and more ethical." That indeed is a big mouthful when one considers how many successive CEOs appeared to have taken the same shortcuts to fortune and fame of sorts that their predecessors had been guilty of.

In an adjoining article in the same issue of the *G&M* ("How a cookie jar crumbled? Check the provisions" by Janet McFarland) we read: "An independent review commissioned by the board of Nortel Networks Corp. offers a lesson in the mechanics of so-called "cookie jar accountancy." Prepared by Washington law firm Wilmer Cutler Pickering Hale and Dorr, it outlines how senior management used excess liability provisions on Nortel's balance sheet to manipulate [the timing of] profits in the first two quarters of 2003.

"Experts say the accounting principles are simple, even if the painstaking review at Nortel required sifting through a complex array of small transactions that ultimately added up to large numbers.

"University of Toronto accounting professor Leonard Brooks says it is not unusual for companies to take provisions if they discover that their assets are overvalued on their balance sheets or liabilities are understated. In either case, a company not only adjusts its balance sheet, where assets and liabilities are recorded, [but] must also simultaneously recognize a new cost on its income statement. Prof. Brooks says the concept is that value that once existed has been eroded.

"The value you have lost is no longer an asset; it has to be expensed on your income statement."

In some cases companies take enormous provisions in one quarter because of a desire to clean up the balance sheet as a result of a dramatic business downturn. Some accountants refer to this as "big bath" accounting, because companies report an enormous loss in a single year.

Big Bath Accountancy

"But big baths risk becoming controversial later, when companies decide their previous provisions went too far. The company revealed Tuesday that its senior managers learned in August 2002, that they had $303 million (US) excess of balance sheet provisions [i.e., in apparent capital losses]. But instead of immediately correcting the financial statements, management chose to wait and use portions of the gains in the first two quarters of 2003.

"While there is nothing wrong with reversing [such] provisions, Prof. Brooks says companies are not allowed to use provisions as a large cookie jar to reach into from time to time to strategically shift profits to preferred quarters [i.e., to quarters when they would become profitable to them because of the vesting of outstanding options or other such arrangements].

"'To present fairly the financial affairs of the company, you need to immediately recognize [such] corrections,' he said. 'If you don't do that, it leads to misrepresentation of the net income. And that can be termed 'income smoothing,' or ' cookie jar accounting,' which is manipulative."

It remains only to point out that the existing globalized and deregulated economic system is to a large extent based on similarly spurious pricing and capitalization. Any real or imagined rate of profit growth gets extrapolated to the remotest future and its alleged present value gets incorporated into the current market price of the stock. Once such valuations have been adopted, a shortfall of the growth in the rate of profitability is penalized by the market in collapse of share values. And since such shares usually serve as collateral for further financing, and credit lines often depend on the market value of the shares and/ or the maintenance of the rate of value growth already attained, considerations of survival frequently leave little elbow room for much morality.

Such accountancy cosmetics can have unpleasant consequences for shareholders who may have been led to buy the shares because of the growth of operating profit incorrectly reported. It may even result in corporation mergers and in general to start wheels spinning that might have more properly been braked if the correct profit picture had been reported. That underlies the perils of concentrating on growth rates rather than on modest but sustainable profits.

There is another neglected aspect to the Nortel phenomenon. Canada's government, as well of those of most of our provinces are in a poor position to cast the first stone at corporations for such cookie jar accountancy.

Where our PM Resembles Nortel

For what the successive Nortel managements were up to is basically very similar to what Prime Minister Paul Martin practised in the name "prudent financial policy" during his years as Finance Minister in the Chrétien cabinet. He hid a few billion dollars in his forecasts of the budgetary results for the year in progress, and then when the results were totted up he trotted out a few billion dollars that he had left out in his forecasts, and proclaimed the result as proof of his prudent management. Meanwhile, the hidden excess of taxes collected "to balance the budget" served to slash social and other essential programs with the plea "Where is the money coming from?," when he himself knew where the unacknowledged revenue was hidden.

Meanwhile the game was not without its costs to Canadian society. Having prolonged the policy of allowing the chartered banks to load up with federal debt introduced by the previous Conservative regime as a means of bailing the banks out of their gambling losses, the deficits or lower surpluses forecast made the resulting dependence on the bond-rating agencies all the more costly, since the bonds marketed through the banks had to show a larger yield. Obviously this was incompatible with the most elementary principles of democracy as well as those of accountancy. The Magna Charta wrested by the Barons from King John at Runneymede had to do with Parliament's knowledge and approval of what taxes were being raised and spent. Our problem is that our current barons have crossed over to side with bad King John.

But there is yet a further dimension of misrepresentation – by far the most serious – in the way our federal government keeps its books. The previous Auditor General, Denis Desautels, in the late 1990s refused to give unconditional approval to two successive balance sheets of the federal government unless it brought in accrual accountancy (also known as "capital budgeting"). When a private corporation acquires a building, builds a bridge, or acquires a machine it depreciates the investment over its useful life. Our federal government and most of our provinces write off such investments in a single year and then carry the asset at a token value of a single dollar. However, the debt incurred by the acquisition is shown at its true outstanding value. Obviously this exaggerated the debt, no small detail at a time when the government to bail out our banks in 1992 from their gambling losses in areas incompatible with banking, shifted some 15% of its outstanding debt to them from the Bank of Canada, where as sole shareholder since 1938, it enjoyed virtual interest-free loans. Moreover, the early 1990s when this shift took place, were a time when the Bank of Canada under John Crow drove interest rates into the skies. Most of our $510 billion dollar debt was run up from those high rates and the end of statutory reserves that along with the *Risk-Based Capital Requirement* guidelines of the Bank for International Settlements had made it possible for the chartered banks to quadruple their holdings of federal bonds without putting up any of their own money.

Moreover, there was still a further costly consequence of the bum accountancy of our federal and most of our provincial governments. If you carry valuable assets at a token dollar, you can privatize them at say 10% of their real value and apply the proceeds of their sale to reducing the debt. The last election both in the US and Canada were run on that misleading promise of reducing the national debt. Whichever well-connected entrepreneur picks up such a bargain, can take it public, screw up user fees and make a killing. That was done federally with the CNR, and provincially with the toll highway 407 which was already built and the original buyers from the Ontario government resold it to a Spanish-led syndicate that raised tolls several hundred percent. It was done with Ontario Hydro. That sort of thing is today one of the supreme rackets that afflict the land.

All these scams make the sponsorship scandal in Quebec appear minor sport, but receive little publicity. Yet the pattern of Nortel and its weirdo books has been applied on a far grander scale both in Ottawa and in many a provincial capital.

Space limitations prevent a fuller account of the bailout of our banks in the latter 1980s and the early 1990s. I will give brief references for further details of the complex accountancy distortions the shift of power from the general economy to the speculative financial sector that these led to and where further information can be found.

But even with this disclosure, we still have not come to the greatest instance of cookie jar accountancy practised by our governments. For example, the value of the physical investments of the federal government written down to a single dollar after year one (except those who are set up as Crown corporations which do use serious accountancy). This bases their argument on spurious net debt – with physical capital assets of government marked down to a single token dollar after year one, It is true that after weeks of pretty harsh argument with the then Auditor General, Finance Minister Martin agreed to adopt in principle accrual accountancy. But the compromise was reached in virtual stealth and the initial phasing in was confined to obligations to aboriginal peoples and to our obligations under the Kyoto agreement.

In last year's election campaign instead of emphasizing the significance of the agreement in principle to bring in accrual accountancy, Mr. Martin was agreeing to pay off half of the existing debt with government surpluses. The fact is that by the time we brought in accrual accountancy and recognized the vast physical capital investments of our governments, our net debt would already be reduced by far more than half of the present figure. And if we extended accrual accountancy to our investments in human capital there would certainly be no net debt at all but a surplus of investment. In the 1960s based on a study of the surprisingly rapid recovery of Germany and Japan from the wartime physical destruction, economists came to recognize investment in human capital as the most productive of all investments. The remaining problem once capital budgetting were brought in would be one of liquidity not of threatening insolvency. And any shortfall in liquidity that might remain could readily be financed through the Bank of Canada on a virtual interest-free basis. That was the original purpose of its founding in the first place. A net debt-free government would have a superb credit rating especially since it owns the central bank.

There is this about investment in human capital – education, health, and social services. Rather than being depreciated, its effectiveness to a large extent gets handed down intact or even with increase from generation to generation. The offspring of healthy, educated parents, tend to be more receptive to education, and healthier than families of uneducated, sickly, impoverished parents. Scrounging on schools and hospitals is not prudent governance. What you save in the proper maintenance of schools and their programs gets spent in building additional penitentiaries and manning them. The extent to which such relationships, escape our governments today is positively Nortelian.

William Krehm

Mayor — Senator — President: "Senate Document 23"

AFTER FOUR OR MORE YEARS of attending to discussions of monetary reform the deepest impression it has left in me is its invisibility to mainstream public policy debate. Major parties seem unconscious of it, smaller parties of dissent focus their indignation on taxation and spending policy. Standard economics literature hardly recognizes the paramount authors of dissenting works on the money and financial system. Many economists appear to go about their work as if the monetary system can be taken for granted, permitting them to use money magnitudes as a convenient and reliable measuring device without paying much attention to the system itself. The reformist issue of who should control monetary policy is not even on the table in university courses in political science (public policy and administration), and economists specialized to money do not seem to find reformers sufficiently provocative to take the time to smite their impudence and ignorance. Money reformers are prone to interpret this silence (indifference?) as conspiracy, and so go deeply into dark and sinister explanations. More sanguine observers, like J.K. Galbraith, offer the tongue-in-cheek interpretation that actors and analysts of the system are perpetrators of "innocent fraud." Part of the problem seems to be an uncertainty among reformers themselves as to how they believe the system should be reformed, and in what direction. The straightforward assertion by such as G.G. McGeer that governments should be in control makes others recoil with shudders and accusations of "fascism" (as noted in January *ER*). Sometimes the issue seems to be as simple as who can be trusted. McGeer (and Galbraith) believe in public servants; Milton Friedman does not (as reported in the book by J. Bakan that I reviewed in September *ER*).

In an age when everything seems to require the expertise of a specialist, it is not only tempting to leave economic policy to the experts but also to wonder just how esoteric money and the financial system actually are or need to be. Governments of today seem to recognize that economies have become "financialized" to the extent that citizens need greater sophistication in the subject in order to survive and so are promoting financial education as an instrument of social security. One is led to wonder who will be in charge of curriculum, and if economic reform literature will find a place in it? And how does one recognize an expert–or more important, distinguish a true expert from a mere specialist? Are bankers the only people who can understand money? Are we safe in leaving monetary management up to the government? Or is government really in charge of money management? Does it matter, after all? Is money just there, "like the earth's crust and the forest primeval"?

Forgotten Prophets

These questions occur to me especially in respect of Robert L. Owen, United States Senator for Oklahoma from its statehood in 1907 until 1925. (The Carl Albert Center at the University of Oklahoma provides a web site with information about Owen and a description of his papers and memorabilia in their collection.) As a young lawyer and banker he experienced and analyzed monetary standards and banking institutions throughout the era of bimetallism, fiat money, heterogeneous banking laws and periodic financial panics that followed on the Civil War. Early in his Senate career he became Chairman of the Banking and Finance Committee and made extensive study of banking institutions in other countries (as part of the major review of the US money system mandated by the *Aldrich-Vreeland Act* of 1908).

From that background, he drafted the initial version of legislation that in 1913 inaugurated Federal Reserve System. His co-sponsor in the House of representatives was Carter Glass. As passed by the House, the legislation left out a provision in the Senate version for assuring the adequacy (sufficiency) of money supply by making monetary policy subject to the wishes of Congress. The Senate tried to put it back in, but the House refused (led by Glass in opposition it seems). Owen appears to have spent the rest of his life calling attention to the defect and to campaigning for its rectification – supported by die-hards like Wright Patman.

When the Depression struck, he was first off the mark in identifying the source of the problem as a contraction of demand deposits. (This was documented in later years by Milton Friedman as *The Great Contraction*.) Although retired from the Senate in 1925, he came back to explain how the defect in Fed legislation had led to the crisis and how it should be rectified. He was called to give testimony before committees of the House and Senate seven times during the 72nd, 73rd, 74th, and 75th Congresses. During that period he had published two books, *Sound, Safe, Sane Money* in 1933 and *Stabilized Dollars–Permanent Prosperity* in 1937. These were both out of print by late 1938, but he had prepared a new one. An item from the Carl Albert Center site mentions a discussion, or possibly a vote, on a *Federal Reserve Act* amendment on January 4 of 1939.

This suggests that Owen's argument was featured in that debate and doubtless circulated among the legislators. One of Owen's allies in banking reform was Marvel Mills Logan of Kentucky who, as a sitting Senator "presented" the draft copy of Owen's new book on "legislative day, Jan. 17, 1939" and it was "Ordered to be printed with illustrations." It is a hardbound book of 108 pages, produced by the United States Government Printing Office and identified as Senate Document 23, 76th Congress, 1st Session, 1939, bearing the title *National Economy and the Banking System of the United States: An Exposition of the Principles of Modern Monetary Science*. (Words in quotation marks appear on the title page.)

From these details it seems that Owen exercised some significant influence in US money and banking issues from before the *Federal Reserve Act* until 1939 at the latest–a period of almost thirty years. As noted in *ER* of May 2004 his book is an impressive argument for "modern monetary science" and "stable money." And he appears to have been speaking with the consent and implied support of leading businessmen of his time, for he described a movement in the 1930s in the US and other English speaking countries identified as the "Stable Money Association...under the leadership of some of the greatest leaders in finance and industry." (See May *ER* for examples.) His list of "Noted Members..." numbers about a hundred, and about half of the total are identified as bank executives. With this kind of experience, influence and profile one might expect that Owen's name would have some presence in literature of the subject. Not much! Carter Glass appears fairly often, but perusal of several textbooks and collections of readings on money and banking policy published since 1950 yields only one reference to Owen. That is a footnote in Friedman and Schwartz, *The Great Contraction*. (They cite his testimony before the House Banking and Currency Committee in 1932.)

The main theme in his book is that the *Federal Reserve Act* as finally passed in 1913 omitted key provisions of the Senate version that would have left ultimate responsibility for monetary policy in the hands of Congress. Owen was critical of Fed behavior in the Depression for not even using the tools it did have to their full potential, and pointed out that if his (the Senate's) draft had become law, Congress would have had the authority to require expansionary rather than contractionary policies. Well into in his eighties by that time, he was taking a very active role in trying to effect change and seems to have had a sense that his message was getting through. On the last page of his main text he expresses belief that a majority of the House in the 75th Congress "were in favor of congressional control and regulation of the volume and value of money. The matter is being debated on the hustings throughout the United States.... Study clubs throughout the country are giving attention to this matter." The reading lists posted to monetary reform sites for Internet access today provide ample manifestations of that grassroots activity, for much of the literature attests that it was prepared for the express purpose of those study clubs of the thirties and early forties.

An Effective One-man Reform Movement

Owen's own relative invisibility as a monetary thinker is not exactly shared by his book, for "Senate Document 23" enjoys fame as the expression of "Lincoln's Monetary Policy." This is due to Owen's endorsement of a policy attributed to Lincoln by the flamboyant Mayor of Vancouver, Gerald McGeer (who by the time of Owen's writing was a Member of Parliament in Ottawa). Owen delivered his own opinion of Lincoln, on page 67 of his book, saying that "Lincoln thoroughly understood the constitutional right of Congress to exclusively create money and to regulate the value thereof." He goes on to say "an abstract of his [Lincoln's] views is given by McGeer in Conquest of Poverty. The views of Lincoln are of surpassing importance. McGeer's abstract will be found in the appendix." That affirmation by a senior statesman and practitioner of monetary policy lends credibility to McGeer not only as an interpreter of Lincoln. It also situates his brief to labor unions and governments (described in January's *ER*) in the mainstream of money and banking reform thinking of his time. The Lincoln policy abstract is not found in that 1933 document, however, but in a later book for which McGeer extended the title as well as the content. *The Conquest of Poverty, Or Money, Humanity and Christianity* was published in 1935 and is ten times as long as the pamphlet (359 to 36 pages). An important distinction of style is the straightforwardly fanciful character of the book. The Foreword is subtitled "The Spirit of Lincoln." There is a substantial expansion of the arguments made in the pamphlet, but the emphasis in the book is on Lincoln, Roosevelt (FDR) and Jesus. His biographers note that McGeer had a thousand books in his den, and that about half of them were about Lincoln, "his boyhood hero." He was also convinced that both Lincoln and Jesus were executed by the money changers and usurers that they each had challenged. A lot of the text is a fanciful exchange between Roosevelt and Lincoln, as the sitting president solicits advice from a predecessor who had faced similar crises. In a chapter that focuses on Lincoln in particular McGeer frankly acknowledges the interpretive nature of his treatise by saying that if Lincoln could speak today "he would probably say...." Then follow ten pages of text, building to the climax with this sentence: "Let us now, from his speeches and his messages to Congress, summarize the monetary policy that Lincoln, at the time of his assassination, was about to more clearly define and establish." Then we get the words that have spread widely as "Lincoln's Monetary Policy." They are on pages 186-7 in McGeer's book and reproduced on page 91 of Owen's "Senate document 23."

Although McGeer was completely frank in acknowledging that he was putting words in Lincoln's mouth and Owen was fully aware that he was endorsing an interpretive opinion, their combined effect was a degree of ambiguity that has given free play to conspiratorial imaginations. For at the end of the "abstract," Owen added this: (The above is an abstract of Lincoln's monetary policy from Mayor McGeer's Conquest of Poverty and has been certified as correct by the Legislative Reference Service of the Library of Congress at the instance of Hon. Kent Keller, Member of the House of Representatives.) The obvious meaning is that since he was no longer entitled to call on the L.R.S. to check his transcription, he got a sitting Congressman to ask for it on his behalf. Careless (or mischievous) conspiracy buffs and reform zealots have represented this scrupulous acknowledgment as evidence that the Legislative Reference Service affirmed that McGeer had himself copied Lincoln's own words, verbatim, and they then imply that McGeer's abstract is the content of *Lincoln's* Senate Document 23. (A notable recent victim being Rowbotham in 1998, *The Grip of Death*) McGeer and his publisher share some culpability in subsequent confusion, for as the host of one website about presidential assassinations pointed out to me, McGeer seems to be claiming that they were indeed Lincoln's words as collected from scattered speeches and messages to Congress, for he precedes them with quote marks but gives no end quotes. That complaint is somewhat justifiable (although not to a careful reader), and a Government Documents Librarian (Robin Hutchinson, St. Lawrence University in Canton, NY) commented to me that McGeer's use of quotation marks is a kind of license that would not be acceptable practice by publishers today, for it does give the appearance of being a direct quotation. (The identity of McGeer's publisher raises an interesting ancillary topic.)

Owen and McGeer died within a few weeks of each other in 1947. McGeer was only 59 and still in full harness. Owen, however, was 91, meaning that he had lived though the Civil War, Lincoln's assassination, the financial sleaze of reconstruction and the gilded age, as well as the Great War and the Great Depression. The "Stable Money" movement he and McGeer represent is not a phenomenon that can be dismissed simply as the theory of a few dissident cranks. Its invisibility in mainstream literature of the past half century therefore suggests questions. Those bankers, industrialists and merchants (not to mention farmers) really were battered by fluctuations in the general price level and they wanted it flattened. But was their concern for *stable* money the same issue that exercises money reformers of our own time? Might central bankers of our own time interpret their contemporary focus on inflation fighting as the triumph of that former movement and therefore as justified by it?

Keith Wilde

PART 2 OF A REVIEW OF A BOOK BY STEPHEN ZARLENGA, AMERICAN MONETARY INSTITUTE, NY

"The Lost Science of Money: The Mythology of Money — The Story of Power"

First published in German translation as Der Mythos von Geld – die Geschichte der Macht, *this first English edition is updated and expanded.*

IN THE FIRST INSTALMENT of this review, I left the reader at the plunder of Constantinople by the Fourth Crusade. That unleashed the gold and silver stocks uselessly hoarded over the centuries in that great quasi-heir to the Roman Empire. I rounded out the piece by noting Zarlenga's masterly summation of both the losses to humanity of the classical treasures accumulated there, and the enormous impetus that the restoration to circulation of so much precious metal was to give to Europe's Renaissance. In a sense it was a dress rehearsal for the conquest of America by the Spaniards that added up to an even vastly greater, more destructive pillage that cleared the way for capitalism and the industrial revolution.

In his Chapter 6 on "Renaissance Struggles for Monetary Supremacy: Zarlenga takes up the threads of his great tale with a closer look at the developing relationship between cities and countryside. This adds depth to his monetary analysis, even though he has not by any means exhausted this neglected historical vein. But let us glimpse at the significant use he does make of the researches of economic historians, especially the Belgian Henri Pirenne. In the later stages of the Roman Empire, the great manors – generally owned by the Church and managed by their *condottieri* – became self-sufficient. A crucial factor in this was the conquest of the Mediterranean lines of communication with the Near East and North Africa by Islam. The Church held the monopoly on literacy, accounting, capital, and management techniques, on which Princes depended.

"Around 1200 the local customs of the towns that sprang up at the centers of these estates became institutionalized by law. One law – 'Stadtluft macht frei' (city air liberates) – gave freedom to escapee slaves from the manors after their having lived in a town for a year and a day. Except for parts of Flanders and Tuscany, towns generally held less than one-tenth of the population and each town's constitution applied only within its walls. Pirenne writes, 'For burghers the country population existed only for exploitation.'" What a cluster of astoundingly transforming institutions for economists to ignore!

"Merchants continued to invest their superabundant reserves in land. In the course of the 12th and 13th centuries they acquired most of the ground in the towns. The steady rise in population by converting town land into building sites sent up their rents to such an extent that from the 2nd half of the 13th century many of them gave up trade and became rentiers.

"Within the towns labor became more specialized and efficient. Capital cities grew up around the Monarch's residence as lesser nobles built residences nearby."

In short, we are brought into the great revolution of urbanization which goes on crescendoing to this day. The ignored implications of this urbanization on price theory – and hence on monetary theory – are vast. As urbanization continues on a mounting scale, it brings a second factor into the price level – life in a great city is more costly in part because of the immensely costlier infrastructures required. On the other hand only in large towns is it possible for liberating ideas and practices to be nurtured. But the price of such urbanization has been almost wholly ignored by economists. The resulting upward price gradient favored the entrepreneur and hence sped the wheels of development. Zarlenga grasps some of these factors. Almost 40 years ago I developed the notion of the *social lien* – a growing stratum of the price level that cannot be attributed to a growing surplus of aggregate demand over supply, or to the greater direct costs of production by the private sector. Rather it is the result of the indirect costs of the human and material investment of a government sector necessarily expanding within the economy and filtering into the price level through taxation on both consumers and producers.[1] Ignoring that and persisting in the search for equilibrium points – identified with a flat price level – as the one concern of official monetary theory has thrown up a wall of obtuseness that favours interests of those who stand to profit from such dogma. That has been so powerful a distorting factor in official economic thought that it can qualify as a twin to the "lost science" that Zarlenga has concentrated on. They intermingle to support a costly monetarist tyranny.

The Trade Fairs

"The principal method of promoting trade were the great trade fairs sponsored by the territorial princes from the 11th century on. These were held at particular places annually or quarterly. The importance of the fair did not depend on the importance of the town where it was held. The greatest fair was at Champagne, sponsored by the Comte de Champagne, an early member of the Knights Templar organization. The fairs were a 'free trade zone.' Taxes were waived, disputes arising outside the fair were set aside, regulations on trading were lifted and merchants were attracted from afar with their gold and silver coins.

"The main monetary feature of these events were payment-clearing mechanisms where merchants' purchases and sales were matched and accounts settled at the end of the fair. If a merchant sold more than he bought, he would receive the difference in coinage. If he purchased more than he sold, vice versa. If his credit were good, he could extend the debt to the next fair.

"At later fairs the clearance mechanism often had reciprocating arrangements with those of other fairs. Bills of exchange and finance bills were payable at fair times. *The fair at Champagne even issued its own token currency.* The fairs reached their height around 1250-1300. Their importance was reduced after bill-clearing mechanisms were set up in money center towns. Finally cities like Antwerp became free trade zones, or perpetual fairs.

"In this period military service became a profession and in the 1400s it required skilful direction and large capital. It was carried on mainly by Swiss, German and Spanish mercenaries. When not at war, soldiers often turned to banditry. The growth of firearms and cannon forced the cities to build defenses, and that usually required getting into debt. A city's credit rating became its most powerful weapon. This gave the cities an advantage over princes, for until the 16th century a prince's debts were not binding on his successors. Cities, with their perpetual existence, were considered safer to lend to." This was another instance of institutions making up for the insufficiency of commodity money.

The institutions of England, developed from the Norman Conquest through the Magna Charta and the Wars of the Roses, served her well. "In England only the King had the power of minting money. In France 300 vassals appropriated the right of coinage; under the Capetians the Crown was constantly trying to recover it.

"The Princes needed revenue mainly for military expenses. Most of the wealth was in the hands of the clergy and the nobles, who were difficult to tax. The result was that the mint became the main source of revenue. From roughly the mid 1300s to the mid-1400s was the period of 'Kingly abuse' of the monetary power, and is still pointed to by banker apologists in their very limited arsenal of arguments against government-managed money. Even real historians have viewed this period in terms of the immorality of monetary 'debasement.' For even when they regained their monopoly over coinage, monarchs continued debasing their coinage. By studying coin debasement as a taxation substitute, Peter Spufford has shown that such debasement could be an effective tax, equitable, unavoidable; and relatively easy to administer. He also noted the necessity of reducing the metal weight of new coinage from time to time to reflect the wear-and-tear loss on already circulating coinage. Otherwise Gresham's law would assert itself. However, the Prince's mixing of taxation with the money system retarded the development of monetary thought and gave the impression that money was merely a commodity."[2]

The Medieval Moneylenders

"From the 10th to the 13th century the Papal collectors were the first Christian moneylenders. Rich monasteries also made loans, but from about 1200 onwards, ecclesiastical establishments rarely lent money. They couldn't compete with the Knights Templars and the Italians, and the Church was enforcing the ban on usury.

"The Knights Templar, with their chain of holdings to the Levant, were the main financial power during the 12th century partly because they found a way to benefit from the East-West dichotomy in the gold/silver ratio. When they were suppressed in 1307, the field was opened to the Italians. The Templars brought double-entry bookkeeping back from the Crusades and the Italians were among the first to master it.[3]

"'Compared with the efflorescence and ubiquity of Italian credit, that of the Jews appears a very small affair. In actual fact the more economically advanced a country was, the fewer Jewish money-lenders were to be found. The revival of Mediterranean commerce in the 11th century made it possible to dispense with them as intermediaries with the Levant. 'The Jews of the West were reduced to mere pawnbroking,' wrote Pirenne.

"Deposit banking arose in the Catalonian region of Spain in the early 1200s at about the same time as the Bank of St. George started in Genoa. Deposit banking was generally intended to perform safekeeping and transfer services, not to make loans. These banks were private enterprises and ran into typical banking troubles, as seen from the banking laws enacted in 1300-1301.

"No moneychanger shall keep a bank in any place in Catalonia unless he shall first have given surety (a bond).

"'No moneychanger who may fail, and none who has recently failed or in times past failed shall again keep a bank or hold any office under the Crown' and 'Until he shall have satisfied all demands, he shall be detained on a diet of bread and water.'

"An appendix was added in 1321: 'If no such settlement is made, they shall be proclaimed bankrupt and disgraced by the public crier in the places in which they failed and throughout Catalonia. They shall be beheaded and their property shall be sold for the satisfaction of their creditors by the Court. In 1360 Fracesh Castello was beheaded in front of his bank.'

"Only the Italians made 'foreign' investments in the 1300s. Their main lending mechanisms were the bill of exchange and the finance bill. Charging interest on riskless loans was generally forbidden by the Church. But as there were merchants who needed to borrow and bankers who wanted to lend, they found semantic ways around the prohibition. One way was to advance a sum in one city's coinage, guaranteed by a bill of exchange in a higher amount in another city's coinage and calling it a foreign exchange transaction rather than a loan."

Early Bank Myopia

"Think of it as a post-dated check in another currency payable after some months. The interest charge was contained in the difference between what was advanced and the amount of the post-dated bill. Finally, the bill may never have been sent for collection. The borrower would pay the money in the local currency. This became known as 'dry exchange.'

"While much is made of the Kings and Princes abusing the money systems, the private bankers often did worse. In 1339 the Florentine bankers were ruined when greatly overextended in loans to Edward III of England who was unable to repay their millions of gold florins when his war with France went badly. Florence was in turmoil. The guilds took over, expelled the bankers, and seized their possessions.

"The clever Florentine bankers (the Medicis) tried again, loaning to Edward IV for the 'War of the Roses' and also loaning to the rebels – just in case. But eventually the rebels were dead and Edward was broke. The London branch went broke. The obvious lesson: [still being learned in every boom] never be overly concentrated.

"The merchant bankers of Lucca, though overshadowed by the Florentines, had been among the first to cross the Alps. They were moderate, kept good relations and neutrality, and outlived the Florentines in both Antwerp and France.

"The Lombards were essentially pawnbrokers making loans on pledges of personal property. They were found throughout Europe but tolerated rather than privileged. Their position was similar to that of the Jews – disliked everywhere, generally expelled from all countries, and occasionally, though much less frequently, massacred. They took time deposits and paid interest on them using the capital for pawnbroking, often going bankrupt to the ruin of their small depositors. Like the Jews, they usually charged 43.5% a year. The medieval pawnshops were an obvious place to 'fence' stolen property. De Roover notes that 'the Lombards were surrounded with so much odium that other Italians did not care to associate with them.'

"In 1400 Barcelona organized a city-owned deposit bank as a department of the municipal government, which guaranteed its liabilities. It was to allow overdrafts only to the city but in fact allowed substantial overdrafts to the city commissioners. In 1468, during the great silver famine, a severe coin shortage forced the bank to suspend payments. It issued a 5% annuity to all depositors willing to accept them. Public officials were personally responsible for the honest functioning of the bank during their terms of office – but they fell behind in their auditing, whereby the prior 6 or 7 administrations were still unaudited! The lesson – independent, timely auditing is essential." That lesson, too, is still being relearned today.

The Great Discovery: Banks Create Money

"It must have soon become apparent to the Templars, the Italian merchant bankers and the great German lending houses that they possessed the power to create money in the form of bookkeeping credits on their books. The bankers sought deposits, on which they generally paid interest and then made loans at higher rates, or used the money to discount bills (cash postdated checks) at a discount. However, the loans would not have to be made in coinage, but could be in credits to the borrower's account in the bank – in bookkeeping entries. The borrower would have the ability to write checks on that account. Such checks might not actually be cashed, but be credited to another account on the books of the same bank." That is the big unmentioned bonus to the banks in bank mergers today, alongside the other unmentioned bonus – the already "too big to be allowed to fail" become even more so by the very merger. And on top of that the increasing power and increasing secrecy of deregulation expose them to taking risks in ever more dimensions.

"In many ways this was a monetary power greater than the King's over the mint. This bank money was a more truly fiat money form and further removed from true barter than the 'precious metal 'coins. But the bankers were usurping a power that derives from and belongs to society and using it for personal benefit.

"The whole process was inflationary, but because it fraudulently pretended that the bankers' paper was redeemable in metal, the system would collapse when too many bills had been written and finally their coinage reserves would be drained away."

There was no lack of resistance to this aspect of banking. But because it threw out the baby with the bath, the positive side of token money along with its exploitative abuses, it was doomed to defeat.

At its height some 180 mostly North German towns headed by Luebeck, Cologne, Bremen, Brunswick, Danzig joined together in a sort of commercial union, and in association with the House of Burgundy and the Teutonic Knights they opposed the incursion of bankers in general and Italian bankers in particular. "Characteristic of the conservatism of the Hanseatic League was that it had no monetary powers whatever, a fact that argues against the assumption that money was originated by merchants.

The Hansa was unable to envisage the unification of the various money systems within her domain, even though the various currencies were a serious obstacle to Hanseatic commerce. The Hanseatic League called itself 'the merchants of the

Holy Roman Empire' and the closely allied Teutonic Knights were the Pope's biggest agents for Christianizing or exterminating the pagan Goths. They had a strong bias against using credit in trade and allowed no trading in futures. They forbade selling herring before it was caught and grain before it was grown and cloth before it was woven. The attitude against futures markets was so strong that aspects of it survived until the early 1990s when most futures contracts in Germany were not legally binding upon the speculator.

"Until about 1400 a major battle raged between the Hanseatic League along with the House of Burgundy using a cash-based trading system against the Italians, south Germans, English and others using credit in trade. One of the oldest features of Hansa policy was its campaign against credit on the grounds that it caused instability of prices which would upset business. Credit was also accused of increasing the temptation to take risks and, even worse, of favoring the dishonest schemes of unscrupulous merchants." They were alarmed by the Italians' command of credit techniques, and the fact that these were catching on among the South Germans.

"The epic struggle against credit raged on the battlefield of Brugge for 150 years, starting in 1389 when the House of Burgundy, in reaction to an extended inflationary period resulting from credit expansion adopted a hard money policy and brought on a severe deflation. The beneficiaries of the deflation were the landed gentry, the clergy, and the rentiers. Rents, which remained constant, were being paid in more valuable money. Finally in December 1390 the Brugge City Treasurer was nearly killed by an angry mob and rents were scaled down by urgent legislation.

"Ten years later Brugge deflated again, ordering that all bills of exchange be paid in coinage and not by crediting an account in a bank. Further it was decreed that all foreign exchange bills were to be paid in gold; silver was phased out in three steps over about a year. The demonetization of silver quickly became unworkable, and was repealed in September, 1401.

"Then the Hansa joined the battle, demanding and obtaining an abolition of all credit transactions in Flanders in 1401. By 1541 some variant of this process was repeated five times."

Calvin's Elevation of Judaism

"An ordinance of 1450 gave the reasons: The banks have wrought utter ruin among all classes of people, but especially among merchants and persons of note. The banks were accused of all kinds of offenses against the common weal and more specifically of picking and culling the currency, of sending bullion to foreign mints and bringing the underweight monies of these mints into (domestic) circulation. The Brugge events had catastrophic results for the Medici banking family in Florence. In 1478 they sold out their Brugge branch to their local partners, and in 1488 the branch was catastrophically liquidated. In 1494 a mob invaded their Palace in Florence and burned the records. Their business tactics, which generally worked in an inflationary environment, had no chance in a deflationary one."

1494 was two years after Columbus set sail westward. The shot in the arm that the sack of Constantinople by the Fourth

Crusade had given the European monetary system had worn off. It was high time that the gold accumulation of the advanced Indian civilizations in the New World were sacked to keep the monetary system of the Old World ballooning.

"It was the followers of Calvin, and especially the Puritans who first elevated the Old Testament into a position of supreme importance,' wrote George O'Brien ('An Essay on the Economic Effects of the Reformation,' London, Burnes, Oates & Washbourne, 1923, p. 126). O'Brien noted that during the Middle Ages, the 'blanks' in the Gospel were filled by Aristotle's work and by natural reason.

"The Calvinist Reformation evolved in a manner that shattered the universality of Christendom and began to alter what was considered acceptable behavior in human relations, especially financial activity. Its seeds took root mainly in northwest Europe where it was nurtured by the effects of two epic discoveries. The Knights Templar had dominated European economic affairs in the 12th and 13th centuries thanks to their financial innovations and their strong trading links with the East, including the gold/silver trade. The 16th to 18th centuries would be dominated by forces set in motion by two navigational feats of the Portuguese Knights of Christ, achieved in their efforts to capture control of this crucial East-West trade. Portugal's ruler, Prince Henry the Navigator (1393-1460), and Columbus were members of the Knighthood, which advanced the art of navigation and map-making. Columbus's voyage to America in 1492 and Gasco de Gama's completion of the route to India around the African Cape of Good Hope became of overriding geopolitical importance. Both discoveries resulted from attempts to engage in the gold/silver trade with the East and to establish an advantageous position in the spice trade. These discoveries diverted control over the East-West trade from the Mediterranean to northwestern Europe and shifted the balance of power to the North Sea area."

Columbus's Gold Fever

"As the Reformation reduced the power of the Catholic Church in Europe, the Church's hierarchy, while professing to view mankind as a brotherhood in Christ, condoned terrible crimes against humanity in the slaughter of untold millions of South American Indians. The instruments of the genocide were the conquistadores sent by the Spanish Crown to loot gold from them.

"Columbus's discovery of America was not only based on bad geography, but on equally defective monetary theory. He was searching for a Western route for Spain to engage in the gold-silver trade with China and Japan. His contract with the Spanish Crown gave him one-eighth of the spoils of the voyage, and one of his first suggestions to Spain was to enslave the Indians. While the monarchy was truly concerned with the religious conversion of native souls, it was brutal in its quest for gold. The Indians were butchered, raped, hanged, and burned, usually on the initiative of the local conquistador operating within contracts structured by the Church's legal talent.

"Sir Arthur Helps in *The Spanish Conquest of America,* estimated that the original population under Spanish control at 32 million and that within less than 40 years the Spanish conquistadores destroyed 15 million of them by working them to death in silver and gold mines."

Europeans Raided Spanish Shipping

"The conquerors were legally required to recite the 'Requerimiento' to any Indians they were about to slaughter. It affirmed that God gave the charge to one man...Peter...that he should be head of the human race. We ask and require that you take time to deliberate upon it, and that you acknowledge the Church as the Mistress of the whole World. If you do so, you will do well.... But if you do not we shall make war against you and shall take you and your wives and children and shall make slaves of them." The Requerimiento had been framed by the famous jurist Palacios Rubios and was normally read in Spanish to the trees, or mumbled by the attacking army. In one case it was actually translated to an Indian ruler Atahualpa of Peru in 1532. After hearing the Requerimiento, Atahualpa said: "Your pope must be a most extraordinary man to give so liberally of what does not belong to him." The conquistador Pizarro murdered Atahualpa as soon as the Inca leader had a room filled with gold for his agreed-upon ransom, totalling 185,000 ounces.

"While Spain did the 'dirty work' on the ground, England and Holland adopted a simpler strategy – they highjacked the Spanish ships bringing the gold and silver back to Europe. Judging from the rise in prices in England and Holland, very large amounts of metals were intercepted. The British Crown gave charters, calling them privateers. The Dutch West India Company was established in 1623 specifically to rob the Spaniards. Piracy was profitable: in its first 13 years the company equipped 800 ships costing 54 million guilders. During that period it captured 540 ships with 72 million worth of cargo and stole another 36 million from Portuguese colonies. Of great interest to Amsterdam was the contract for supplying Negro slaves to the Spanish colonies of America. From 7 to 18 million slaves were brought to South America from Africa; about 400-500,000 were brought to North America.

"While the effect of the precious metals created a 'renaissance of the north,' the effect on Spain was negative. Spain plundered the Americas and mainly enriched her 'Nobles.' [The conquistadores were actually recruited disproportionately from amongst the pig-herders of the impoverished Western province of Extramadura.] Spain produced little of anything after the conquest, and the ill-gotten, blood-stained gain, which flowed to her shores from America served only to feed impractical vanity. Finding she could purchase anything and everything with gold and silver, she threw herself into her work of conquest and let commerce go" (W.A. Shaw). [It gave rise to the literary genre of the 'picaresque novels,' where a stock character, too impecunious to sup, nevertheless picks his teeth ostentatiously on the town square to prove to his peers how well he has dined.]

"This Spanish evidence provides additional support for the viewpoint that money is not productive capital. We noted that Naples and Venice had begun using milled copper coinage for smaller transactions in 1472 and 1473. However, the plunder of the precious metals from America retarded the development of money systems and though away from Nomisma and back to commodity money, which is essentially just an advanced [three-way] form of barter."

A "Crime-stained" Money System

"In 1902, Alexander Del Mar, in *The History of Precious Metals*, 1902, estimated: 'About half the existing stock of precious metals was obtained through conquest and slavery. The value at which this crime-stained metals has entered the exchanges of the world keep down the value of the portion produced by free labour; so that the latter is sold to the minter at less than its average cost,' wrote Del Mar. In fact such slavery has reduced the value of all free labor, not just that engaged in mining.

"From at least the time of Alexander the Great, whoever controlled the gold/silver ratio trade with the East was paramount in the West. We have seen how it consecutively benefited the Ptolemies, Rome, Constantinople. Venice, the Jews, and the Knights Templar. After the 1307 suppression of the Templars, Venice once again dominated the ratio trade up till 1500. Opening the Cape Route allowed Portugal to dominate trade with India and points east from the beginning of the 1500s. Between 1565 and 1625 Portuguese traders stripped Japan of two-thirds of its gold, approximately 250 tons. Japan, valuing the gold/silver ratio at 6 to 1, was unaware that the ratio in Europe was 15 to 1 at that time. The Portuguese channeled the pepper trade though the city of Antwerp, which quickly became Europe's greatest trading port. The Cape Route also reduced Moslem economic power as a go-between for Venice and India."

W.K.

End of Installment Two of the review of Zarlenga book. Further installments to come.

1. Krehm, William (May, 1970). *La Revue Économique*, "Le Secteur Public et la Stabilité des Prix."

2. Krehm, William (1975). *Price in a Mixed Economy – Our Record of Disaster*, Toronto. Significantly, when COMER finally dug up and put together the details of the surreptitious bailout of the Canadian banks from their immense losses in financing major speculations in gas and oil, real estate, and an Ottawa builder's sudden fantasy to start collecting US department store chains, the bank spokesmen cried that the statutory reserves, the core of the bank bailout, had been an unjust tax levied on the banks. In fact the statutory reserves had been a modest quid per quo for the government assigning to the banks a major part of its powers of money creation, while remaining responsible through the central bank as their lender of the last resort, The statutory reserves varying from 8 to 10% for some years were the portions of deposits received by the banks from the public in chequing and other short term accounts that had to be redeposited with the Bank of Canada on an interest free-basis. They provided an alternative to influencing the volume of lending by raising interest rates. The same illusions and misconceptions crop up concerning money over the centuries and millennia.

3. Distinguishing as it does between capital investment which is depreciated over its useful life and current spending, it is basic to double-entry bookkeeping. When they apply a bit of it here and there to produce a better statistic for impressing the bond-rating agencies, governments in our day hide what they are doing. With a total write-off of bridges buildings, and human investment in a single year governments are driven to raise more taxation in that year than is strictly necessary, and when the excess taxation shows up in a higher price level, they now proceed to pushup interest rates "to lick inflation." What they need to lick is their stubbornness in resisting their auditors and refusing to adopt accrual accountancy, On the other hand excluding the depreciated value of their capital investments from their assets but including the debt incurred by financing them through the private banking system, leads to an exaggerated net deficit (i.e., the excess of debt over assets). This serves as a pretext for selling private assets that appear on their books at a token value at a small fraction of their real worth, to well-connected investors, who apply accrual accountancy to their acquisition, list it on the stock market, and by driving up user fees for what the taxpayers have already paid for in taxes, now pay for them a second time in users' fees.

Mail Box

THE EXCHANGE between Bill Krehm and the Cambridge Journal of Economics highlights what I have come to call the "How do we get from here to there?" syndrome. Any significant departure from a status quo norm discovers this syndrome. I discovered it early in a career as an innovative research scientist introducing new ideas and equipment to the Paper industry. Developing such ideas and their applications was reasonably straight forward. Convincing the industry to try out the resulting products was an enormously challenging task. Although ultimately successful, the cost in time and money to make an impact far exceeded the actual development costs. Finding publication space in refereed scientific journals was difficult because reviewers were typically established scientists with a huge bias toward the viewpoint of their own output (frequently from years long passed. I was told that the first thing such referees do is check the list of references to see how often their own work has been quoted. Note the referee's comment reported in COMER): "...It makes no systematic use of the academic literature at all, and there is no list of references." (Read – I am not quoted.) When the "how do we get from here to there?" syndrome represents a major obstacle to introducing relative simple new ideas into a small well-defined industry, think about the COMER challenge! The whole economic structure of our modern society is fundamentally rooted in an acceptance of the validity of the economic models which all modern-day economists absorb as the mother's milk of their academic training. The financial beneficiaries and through them the large corporate community are huge beneficiaries of the status quo, and are incestuously connected into the political system. For those who are not brain-washed by academic training and are willing to spend the mental effort to bring the COMER economic ideas into a broad focus, these ideas are clearly very powerful. Nevertheless they are by no means simple ideas, but require substantial background study to fully appreciate.

How to overcome the huge obstacle established by the "how to get from here to there?" syndrome is indeed mind-bogging.

Wavell Cowan

Chasing the Tails of Historians, Economists and Other Evangelists

A TELEVANGELIST (who looks rather like George Bush) was praising the Geneva of John Calvin and the Scotland of John Knox, where democracy was the rule of the day. Though this brace of former lawyers provided great spiritual guidance to Protestant Reformers, their political attempt to impose the rule of Christ by law was a contradiction in terms. John Milton, a redoubtable reformer himself, said: "Whoever knew truth put in the worst in a free and open encounter?" That is to say, you can't legislate truth away. The same is probably true for immorality.

The Christian Republican constituency in the US (and Canadian branch plant churches of the big American denominations) want to capture the levers of political power in order to legislate their brand of morality for all. In their terms to legislate immorality away. They may be naive about the horse they have bet on.

A Sin Becomes Virtue

They do seem to have a somewhat limited range of immorality in their sights, too. Abortion, evolution, and gay "marriage" seem to be the Big Three. But for every reference in the Bible to these three favourites, there must be a hundred references to another, unmentioned one – greed.

For the mediaeval Church, greed was one of the Seven Deadly Sins. They called it *avaritia*, Avarice. It is not a big topic in American Republican Christian preaching today. In fact, it is funny to note how often the prosperity gospel ("God wants you to be rich") comes from the same pulpit as the prediction that Muslims and other pagans will soon be destroyed (along with all those "liberals"). Funny, because Islam still has a proscription against usury (lending for interest), while Western Christians have largely embraced that former sin. Granted, some Muslims get around their law by permitting service fees for a loan. Christian and Jewish bankers, of course, have the best of both worlds – interest *and* service fees.

If, in the second G.W. Bush term, the Christian Republican constituency becomes the "Established Church," its interests advanced by the state, the US will have come a long way from its origins. The Pilgrim Fathers, the Quakers of Pennsylvania, the Catholic settlers of Maryland, the independents of Rhode Island, and thousands of others came to this continent chiefly to escape the tyranny of an Established Church.

But fear not: for after all, if the Second Coming is imminent, as the evangelist hinted, it may arrive before the Re-Establishment does. Consider that for a moment. When the End comes and the faithful are raptured away, as one millennialist version predicts, what will those "left behind" do? Probably breathe a sigh of relief and go on with their sinful practices – especially the greed group.

Greed, by the way, is not a prerogative of the rich. True, it shows up prominently in the bankers and mutual fund managers who are competing to gobble up those big pools of capital in the insurance companies. Also, we may detect minute traces of it in the remuneration contracts negotiated by hot-property CEOs hired to "enhance shareholder value." But it also affects the common folk, who maxed out their credit cards again this past Festering Season. For rich and poor alike, too, it shifts over into Gluttony – another of the Seven Deadlies – labelled for all to see in the silhouettes of some of your neighbours. If we ever want to look at a set of more virtuous silhouettes, of course, we can look at the photos of Sub-Saharan Africans.

Money Goes Where Money Is

The prevailing economic orthodoxy about them, however, is that, if the rich are left free to get richer, the poor will get richer, too – eventually. "A rising tide lifts all boats," as some owners of large yachts are fond of saying. That is a neat nautical image, to be sure, but as an economic law it sinks like a torpedoed tanker. The truth in the real, as opposed to the theoretical world, is that the financial rising tide lifts only the big, most buoyant boats. The rest get swamped. Without redistributive mechanisms – such as *noblssse oblige*, graduated income taxes, or free collective bargaining – the Law of Money will prevail, for "Money goes where money is." And money stays there, often for generations, as the history of the last century demonstrates. Though corporations have risen and fallen, moneyed families have remained, by nimbly switching their resources from fallers to risers.

Now are we here talking economics or history? The question is a relevant one, and one raised by the CBC broadcast of the 2004 Massey Lectures, Ronald Wright's *A History of Progress*. A review of the Lectures in the *National Post* (1/12/04, "CBC Radio's Marxist Masseys" by Peter Foster) dismisses them in a burst of rhetoric with the charge that Wright has not "the slightest clue about how economics work." The writer identifies the command post he is firing from in the next breath: "or how, by their fundamental nature, markets are both moral and 'sustainable.'"

Clearly we are listening to the voice of one who considers himself an economist, and a theoretical one at that. But at the same time he writes like a journalist – or perhaps like an evangelist? He concludes "What really needs some psychological excavation is Ronald Wright's mind, which carries a set of inflated, emotionally based moralistic assumptions derived from the structure of his primitive ignorance about markets and economics."

Was the world invented yesterday?

How I wish I could write as persuasively as that! But, alas, I do not have the economist's profound and penetrating understanding of how the world really works. Still, as a sometimes historian and a once-upon-a-time student of rhetoric, I can be of service to Mr. Wright's cause by suggesting a tentative comparison of the economist and the historian.

Economics has been called "the dismal science – justifiably if we are to judge by the *NP* article, which contains barely enough science to half-dot a microscopic slide.

Both history and economics reside in university calendars

among the "social sciences." Economists work with the quantifiable; if it cannot be quantified, it is not relevant to economics as at present constituted. That is their scientific side. On the social side, though, most economists seem to want no truck with human foibles, morality, ethics, or the art of democratic government. That surely is their dismal side.

Some historians also profess to be scientists, but their social side is more broad-ranging. Both historian and economist deal with the past, in order to predict the future. The economist resides mainly in the immediate past – call it the recent present – and attempts to see the future from there. The historian deals often with the remote past. His field, in fact, by definition, begins with the written record, that gives him about five millennia. The economist has no interest in anything so remote; the statistics are unavailable. Besides, the current generation of economists seem to be stuck with the view that the world was invented yesterday, but that even if it was not, today's world is totally different from anything in the past.

Both specialties use geometry. The economist touts the current trends – upward, or downward – and projects upon a jagged, upsy-downsy graph, the illuminating clarity of a straight trend line. The historian, conducting a similar assessment, over a millennium or three, tends to find the pattern cyclical, or, perhaps better, helical.[1]

Economists are fond of the word "engine," as in "the auto industry is the engine of the economy," or "housing is the engine of the money supply," or economics is the engine of civilization." It's a good metaphor. May we play with it a little? Economists, we might say, are like experts on engines; they can rest on their specialty without regard for the rest of the vehicle. They care not for how comfortable the seats are, and how fast the vehicle is travelling, nor if the brakes are functional, nor whether the roads are passable or even where they lead, nor how clear the driver's eyesight is, nor how exact his/her hand-eye coordination. They need not be concerned with the driver's purposes, that is, from what presuppositions or to what destinations the steering is directed, for, after all, without the engine those things are of no consequence whatsoever.

The historian, in addition to being a scientist – a collector of quantifiable data, and not unfamiliar with the economics engine – taps a wide range of data, drawn from the whole vehicle of civilization, and its road grid, and, yes, its destiny. Toynbee's great *Study* was praised by many historians with the format: "it is a great work, except in the area of [here, fill in the writer's personal specialty]. It's the eternal misunderstanding between the specialist and the generalist. For comment on it, we might call on the Apostle Paul, who explained (1Cor.12:14-26): "Now the body is not made up on one part, but of many…. The eye cannot say to the hand, 'I do not need you! And the hand cannot say to the feet, 'I don't need you!'"

To be continued.

Gordon Coggins

1. Arnold Toybee's final response to Oswald Spengler's great cyclical theory of the rise and fall of civilizations was contained in a metaphor: the cycling civilizations are like the wheels on a chariot which is moving steadily upward.

Pay Dirt in Other Cultures

RIVERS, crossroads, oceans, skies, have a way of recurring in humanity's great legends. It is when we leave home and travel, that we may forget what our father and mother looked like, and risk becoming entangled in the traditions of other cultures that we do not necessarily understand. Worse still, we may try to impose our own hangups on those faceless aliens we encounter at the crossroads.

Increasingly, it seems that will be the great lesson that we still have to learn from Globalization and Deregulation. Especially in our relations with China. China is a country, not only of vast population, but of great traditions that should warn us of too facile solutions. Many of our basic inventions can be traced to the Chinese: paper, printing, gunpowder, innovations in navigation. Her system of writing and even her language were seminal for other cultures in the Far East. But she somehow got colossally mired down. When her wealth of knowledge attracted too many aggressive outsiders, she simply closed all her frontiers. That didn't help much, because it led to an ingrowth of ignorance that left her defenceless against her invaders. She was finally awakened by the intrusion of a series of alien economic systems.

The most recent were the taking over of economic and even political power under the system of territorialism, when European traders cut pieces out of the Central Empire as formal colonies or de facto ones. Then came the Communist regime, that used the vast population and land mass to erect a massive military power, devoted to quick quasi-solutions that made short shrift of the country's great inheritance. But in many ways that led to her great reawakening. The very political refugees from the Communist dictatorship, were driven by their strong family ties and Confucian reverence for discipline and learning to sop up Western technology and science in the universities of their exile. And when they returned to China they brought back with them untold treasures to a country that had come to blend some of the least humanitarian aspects of Communism with the scratchiest dogmas of capitalism. And with by far the greatest population base – and one with unspoiled "expectations" – they are in a unique position to eventually challenge the American world hegemony. Their insights into the weaknesses of capitalism acquired during their Communist apprenticeship occasionally gives them great advantages in doing so. Obviously the preemptive strike mania in Washington's foreign policy strengthens their position. However, the social problems stirred up in China by the massive infusion of raw capitalist appetites are as intimidating as the availability of an excess of dirt-cheap labour power. And if these problems give rise to a technologically equipped taste for military adventure in the Washington style, the outlook for survival of humanity will hardly be enhanced.

Meanwhile the input of fiction in the information that China has to offer about its material progress is documented on the same front-page of *The Wall Street Journal* that we have been dealing with in this little survey ("China Stocks Evoke the Ghost of Bubble Past" by Craig Karmin and Joel Baglole):

"When clear-headed investors sounded the alarm about the technology-stock bubble in the late 1990s, they were soundly ignored. Today, another group is raising the same call about China. And many investors, who have apparently wiped their tech-stock losses from their minds, don't seem to be listening. 'China looked like a bubble at the start of last year,' says Mark Madden, manager of Pioneer Emerging Markets Fund.

"The Chinese market as measured by the Morgan Stanley Capital International China Index gained 81% in 2003. Chinese stocks that trade in Hong Kong rose 152% last year. The Chinese market is up 6% this year [so far]. The list of most outrageously overpriced companies must by tradition be led by Internet companies such as China's top three portals – Sina Corp., Sohn. Com Inc. and Netease.com Inc. – each rose between 220% and 420% in 2002.

"But the real proof that valuation is out of kilter is the prices investors are paying for mundane industries such as beer producers and car-makers. Typically, a new and volatile market such as China would trade at a valuation below the 15 times trailing 12-month earnings that is the average for emerging markets. But China now trades at 17 times trailing earnings.

"There's often a gray area in terms of property rights when you're buying Chinese companies,' says Chris Lively, a portfolio manager at Citiesgroup Asset Management. Not a comforting thought."

William Krehm

Dearly Bought Lessons Out of Argentina

WHEN YOU LAST HEARD of Argentina it was probably as a basket case hopelessly enmeshed in debt and government changes as though by revolving doors. And what emerged as even worse by official logic was that since it was thumbing its nose at the advice of the International Monetary Fund and refusing to put its debt into better shape, there was no chance of recovery.

But listen to this front-page story in *The New York Times* (26/12, "Economic Rally for Argentines Defies Forecasts" by Larry Rohter): "Buenos Aires – When the Argentine economy collapsed in December 2001, doomsday predictions abounded. Unless it quickly cut a deal with its foreign creditors, hyperinflation would surely follow, the peso would become worthless, foreign investment would vanish and any prospect of growth would be strangled.

"But three years after Argentina declared a record debt default of more than $100 billion, the largest in history, the apocalypse has not arrived. Instead, the economy has grown by more than 8% for two consecutive years, exports have zoomed, the currency is stable, investors are gradually returning and unemployment has eased from record heights – all without a debt settlement or the standard measures required by the IMF for its approval.

"Argentine's recovery has been achieved at least in part by ignoring and even defying economic and political orthodoxy. Rather than moving to immediately satisfy bondholders, private banks and the IMF, as other developing countries have done in less severe crises, the Peronist-led government chose to stimulate internal consumption first. It told creditors to get in lines with everyone else."

"'This is a remarkable historical event, one that challenges 25 years of failed policies,' said Mark Weisbrot, an economist at the Center for Economic and Policy Research, a liberal research group in Washington. 'While other countries are just limping along, Argentina is experiencing healthy growth with no sign that it is unsustainable, and they're doing this without having to make concessions to get foreign capital inflows.... More than two millions jobs have been created since the depths of the crisis in 2002, and inflation-adjusted income has also bounced, almost to the level of the late 1990s.'"

In short the Argentine has not turned out the basket case almost universally predicted. The basket involved, it turns out, had been largely woven by the IMF. Or if we may change our metaphor it turns out that in the run for the exit the fat guy – the IMF – representing the foreign bondholders ran ahead of the crowd and got stuck in the door, blocking the exit for everybody else including productive workers. The government – of populist if not always democratic tradition – opened a few windows and let in some fresh air.

No black magic was involved. It simply applied something very obvious because it is usually applied in any major war by the developed creditor countries themselves – their first concern on the outbreak of war is not to pay off the debt and settle with the creditors on the creditors' terms – highest interest rates. It is to get production humming. And that usually produces the revenue before long to handle its debt. It is only because the world has been brain-washed to the point of our having to figure out why this can be done under the pressure of war when production goes largely for destruction, but we are told that we cannot do so when production could be applied for socially useful purposes.

The Twisted Agenda of Bretton Woods

This is not the first case where the wisdom of the IMF and the international official credit-managing bureaucracy has been questioned. Malaysia did so in controlling the free movement of capital across its frontiers. Chile – made safe for Wall St. by the Pinochet coup backed by Washington – on getting rid of that murderous and arch-corrupt regime, restricted the free flow of speculative capital. Short-term inflows of speculative capital were taxed heavily. Only foreign money was allowed free access if it undertook to stay in the country for at least a year. Governments through the emerging world are likely to follow the Argentine lead. And as that happens, the whole rigged perversion of the international financial institutions will come up for reexamination.

The IMF and the World Bank were founded at the Bretton Woods Conference in 1943 while WWII raged. Its original goal was to find a fair way of applying the lessons of the 1930

Depression made crystal clear by the financing of the war itself. As proposed by the British delegation headed by John Maynard Keynes, the international credit institutions created were to make the handling of international debt the responsibility not only of the debtor nations but of the creditor nations as well. The latter would do their part by allowing their currencies to strengthen to help create a better market for the exports of the debtor nations, and by making productive investments in the debtor countries. If they failed to do that, part of their credits – after a reasonable period – would become forfeit to the United Nations to be used for development of the debtor countries. Unfortunately Bretton Woods turned out to be a power test and the American delegation – the one great creditor nation, simply steam-rollered Britain and the other heavily indebted countries to set up the new world financial institutions as what became collection agencies for the powerful financial interests. Growth became a privilege of only the developed countries – more wealth was sucked out of the emerging and third world countries at punitive rates, than went into them as new investment on terms that would open the possibility of their ever leaving behind their role as sources of ever cheaper labour.

But back to the *NY Times* article:

"Some of the new jobs [in the Argentine have resulted] from a low-paying government make-work program, but nearly half are in the private sector. Unemployment has declined from more than 20% to about 13%, and the number of Argentines living below the poverty line has fallen by nearly 10 points from the record high of 53.4 percent early in 2002.

"Traditional free-market economists remain skeptical of the government's approach. While acknowledging that there has been a recovery, they attribute it mainly to external factors rather than to the policies of President Nestor Kirchner, who has been in office since May 2003.

"'We've been lucky,' said Luis Bohr, chief economist at the Latin American Foundation for Economic Research here. 'We've had high prices for commodities and low interest rates. But if we want to grow in 2005, we're going to have to settle the debt question and have foreign capital come in.'

"The IMF, which Argentine officials blame for inducing the crisis in the first place, argues that the current government is acting at least in part as the IMF has always recommended. It has limited spending and moved to increase revenues, a classic prescription when an economy is ailing, and has built up a surplus twice the size of what the fund had asked before negotiations were put on hold several months ago.

"But some of the record budget surplus has come from a pair of levies on exports and *financial transactions* [our emphasis] that orthodox economists at the IMF and elsewhere want repealed. About a third of government revenue is now raised by those taxes.

"The IMF [also] wants Argentine to improve the offer to creditors and also pay back its loans fund so that can reduce its own exposure. 'In other words,' said Alan Cibils, an Argentine economist of the Independent Interdisciplinary Center for the Study of Public Policy here, 'You have to pay more and take in less,' which is a sure prescription for another crisis." Note the

"Interdisciplinary" in the title of that organization. That is the new buzzword that is surging across the horizon, a sure sign of the growing realization that degenerate economic theory has become a tool of the international financial sector.

Revived Capital Influx

"Because of the absence of a debt accord and a stalemate over utility tariffs, some investors, mainly Europeans, continue to shun the Argentine, citing what they call the lack of 'judicial security.' But others, mainly Latin Americans used to operating in unstable environments or themselves survivors of similar crises, have increased their presence here amid expanding opportunities.

"'These are slogans that people repeat without thinking, as though, they were parrots,' Roberto Lavagna, the minister of the economy said when asked about the predictions that investment would disappear. 'So why are they investing? Because today clearly they can get a very good return.'

"The Brazilian oil company Petrobras bought a stake in a leading energy company. Another Brazilian company, AmBev has acquired a large interest in Quilmes, Argentina's leading beer brand, and a Mexican company bought up control of a leading bread and cake maker. Asian countries with China and South Korea in the lead, have begun to move in. During a state visit last month, the Chinese president, Hu Jintao, announced that his country plans to invest $20 billion in Argentina over the next decade. For the first time in three years more money is coming into the country than is leaving it. That has given Mr. Kirchner the luxury of taking a hard line with the IMF and with foreign creditors clamoring for repayment. 'The thing is that Argentina has a current account surplus, so that they don't really need so much foreign investment,' said Claudio Loser, an Argentine economist and the former Western hemisphere director for the IMF. Just this week, the government announced that reserves of foreign currency have climbed back to $19.5 billion, more than double the low point recorded in the middle of 2002 a year with a net outflow of $12.7 billion. The peak of investment in the 1990s was 19.9% of the GDP annually, and today it is at 19.1%, having risen from 10.1%. The Kirchner administration continues to seek an accord on the $187 billion in debt, and plans to make what it calls its final offer early next month. But the turnabout here has inspired such confidence that the government is not only talking about cutting the last ties with the IMF, but also insisting that any payback to the bondholders be linked to Argentina's continued good economic health."

W.K.

The Bank of Canada to the Aid of our Stressed Municipalities

January 21, 2005

Mayor David Miller
Toronto City Hall

Dear Mr. Mayor:

I refer to your recent appearance on CTV in which you pointed out that it will be years before the Toronto subway system is extended to our airport, I note, too, the letter to you of Richard Priestman of Kingston and a leading member of the Committee on Monetary and Economic Reform, in which he referred to the use of the Bank of Canada, and its provisions under guarantee of either the Federal or Provincial governments to finance essential investments by municipalities. Since 1938 when a Liberal government nationalized the Bank of Canada, the interest on such loans, less the overhead of the BoC in handling the arrangement, would revert to the federal government as dividends. The extension of Toronto's subway you mentioned would indeed be an investment from which the entire nation, including the federal government would benefit. Not only would it allay the congestion and pollution on our highways, But bring home a bit earlier to their children the two wage-earners that have become necessary to support a family in recent decades. Moreover, given the long depreciation periods of much of the tunnelling structure involved in extending the subway, the corresponding investment could claim particularly lengthy depreciation rates.

This matter of depreciation is of particular relevance to the financing of an extension of Toronto's subway system, in view of its belated recognition by the federal government when the previous Auditor General Denis Desautels in 1999 refused to give unconditional approval of two federal balance sheets unless the capital investments of the federal government were treated as such instead of being written off in a single year as a current expenditure. Little explanation of the immense significance of this step was given to parliament let alone to the general public. Nor has the provision of the act in question have had time to work itself through to show up in the governments accountancy. When it will, the entire net debt will be shown considerably less – the money owed by the government less the depreciated assets of the government that up to now had been carried on the books at a token dollar. Moreover, the investment of government in human capital – education, health, social services – was not even mentioned during the long wrangle between our Prime Minister, at the time Finance Minister in the Chrétien government. And yet such human capital had in the 1960s been widely recognized by economists as the most fruitful investment government could make. In short, there are powerful arguments to support your emphasis on the need for an extension of our subway system. The question is can we afford not to make that investment rather than can we afford to make it? Once that question is answered, the means of financing the project can be found in the *Bank of Canada Act*.

Obviously, you are going to need the full support of your own citizens to make that point of view prevail in Ottawa and Queen's Park. Our organization, the Committee on Monetary and Economic Reform (COMER) had been prominent in getting approval for initiatives urging the federal government to use the central bank for the purposes for which it was nationalized in 1938. That is why COMER has appointed three of its senior members – all from Toronto to lay before you the documentation on the past use of the Bank of Canada in war and peace for the purposes set forth in its preamble.

So long as we have valuable capital investments carried on the government books at a token dollar, we shall continue witnessing the unloading of these assets for a song, privatized and listed on the stock markets they give rise to speculative profits while the taxpayers pay a second time in user fees what they have already paid for as taxpayers.

I am enclosing a copy of COMER's monthly newsletter which is now in its 17th year of publication.

Your truly,

William Krehm, Editor, Economic Reform, *the monthly periodical of COMER*

January 15, 2005
Mayor David Miller and Council
City of Toronto

Dear Mayor Miller:

Re: Funding public transit and other public capital expenditures

Your recent appearance on CTV stating that it will be years before the Toronto subway system will be extended because of the lack of funds leads me to ask if anything has been done since my letter to you of December 22, 2003, in which I spoke of using the Bank of Canada to finance public capital expenditures. I am aware of the arguments against this put forward by your Chief Financial Officer, Ms. Wanda Liczyk, and I am also aware that these arguments were thoroughly discounted by William Krehm, Director of the Committee on Monetary and Economic Reform. I won't take space here to repeat Mr. Krehm's statements, but if you do not have his information on file I will be glad to send it to you.

Suffice it to say that the Bank of Canada could finance public capital expenditures IF the government saw fit to instruct it to do so. It is a purely political decision. The *Bank of Canada Act* provides all the authority needed. A separate Act, the *Bank Act*, which was amended under Prime Minister Brian Mulroney to eliminate the statutory reserves, would have to be amended again to reinstate the reserves in order to control the amount of money created and avoid inflation.

While funds for essential services are slashed and the infrastructure deficit climbs, the federal government continues to spend billions (currently about $35 billion) annually on unnecessary interest. On top of that provincial governments also spend billions on unnecessary interest (about $10 billion in Ontario), and the City of Toronto cannot carry out necessary capital projects.

As mentioned in my previous letter, for 35 years from 1939

to 1974 much of the government's capital expenditures were financed by the Bank of Canada. The advantages of using our publicly owned bank can be enormous. Not only could debt be carried for the cost of administration (which for the Federal Government has been as low as 0.37%), but it could also be carried for the expected life of the asset so that the debt is always offset by the depreciating value of the asset. For example, if a given capital acquisition has a life span of 50 years and costs $100 million, payments would be $2 million a year plus the cost of administering the loan – less than half of 1%. Contrast this with borrowing $100 million at, say, 6% for 20 years. Payments would amount to $8.5 million a year and the total cost would amount to $170 million.

The City of Toronto adopted a resolution pertaining to the Bank of Canada at its regular meeting held on April 23 to 27 and its special meeting held on April 30 to May 2, 2001. It requested that "the Federal Minister of Finance, in conjunction with the Province of Ontario, provide low cost, below prime, long-term loans to municipalities, such as through the Bank of Canada." The resolution was sent to the then Minister of Finance, the Hon. Paul Martin as well as to the Federation of Canadian Municipalities and the Association of Municipalities of Ontario.

The City of Windsor is the latest municipality to adopt a resolution in support of using the Bank of Canada to provide financing for public capital expenditures, bringing the total number of municipalities to do so to 17. Will the City of Toronto provide leadership and press the government to act on this issue?

Richard Priestman, Committee on Monetary and Economic Reform, Kingston

January 15, 2005
Gilles Duceppe, Leader
Bloc Quebecois

Dear Mr. Duceppe:

The Committee on Monetary and Economic Policy (Kingston) would like to know what the Bloc's position is with respect to using the Bank of Canada for financing public capital expenditures or, to put it another way, to carry federal public debt. As you may be aware, Canada's federal public debt ballooned over the short space of twenty years reaching a high of more than $588 billion in 1997 and consists almost entirely of interest (94%). Today it is still over $500 billion.

This state of affairs has occurred because during this time the government has been using the private sector to finance its long-term capital needs instead of using its own bank, the Bank of Canada, where any interest paid by the government to it is returned as dividends less the cost of administration. As a result of this huge debt the government has paid hundreds of billions of dollars in unnecessary interest, and uses the debt and debt servicing costs as an excuse for slashing its funding for health and other services, infrastructure and transfer payments to provinces. It is one of the most important issues facing us because other problems are made worse by the lack of adequate funding.

In spite of numerous letters to Paul Martin as Minister of Finance, and now to Finance Minister Ralph Goodale, the government has not moved to increase its use of the Bank of Canada to finance capital expenditures as it did prior to 1974.

Few Canadians know about this because few politicians talk about it publicly. It needs to be brought into the open! It needs to be raised in Parliament! And the government must be pushed on this issue again and again and again, or it will be left to die. Henry Ford was quoted as saying that if people really understood how money is created we would have a revolution. If Canadians really come to understand how our government has spent hundreds of billions of dollars unnecessarily on interest, that the cut backs which occurred during the 1990s were unnecessary and all the resulting pain and suffering could have been avoided, there would be a revolution – a revolution of ideas about how money is created and controlled.

I look forward to your reply.

Richard Priestman, Committee on Monetary and Economic Reform, Kingston

A BOOK BY JAMES GIBB STUART, OSSIAN PUBLISHERS, GLASGOW, UK

"Fantopia"

THIS IS A WORTHY SEQUEL to the first of the series, written with the same dry, uplifting mockery, tongue ever in cheek but never bitten. To begin, Gibb Stuart neatly disposes of the eternal evaders, who slip out of the back door of any serious discussion pleading that they "are not economists" – as though being an "economist" were a blessed estate "Like Nelson at Trafalgar, they put the telescope to the blind eye, and thereby manage to ignore the obvious." Instead, Stuart betakes himself to his beloved never-never land, and invents a new set of characters for the occasion. "Once upon a time there lived a Talented Engraver who worked on specially etched and watermarked paper to produce beautiful designs which became highly prized and admired. And because he was concerned for the happiness of the society around him, he bestowed some of his coveted designs upon distressed areas of the community, and soon discovered that they could trade the engravings for food and shelter and all things a poverty-stricken environment would most require.

"In response to increasing demand, the Engraver moved on to produce a range of designs that were even more remarkable than the first, and stamped them with denominations in Fantopian paper crowns, so that the recipients would know what value to put on their acquisitions when they exchanged them for necessities of life. The engravings spread far and wide across the queendom, were universally accepted, because they put purchasing power in the hands of the erstwhile deprived and sought out the otherwise unused resources within the community.

"Only the bankers and economists were worried. They said the design notes had become a new kind of currency which would be *vastly inflationary* because it increased the money supply, and encouraged excess activity within a monetary system whose checks and balances depended upon a continuing measure of unrequited demand."

There you have the naked essence of a hangup laid bare in terms that can be fully grasped by even those without a Ph.D.

"They tried to have the Engraver arraigned as a forger and counterfeiter, but failed to substantiate the charges because he was shown not to have peddled his notes deceitfully, and deriving no personal benefit from the distribution of his handiwork beyond the cost of paper and printing.

"In retaliation, the various private banking houses seized and sequestered the design notes whenever they came into their hands, using them as collateral for the issue of negotiable bank credit which was loaned out at the going rate of interest." Bull's eye.

But isn't this a fairy tale? To meet that objection, Gibb Stuart, like the Talented Engraver punctuates his wonderful story-telling with quotations in red ink: from Plato: "I wonder if we could contrive some magnificent myth that would in itself carry conviction to our whole community (from Smith, H.N., MP (1944), *The Politics of Plenty*, G. Allen & Unwin Ltd., London)."

Two Monies in Conflict

"As long as money has to perform two functions – that of 'tickets to consume' and at the same time that of a store of 'wealth in itself' available for saving and investment – there will inevitably be a shortage of purchasing power in the consumers' market.

"This was not a threat to be taken lightly, for the bankers had much power in Fantopia. At the advent of the New Era a benign Chancellor of the Exchequer had bestowed upon them total control of interest rates and money aggregates. They were to be his champions in the battle against *inflation*, and few could agree about its effects and causes. In the old days of strikes and industrial disruption it had been diagnosed as a situation where *too much money was chasing too few goods*. But when automation and technology had solved the manufacturing problem, and the shops and supermarkets were packed with many more goods than the public could want or need to buy, there had to be another reason.

"The economists said that the matter was more complex, much more so than the ordinary person could be expected to understand. The trick, as they explained it, was to see that a certain level of demand was never satisfied. It meant lowering the expectations of certain sections of humanity, deferring their prospects of social and material uplift so as to cultivate a pool of idle resources which could always be used to soften the impact when there were signs of increased activity within the economy.

"'*The poor are always with us*,' said the dignitaries of Church and State, and if they said it with regret and piety, and accompanied it with a prayer for the ultimate salvation of all mankind, the dictum was generally accepted without qualm or question. People just had to realize that everything from the food they ate and the water they drank, perhaps one day even the air they breathed, came at a price that would have to be paid if this *inflation* monster was to be fought to a standstill."

Tumbledum and Tumbledee

Since the public has through advertising been led to overdevelop their taste for fair tales, Gibb Stuart gives his tale a turn at this point that, though couched in mythic language, becomes very concrete and practical, the sort of thing you can knock your knuckles against even while your exhausted mind takes a holiday.

"The controversy was still raging when two major construction projects began to attract nationwide attention. Tumbledum and Tumbledee were two similar towns situated at extremities of the queendom, each built upon broad river estuaries which, with the rapid development of motor traffic, eagerly required bridging.

"But whereas the town fathers of Tumbledum proposed to pay for the entire outlay by means of sound city finance – and engaged a renowned firm of merchant bankers to guide and advise them – the inhabitants of Tumbledee were electrified by the news that *their* elected members had been in touch with the Talented Engraver, who was promising to produce a unique range of designs which, stamped in appropriate denominations, would be presented as collateral for free, stage payments and all other costs and expenses that would fall due during the various stages of construction.

"There was surprise and fury, disbelief and derision all at once in the City. They had accepted the design notes circulating amongst the poorer communities, stimulating a certain amount of enterprise and commercial activity where none had existed before. But to consider such unorthodox methods for funding a major infra-structural project costing in excess of a million paper crowns? It was absurd. It had never been done before. It would make a nonsense of Exchequer constraints on the economy. It would destroy the value of the Fantopian crown on the international exchanges. The bridge would never be finished. Its approach works would lie mouldering and rusting, waiting for some wiser heads to assume responsibility.

"By contrast, said the market analysts, Tumbledum would have its bridge on time. It would be up and functioning, and beginning to pay for itself, the citizens of all Fantopia would come to rue the day when even a tiny minority of their number had been tempted to pursue the illusory benefits of *maundy* money, as the Engraver's notes had come to be called. *Maundy* was a medieval distribution by the monarch to the poor.

"Only in the manner of financing did the contracts differ. At Tumbledum, when staged disbursements were due, there were simply credited in bank drafts drawn upon one of the most highly respected of City institutions. For the progress payments at Tumbledee, the Engraver produced designs of such artistry that they immediately commanded their face value in the market, and the construction work went on unhindered. *Both bridges were completed on time.*

"For the Tumbledeenies traffic rolled freely across the estuary as soon as the visiting dignitary could deliver his speech and cut the red tape at the opening ceremony. For the Tumbledummies there was a short delay as the builders hurriedly installed toll booths at each end of the approach roads. This was necessary to cover the cost of the bank interest, which had been levied progressively on each of the stage payments, and was now accumulating."

However, it is doing our readers no favour giving them a disjointed second-hand version of something that in the original is pure delight. It sheds light on a broadly misunderstood subject that holds a headlock on all of society's aspirations. You will shortly be able read the original and enjoy Gibb Stuart's cast of characters, chosen to illuminate the amazing phenomenon of the engraver's miraculous designs. The panel consisted of a Banker, an Economist, a Politician, a Journalist, and an Antiquarian. It was the Antiquarian, undoubtedly because of his professional knowledge of history, who peered best into the future, and understood what was needed in the present. How the panel members interacted is a rich study in psychology that confronts us every day in whatever political arena.

The book is a little marvel, quite the equivalent of painless dentistry, but completely living up to its claims. With one tiny lapse. The quotation from Abraham Lincoln on monetary reform was actually not said by him, but has long since been proved to have been a translation into words of what he did with his issue of unbacked Greenbanks that made the Civil War a struggle against not one but two forms of slavery. Our American cousins have a weakness for exaggeration, and we rely on the Scots to keep the record straight.[1] With that little reservation, I highly recommend the sequel to the original Fantopia for delightful learning. Further information can be gotten from Ossian Publishers Ltd., 268 Bath Street, Glasgow G2 4JR, UK.

William Krehm

1. Our conscientious research department pulled me up on this bit of unconscious jingoism. As Keith Wilde so well set forth in our last issue, one of the most effective promoters of the unauthentic Lincoln quotes was actually a heroic Canadian monetary reformer, G.G. McGeer. In his enthusiasm he actually translated Lincoln's great deed in issuing unbacked Greenbacks to finance the Civil War into a direct quote. As Mayor of Vancouver, and eventually a federal Senator, his tremendous efforts were largely responsible for the nationalization of the Bank of Canada in 1938.

Perks of Altruism

THE WILES of evolutionary adaptation for species survival once inspired the faith in a Creator who blessed the chosen with progeny as numerous as the sand on the seashore, and punished tribes of stubborn sinners with extinction. Today the tsunamis have brought the two-faced miracle into the headlines again in terms more accessible to us. And, for us, good deeds and biological rewards almost have to have a scientific link. And the latest evidence suggests that they do indeed.

In *The Globe and Mail* (15/01, "Doing good deeds can improve health, make you happier, scientists suggest" by Erin Anderssen) informs us: "If Canadians are finding it easier to fight off the sniffles lately, feeling lighter in their step, or sleeping like a dream, a batch of new science has proposed a possible explanation. Good deeds are good medicine.

"In the past three weeks, Canadians have performed more than their share of generous acts for strangers, from assisting the presidential election in the Ukraine, to donating their time and money – more than $147 million – to victims of the tsunamis in Asia.

"Overdosing on altruism may have a hidden perk.

"Researchers call it the 'helper's high,' the same kind of endorphin rush that runners get loping along a trail. A growing number of studies suggest this high can give the immune system a boost, speedy recovery from surgery and cut down on those restless nights.

"The science suggests that the old saying, 'It's better to give than to receive,' is literally true, said Jeffrey Schloss, an evolutionary biologist at Westmount College in California. 'It's not just an oral cliché.'

"Using brain scans, scientists have found evidence that human beings are 'hard-wired' to help each other."

"Experiments show that thinking about someone else's problems lights up the same part of the brain that gets activated when we reflect on our own, while compassion registers in the brain's pleasure zones.

"Good deeds make us feel more secure in our communities and reduce stress – two keys to the health benefits of philanthropy,' said psychiatrist Greg Fricchione who studied altruism at Massachusetts General Hospital. 'We are born to find social solutions for our problems,'

"When researchers sampled the saliva of Harvard students watching a videotape of Mother Theresa, they found evidence of temporary spikes in immunity-boosting chemicals. Women considered good neighbours in their community have been found to have higher levels of oxytocin, a hormone linked to a feeling of well-being – although scientists have not established which comes first, the feel-good hormones, or the good deeds.

"Stephen Post, director of the Institute for Research On Unlimited Love, which financed a scientific study of altruism, points out that how long the pick-me-up lasts depends on the extent and nature of the good deeds.

"Performing them for good press only is believed to slash the health payoff. In the same way that it pays to eat broccoli several times a week, research suggests you'll be healthier offering up regular servings of compassion. One study even puts a number on it – after tracking the moods and activities of subjects, it proposes that five acts of altruism a week is what it takes to substantially increase happiness."

This mental and moral shake-up that is emerging from the salvage effort in the wake of the Asian Tsunamis is putting in a new light the neglected work of the American economic historian Douglass C. North. We have dealt with him in connection with the soul-searching of two youthful leaders of the 1989 Tianamen Square pro-democratic demonstration so savagely repressed by the government. They met again in Taiwan after one of them, Wang Dan, was finally released from six years in prison, and the other, who had the good fortune to escape, and was able to pursue his studies in Europe and Harvard. Into the next morning, they discussed whether they had been justified in encouraging demonstrations for democracy that led to such killing.

Is Altruism Rational?

They were haunted by the dilemma, "Was it right and helpful to have exposed themselves and countless others to such "irrational" sacrifices? In an article in the October, 2004 *Economic Reform* ("Heroism or Foolhardiness") I brought in the writings of the American economic historian Douglass C. North who had been awarded a "Nobel Price for Economics "for his work on the role of "irrational" self-sacrifice in economic progress. The very subject clashes with the official belief in the maximising of selfish money-making as the only "rational" economic activity.

I quote from the passage on North's work: "Though of a Marxist background, for lack of anything better, North takes as his point of departure the standard neoclassical model to show how it misleads. This he achieves by extending that theory far beyond its traditional bounds. For example, he defines social capital as 'human capital, natural resources, technology and knowledge.' What a gush of fresh air! It contrasts with the view of equilibrium theory where government capital is not recognized, and the destruction of non-marketed capital is not reflected in government ledgers. To this he applies the maximising postulate [which] will result in investment in whatever part of the capital stock has the highest rate of return. New types of physical and human capital will then be invented and types of natural resources discovered when the rate of return to be earned by investing forgone consumption in invention and natural resources exceeds the return in the existing machines and skills.

"This neoclassical formulation begs all the interesting questions. Its world is a frictionless one in which institutions do not exist and all changes occur through perfectly operating markets…. However, throughout history, many resources are closer to common property than exclusively owned. As a result the necessary conditions for achieving the marginally efficient solution have never existed. He brings in the 'national heritage' of Major Douglas without even intending to."

"Individuals may ignore a personal calculus of cost/benefits. Mansur Olson in *The Logic of Collective Action* (1965) demonstrated when large groups were organized to create change but did not possess some exclusive benefit to members, they tended to be unstable and disappear. In essence, rational individuals will not incur the costs of participating in large group action when the same benefits can be received as a *free rider*.

"North goes on: 'The Marxist finesses the entire issue by arguing that classes are the initiators of structural change. The best evidence that this is not standard behaviour comes from Marxist activists themselves: they devote enormous energies attempting to convince the proletariat to behave as a class.

"Could it be that humanity up to now has survived as a species, because of a 'rogue gene' that violates the 'natural law' of the self-balancing market. That gene apparently occurs often enough to produce sufficient individuals ready to risk their lives that the tribe may survive."

The scientific studies mentioned in the *G&M* article suggest that the tongue-in-cheek hypothesis of "rogue genes" may no longer be needed. There would seem to be deep psychological and even physical advantages to the individual in making sacrifices on behalf of his fellow-man. And from the evolutionary logic of species survival that does make sense.

In his remarkable *The Lost Science of Money*, Stephen Zarlenga. establishes the continuity of an underground tradition of the key role of token as distinguished from commodity money. He traces it back at least three thousand years. Though repressed over long periods, it resurfaces as an important tool for the management of trading societies. The costs of keeping that chain unbroken are immense in terms of personal sacrifice – to the point that the efforts of small groups to do so are considered by many as a form of madness. It is consoling to have confirmed that there are even some personal advantages to efforts not always evident to the naked eye.

William Krehm

Defending the Framework that Nested Society's Gains

SOMETHING has been bothering me, deep at the back of my mind. So far back, indeed, that I must be excused for thinking out loud about some basic thought processes, that were better at this stage kept private. I note that Gordon Coggins by a different approach is aware of the same troubling bass figure in contemporary thinking – persistent to the point of intrusiveness.

All past achievements in theorizing and policy-making tended to be achieved within a very local framework. "Local," moreover, is a highly relative term. The very success of your "local effort" is likely to bring you onto a broader, most universal stage, which will turn out still local vis-a-vis the next pushing back of horizons. Noting the progression, is it not a fact that rhetorical convictions creep up on us that broader visions are better than mere "local" ones?

But it is a stubborn truth that we ourselves are local phenomena, as are our wives and children, and the meals they need, and the clothes they wear.

And if we abandon the local framework in which our achievements were originally conceived, do we not risk surrendering what has already been achieved and blocking future progress on strictly ideological grounds? Are we not risking abandoning solid past achievements, by grasping blindly at the unanalyzed potentially more universal setting? May the more ambitious sweep not prove a pitfall rather than an aid to further advance? And may they not be staked out as a "local" playground for some transnational corporation? Must we not carefully check to make sure we have not been sold someone else's ideology?

Of all places, I found help with my half-articulated problem in the following passage of Arnold Schoenberg's *Theory of Harmony*, published in the original German in 1911, translated by Roy E. Carter, Faber & Faber, 1978. For those not familiar with this province of music, let me note that Schoenberg was the essentially self-taught composer who brought down the tyranny of scale systems, conventional or otherwise, and brought forth the relation of any note to any other note as important for the freedom of creation beyond the prearranged relationships in a predetermined scale. That opened up the resources for expressing new needs of a rapidly changing world. For years while revolutionizing musical thought and creativity – and perhaps because of it – he had earned his living as a bank clerk. Here is his electrifying passage that I wish to share with you:

"It is entirely possible that in spite of an observation falsely construed as fundamental, we may, by inference or through intuition, arrive at correct results; whereas it is not at all a proved fact that more correct or better observation would necessarily yield more correct or better conclusions. Thus, the alchemists, in spite of their rather poor instruments, recognized the possibility of transmuting the elements, whereas the much better equipped chemists of the nineteenth century considered the elements irreducible and unalterable, an opinion that has since been disproved. If this view [of 19th century chemists] has now been superseded, we owe this fact, not to better observations... but to an accidental discovery. The advance, therefore, did not come as a necessary consequence of anything; it could not have been predicted on the basis of any particular accomplishment; it appeared rather in spite of all efforts, unexpected, undeserved, and perhaps even undesired.

"Now if the correct explanation must be the goal of all inquiry, even though the explanation does almost always turn out to be wrong, we still do not have to allow our pleasure in searching for explanations to be spoiled. On the contrary, we should be satisfied with this pleasure as perhaps the only positive result of all our trouble."

Apply this to the current assumption that because broader more universal frameworks are assumed to have been the highway of past progress, that abandoning special limitations is in itself a guarantee of progress. Such thinking – mobilized to justify the outsourcing of vital industries and innumerable jobs, the importation of a degree of unemployment and reduced living standards unknown in the advanced countries for decades; the preemptive war in Iraq; and Washington's uncontrollable craving for the ultimate space weapon. All are presented as aspects of the one irresistible onslaught of progress against local restrictions.

But let me pass from the unlimitedly great to the other end of the spectrum to make the same nagging point. *The Wall Street Journal* (07/01, "Drivers Deliver Trouble to FedEx By Seeking Employee Benefits" by Monica Langley): "Madison, Tenn. – As a driver for FedEx's ground division, Brion Butterhaugh, must wear a full FedEx uniform, a long list of delivery and pick-up times and hook his truck keys on the finger FedEx tells him to when walking to doors to deliver packages (the little finger of the nonwriting hand).

"Mr. Butterhaugh, 41 years old, isn't a FedEx employee. He's one of 13,000 'contract' drivers who operate their own trucks and pay for their gas and other expenses. The company says these drivers are 'independent' and has advertised that becoming a contractor is a way to 'be you own boss.'

"But some contractors have set off a high-stakes battle with FedEx by contending the company calls all the shots in their operations. They say rules such as the little-finger requirement show they're essentially employees of FedEx, with all the risks and none of the benefits, such as health insurance and a retirement plan.

"In July 2004, FedEx Ground drivers who had filed a class-action lawsuit against the company won a victory when a California state court ruled that they are employees because of FedEx's 'close to absolute actual control' over drivers."

The Giants as Champions of Small Enterprise?

"The Internal Revenue Service is also investigating FedEx's driver classification, prompted by driver complaints, according to people familiar with the situation. The tax agency will examine whether FedEx has 'pushed the envelope of control so far' that it's no longer in compliance with an earlier agreement under which its predecessor company was permitted to count drivers as independent contractors, according to one knowledgeable person. An IRS spokesman refused to comment. FedEx isn't aware of any IRS probe.

"The issue has become potentially serious for FedEx over the past year as it battles United Parcel Service Inc. In the fast-growing parcel-delivery business.

"The US companies have long sought to get an edge by treating workers as independent contractors instead of employees. Employees receive benefits such as health care, paid vacations and pensions. And the law requires companies to pay 6.2% of the first $90,000 of an employee's salary in 2005 for Social Security taxes as well as 1.45% of all salary for Medicare taxes.

"From coal miners in the 1940s to Microsoft Corp. programmers in the 1990s, hired hands seeking to be classified as employees have clashed with companies. In recent years the IRS, courts and state agencies that determine worker classification have focused on one key issue: how much control the company exerts on the day-to-day activities of the worker. A worker is likely to be considered an employee if he or she works set hours, is required to follow instructions on how to do the job, receives training from an employer and works on the employer's premises.

"The IRS has estimated that in 2001 'sole proprietors' – people such as the contract drivers who report their business income on their personal tax returns – failed to pay $81 billion in taxes they owed. The Government Accountability Office, the investigative arm of Congress, has estimated that 38% of employers examined by the IRS have misclassified workers as independent contractors.

"FedEx, which originally focused on shipping packages by air, got into the ground delivery business in 1998 to compete directly with UPS. It acquired a ground-delivery company, Caliber System Inc., that had fended off a string of challenges, including on from the IRS, seeking to designate its drivers as contractors.

"Luis Espinoza of Santa Cruz, Calif., says becoming a FedEx Ground contract was a good outlet for his entrepreneurial drive. Mr. Espinoza worked odd jobs at minimum wage for a construction company until he signed up to drive for FedEx Ground. With a $5,000 investment and a $700 monthly rental of a van, he started a route and now had three routes. He says he earns about $90,000 a year on revenue of $200,000.

"Some current and former FedEx Ground drivers say FedEx terminal managers set rules for nearly every facet of their work says William Beattie of Mentor, Ohio, a driver for 15 years. 'I can name only one business decision I'm allowed to make without FedEx approval – where to get my gas.

"John Marcellino, who drives in the area around Yosemite National Park in California and is also a plaintiff, says a FedEx manager told him to cut his hair and take off his earring. 'I'm even told when to change my truck's tires and get an oil change."

Our life style in an increasing number of respects is becoming a mere by-product of corporations' drive to maximize their growth. And inevitably the goal of universal independent private property is touted to make possible its exact opposite. Whether big or small is beautiful increasingly depends on the power of whoever has an interest in saying so.

William Krehm

Derivatives and Hedge Funds — How They Do and Don't Work

THIS EFFORT had a remarkable beginning. Last September Robert Mathews of Chase, BC, sent us a note: "I want to renew my membership to COMER and a subscription to *ER*. I recall seeing mention of a 'lifetime membership.' Is that still available?"

To which your editor replied: "I am flattered indeed by your enquiry re a lifetime membership. I suppose I should enquire 'Whose lifetime?' I am 90, but you may have noted that we are recruiting and developing a bevy of talented writers so that *ER* is the product of more people spanning several generations from a 17-year-old high-school student's meditations on the two 11/09 black anniversaries – the Twin Towers but also the Washington-backed coup of General Pinochet in Chile. There are also a growing core of devoted writers closer to their physical prime than the original founders of COMER. We appreciate your enquiry far beyond the money involved.

Robert's reply came: "On the basis of my belief that you will still be thinking, analyzing and writing for *ER* for at least another 8 years, I am enclosing [the corresponding cheque]. Thanks to COMER for opening the obscure world of economics and shining light on the control levers of G&D."

We are determined to build *ER* to an excellence that will smash the inverse metric that has tightened around any independent assessment of the failed official policies: the greater the scale of their disasters, the less the possibility of voicing dissent from their wrongheadedness. We are determined to bring our publication and interventions in conferences throughout the world to a cogency that will break through this wall.

A few days ago I received another note from Robert that asked in part, "Could you write for *ER* explaining the mechanics of hedge/derivative funds, e.g., 'Who puts whose money where, with what leverage, and under what circumstances, what are the main risk factors, etc.'"

Let us begin with the article in *The Globe and Mail* (20/01/05, "Bankers raise red flag over hedge funds" by Sinclair Stewart). "Canada's major banks are calling for greater regulatory scrutiny of the burgeoning hedge-fund industry, an area of the market that has increasingly found favour with retail investors looking for an alternative to mutual funds.

"Gordon Nixon, CEO of Royal Bank of Canada, said the sheer size of the hedge fund market, coupled with the speed at which it is growing, is cause for concern in financial markets.

"'I think it reinforces the importance of sound and increased regulatory scrutiny,' he said during a panel discussion of banking executives at an investor conference yesterday. We all worry about it. It's a very complex market. Certainly the regulators are starting to look at the whole hedge fund market a bit more carefully and that's something we would very much encourage."

Managing Risk by Keeping It High

Yet for some two decades bankers, central and commercial, raised every possible obstacle to prevent the registration and control of derivatives and thus of hedge funds. That rhetorical turn-around needs some background. But that requires no great amount of new excavation. I merely turned to the COMER book *Meltdown*, published in 1999 that contains key extracts from ER during the first ten years of its publication. So readily was the material available, that I concluded right there that it was time to start planning a sequel of that volume covering the next few years of valuable critique that we and others have made since the original volume appeared.

And such a disingenuous statement from the head of one of Canada's largest banks must be taken seriously. For our banks not only had been bailed out of their speculative losses in areas incompatible with banking in 1991, but the manner in which this happened – the phasing out of their statutory reserves – vastly increased the leverage of their powers of money creation. Shortly afterwards, they were further deregulated to allow them to take over brokerages, merchant and investment banking, derivative boutiques, insurance companies. This combined the new higher leverage of their powers of money creation with access to the capital pools essential to these new business this deregulation allowed them to take on. When this was underway the banks justified it by the need for them to acquire the size and power of their Japanese competitors to match and even outstrip them in the glorious "kick-ass" contest (an elegant expression much used by them in those heady days). We pointed out – to no effect – that much of those great banks had already lost much or even more than their capital in the euro-dollar speculative market and were no longer lending.

Confirmation of an official change of attitude towards unregulated derivatives has come from the federal budget just brought down in Canada. But again the dogged refusal to come clean with the full extent of the disaster of the policy being abandoned informs us that power is still being clutched in the same hands. And that will guarantee us against even more outrageous extensions of these same policies in the future. Meanwhile, in *The Globe and Mail* (25/02) Andrew Willis has this to say in a column headed "Derivatives – Banks lose on budget's foreign investing changes": "For 34 years, it was the sweetest of jobs. Two generations of Canadian derivative specialists came to work each day, found new ways for investors to get around Ottawa's ridiculous restrictions on foreign investing, banked sweet fees, and went home. Helping both the institutional and retail crowd get better returns, with less risks, was a great way to make a living.

"However, this sophisticated and total legal use of derivatives made a mockery of the federal foreign content limits, while adding needless costs to pension plans and various species of mutual fund. To his credit Finance Minister Ralph Goodale put a bullet in the whole concept yesterday.

"For the banks and a few fund managers, Mr. Goodale's move was one of those be-careful-what-you-ask-for situations. 'The big losers in this budget move are those banks that were counterparties in the derivative contracts that got around the content limits, along with those innovators who came up with these structures,' said John Hall, a top fund lawyer at Borden Ladner Gervais.

"All the big banks were in this game earning fees that likely averaged about 20 basis points (there are 100 basis points in a percentage point) to supply these derivatives. It was a low-risk way to make money renting out the balance sheet, and now that income is gone. Over time, those 20 basis points and the other potential gains from unfettered investing will make a big difference on multi-billion dollar portfolios. The pension crowd is already looking at ways to undo existing derivative contracts, and cut costs on their foreign investments."

Fashioning the God of Clay

This remarkable way of avoiding coming clean on a reversal of long defended policy calls for two comments.

(1) The design and peddling of derivatives to keep vital information off corporation balance sheets was far less innocent than Willis seems to know or care to tell. Three of our six largest banks were fined a total of some hundreds of millions of US dollars for having designed the notorious partnership scams that kept side deals off Enron's books. Derivatives likewise led to the bankruptcy of Barclays Bank in London when a junior official of the bank in Singapore had his day with derivatives. This not only cost the Canadian economy hundreds of millions of dollars but left it with a moral black eye. Without derivatives George Soros could not have outgunned the Bank of England to shoot down the British pound in the early 1990s and then gone on to do the same with the Italian lira and other currencies.

(2) In its day the economic authorities beginning with the Bank for International Settlements and the world's central banks resisted any suggestion of regulating Over the Counter derivative markets as an intrusion into the "free market." Now the use of derivatives to get around Canadian foreign investment ceilings is applauded as an assertion of the same "free market." The essential story on derivatives – let alone the full one – is still not told. But the indications are that there is enough explosive material behind the scenes to blow up in the faces of those in power.

What is vital is that the full facts be aired, so that we can learn from an experience highly costly in wealth and morality.

Unquestionably, the new stance of the Royal and other banks on this matter today indicates that we are on the very edge of a new financial blow-out that could well put that of the late 1980s in the shade. To establish a bit of that record, I will quote from *ER's* coverage out of *Meltdown* (10/1996, p. 226).

"We hear a great deal about the omnipotence of the money market. Our central bank in particular professes its helplessness to do anything but consult, indeed anticipate its wishes. It is presented as the embodiment of deeper natural laws that elude ordinary mortals.

"It is surprising therefore that the money market should in fact have been a creation of our central bank, and that it required a great deal of effort, artificial respiration and intravenous feeding to keep it alive before it was able to take over our destinies. Listen to the testimony of George S. Watts who served as archivist of the central bank for many years. The introduction to his book was written by Gerald Bouey, a former governor of the Bank of Canada (*The Bank of Canada – Origins and Early History,* ed. Thomas K. Rymes, Carleton University Press, 1993).

"During the war years and immediately after, the program of controls meant that there was less need for a market mechanism. However, by the end of the 1940s it had become apparent, with the return to peacetime conditions, that not only was the need for innovative steps becoming pressing but that the strong postwar expansion of the economy was creating an environment in which efforts to foster a money market could have prospects for success. For several years, the Bank in trading in treasury bills, had progressively widened the spread between its buying and selling levels to create an incentive for the chartered banks to look elsewhere for buyers.

"These efforts had met with little success and in early 1953 a number of new steps were taken. The principal objective was to broaden the market for treasury bills and other short-term paper by encouraging some of the larger investment dealers to act as 'jobbers,' that is to hold an inventory of short-term securities and other paper and to stand ready to buy or sell. With this end in view, the regular auction of treasury bills was changed from a fortnightly to a weekly basis, a nine-month issue was offered in addition to the three-month issue and the amount outstanding was gradually increased over the next few months from $450 million to $650 million. Concurrently, the Bank of Canada undertook to provide investment dealers who were prepared to take a jobbing position with an alternative means of financing inventories of short-term Government securities through Purchase and Resale Agreements (PRA). Under these arrangements, the Bank would, if required, provide dealers with short-term accommodation by purchasing treasury bills and/or short-term Government bonds under an agreement to resell the securities at a pre-determined cost to the dealer. Initially these facilities were made available to approved dealers at a rate lower than that charged by the banks for call loans, but it was hoped that a true call loan market would develop and that the Bank would become a lender of the last resort.

"It soon became apparent that the steps taken in early 1953 were proving more attractive, and as a result the investment dealers that had been given PRA privileges were shifting their borrowing to the Bank of Canada.... A non-bank market had not developed and the amount held by the general public was about the same as a year earlier. However the BoC's holdings of PRA had risen from nothing to between $15 and $25 million toward the end of 1953 and continued to rise to more than $70 million in June 1954.

"By June 1954 it was possible, with the cooperation of the banks, to take a further decisive step. The BoC had developed a group of approved dealers who were prepared to act as jobbers and the chartered banks agreed they would provide day-to-day accommodation to these dealers, within the limits of their PRA arrangements with the BoC, on the pledge of the same type of securities that were eligible for PRA. call money arrangement with the chartered banks.

"That was the way the BoC fashioned the clay god – the money market – before which it bows in reverence today."

Did the Emperor Ever Wear any Clothes?

ER, 03/1998, p. 309, from an interchange with former Governor of the Bank of Canada in *The Globe and Mail*, 3/02, 1998):

"Mr. Crow's letter abounds in quasi-facts that do not stand up under inspection….

"[For example] "The banks financed this acquisition [of the $60 billion increase in government debt] by raising deposits from the public."

Not so. When a bank takes in $1 as a deposit it appears as an asset in its till and as a debt on the other side of the ledger. It in no way changes its capital position (and thus the amount of bank capital that the Bank of International Settlements *Risk-Based Capital Requirements* of the loans it allows it to make). Those BIS Guidelines declared the debt to be risk-free, which they most certainly are not, because whenever the BoC raises interest rates, the market value of preexisting government debt with lower rates drops. It in no way changes its capital position.

Mr. Crow: "What Mr. Krehm appears to be proposing is that the overall rate of Canadian money creation be determined by the pace at which the supply of government debt expands."

Krehm: "It is odd that Mr. Crow should think so when he is defending money creation [by the banks] by a ratio of assets over legal tender whose denominator is approaching zero, while the numerator is a rapidly shrinking finite number. [This statement is based on their own figures.] Phasing in reserves again would in fact discourage the banks from holding their present mountain of government bonds. That ratio in 1946 was 11:1, In the second quarter of 1997 it had attained 347.1."

That in turn would make the public purse available for pressing human survival needs rather than to fund the casino indulgences of our financial institutions.

The Incredible World of Derivatives

ER, July, 1998, p. 344, *Meltdown*, quoting from an excellent paper by Adam Tickell, Professor of Geography at the University of Southampton:

"The development of modern derivatives stems back to 1848. [In that year] the development of 'to arrive' contracts and men who don't own something are selling that something to men who don't really want it.

"In 1972 the Chicago Mercantile Exchange created the International Money Market which permitted trading in currency futures (the first derivatives contracts not based on physical products). That laid the basis for the development of more esoteric and abstract contracts later on.

"The most basic form of derivative is a variant of the form that developed in Chicago in the 1860s – the 'future.' A buyer of a future agrees to pay a given price on an agreed date for an asset (ranging from agricultural commodities to foreign currency), while the seller of a future agrees to sell on the same terms. Futures enable a buyer to lock into a given price and provide certainty. To ensure that buyers of futures can afford to meet their commitments, they are required to deposit an initial margin payment before they are allowed to trade on an exchange. [The payment varies] according to the volatility of the market and type of asset being traded. For example, trading government securities requires smaller margin payments than trading futures based on equities.

"A swap is an agreement to exchange cashflows between two parties and is effectively made up of a series of futures contracts. Interest rates swaps dominate the market and typically involve the 'counterparties' to exchange their interest rate liabilities. For example, if Firm A is borrowing money at variable interest rates it may wish to protect itself against rising rates. It can then agree to pay fixed interest rates by swapping its borrowing for fixed interest rates with Bank II."

Long Live the Options and Swaptions of the Free Market

"The third common derivative tool is the 'option.' In exchange for a premium, options give buyers the right to buy in the case of a 'call option' or to sell (in the case of a 'put' option) at a predetermined price. Buyers will exercise that right if – and only if – interest rates move in their favour. Sellers, on the other hand, expose themselves to theoretically unlimited risk in exchange for a premium paid and will therefore hedge their exposure themselves. Sellers of options receive premium income for potentially limitless losses and for this reason most sophisticated options traders both assume that they need to trade sufficient options for premium income to be able to cover inevitable losses in the same way as household insurance companies pay for claims by pooling the risk.

"Banks and brokers have developed these three basic forms of derivative instruments into more complex variants, largely by combining features of each. Swaptions, for example, are options to buy swaps and allow purchasers flexibility effectively to terminate another swap contract. For example, if a firm has a ten year swap A which it believes it might want to end after five years, it could buy the options to buy a swap it believes it might wish to end after five years, it could buy the option to buy a swap (a swaption) which has the opposite characteristics of its original swap A and would therefor cancel the costs of A. However, if circumstances determine that it wishes to continue with its original swap, then it will not exercise its swaption. Other more complex derivatives include exotically named instruments such as butterflies, differential swaps, 'strangles' and 'straddles.'

"Derivatives provide institutional investors, corporate treasury departments and bank risk management departments with a number of significant benefits over trading the underlying asset. The principal benefit is that it allows investors to hedge risk, in effect providing insurance against adverse market movements Second, some derivatives provide signals to the wider financial markets which advocates claim, reduces uncertainty. In the case of commodities, rising future prices may be a stimulus for increased production. Third. Derivatives significantly reduce the costs of diversifying portfolios, because investment managers can expose themselves to derivatives based on baskets of stocks rather than on a smaller number of more volatile stocks. Fourth, derivatives are relatively cheap because they effectively operate on leverage. US Treasury futures, for example, require an initial margin payment of only 1.5% of the value of the Treasury Bond.

"Derivatives are more prone than other financial products to liquidity and credit risks. Credit risk is more common and occurs when the counterparty to a trade is unable to meet its obligations. The capacity of some derivatives for high gearing and the implicit non-linear risk structure mean that credit risk is a particular problem of derivatives. As an IMF study put it, derivatives reinforce the on-going process of global financial integration."

A Cheap Way to Circumvent the Law of the Land

"Derivatives are traded in two ways: on organized and regulated exchanges, and 'over the counter' OTC. Exchange-traded derivatives are less flexible than OTC products, have standard structures, require that money be placed with the exchange as a guarantee and that extra margin payments have to be made against adverse market moves. In effect, the exchanges become counterparties to the trades.

"OTC derivatives are tailored products which have no protection from the exchanges and are held off balance-sheet. As a result they are cheaper and their risk profile is higher. The nimble nature of the OTC markets actively encourages the introduction of new products.

"However, concern about the absolute and relative growth of the OTC markets is not confined to left-wing commentators, but include senior investigators, and participants on organized exchanges. That is because the OTC markets are less liquid than exchanges and during periods of turbulence they have enhanced the potential for a widespread collapse of market liquidity throughout the whole financial system.

"One of the contributory factors in the collapse of Barings, for example, was the lack of clarity in the reporting liens. Second, an increasing share of international financial transactions is dominated by a small number of institutions from a small number of countries which have the geographical networks, specialist knowledge and technological expertise to command market power and manage internal risk. In foreign exchange, for example, the top-end dealers have increased their market share from 31% in 1990 to 43% in 1997 and by the end of the century over 75% of the market is expected to be controlled by the top 15 firms. If one of the dominant institutions were to get into difficulty the effect would be serious.

"The collapse of the postwar financial order, when money

was largely national in character and currencies were little traded and largely at fixed exchange rates, undermined the basis of the international regulatory environment. From the development of the Euro dollar markets, in which banks could evade USA regulatory jurisdiction of their dollar holdings in London in the 1960s, international banking ceased being solely an ancillary in trade and investment and began to develop its own dynamic. In the USA these pressures, as well as intensified competition from non-bank financial institutions that had been stimulated by the deregulation of the NY Stock Exchange in 1975, encouraged banks to lobby Congress to relax the regulatory 'burden.' The lobbying was hugely successful, leading to the dismantling of bank regulations, and the establishment of international banking facilities (IBF) in 1981 as a direct challenge to the Euromarkets.

"As Eric Helleiner has emphasized, the failure of the Federal Reserve to dictate the US regulatory environment was a seminal moment in the history of international finance for three reasons. First, it demonstrated that financial institutions could now arbitrage between national regulatory systems and choose the one most conducive to their business aims. Second, the establishment of IBFs, free from tax and domestic US regulatory restrictions, led directly to competitive deregulation in countries which wished to compete with the US and UK as host for financial institutions. Third, the failure of a conservative approach to bank regulation and macro-economic management heralded the development of neo-liberal financial regulation.

"As Helleiner points out, 'the regime's strength should not be overstated. It was focussed only on the narrow task of preserving global stability through lender-of-last-result, regulatory and supervisory activities.'

"Indeed, as derivatives were the fastest growth component of the financial sector, supervisory authorities positively encouraged product innovation in the exchanges within their jurisdiction at the same time as promoting exchanges internally."

The "Washington Consensus" Knocks Out the Windsor Declaration

"The collapse of Barings Bank in 1995, when a single trader managed to evade both internal controls and external supervision to effect a series of disastrous derivative trades, proved to be a seminal moment in international approaches to derivatives regulation. Although the British authorities initially attempted to isolate the impact of the event by claiming both that it was unique to Barings and that the involvement of derivatives was incidental, less publicly oriented supervisors began to take the potential threat from derivatives far more seriously. Within three months of the Barings incident, regulators of the major financial centres issued the 'Windsor declaration' which signalled their willingness to force greater disclosure of information about derivatives exposure, and to develop cooperative structures so that regulators could successfully intervene during emergencies.

"[Yet] it is important to recognise that pro-market regulation is inscribed with a series of ideological understandings about the role of the state. The development of an international policy community in finance centred on the BIS, which is largely technocratic and free from democratic accountability, serves not only to set the tone for international cooperation, it also sets the parameters of thinking. In response to Congressional moves to increase the supervision of over-the-counter derivatives, Alan Greenspan, chairman of the Federal Reserve Board, argued that 'there appears to be no reason for government regulation of off-exchange derivative transactions between institutional counterparties.'

"Credit rating agencies have increasingly assumed a governance role in international finance. Yet it is a form of governance which may be fragile, is unaccountable, and excludes alternate ways of seeing the world. Shortly before the bankruptcy of Orange County (California) in 1995, both Moody's and Standard and Poor's issued very strong grades for the municipality; while high grades were also issued on the sovereign institution and corporate debt of East and South Asian countries prior to the crisis of 1997."

To substantiate this diagnosis from my recent personal experience, I need only add this note to supplement my "Cambridge File" that appeared in *Economic Reform* (10/04): "At the final plenary session of the Cambridge conference of June that I reported on, three most distinguished critics renowned in the academic community for their disbelief in an automatically self-balancing market and other official myths spoke on the subject of derivatives. From the writings of one of these I had learned much of what I know about derivatives.

"Nevertheless, there was a strange omission in what they had to say: it was not made clear whether they were for the regulation of derivatives or not. I asked what their position on that crucial matter might be. From each in turn came the reply that could be summed up 'Such a regulation was not likely.' I could not help myself and interjected: 'I didn't ask whether the regulation of derivatives is likely to happen. I asked "Ought it to happen?"'

"The persistent absence of an answer to so vital a question was more eloquent of the crisis in economic thinking than anything else in the entire conference."

The author of one of the best studies known to me on derivatives and the problems of their regulation, remarked to me some years ago: "the academic community is simply irrelevant to the making of policy in this world." And, understandably, he was not in a position to challenge that verdict, since he is a young man with a family whose future he cannot ignore.

But unless it is seriously challenged by those who feel free and equipped to do so, it is a death sentence – a moral tsunami – for society as we know it. That is why COMER with its limited resources proposes focussing by every means available on setting up the warning signals that society stands in need of.

We propose continuing our presence at as many world economic conferences as seem to hold some promise for addressing this survival issue. We propose using every resource of tact and discretion in getting our message across. Obviously academics who have done important work in the field but cannot endanger their livelihood, are an important part of the bridge that must be thrown up between academia and non-academic economists knowledgeable in the field.

Meanwhile let me complete my answer to the important question of Robert Mathews:" Can you write an article explaining the mechanics of hedge/derivative funds? We have dealt with the essence of the role of derivatives, and these are the farthest-ranging tools with hedge funds tools are constructed. I will therefore confine the balance of my answer in quoting from recent pronouncements of bank chieftains in reversing their long established advocacy of complete global freedom for the use of derivatives.

Wall Street's Darkening Corner

In *The Globe and Mail* (10/01, "Mutual Funds – Market Timing shortchanged investors in 54 funds" by Karen Howlett): "The four companies swept up in market timing scandals revealed that they allowed rapid, in-and-out trading in 54 mutual funds, confirming that the controversial practice cut a wide swath through the Canadian investment community. The trading primarily took place in the companies' international equity funds. There were roughly 500 international equity funds managed by Canadian firms in 2003, the year all market timing activity came to a halt."

[Market timing with respect to such funds allows privileged traders to buy or sell after hours at the closing quotes, possibly after having taken advantage of news customarily released after closing stock exchange hours). Profits earned in this way are at the expense of the non-privileged fund members who can only trade during exchange hours.]

"As part of a settlement agreement with the Ontario Security Commission last month, the four companies – Investors Group Inc., CI Fund Management Ltd., AGF Management Ltd., and AIC Ltd. – have acknowledged that they routinely gave preferential treatment to a select few clients at the expense of long-term investors. About 1.4 million clients in 24 separate funds were affected, CI CEO William Holland, said."

"Canadian-sponsored hedge funds held $14.1 billion in assets as of last June, compared with just $2.5 billion in 1999, according to Investor Economics, a Toronto consulting firm, that is releasing a report on the hedge fund sector this week. Although the industry is dwarfed by the mutual fund business, it is gaining ground at a fast clip. The 46-per-cent compound annual growth rate for hedge funds is 10 times the 4.6-per-cent rate for mutual funds. The numbers are even bigger when you include pension plan money invested in hedge funds.

"The funds – recently referred to as 'the dark corner' of Wall St. by a top US securities regulator – have traditionally catered to wealthy individuals and required minimum investments of hundreds of thousands of dollars. Part of the reason for these limits is that they rely on arbitrage, short selling and other complicated investment techniques. But recent alternatives such as hedge fund 'funds of funds' and 'principal protected' products have provided regular investors with a more affordable way into the sector." Clearly this involves a further level of aggregation which means an additional level of handlers to be paid no matter what the effect on the investment thus accommodated.

But more serious is the following factor: "Hedge funds have

been large buyers of corporate loans and derivative instruments from banks, which have been mopping up their balance sheets after getting scorched by a credit flameout a few years ago. This raises another concern. The same investors who are scurrying to get into the hedge fund game could end up shouldering some of the risk that banks are looking to unload."

This means that the deregulation of banks that allowed them to take over just about all other non-banking finance firms, is now backing up to the peril of other firms and of course individuals who were promised to benefit by from "one-stop banking" which could deliver them directly to the poorhouse.

"There's been a tremendous transfer of risk from the banking financial institutions to other institutions, whether they're pension funds, or insurance companies, or to the individuals via the hedge funds,' said TD Bank CEO Ed Clark."

Our Banks are Teaching Chinese Banks How to Unload Bad Debt

"When corrections occur how does that risk rebound? Does it end up rebounding on us? Mr. Clark said banks face potential reputational problems if average investors are exposed to too much of this risk through their participation in the hedge fund market.

"Are people going to say, 'Well, you guys should have understood that there was this transfer of risk and the consumers couldn't understand the risks they were absorbing,' Mr. Clark asked. 'The banks as a whole sit and worry about this.'

"The purchasing appetite of hedge funds, coupled with their buying clout, has provided much needed liquidity for banks intent on cleaning up their loan books. At the same time the size of these funds is unprecedented, and bankers worry what sort of consequences there may be in the derivatives market when financial conditions sour.

"The US Securities and Exchange Commission, concerned that the opaque nature of the industry could attract fraudsters and other market manipulators, is introducing rules aimed at bringing more transparency to the sector. They are expected to go into force next year."

While the authorities most belatedly have moved themselves to do something about abuses that almost brought down the world financial system less than a decade ago, new designs of crookery have risen. But their deepest roots are in the credo of a self-balancing market that has not been disturbed.

Postscript to Hedge-Derivative Inquiry

Since writing the above, our banks' change of heart on the subject of derivatives and hedges and the causes prompting it are pouring forth in the public prints. On a single page of *The Globe and Mail* (22/02) we have two revealing articles. "CIBC learns costly lesson in hedge funds" by Susanne Craig from *The Wall Street Journal:* "On Wall St., hawking hedge funds has become highly profitable. But a recent arbitration award against the Canadian Imperial Bank of Commerce shows the downside of marketing these lightly regulated vehicles.

"A three-person arbitration panel this month ordered the bank's brokerage arm, CBIC World Markets Inc. to pay almost

$3.6 million US to 11 wealthy investors who lost $5.5 million investing in a NY-based hedge fund marketed by the firm. The funds sometimes make high-stakes bets on stocks and other investments, often using borrowed money to boost returns. In the CIBC case, the aggrieved investors claim the banks' brokers conducted almost no 'due diligence' or research on the fund it sold to its client, part of a hedge-fund family known as Red Coat, and failed to disclose that some of Red Coat's other funds were losers. Then, after they learned the fund was tanking, they weren't allowed to cash out – even though a CIBC employee involved in the marketing efforts for Red Coat was allowed to pull his money.

"Most people who put money in hedge funds have few legal options if they feel they were wronged when the investments go sour, other than the costly process of suing. Brokerage clients, however, agree to settle any disputes through arbitration, usually overseen by the National Association of Securities Dealers. That provides a lower-cost alternative.

"The CIBC case is one of the first big ones involving a hedge fund to snake its way through the arbitration process. Traditionally hedge funds have required an initial investment of at least $1 million. But some of the clients who invested in Red Coat through the CIBC World Markets put down as little as $75,000.

"Red Coat charged investors a 1% management fee, plus 20% of any profits the fund earned. CIBC World Markets got one-fourth of both fees for clients it steered toward Red Coat. CIBC shared those proceeds with its brokers.

"'Red Coat also steered stock-trading business – and the commissions it paid for such services – to the CIBC brokerage. That provided an added incentive for CIBC brokers to steer investment clients to Red Coat,' Philip Aidikoff, the investors' lawyer said."

Was it for such scams that our lordly banks were bailed out of their gambling losses of the 1980s and further deregulated?

Another article – on the same *G&M* page (from Reuters News Agency, "Bankers warned of credit-crunch litigation" by David Wigan, London) – suggests how close we are to the next credit crash.

"A decline in credit markets could prompt a wave of lawsuits against investment banks, as investors ratchet up losses on risky credit derivatives, lawyers said yesterday.

"The warnings come after Barclays Capital last week settled a claim by Germany's HSH Nordbank over a $151 million (USA) collateral debt obligation (CDO), while Italy's Banca Populare di Intra sued Bank of America Corp. for selling credit-linked notes at what it called an 'excessive price with respect to their risk level.'

"Low volatility in the past two years has encouraged investors into highly leveraged investments, such as CDOs. But many do not understand the pitfalls, lawyers say, and will blame their bankers should the bets go wrong.

"'Spread reversal will produce large losses, which inevitably will lead to lawsuits,' said Claude Brown, a partner in the CDO group at Clifford Chance LLP. European and US credit spread are hovering near record tight levels after a sustained period of interest rates and stable ratings. With global growth slowing, however, and interest rates predicted to rise, spreads could widen in coming months, analysts say.

"Collateralized debt obligations are structured assets that can be divided into tranches. Returns are higher than on single-name investments, but lose more when spreads widen or underlying credits default." The first call on securities that support other debt is for that prior purpose. When interest rates are pushed up as our central banks are straining to do, the likelihood of that supported debt being discharged diminishes, and hence those who have bought the securities serving as collateral stand to lose their investment. In a sense it is like a second mortgage.

"Further, says Mr. Brown their complexity makes them fertile grounds for legal machinations. Litigants will argue either they were sold something they didn't want, or were sold a toxic product or exposed to some risk that was hidden from them.

"Among innovations heavily marketed this year are CDO-squared – or CDOs of CDOs – and options on credit default swaps. The credit derivatives markets reached $5 trillion at the end of 2004 and is expected by the British Bankers Association to hit $8 trillion by December, 2006.

"Such is the level of concern among regulators that the Bank for International Settlements last month warned investors to beware of credit ratings on structured products."

Such is the witches' sabbath that Globalization and Deregulation have prepared for us.

William Krehm

From Our Mailbox

17/2/05
The Editor
The Star

Attention: Carol Goar

Carol Goar's well-written summary of Ellen Russell's new study, "What Should We Do with the Federal Budget Surplus?" will, hopefully, stir some to think, but it will be hard for many to break away from the idea that we should reduce interest payments in order to use the money for more worthwhile things. I am one of those, not because I believe that government should reduce interest by "paying down" the debt, but by transferring it in manageable amounts to the Bank of Canada where it can sit at almost no cost to the government until it does become prudent, if ever, to "pay it down." Currently, Canadians are paying about $65 billion a year in interest through our three levels of government – an amount which could go far to improve health care, education, infrastructure and much else.

I believe Ms. Russell is right on the mark. She shows that the federal debt to GDP ratio will fall as a result of economic growth alone – "even with absolutely no debt repayment." She shows that the rate of return on using the surplus to pay down the debt (5.5%) is less than investing it in education (7% to

12.7%), and that "every dollar spent on comprehensive public child care programs produces about $2 worth of benefits." She states that the government should spend the surplus to enhance Canada's economic potential, to reduce poverty, to use it for social programs such as health care, education and affordable housing for example. I agree with all that, but why stop at making better use of the surplus? Why not make better use of the Bank of Canada as well?

If an amount equal to the surplus was transferred to the Bank we would benefit from reduced interest payments and still have the surplus to use as Ms. Russell suggests. The financial community would not like it, especially the chartered banks, but is that a good enough reason for not doing it? Is our government there to benefit a handful of wealthy investors, some of whom don't even live in Canada, or to serve the interests of Canadians as a whole?

To do this, the government would borrow the necessary funds from the Bank of Canada to buy the private sector debt just as it uses its surplus to do the same thing. To avoid inflation from the increased money supply, the Bank could require the chartered banks to put the same amount in reserve (called "statutory reserves") unless it ascertained that the increase in the money supply was appropriate for the growth in the economy. Some will point out that statutory reserves were eliminated from the *Bank Act* by Brian Mulroney in 1991, but what the government takes out, it can put back in.

Some think that the question of using our public bank, the Bank of Canada, to finance public debt is too complex for the "average person" to understand, but it is as simple as getting the cheapest interest rate. If you owned a bank, would you go to your competitor's to make a loan? The government owns 100% of the Bank of Canada. Does it make sense for it to borrow from private interests instead of its own bank?

Richard Priestman

Uncertainty and Correspondence in Economics

The Epistemology of Modern Economics

During the early part of the twentieth century physicists realized that many of the new discoveries their science made could not be adequately described by Newtonian physics. As a result, the theories of relativity and quantum mechanics emerged, and gave rise to important new conceptions, some of which – such as complementarity and the correspondence principle – have implications for other sciences.

Economists, however, have ignored these developments. To this day, they go on embracing an epistemology that holds the world to be fully predictable and peopled by rational economic men.

That leaves economics littered with unrealistic assumptions. Perfect markets are joined by perfect competition, free entry and exit from markets are always possible, and rational agents possess complete information equally available to everyone. Externalities are gotten rid of by cost-free Coase litigation, and, finally, monopolies are aberrations bound to wither away as competition – always trending towards perfection – applies its pressures.

However, few of these assumptions can be supported by the observed facts. For example, in the ubiquitous malls, where the bulk of consumer transactions take place, the trend is growing market corporatization into large, often multi-national firms. It is the small independently owned businesses that wither away, not the monopolistic competing corporations.

Informal Interests

The assumption of fully rational individuals is also highly problematic, seen from the angle of the behavioral sciences. The corporations' willingness to spend almost unlimited sums on marketing, which contains little informative value but a lot of subconscious triggers, suggests that the corporations' also have their doubts about the rationality of economic man.

In a narrow sense, the motivations driving economic activities originate from supply-demand relationships. For instance, when I work for a firm, it is willing to pay me money in exchange for my efforts. Modern economists generally make the assumption that the supply-demand rationale covers all aspects connected with economic activity.

This view glosses over the fact that relations originating in economic interests, such as job situations, also create contexts that interact with other social and cultural aspects. Complicating matters is the fact that such relations are perceived through each individual's filter of beliefs and attitudes, conscious as well as subconscious.

In organizations engaged in economic activities, employees establish networks of work relations as required by their functions. Such relationships will however also develop on the personal level, based on personal likes or dislikes, common background, and other similar factors. Within larger organizations networks of personal relations often turn into informal groups, which can be a significant factor determining how work is organized. For instance, during work group meetings participants' attitudes to proposals might not only be based on the proposals' merits, but also on the personal ties to those making them.

What results may be a complex web of conflicts between the stated function-roles, individual interests, and informal group interests. All such factors play important roles in how organizations reach their goals.

The Uncertainty of Economic Motivations

Such aspects of human behaviour cannot simply be shrugged away. The latter, however, is the approach of the current discipline of economics. Its fundamental theories rest on the principles of rationality and perfect states. However, since the individuals on both sides are driven by mixed motivations, it is impossible to separate exchange sequences from their non-economic context that this approach warrants.

Accordingly, fields of cause-effect uncertainty surround all economic micro events. However, while the uncertainty prevents the outcomes to be fully predictable by value calculations alone, if data of comparable events is available, it becomes possible to express them as statistical probabilities. For instance, no shop owner can accurately predict which customers entering his shop will buy something. But with data recording daily sales and the number of customers entering the shop, he can calculate the likelihood of a sale as a statistical percentage.

Experienced operatives can recognize recurrent patterns as they appear within areas of their expertise and use probability functions to describe them. For instance, the assumption that higher prices sell less and lower prices more – the most basic axiom of current economic theory – is ultimately nothing more than a probability function that changes with specific circumstances. A Christian Dior executive knows that in his company's particular market segment the axiom is very weak – even sometimes turning completely around so that lower prices reduce sales and higher enhance them. Therefore, he intrepidly keeps prices well above the supposed equilibrium point where marginal cost and revenue meets.

Micro and Macro Level Correspondence

One of the new conceptions that arose from the quantum revolution was the correspondence principle, connecting the phenomena of the sub-atomic world to the macroscopic world of everyday life. In economics there also exists a well-recognized dichotomy between microeconomic events and macroeconomic aggregates. What differs is that in the case of economics our field of vision is the micro level, from where we extrapolate the phenomena of the macro level. Thus a macroeconomic phenomenon, such as inflation, only exist as a conceptual construct that we form on the basis of data observed on the micro level.

When interpreting economic events, the nature of the correspondence between the two levels must be taken into account. On the micro level, individuals' interests divide between the supply-side and the demand-side dependent on their function-roles in given contexts. We are however not bound to one-sided function-roles; depending on changing contexts we switch in and out between supply-side and demand-side roles. For example, at my workplace my function-role is supply-side, since I supply my labor to the firm. When I on my way home stop by the local supermarket my function-role switches to the demand-side.

On the macro level the supply-demand dichotomy disappears, since aggregated data are outcomes that fuses the supply and demand interests without telling us anything about their initial distribution. However, the correspondence existing between the two levels means that the causative uncertainty is not resolved when we view phenomena from the macro level, it continues to exist as a submerged condition that will to blur all attempts to pin down the exact causes for observed trend changes.

The Role of Governments

The role of governments in the economy is a heatedly contested question, but in reality much of our interest in macroeconomic phenomena is spurred by the existence of governments. In general, individuals or firms operating on the micro level cannot purposely change macroeconomic trends. Only government can do that.

Government actions, such as a sales tax, change the probability vectors for the affected micro events. But discussing the desirability of a sales tax from the view of the affected private interests lacks the overall macro context needed to make a proper judgement. Such a context, for example, might include providing market places with adequate infrastructures, or the individuals with the social skills they need to work effectively.

A pragmatic approach to governments' role in the economy mainly focuses on analyzing policy alternatives. However, macro variables, such as for example 'economic growth,' are ambiguous with respect to the supply-demand divide on the micro level.

Governments' actions cannot replicate this ambiguity, since their actions are impacts affecting the flow of real variables. Therefore, if a trend is observed in the data aggregates – indicating for instance a looming depression – it is faced with a dilemma: while it can never fully ascertain a trend's exact causes, it has to make a choice of what specific variables it should impact.

The direction of a policy's macro effect is a structural question that can be ascertained by analytical means, but its magnitude depends on motivational factors that drive the individual micro events. The uncertainty regarding the distribution of these at any specific moment makes it impossible to gauge the exact magnitude effect of different policy alternatives.

Government policies that affect macro variables also have income effects, where their impact on the direction of income distributions is a structural question that can be answered by analysis. For example, expanding government's expenditures affect demand-side variables, while cutting personal income taxes effects the supply-side. Both support growth but have different income effects. In situations where it is impossible to make clear-cut cause-effect determinations of the growth impacts, such economic policy differences in a practical sense are reduced to the differences in the income effects they create.

Growth effects dissipate over time as new motivational forces arise at the micro level, caused by new trends in variables such as production methods, consumer habits, and trading patterns. In contrast to this, income effects have cumulative tendencies. Although short-term income effects may seem small, in the long term they can cause significant changes in income distributions. In that case, policy choices become largely dependent upon which interests they serve, and the answers to these questions are not found within the realm of economics but belong to interest-driven politics.

Dix Sandbeck

Cross-currents

WHILE PRESIDENT BUSH is proclaiming the democratization of the world by higher military budgets, counter-currents are gaining momentum. These raise a troublesome question: can democracy prevail by merely increasing the clout of a lone overweening superpower?

Deep doubt on this is spreading into areas that Washington takes for granted. Thus, most of Spain's former colonies are considered as almost protectorates by the US. That was the sense of the Monroe Doctrine and the conquest of the Philippines. Over the years, however, the Monroe Doctrine was kept fresh with more than a sprinkling of gunpowder. In Mexico there were the not always successful interventions into the civil wars of the early 20th century. In Central and South America during and after World War II, Washington set up or supported particularly savage dictatorships. Agents for the purpose were trained in torture at a special school of the US army. In Panama.

Hate or Like Him — The World is Intrigued by Castro

The Latin American countries whose contribution in delivering vital raw materials to the American war machine at prices set by Washington, were denied the closure of that regime when victory was won. Instead, they were excluded from the Marshall Plan or some similar compensation. What came their way instead was brutal military action to enforce the continued low prices for their exports. Like him or hate him, it is no accident that Fidel Castro has been regarded by the Spanish-speaking world not without admiration for having stood up successfully to Washington. Without that he could never have survived the collapse of his Soviet backer.

That appeared centre stage in Spanish politics early in February when the local press reported that the Cuban Foreign Minister, Felipe Perez Roque, would travel to Madrid to advance the arrangements for a visit in 2006 to Cuba of the Spanish King and the president of the Spanish government. Significantly, the announcement was made by the president of the regional council of Andalucia, Manuel Chaves. Chaves himself back from a meeting with Castro, declared to the press that he had found him a 'fascinating personality.' For days there were half-denials and denials that anything had been definitely arranged. for 2006. but what emerged was a practical confirmation that the King of Spain and his Socialist chief of government were headed for a meeting with Fidel Castro. This added to the unpopularity in Washington of the Madrid Government that had already withdrawn its troops from Iraq.

As the ex-colonial power, against whom the legendary victories of the Latin America's War of Independence were won, that proves the immense determination of Spain to live down its past and rally its former colonies around its current international policy. And given Spain's highly successful experience within the European Union, that puts Spain in a unique position as bridge between Latin America and Europe for countervailing Washington's unilateral urges. Not surprisingly the new Secretary of State, Condolezza Rice, gave Spain a wide berth in her recent European travels. The Spanish Foreign Minister,

Miguel Angel Moratinos, did manage a 4 or 5 minute conversation with her at the recent Brussels NATO ministerial meeting, but the deepening chill was evident. Some 19 meetings of the Spanish monarch, president and Latin American heads of government have already taken place.

Spain as Bridge between Europe and Latin America

For all this a vast cultural and political preparation has been necessary. As never before, Spain has come to appreciate the richness of her own vast cultural heritage from a more peaceful Islam; and the sheer crassness with which the Pentagon handles such background. Thus its failure to prevent the looting and destruction of the irreplaceable museum treasures in Baghdad at the beginning of the war. That could hardly be lost on Spaniards who themselves are excavating their local equivalents with reverence. Such factors, as well as their share of Islamic and more local terrorism, all contributed to the withdrawal of Spanish troops from Iraq once the new Socialist-headed government of Rodriguez Zapatero came to power.

Having itself settled the choicest portions of a rich, under-populated continent with disillusioned emigrants from Europe, the United States developed a peculiar insensitivity to other cultures. And left a lone superpower by the demise of the Soviet Union, it fell victim to the temptations of this background. It has, moreover, succumbed to an aggressive commitment to unbounded economic growth. The very scale of its financial and military operations is seen by others as a menace. It has led to imperial plans in high-tech armament in heavens once reserved for the worship of an even Higher Authority. It is overplaying its privilege of churning out debt acceptable as money by an increasingly impatient world.

Today, in fact, the skies are darkening with chickens homeward bound. China has battened on technologies that it has out-maneuvered the United States to trade for leveraged access to its own low labour standards and vast underemployment.

The European Currency Unit is tending to become transformed into a barrier to Washington's boundless ambitions. To this Spain is making a unique contribution.

Patterns within Patterns

But there are patterns within patterns, and to ignore them would leave us unprepared for further surprises. We have been led to put absolute faith in the unique virtues of bigness. It began in financial policy, but tends to move into all other areas including world politics. As in economics, however, "larger" does not necessarily imply "better." Much of what society has done best was nested and nurtured within quite local limits. Sacrifice more modest structures to unlimited growth and you risk undermining the well-being of society itself. That is why growth and globalization must be accompanied with an active concern about keeping essential grass-root structures in a working state. And in this, too, Spain today provides some striking lessons. Many of these arise from the circumstance that apart from Spanish, three other regional languages are spoken in Spain – Catalonian, Gallego akin to Portuguese, and Basque definitely related to no other known tongue. With the restora-

tion of democracy this has given rise to a considerable demand for the autonomy within the Spain of such local linguistic regions. This is taking place at the very time that the European Union is preparing the acceptance of another 15 nations into its midst.

Thus the Spanish rightist paper *ABC* (8/2, "Notas Clinicas" by Jon Juaristi) writes: "The introduction of the formula of 'national communities' into our political vocabulary of progressive revolution presently under way has raised confusion to a level that touches on semantic catastrophe." What is more, the already achieved settlement between the Catalan government and the central Spanish authority is being reopened by the Catalan leader Pulcercos under the stimulus of the aggressive position of the Basques in their current negotiations with Madrid. "The spokesman of the ERC (the Catalan political centrist party) threatens taking Catalonia out of Spain, and proposes a 'friendly relationship with Spain' as does the *lehendakart* (Basque chieftain) Ibarreche." There is thus a reshaping of the relationship between the peninsular cultures and peoples even as political consolidation proceeds. There is nothing inevitable or even absolutely useful in globalization and deregulation. If you take even consolidation on a national scale, let alone on an international one as sole criterion, you risk creating more problems than you solve.

That is a basic lesson of Canada's surrender in accepting North American Free Trade Alliance that we may have to re-learn as Europe is beginning to cope with it.

A further important point: To make possible education and public life in a second language and culture inevitable gives rise to substantial additional costs. These would include what should be considered investments rather than just current spending. There is no way of estimating the monetary loss when a language and a culture are allowed to disappear. And in our own case as a historic immigration country, a modest amount of education of the newcomers directed to preserving and developing their command of their ancestral tongue and cultural would not only enrich our domestic public life, but be of immense value in a world where globalization is being thrust down our throats. That means that access to cheap central bank financing must be allowed for financing such investments.[1] Ottawa owes us comparative cost studies of the surrender of our money creation to our commercial banks that we had just bailed out of their gambling losses in 1991 and what it would cost to institute classes of European and Asiatic immigrants in their mother tongues. Has our Minister of Finance ever ordered research on the cost of educating an Anglo- or French Canadian to proficiency in Japanese or any other Asian language?

Obviously the European Union some of whose members are giving special attention to the needs of such minority cultures must consider a similar course. The current inflexibility of the European Union's central bank is likely to be challenged by the cross currents that are beginning to appear in the world's affairs.

The comparative benefit studies proposed would compare the cost to Canada of deregulating and subsidizing our banks to permit no less than three of the largest to feature in the settlements with the regulatory authorities in the US in connection with the Enron scandal alone, with a program of preserving and nurturing our aboriginal and immigrant cultures for domestic as well as trade benefits.

William Krehm

1. In Canada that would be a further argument for putting into practice an arrangement that is still in the *Bank of Canada Act* (Article 18(c)): "The Bank may buy and sell securities or guaranteed by Canada or any province." Since the federal government is the sole shareholder of our central bank, that means that the interest paid to the Bank of Canada by Quebec or any other province to preserve French culture or a native language and culture could be financed through the Bank of Canada. And the interest paid on that would return (less the Bank's overhead costs for such financing) would end up with the federal government. All that is needed is an agreement with the provinces for a negotiated part of such dividends be passed on to the junior government in question.

Debt Rising

A NEW REPORT from CIBC World Markets (not available to the public) gives cause for alarm. Household debt rose 7% last year (20% over the past decade) and now stands at 110% of disposable income. Debt has been rising faster than assets despite the run-up in home prices.

Interest payments on the debt are about 8% of disposable income. However about 40% of Canadians have little or no debt, and they hold about $40 billion in cash. This means that the debtors must spend an average of 14% of their disposable income on interest. When we add in the interest paid on corporate and government debt, the burden rises much higher. And it is constantly increasing.

The CIBC report says this is no big deal as long as interest rates stay low and there is no recession. The problem, apparently, is not excessive credit, but a lack of income growth which is attributed to a "significant drop in the quality of employment in the Canadian labour market over the past 20 years." There is however no indication that trend is about to change. In fact, given free trade, outsourcing, etc., it seems likely to get worse.

As the report makes clear, but never overtly recognizes, most of the credit and debt is coming from the banks. They of course must put the blame on workers who borrow to try to maintain their standard of living. But what if these workers stopped borrowing? Where would the money come from then?

The simple truth is that we have so structured our monetary system that a large proportion of the population must assume ever increasing debt. As a society we must take on even more debt if the economy is to grow. But this trend is unsustainable. There is a limit to the amount of interest people can pay. It's a crazy way to run an economy and the day of reckoning must come.

David Gracey

Municipalities — A Critical Level of Government

M UNICIPALITIES across the world have been getting the wrong end of the big stick. In a rapidly urbanizing, high-tech world much of the responsibility of running our society is downloaded onto them, without the funds to pay for it. Thus *The Wall Street Journal* (7/12, page B1, "Economic Time Bomb: US Teens Are Among the Worst at Math" by June Kronholz) brings the shocking tidings that "…[teenagers] in the US rank near the bottom of industrialized countries in [student] maths skills, ahead of only Portugal, Mexico and three other nations, according to a new international comparison. Economists say it is bad news for long-term economic growth.

"Two of the study's most unsettling findings: the percentage of top-achieving maths students in the nation is about half that of other industrialized countries, and the gap between scores of whites and minority groups – who will make up an increasing share of the labor force in coming decades – is enormous. The US ranked 24th among 29 countries that are members of the Organization for Economic Cooperation and Development, which sponsored the study. Using the OECD's adjusted average score of 500 points, the US scored 483 – 61 points behind top-scoring Finland and 51 points behind Japan. In a wider group that also included 10 non-members, many of them developing nations, the US tied Latvia for 27th place. The OECD study, called Program for International Student Assessment or PISA, also looked at reading and science skills, where US students scored slightly higher than in maths, and at general problem-solving skills, where they scored close to the bottom. In science, US youngsters scored 491 points, in reading they scored 477, all using a 500 point average."

The important detail is that not only application, talent, and teaching standards determine these results. Hardly less important, will be the earnings that help determine the presence of the mother in the home or her absence helping to earn the family's living. Highly relevant as well is the cultural level and quality of family relations, in general influences outside the schools. Squeeze municipal budgets like a lemon to provide statistics to keep Wall St. in a perky mood, and education, and other social services take a beating. In the long run, of course, that does the financial markets no good. A swarm of parasites too gluttonous of their victim's blood, may have a merry future, but hardly a lengthy one. That is the message of these statistics. They show that a country whose elite has taken upon itself to set the world aright by futuristic military means is not able to educate its young generation better than the tiny ex-Soviet republic of Latvia.

Bridging the Digital Divide

A complementary message from another angle comes from another recent issue of the *WSJ* (23/11, B1, "Telecom Giants Oppose Cities On Web Access" by Jesse Drucker): "Dozens of cities and towns across the country are rushing to offer low-or no-cost wireless internet access to their residents, but the large phone and cable companies, fearful of losing a lucrative market, are fighting back by pushing states to pass legislation that could make it illegal for municipalities to offer the service.

"Over the past few months, several big cities – including Philadelphia and San Francisco – have announced plans to cover every square block with wireless internet access via the popular technology known as Wi-Fi, short for wireless fidelity. Cities say these plans will spur economic development and help bridge the digital divide, making Web access nearly ubiquitous." Ponder that expression 'the digital divide' – it decides who may have access to vital skills for earning more than a pariah's living, or have enough information to know whom he/she is voting for, and who remains completely outside the social loop. The importance of this for raising educational levels not driven by deadbrain commercialism should be evident.

"But that is bad news for the large Bell telephone companies and cable operators, who are looking to their digital-subscriber-line (DSL) and cable-modem businesses for growth. Wi-Fi, technically known as 802.11, takes existing high-speed internet connections and wirelessly extends them by several hundred feet, allowing dozens or even hundreds of people to share one subscription."

That sounds to my ears like increased productivity of the sort that is supposed to keep the creaky market system churning.

"Philadelphia announced during the summer that it would hook up the entire city with Wi-Fi. Its current Wi-Fi service is free, but it hasn't decided whether that would continue with wider deployment. 'There are some very specific goals that the city has that are not met by the private sector: affordable, universal access and the digital divide,' says Dianah Neff, the city's chief information officer. She says that less than 60% of the city's neighborhoods have broadband access.

"However, last week, after intensive lobbying by Verizon Communications Inc., the Pennsylvania General Assembly passed a bill that would make it illegal for any 'political subdivision' to provide to the public 'for compensation any telecommunications services, including advanced and broadband services within the service territory of a local exchange intercommunications company operating under a network modernization plan. Verizon is the local exchange telecommunications company for most of Pennsylvania, and it is planning to modernize the region using high-speed fiber-optic cable. The bill has 10 days for the governor to sign it or veto it.'

"The Pennsylvania bill follows similar legislative efforts earlier this year by telephone companies in Utah, Louisiana and Florida to prevent municipalities from offering telecommunications services which would include fiber and Wi-Fi.

"Critics denounce this legislative tactic, arguing that the US lags behind other countries in broadband internet access because the phone and cable companies have been able to roll out the service in some areas.

"'We should be encouraging our municipalities to take a major role in broadband, the way other countries are doing,' says James Baller, who represents local governments on telecommunications issues.

"The telecom companies argue that it is unfair for them to have to compete against the government. They say that the legislation enables them to improve service to their customers by investing in their networks. If we put that money at risk and here comes the government to compete against us, with advantages that government has – not paying taxes – access to capital at good rates."

But are they really providing the same services? The international figures on the scholastic achievements of US scholastic would not say so. We assume that municipalities would provide internet services affordable to most families that would be less soaked with advertising, sex, violence. Besides was it not a basic principle of anti-trust doctrine of the late last century that where a monopoly service is being provided, there should be at least a measure of control – or another competitor – to keep the lone private actor straight? In any major scam the first concern of the miscreant is to bury the nation's history. The whole matter reduces to this: will the private sector and the municipalities really provide comparable services? But why is that not so much as mentioned even by the usually savvy *Wall Street Journal?*

William Krehm

Science and Economic Reform Consilience and Economic Reform

AN ISSUE that seized my interest as a graduate student was launched by the 1959 publication of C.P. Snow's essay *The Two Cultures and the Scientific Revolution*. I later assigned it as reading material for my students in Economics 101 (in its 1963 re-issue as *The Two Cultures and a Second Look*), for it seemed to me that political economy was (is) the quintessential bridging discipline. Recently, two distinguished scholars of my generation have revisited the subject with substantial and impressive approaches to the problem that differ on a fundamental point. That point is central to the subject of economic reform.

Edward O. Wilson, *Consilience: The Unity of Knowledge*. Alfred A. Knopf, Inc., New York, 1998. (Random House Vintage Books edition, 1999).

Stephen Jay Gould, *The Hedgehog, the Fox, and the Magister's Pox: Mending the Gap Between Science and the Humanities*. Harmony Books (division of Random House, Inc.) New York, 2003.

Wilson, an evolutionary biologist, argues for one way of knowing; Gould, a paleontologist, celebrates multiple ways. Their two approaches are significant for a great divide that separates political economic writers between those who believe governments should control money power and those who are content that money power control governments.

Faith in *the* Method of Science

Wilson proposes that all of the questions that have puzzled mankind from as far back as we can trace conscious thought can be answered through application of the method that natural scientists have tested and honed successfully over the past 300 years. If this *reductionist* approach is supplemented by *consilience* he believes that even the perennial "greatest enterprise of the mind – the attempted linkage of the sciences and humanities" can be achieved. Wilson acknowledges that this entails belief in the material basis of the world and "a conviction that the world is orderly and can be explained by a small number of natural laws." Not only will this approach lead understanding and guidance of the instincts of workmanship and artistic endeavor, it also will demonstrate that the religious hunger for understanding the meaning and purpose of life is satisfied more effectively through the search for objective reality than by revelation. Wilson is confident that "when we have unified enough certain knowledge, we will understand who we are and why we are here." With this kind of knowledge, public policy analysis and social engineering will become a trivial pursuit.

Gould shared the aspiration for progress through knowledge growth and application, but disagreed that the means proposed by Wilson are sufficiently powerful to bring the tantalizing fruit finally within our grasp. I wish to record here an appreciation to Gould for having given us this rejoinder to Wilson as one of his last acts as a premier scientist and communicator, for otherwise I and others of similar persuasion would have to struggle against the masterful brief of another front-rank scientist that fails to persuade me. In particular, Wilson boldly asserts that knowledge of what *is* can pass seamlessly to judgments of what *ought to be*. (This is the ultimate justification for the 'trickle-down' benefits of economic growth.)

Resurrecting the Enlightenment

Wilson's purpose is to revive our faith in the Enlightenment vision of moral and esthetic progress through science. For an epitome of the project he turns to its last great representative, the Marquis de Condorcet, who "wrote as though social progress is inevitable…. His serene assurance arose from the conviction that culture is governed by laws as exact as those of physics…. The sole foundation for belief in the natural sciences is the idea that the general laws directing the phenomena of the universe, known or unknown, are necessary and constant. Why should this principle be less true for the development of the intellectual and moral faculties of man than for other operations of nature?" (21) The laws that govern culture can be adduced from a study of past history, said Condorcet, and we need only understand them to keep humanity on its predestined course to a more perfect social order ruled by science and secular philosophy.

To reinforce his argument that the method of science is adequately comprehensive for linking humanities to the sciences, Wilson introduced the concept of *consilience*. Credit for the word and the idea goes to William Whewell in an 1840 work on the philosophy of science. Whewell described it as a "jumping together" of knowledge, "linking facts and fact-based theory across disciplines to create a common groundwork of explanation…. The Consilience of Inductions takes place when an Induction obtained from one class of facts coincides with an In-

duction obtained from another, different class. This Consilience is a test of the truth of the Theory in which it occurs."

Who Was Whewell?

Gould's book provides considerably more detail about Whewell than Wilson's, and a more digestible (for non-scientists) explanation of induction, reduction and consilience. For one thing, we learn that Whewell (as in *hew* or *hue*) was a prodigious and important Cambridge scholar of the 19th century, who wrote the founding works in historiography of science and contributed the word *scientist* to our language also. An example of induction is the inference from repeated experience (not always by deliberate experiment!) that water expands when frozen. By Consilience of Inductions Whewell meant the inference of a much more general principle from many individually induced conclusions that do not appear to have any connection with each other. This is an activity of synthesis, in contrast to the "normal science" procedure of *reduction* which focuses on a micro-phenomenon to abstract a generalization (induction) that may potentially explain it and be amenable to deliberate test. (This procedure was re-named by Karl Popper as *hypothetico-deductive*.)

Whewell inferred the *consilience* function after voluminously documenting the thoughts, experiments and explanations of productive scientists. Gould suggests that the greatest example of consilience is Darwin's inference of *The Origin of Species* from "thousands of well-attested facts drawn from every subdiscipline of the biological sciences… through thousands of equally firm and disparate facts. Only one conclusion about the causes and changes of life – the genealogical linkage of all forms by evolution – can possibly coordinate all these maximally various items under a common explanation. And that common explanation must, at least provisionally, be granted the favor of probable truth." The explanatory power and hence probable truthfulness of this generalization is increased as further inductively generated principles are seen to fit under it. (Historians' work is similar in the synthetic aspect, but differs in that the explanation of past events does not permit of experiments to promote repeat events.)

Wilson's Confession of Faith

Although Wilson provides a volume of highly persuasive supportive argument for the Enlightenment vision, he is frank in acknowledging throughout that "consilience beyond science and across the great branches of learning…is a metaphysical world view" and not widely shared. "Its best support is no more than an extrapolation of the consistent past successes of the natural sciences. Its surest test will be its effectiveness in the social sciences and humanities." Wilson's explanation for how and why the Enlightenment program lost support and was replaced by Rousseau and Romanticism is persuasively informative. In brief, the "dreams of reason" for a better social order entailed an examination of human mental life and implied that ultimately we are not free to choose. Natural scientists abandoned such questions to concentrate on areas of research that did not get them into metaphysical controversies. Philosophers and poets retained primacy in that realm, while the social sciences arose and "vied for territory in the space created between the hard sciences and the humanities." Rapid progress in the natural sciences in contrast to the other fields led to the situation described by C.P. Snow which "all but erased hope for the unification of knowledge with the aid of science." Knowledge expanded far beyond what could be embraced by young scientists, and in the era of specialization, scholarship for wisdom was progressively devalued. Finally, says Wilson, we get the polar opposite of the Enlightenment – the radical Postmodernist philosophy that we can know nothing.[1]

His Refutation of Postmodernism

Giving voice to the impatient scorn of scientists for the Postmodern perspective, Wilson turns it neatly on its head by invoking the deconstructionists' own line of reasoning. For in their solipsistic worldview, they turn to psychology for an explanation of how "root metaphors" get implanted in the minds (brains) of individuals and thereby color their creative output. "Modern psychology is dominated by the metaphor of human beings as machines" (45). (Wilson elsewhere cites Auguste Comte, founder of sociology, to the effect that "if people are just extremely complicated machines, why shouldn't their behavior conform to certain still-undefined natural laws?" (33). "Put briefly…psychology is at risk of becoming a natural science" (46). With this jab at his adversary, Wilson launches us into a trip through what has become known of human mental life by means of explorations in scientific fields linked to neurobiology and experimental psychology. Along the way he points out that logical positivism was "the most valiant concerted effort ever mounted by modern philosophers" to divine the general formula for objective truth. "Its failure…was caused by ignorance of how the brain works" (69). It is through neuroscience, then, that Wilson foresees fulfillment of the Enlightenment project of understanding the natural bases of morals, esthetics and the creative process. For readers who enjoy histories of science, his exposition is an unmitigated pleasure.

The empiricist approach to investigation of the brain and mental processes provides Wilson with a refutation of the argument (attributed to philosopher G.E. Moore) that an *is* cannot be logically converted into an *ought* without the interposition of some explicit statement of values. For what is *ought*, or whatever can it be, Wilson asks, other than *what is*? (273) For what is morality other than the translation of millennia of human experience into generalizations of principle?

A Challenge to Economic Reformers

By this extension of his thesis Wilson implies the impossibility of policy analysis and advice as an intellectually honest profession. I therefore respond by observing that while he may have a plausible explanation for the *content* of moral codes, I do not see it as a compelling criterion of what morality *is*. It implies that morality is *whatever works*, which begs the question *works to what end*? In Wilson's explicitly Darwinian context the answer to that question seems inevitably to be some qualified variation on *the thriving of the human species*. And that answer

may imply a different explanation for what morality is today than what it will be if our species survives for another century or more. What does it mean for the ecological-economic conundrum of our own time? Does it mean that Social Darwinism should be our moral code, or that humanity should voluntarily self-destruct in the deepest interpretation of deep ecology? Can nihilism be part of a natural set of instincts? This seems unlikely, and therefore leaves us looking for the ultimate answers to what is good for humankind, which has to entail some ideal of ecological balance.

For readers curious about the implications for science as an arbiter of esthetics I simply affirm that Wilson does have a chapter on The Arts and Their Interpretation.

Whewell Did Not Agree

As champion of more than one way of knowing, Gould made some important counters to Wilson's hopes for consilience. For one thing, Wilson adopted Whewell's concept of consilience to buttress the credibility of reductionism as *the* way to unify all knowledge into a few clean principles. That entails a new and modified usage of consilience, for Whewell explicitly denied that "moral rules can either flow from or contradict the mechanics of empirical nature, because ethical discourse rests upon another foundation altogether, with validation achieved by different criteria." "If anything, Whewell stated clearly, over and over again, that he had carefully analyzed the ways of science largely to show why this enterprise had been so stunningly successful *in its own domain* of factual nature, and why such an apparatus of explanation could not, in principle, regulate the defining subjects of different logical standing in other magisteria." The message is reinforced in an ironical footnote: Whewell was an ordained Anglican minister as well as Master of Trinity College. He could not abide Charles Darwin's theory, even though acquainted as master and student. "In a famous incident and anecdote, the powerful Whewell…even barred Darwin's book from the college library" (249).

Gould Dethrones Reductionism

Gould goes on to point out that reductionism has important limitations even in the natural sciences. His argument concerns two phenomena that occur in the investigation of the extra-human world. One of these is *emergent properties*. To explain it, Gould first observes that:

"Reductionism works by breaking down complex structures and processes into component parts and then ultimately explaining the complexity as a consequence of properties and laws regulating the parts" (221).

It yields satisfactory results, however, only if the component parts can be *added up* into an explanation that works reliably. An "additive" or "linear" principle is therefore required of the parts. It sometimes happens, however, in complex systems, that the relationship between two parts depends on the presence of third or fourth parts, and that the outcome cannot really be forecast with accuracy unless every detail is accounted for. If general principles about the nature of their interactions can only be formulated at the level of their direct occurrence (i.e., if they are "nonadditive" or "nonlinear") then a reductionist explanation is precluded.

"Properties that make their first appearance in a complex system as a consequence of nonadditive interactions among components of the system are called *emergent*.... Emergence is a scientific claim about the physical nature of complex systems. And if emergent principles become more and more important as we mount the scale of complexity...then the reductionist research program...will fail...as a heuristic proposition for advancing scientific knowledge" (223-4).

The other barrier to the reductionist approach is *contingency*. This refers to unique events that, although they can be explained after the fact, could not have been predicted.

"Unique historical events in complex systems happen for "accidental" reasons and cannot be explained by classical reductionism.... The central importance of contingency as a denial of reductionism in the sciences devoted to understanding human evolution, mentality, and social or cultural organization strikes me as one of the most important, yet least understood principles of our intellectual strivings."

In these circumstances, the narrative approach of historians is the best or only way of finding the desired explanation.

Wilson Accepts Establishment Economics

With that context, visit Wilson's chapter on the social sciences where economics is recognized as the social discipline approaching most closely his reductionist prescription. In particular, he approves an adding up, from the micro level of marginal analysis to general equilibrium at the macro level. And although he is fully aware of the limitations of economics as a predictive science, there is no acknowledgment that a "fallacy of composition" might be at work. This gives a distinctly pre-Keynesian flavor to Wilson's treatment, and no room for the thought that *emergent properties* might be the source of the obvious failures. His commentary reflects uncritical acceptance of the notion that economic growth and trickle-down are the inevitable path toward, indeed the meaning of, increased general welfare. And further progress via reductionist research will add up to more successful fine-tuning of money supply (by implication, the ultimate and only legitimate instrument). The aspiration for an eventual Newtonian triumph of general equilibrium is assumed to be a given rather than an esthetic vision of utopia.

An explanation for this performance is suggested by the *contingency* that Wilson relied for his information about the frontiers of economic thought on the committee who award the Bank of Sweden Prize in Economic Sciences in Memory of Alfred Nobel. As of 1998, he apparently did not share the complaint expressed by many scientists that the Bank prize was diluting the value of the real Nobel Prizes. This criticism seems to be gathering momentum, as reflected in this comment by a Norwegian observer:[2]

"What is new...is that there is now open Swedish criticism.... [With the latest award, to Prescott and Kydland] the Swedish Bank...is bolder with the Prize than ever before, since it is an outright myopic homage to the financial bureaucrats

and a degradation of politicians. It is therefore a degradation of democracy as such. The big irony is that the conservative politicians are praising this degradation of themselves. So, at a time when criticism is presumably stronger than ever, the nomination is bolder than ever." It seems that Wilson has been "neo-conned," but in fairness, where *should* he have turned for an authoritative judgment on the state of the art?

These comments provide only a sketch of the important issues that the two books raise on the topics of interest to economic reformers. And as an encouragement to potential readers, let me say that I feel I should apologize to Wilson and to the memory of Stephen Jay Gould for confining my remarks to such a narrow perspective on the value of their inspiring treatments of the human achievement and prospect.

Keith Wilde

1. A more positive perspective on Jacques Derrida is an obituary essay in *The New York Times* of October 14, 2004, parts of which I quoted in my report on the BIEN conference, November *ER*.

2. Arno Mong Daastoel, economic policy analyst and moderator of an Internet forum on Creditary Economics.

Chasing the Tails, of Historians, Economists and Other Evangelists

IN THE 1940s Robert Maynard Hutchins at the University of Chicago, disturbed at the divisive effect of academic specialization, proposed a curriculum built around "The 100 Great Books." Its goal was to enable specialists to talk to each other through a common participation in "The Great Conversation" from Homer to Dante to Darwin to Weber (and ninety-six other writers and works.) The concept migrated to St. John's College in Annapolis, Maryland, and, in the 1980's was exported to Brock University in Ontario. Unfortunately, it has not overcome demands of the established academic disciplines, particularly the sciences and social sciences, for exclusive control of their students' timetables. "We have so much within the discipline which is absolutely necessary to qualify them" [for degrees as chemists, economists, sociologists]. Jane Jacobs (*Dark Age Ahead*, Random House, 2004), labels it "credentialing" – the granting of degrees and diplomas which guarantee that the graduate has a grounding in X, Y, or Z discipline, but which also guarantee that the he or she knows nothing about logical or commonsense thinking and can seldom grasp a bigger picture than the one on the side of the discipline box.

Wright's Bigger Picture

Ronald Wright's *History of Progress* is a refreshing window on the bigger picture from a non-traditional historian. His main theme, as he examines the past civilizations with an archaeologist's bias, is that civilizations rise on the strength of some technical problem solved. They then succumb to a surfeit of success in that solution (say that three times fast). A village in the middle of a fertile landscape masters agriculture to provide for its needs. It succeeds so well it becomes a city. Then having paved over its most fertile land, it must go farther and farther afield to poorer and poorer soil to meet its increasing demand for basic maintenance. The outcome is decline. The early civilizations of the Fertile Crescent of Mesopotamia (somewhere in the vicinity of modern Iraq and Iran, you know), were built on a mastery of irrigation. But the constant evaporation of the water left the land saltier and saltier, with lower and lower yields. The outcome was decline. Until oil was discovered. Other examples make the same point.

Is this process of rise and fall inevitable? the historian asks. Or is it due, in Wright's phrase, to "inertia, greed, and foolishness?" A pessimist would answer, both. Looking at contemporary Western civilization Wright is slightly optimistic that knowing history we may not fall into our own version of the success trap.

Our Surfeit of Success

Western civilization has been successful in so many ways: in food production, through high-speed cultivation and fertilization of the deteriorating natural farmland; in manufacturing useful goods (one trillion plastic bags per annum, according to one researcher); in energy production, from dams which flood land, and from coal, oil and gas from a supposedly inexhaustible supply; in transportation, with personal SUVs and just-in-time delivery in half-empty transport trucks (with a touch of CO_2 emission as an externality.) Above all, perhaps, in money-making, through private bank control of money creation as debt, on which interest must be paid, and also through requiring by law that those highly-rewarded CEOs enhance shareholder value (in the short term), even if it bankrupts the enterprise in the long run.

Are there traps in any of these successes in which common-sense economics or "inertia, greed, and foolishness" might do us in? There is certainly no end of awareness of the problems, from global warming due to CO_2 emission, to monetary collapse. We have also been very successful in another area, which may, in fact, be the one to decide the issue: that is the arts of persuasion, demonstrable in election rhetoric and television programs. The key question is which persuaders will be the successful ones, economists, or historians, or evangelists of one sort or another?

Consensus: Washington to Copenhagen

One aspirant is Bjorn Lomborg (*The Sceptical Environmentalist*). He is on tour, explaining to economists, politicians and environmentalists, and anyone else who will listen, just how a rational (economists') assessment ranks a set of current proposals for addressing world problems The substance of his talks is the report of a conference held in Copenhagen. The proposals, which ranged from dealing with climate change to reducing government corruption, to lowering subsidies and trade barriers, were subjected to a three-step process. A set of papers by well-credentialled experts were assessed by a super-committee

of eight highly-credentialled economists (predominantly white, male, average age 70+), who applied a cost/benefit analysis to each proposal – which would give the most bang for the buck? – "because prioritizing is what economists do." Finally, the hoi polloi were given a voice in the form of a panel of young people, varied by race, colour and creed, who also listened to the conference papers and did their own prioritizing. Not surprisingly, they came to a somewhat similar listing of priorities as the gold panel economists. It is necessary to note, however, that the pure cost/benefit analysis was adjusted for another factor – here the economists ventured outside their field – the political viability of the proposals.

The result is titled the Copenhagen Consensus. Notice any resonance? High on the list is reducing subsidies and trade barriers, which would have "low costs" (for some people) but "amazing benefits," and only "short term political costs." Low on the list is addressing global climate change. In the middle are reducing malnutrition and hunger and, specifically on the health front, eradicating malaria and controlling HIV/AIDS. In the malnutrition and hunger category, a favourable nod goes to providing mineral and vitamin supplements (manufactured where?) and developing agricultural technology including GMOs (patented by whom?).

Monetary Reform Postponed Indefinitely

Monetary reform, under the heading of "financial stability," included regulating financial transactions, imposing capital controls, establishing a single world currency, and making borrowing cheaper for developing countries. It was dismissed as "good, but not now."

It is hard not to suspect that the Copenhagen "Consensus" was named not just as an echo of the tarnished "Washington Consensus" but to assure the beneficiaries of the latter that this is a safe new packaging of their old agenda. But we'll have to wait for more than the superficial summary given in the Lomborg presentations to confirm that..

Lomborg does claim that the Copenhagen package is something new, but peer review is a virtue that comes with a dark side, the stultifying hand of conformity. Economists are not exempt.

Fukuyama Undresses the Emperor

Francis Fukuyama's latest book, however (*State-building; Governance and World Order in the 21st Century*, Cornell UP, 2004), shows that even the leopard can gradually touch up his spots to a different hue. Fukuyama does not renounce his earlier conviction that American democracy/free market capitalism is the concluding nirvana of historical development for the human species, and he calls economics "the queen of the social sciences," but he does challenge the simple-minded "government is bad; private is good" mantra of the "Washington Consensus."

He does more than that. State-building is what the Bush administration claims it is about in Iraq. Its stated aim is to build a strong democratic state with liberal institutions. Fukuyama may be scuttling his favour with the powers-that-be by not only suggesting that they do not know how to do it, but arguing that it may not even be possible, either from without or as an occupying power, to engineer the state-building necessary for a stable pro-liberalization polity. Is the emperor's underwear about to be revealed?

Fukuyama will not endear himself to the Christian Republican constituency, either, because he eschews discussion of government with a "moral" agenda.

But the times they are a-changing, as any historian will tell you they always do, usually by repeating the same old staggering steps from zenith to nadir. Jane Jacobs proposes that the trademark symptom of decline is "memory loss." Memory loss? Help, isn't there a historian in the house?

Gordon Coggins

PART 3 OF A REVIEW OF A BOOK BY STEPHEN ZARLENGA, AMERICAN MONETARY INSTITUTE, NY

"The Lost Science of Money: The Mythology of Money — The Story of Power"

The Bank of Amsterdam

"Some of the Jews emigrating from Antwerp had set up an exchange banking operation, a '*wissell bank*,' changing money and discounting bills of exchange, taking deposits and making loans. The city fathers created the Bank of Amsterdam in 1609, and forbade the Jews and all others from engaging in banking. The Bank of Amsterdam's most vital feature was that it was a civic and not a privately owned institution. In theory it was not a bank of issue, and not supposed to make loans, and was considered a precious metals system.

"The City required that all bills of exchange above 600 Florins (later 300) had to be changed at the Bank. Accounts could be debited by withdrawing coinage or mainly by transferring it to another account at the Bank." The monopoly of banking showed an early appreciation of the profitability of a banking monopoly or nigh-monopoly. These increased the proportion of transactions that would become mere bookkeeping entries – an entirely internal matter.

"No interest was paid and no overdrafts or loans were made. The Bank did not discount bills – that is accept bills on other institutions or merchants at a discount, and then send them for collection. Deposits at the bank could not be attached. The City itself was responsible for the deposits. The Bank made profits on money-changing and gold and silver purchases, charging up to 2.5%.

"*All profits of the Bank belonged to the City of Amsterdam. The message to merchants was clear: make profits in commerce and industry, not in money-changing games or clipping or culling the coinages.* [Our italics.] And the Bank helped them earn money, removing one of the uncertainties in trade – the quality of payment. The very vaults of the Bank were in the basement of the old City Hall."

Many of the key features of central banking were incorporated. But the basic feature of banking itself was oddly omitted. The multiplier whereby modern banks lend out multiples of the money they keep in their vaults to meet the claims of depositors did not exist. It made its profits as money-changers, guaranteeing the quality of the currency. But for every amount of money it gave out it received an equivalent amount of money. The money in question was commodity money, and the Bank's contribution was to provide a dependable equivalent in Amsterdam coins as the coins in exchange for the foreign coins it received.

"The Bank made three exceptions in granting overdrafts: to the City of Amsterdam, to the Dutch East India Company, and to fund a city loan bank, the Bank Van Leening in 1614.

"The overdrafts to the City began in 1624. At first Amsterdam paid interest of 3 to 4% on its debt to the Bank, then reduced it to 0% when they realized they were paying interest to themselves."

In doing so they proved more alert than our federal government that has still not awakened to the fact or forgot what it had already learned.

"The Bank of Amsterdam's great success was that it was a public institution run by the City for the benefit of the country and its merchants, and not for private interests. This enabled it to raise the credit to make good on all of its deposits when it got into trouble. As such, its operation and policies were generally fair, but only to the Dutch."

The Dark Side of the Bank

"The Bank engaged in nefarious activities similar to Venice's vicious 14th and 15th century exportation of Europe's silver money to India. 'Already in the 1620s we see the Amsterdam Bank carry on the prohibited trade in precious metals,' wrote J.G. Can Sillen (*History of Banking and Credit*, reprinted by A.M. Kelley, New York, 1967, p. 73). 'The Netherlands attracted the silver coinage of her neighbours by frequent changes in her gold/silver ratio, just enough to make it profitable for the silver coins to be sent to her. Above-average weight English and French coins, as well as the clippings from them, also found a market in the Netherlands, where they were minted in underweight coins and sent back abroad. Officials of the French mint and the English Privy Council complained about this.

"Assisting these coining operations was Holland's enactment of the first 'free coinage' law in Europe just after 1575. This allowed metal to be passed easily between bullion and coinage.

"The Amsterdam stock exchange was built in 1611, modeled on that of Antwerp from 1531. Commodities as well as stocks were traded, with specific areas ('pits') designated for trading in different items. Amsterdam from the 1600 onwards was the direct origin of our present exchange mechanisms and procedures. She got them from Antwerp, which is said to have gotten them from the Levant."

Anticipating Our Derivatives

"In the 1980s and 1990s attention was focused on the 'innovations' known as derivative products: stock market indexes and futures and options contracts based on them. Nearly all of these 'innovations' were in use on the great Amsterdam Stock

Exchange in the 1600s and 1700s. We find the same types of contracts, the same general rules of trading, the same methods of cheating the public and manipulating markets: stock sold on margin up to 80%; monthly settlement dates; put and call options with premiums payable immediately at the Bank of Amsterdam; the 'ducatoon' – an imaginary share representing 1/10 of a Dutch East India Company share, with a monthly settlement price.

"The primary security traded in Holland was [of] the Dutch East India Company (DEIC) In its first six years it paid a dividend of 25-30% a year. Then in 1612 it paid 57% and in 1613 another 42%.

"The company had been formed in 1602. By 1607 its shares had risen to 100% over their original par value. However by 1607 its shares fell to only 30% over par value. The blame for the drop was placed on short selling, and in 1610 laws were passed against short selling. By 1688 the DEIC shares rose to 380% over their par value, not counting the tremendous dividends paid on the stock, totalling 1,482% of the par value.

"There were two types of brokers on the Amsterdam exchange: officially appointed 'sworn brokers,' of which there were 375 Christians and 20 Jews; and more than 700 unsworn brokers, or 'free' brokers who were mainly Jewish. The free brokers were sometimes wild and not proscribed from engaging in 'dual trading.' This means they were free to execute orders for their own accounts as well as for their clients, and could 'front run' their clients as well as orders they could see entering the pit through the 'sworn brokers.'" In a many ways such practices are still in the repertories of brokerages – not excluding those of our mightiest banks.

"In 1688 Joseph De La Vega, a Jewish stockbroker in Amsterdam wrote a book called *Confusione de Confusiones* describing exchange activity. [The title was a play on the celebrated theological work of the 12th century Spanish Jewish philosopher of Cordoba, *Maimonides*.] He gave a detailed description of how manipulators would launch a bear campaign to lower prices. At the beginning of the campaign the syndicate borrows all the money available at the exchange and makes it 'apparent' it wishes to buy (!) shares with the money. They actually start their campaign to drive prices down with purchases to raise prices. Then they start selling. They strike their first blow selling futures, reserving the cash sales for the moment of greater distress."

Their 5th stratagem of a total of 12 listed is to sell the largest possible quantity of call options.

The 6th is to buy the largest possible quantity of put options.

7th loan the bulls money, taking their shares as collateral. Then sell their shares.

8th Spread false news by dropping a letter "at the right spot."

10th Whisper loud enough to be heard.

12th Sell government bonds to shock the general situation.

"The manipulation of news was also important. The small boats which were supposed to meet the English ships and speed back to harbour with news, in reality merely took a turn outside the harbour and having invented their own plausible gossip, came back and sold it to the feverish crowds of speculators."

[This is the equivalent of false reports on promoted stocks by e-mail in our enlightened age.]

"The ducatoons – one tenth of a share of Dutch East Indian Company which served as a sort of index for the entire market – allowed structurally unsound trading, because any shorting of ducatoons would be paid for once a month, with cash rather than by returning ducatoons. That made it equivalent to index futures because debt in ducatoons was cancelled with a cash payment rather than with ducatoons or DEIC shares. That constituted a structural flaw because wiping out ducatoon shorts would not increase the purchase of Dutch East India Company shares." [One cannot meditate on the fact of Albert Einstein being hired at $35 a week when he managed to get out of Germany and arrive in America and the hundreds of millions of dollars available to executives and their accountants on Wall St. from practising such scams – particularly in unregulated derivatives.]

Concentration on such financial activities and speculation to the neglect of actual production led to the decline of the Dutch economy as early as 1660-1690, presaging what is overtaking the developed lands in our day. Dutch financiers of Christian and Portuguese Jewish stock helped establish the British banking system and stock exchange. One third of English debt came to be held in Holland. That led to the decline of Holland's influence in Europe.

"England had two advantages over continental Europe: as an island it profited from a degree of isolation and oneness. And as the westernmost outpost of the Empire, distance made her less subject to the whims of the Imperial, and later the Papal will. When the Western Roman Empire had degenerated, England's money system totally collapsed back into barter with no coinage circulating for about two hundred years from about 430 to 630 AD.

"As silver reappeared in Europe, coinage also revived in England. Many mints were established from 800-900 AD. Consistent with the sacred control of money, Anglo-Saxon mints seem to have been run mainly under ecclesiastical dominion. In 930 Athelstan's Law decreed that only one coinage should circulate in England. Mining thrived in the 10th century and the abundance of silver is indicated by the large tribute payments of Danegeld to Denmark: 10,000 pounds in 991 AD and 82,900 pounds in 1018.

"'Anglo-Saxon pennies were of token rather than intrinsic value. They fluctuated in weight and finesse from one issue to the next and yet their [monetary] value was constant since it derived from the word of the King,' wrote the monetary historian Peter Spufford. The Anglo-Saxon kings recoined the money about every six years, calling in all the coins and issuing three pennies for every one taken in. This represented a 25% tax or about 4% a year. Spufford maintains that this revenue provided the strength of the late Anglo Saxon and early Norman kings, who adopted their money system."

England Draws Strength from New Token Pennies

"Some religious officeholders attempted to continue exercising the money powers. We hear of them mainly through the record of their arrests. The first English gold coinage was in

1257 at a gold/silver ratio of 10/1. Silver, however, remained the mainstay of the coinage."

The issue of commodity vs. token money was further confused when it was preempted by the merchant class to deprive the monarch of his privileges.

"The landmark Mixt Moneys of Ireland case during the reign of Elizabeth I is still cited in 20th century court decisions. Elizabeth issued base metal coinage as legal tender in Ireland in May 1600, annulling all other coins there and requiring they be returned to the mints. An Irishman then paid a 100 pound debt to a London merchant in the new coinage. The merchant sued for the 100 pound in gold and silver coin.

"*The nature of money was identified as a societal institution rather than merely metal.* According to Del Mar the decision was so detested by the merchant classes, the goldsmiths, and later the British East India Company, that they worked incessantly to destroy it.

"This occurred in two stages: The first stage *was to destroy the British Crown's monetary prerogative, throwing the control of money open to the merchants and financiers.* This was done by undermining the Crown and then passing the free coinage act of 1666, opening the way for the foreign element to establish a new Monarch, *and to reconstitute the money prerogative in the hands of a specific group of financiers* – not elected, not representing society, and in large part not even English."

[This parallels the bailout of Canadian banks from their heavy speculative losses by shifting money creation from the central bank to the commercial banks by doing away with (or in other countries such as the UK and the US reducing the statutory reserves to near insignificance).]

Sanitized Monetary History

"The sanitized Whig histories of this period misrepresenting Charles II as a spendthrift, and London's goldsmiths as good businessmen, are still swallowed by economists. Christopher Hollis presents a very different pictures in his book, *The Two Nations* (London, 1935, reprinted Gordon, 1975).

"When Charles II returned to England, he needed a standing army to ward off continental threats, but Parliament refused to vote the funds and delivered only £800,000 of the £1,200,000 money that was voted, forcing Charles to use his wife Catherine's dowry for expenses of the state. Dutch financiers appeared willing to finance him but when he allowed legislation to pass contrary to Dutch merchant desires, they concluded that 'the King could not be made serviceable to his creditors.' Charles was forced to borrow from the English goldsmiths at 8%, giving as security the first taxes later to be voted by Parliament. As this 'security' became postponed, they demanded 20% to 30% per year.

"Charles considered issuing debased coinage to pay the army, but the merchants immediately raised prices 10% 'in anticipation' of a debasement! He offered to drop all talk of debasement if they would loan him £200,000. They refused.

"The merchants kept some of their money stored at the Tower of London. Charles finally blocked the funds – £130,000 – refusing to release them until they agreed to lend him a pitiful

£40,000. This led to a flight of coinage to the goldsmiths, who had secure premises and accepted deposits from people who no longer trusted Royal safekeeping at the Tower.

"According to Hollis, the London goldsmiths who play such a large part in the story of Restoration England were to a great extent mere agents operating with Dutch money. Finally in 1667 Charles II began to issue a kind of paper money to pay state expenses. It was almost true money, and took the form of Royal Exchequer Orders to Pay, good for coinage after one year. Taking one more step would have made them true money – that is, that is not having them payable in 'money' but be the money themselves."

The Nonsense Printing on Bank of England Bills

The UK has still not taken that decisive step. I have before me a "Canada Ten – Dix Dollars" or whatever the denomination. On the other hand £10 note of the Bank of England, the sole shareholder of which is the Government of the UK. On it, the Chief Cashier of the Bank of England commits the Bank "to pay on Demand the sum of Ten Pounds."

Canada on its currency, like most developed countries today, dispenses with such nonsense, and merely entitles the bills that their government (via the Bank of Canada) issues. Our election campaigns are, unfortunately, less sophisticated. Our Prime Minister and the heads of the major opposition parties make a major promise of paying down and even "paying off" the national debt. Looking after the deepening potholes in our health care, transport systems, education and much else must apparently wait until that is achieved. But even the government no longer implies that it is possible on our banknotes. Carefully these omit to reveal what currency they propose using to pay off the debt, other than the very identical debt of the federal government. For that is the only legal tender that has existed for at least thirty years. There is not the slightest attempt of the government to explain or of our parliamentarians to demand an explanation of what they would use to pay it off with. Presumably bills of a different colour. Meanwhile they are cheating the nation by ruling out elections that would address the country's crucial issues to talk of imaginary ones.

The destruction of a key taxation arm of the monarchy by the "revolutionary" speculative proto-banking interests has two vital implications both of which have been ignored by economists.

The first of these resembles Karl Polanyi's treatment of the role of the local Speelhamland laws in early industrializing England as a social brake to prevent too rapid a transition to a labour market before some even temporary social system had been set up to take care of the peasants thrown off their lands by the enclosures. Though the Stuart monarchy may have represented a "reactionary" force by both Liberal and Marxian logic, it was entrusted with the provision of key functions necessary for society's survival. These could not be discontinued overnight until some successor government had made provisions to take them over. At its most promising revolutionary junctures the Dutch monetary speculative band could hardly be relied upon to provide the brake to slow down the necessary transition. Charles II's monetary improvisations addressed this need.

There is a nexus with another suppressed aspect of monetary evolution that concerns working the cost of government services into the monetary equation. Under centralized monarchical governments this was largely achieved by the monarch's recoining the token monetary medium.

The Other Suppressed Monetary Secret — The Growing Layer of Taxation in Price

Under our modern pluralistic society – in a strange mirror relationship to the recoining operation of yore – it takes the form of an ever deepening layer of taxation in price which has nothing to do with an excess of aggregate demand over supply and everything to do with the essential growth of public infrastructures and services within the total social product. This latter phenomenon I have called "Structural price rise" to contrast it with "market inflation" which can be related to an excess of aggregate market over aggregate supply. This I first described in the then leading French economic publication *La Revue Économique* (05/1970, "La stabilité des Prix et le Secteur Public").

This tracks not the monarchical clipping of the monetary token coins as a necessary substitute for unavailable taxation due to the exemptions enjoyed by the church and/or the feudal landowners, but the erosion of market price structure to reflect the growing layer of taxation that finds its way into prices reflecting the cost increases of unmarketed public services. There is another aspect to this mirror symmetry of these two monetary relationships. To both of them official economists of every school have been willfully deaf, blind, and dumb. To fight "inflation" which covers both highly dissimilar components of our price rise, they have chosen higher interest rates as "one blunt tool." That has surrendered the conduct and profits of our hypertrophied monetary system to speculative finance. Economic historians like Fernand Braudel have been more sensitive to these relationships. See William Krehm, *Price in a Mixed Economy: Our Record of Disaster*, Toronto, 1975, ISBN 0-88963-000-3.

The Free Coinage Act of 1666

"According to Del Mar, the British East India Company, carrying on the metals trade with India used heavy bribery to help pass the *Free Coinage Act* of 1666. The Act provided that anyone could bring gold or silver bullion to the mint and have it refined and stamped into coins for free. In practice this placed the power to increase or decrease the money supply into the hands of the merchant financial classes rather than the Crown [acting for the nation]. Thus if the merchants were in debt they could reduce the value of their debt by having more bullion turned into coins. If they were creditors they could increase the value of what was owed to them by hoarding coinage or melting it into bullion and having it turned into coins again later, free of charge. Del Mar considered this act a watershed event in monetary history.

"The *Free Coinage Act* specifically destroyed the royal pre-rogative of coinage, nullified the mixed moneys case and inaugurated a future series of commercial panics and disaster which to that time were unknown. The conception of money which has grown up since the *English Mint Act* of 1666 and the *French Mint Act* of 1679 is that of two different things designed to measure one relation called value: (1) A commodity whose value conforms to an unknowable cost of production; and (2) A series of coins, notes, etc. the value of each of which is in inverse ratio to their aggregate number and which can therefore have no relation to the cost of production" (Del Mar, *The Science of Money*, NY: Cambridge Encyclopedia, 1904, p. 79).

We might add that the Crown itself had a very parallel duality of social significance. On the one hand it was by its very origins the apex piece of the land-owning nobility. On the other hand in other respects as well as in its monetary function it was the symbol of the national interest and as such had an important function in creating and backing token money.

Del Mar sums up that chapter of English monetary history: "The appropriation [by] the goldsmith class of the Royal prerogative has been accomplished in so stealthy a manner that scarcely a trace of it appears in historical works; and none at all in works devoted to political economy – a glaring proof of the prejudice and one-sidedness which have hitherto animated the teachers of that science" Zarlenga adds: "Del Mar is right. The only other source this author has found, which discusses it meaningfully is W.A. Shaw's *History of Currency, 1252-1896.*

"The operators on Amsterdam's Stock Exchange grew more powerful based on a metallic monetary system, obtained in large part by two centuries of genocide against the American Indians. Still, the inadequacy of this abundant gold and silver was indicated by the Bank of Amsterdam's secret credits to the Dutch East Indian Company for over a century.

"While the Bank of Sweden was the first western bank of issue, in 1661, it was the formation of the Bank of England that signaled a recovery of the lost science of money. However, since it was organized for the private power and profit of a small group, it was an illicit misuse of the science for private gain, instead of for societal use, as its true nature requires. While creating abstract money, they put forward a backward commodity concept of money as gold and silver, pretending the necessity of converting the abstract money into metal.

"Coin clipping was almost unknown in Venice but appears to have been a primary activity of merchants in Northern Europe. In the mid-1690s the English coinage was again in dreadful condition, being clipped and about 50% underweight. There was a £40 reward for denouncing a clipper, and the clipper could go free if he denounced two more clippers. Hangings were held regularly. On just one day, seven men were hanged and one woman burned at the stake for coin clipping.

"The goldsmiths were charging 30% to 80% yearly on small loans. The public therefore wanted a bank to regulate currency and to lower interest rates. From about 1650 to 1710, J. Keith Horsefield's study, *British Monetary Experiments*, counts at least 60 monetary proposals of various types including nominal money, land banks, glorified pawnshops, and tax anticipation notes. There were even two proposals for a negative rate of

$\sim$ 265

interest, anticipating theories of Silvio Gesell. William Paterson had made at least four proposals.

Paterson's Proposal, Montagu's Bank

"However, it was not until the takeover of William III that the plans for a bank by the Scotsman William Paterson, a relative of John Law, were adopted in 1694. Though brilliant, he received little education. In 1685, in Amsterdam, he became involved in William III's 1688 revolution. Returning to London with William's army, he became rich and influential organizing the North London Water Company, with the help of Charles Montagu. That Paterson's plan was even adopted can be explained only by his being sponsored by Charles Montagu, whose family had held positions of importance in England for five centuries. Montagu should be considered the true founder of the Bank of England.

"Paterson was more than a front man, though. His biographer Saxe Bannister says he enjoyed 'intimate relations with the rich Hebrews of London and probably Amsterdam and Germany.' He was an interesting man and not the 'evil genius' some have made him out to be. He was trying to aid society and make a fortune while doing it. Montagu was a friend of Isaac Newton, and of Edmund Halley (of comet fame)."

Hatching the Bank of England

"The ostensible reason for chartering the Bank was to obtain a loan of £1.2 million of gold for William III's government. The shares for this were to be subscribed by the public in gold coin or bullion. The entire proceeds were to be loaned to the Crown at 8% interest. Once operating, the Bank would accept deposits, paying 4% on them and should issue its own bank notes which would circulate as money and which the Bank would keep redeemable in gold. At first these notes were to have no legal tender power but were to be acceptable and payable by the crown for all things.

"The Bank was to be allowed to create bank notes in an amount equal to the money it lent the government. This is another way of saying that it could use government debt as its reserves or collateral. What the promoters argued was that the Bank would be 'founded upon a reserve that cannot fail but with the Nation.'

"What they did not point out was that although the Bank would be paid interest on this created loan, the Bank was completely unnecessary in this money creation process. The Government could have created its own paper notes on the same security and not paid interest on it to anyone! And unlike the Bank of Amsterdam which was owned by the Government, the Bank of England was owned and controlled by private individuals.

"Substantial opposition to the Bank arose immediately. Some came from coin clippers such as the goldsmiths, who wanted no competition from the Bank, The Tories, England's landowners, opposed it as they saw the power it would give to their commercial political opponents. Others opposed it for sound, moral reasons.

"One of the monetary thinkers of the time, William Lowndes,

said, 'who can think that posterity will be willing to pay a tax of £110,000 per annum (on the original loan), to go into the pockets of private men, when it will be in their power to acquit the public of such a burden?'

"Lowndes didn't realize that through constant warfare vast amounts of new debt would be piled onto the original, making it impossible to pay in gold and silver."

The Bank's Charter

"The Bank was given a charter for 12 years. Of the £1.2 million share subscription, no one person was to own over £10,000 (later 20,000) though nominee ownership through another person couldn't be stopped. The whole capital was subscribed in gold within three days. The shares had a provision whereby an additional 40% of par value could be called from the shareholders in gold, by the Bank's Directors. At first it would only lend its paper notes to the Government at 8% interest plus £4,000 annually for expenses.

"The Bank also took deposits, paying 4% on them, and discounted bills for merchants. The Bank of England was not even given the monopoly of note issue until 1844. Other banks could issue their own paper notes until then. The Bank's notes had the one supreme advantage of being accepted by the Government for all payments due, and of being paid out by the Government for all state expenses. Thus they came to be identified with the Government.

"The Tories formed a competing bank in 1696 – Chamberlain's Land Bank. It would use land as a reserve asset. It would liquefy the Tories' main holding by issuing an equal amount of paper notes for the value of the pledged land. This was based on the flawed concept of liquefying property. The flaw: as new money is created to liquefy property, the value of property keeps rising with the additional liquidity, so even more money is created, etc. Eventually the bubble must burst, as interest costs grow.

"Bank of England shares plunged from £108 to £83 in two weeks on this development. But the landowners were hopelessly out of their element. Within a few months the Chamberlain Bank, attracting only a few thousand pounds, was abandoned.

"Also affected by the recoinage, in 1696 the Bank failed for the first time, just two years after its founding, when it could no longer redeem its notes in coinage. Paterson insisted that the Directors use their power to call for more gold from the shareholders. [When the Directors refused] Paterson scolded them and resigned over such disagreements within a year.

"The Bank of England succeeded where others failed because it took on each new situation as it came, without ideological commitment. Its main protection was that its complexity kept people from understanding the true source of its power – the money creation process."

That has passed down as a banking tradition. People are kept in the dark about banking – even when the banks are not in stress – because that public ignorance is in itself a principal asset of the bankers. It is particularly so when the banks have been deregulated as today to allow them to engage in just about every non-banking sphere of finance.

Ricardo Speaks Up

"One man who exposed the Bank's essence was an English Jew named David Ricardo (1772-1823). His clear thinking (on the Bank, not economics), simplicity of statement and courage stands out as an important contribution. In 1815 Ricardo wrote to Malthus, 'I always enjoy an attack on the Bank and if I had the courage I would be a party to it. They have the power, without any control whatever of increasing or reducing the circulation in any degree they may think proper: a power that should neither be entrusted to the State itself, nor to anybody in it. When I consider the evil consequences which might ensue from a sudden and great contraction of the circulation as well as from a great addition to it, I cannot but deprecate the facility with which the state has armed the Bank with so formidable a prerogative.'

"By 1823, Ricardo had worked up the courage to propose establishing an English National Bank. He explained why the government should issue its own money: 'Suppose that a million of money should be required to fit out an expedition. If the state issued a million of paper, the expedition would be fitted out without any charge to the people; but if a bank issued a million of paper, and lent it to the government at 7%, the country would be charged with a continual tax of 70,000 per annum…. The only difference would be with respect to interest. The Bank would no longer receive interest and the government would no longer pay it. It is said that the Government could not with safety be entrusted with the power of issuing paper money – that it would certainly abuse it. I propose to place this trust in the hands of Three Commissioners.

"As a member of Parliament and successful stock trader, Ricardo's observations were hard to ignore. In 1844 several factors forced the note-issuing function to be placed under a separate department of the Bank under some safeguards, and England was no longer required to pay interest on her debt to the Bank.

"William Paterson himself saw the inequity of the National debt. In 1715 he had been living in poverty when Parliament voted him a huge £18,000 payment in appreciation for his contribution in founding the Bank. Nevertheless he remained opposed to the Bank's building up debt and in 1717, no doubt using some of the money Parliament gave him, he published a proposal for paying off the national debt.

"It gave so much offense to the stock jobbers that some of the meaner sort caused the book to be burnt before the Royal Exchange. The Bankers did not want the debt paid; just the opposite. They wanted to build up a real interest charge into perpetuity on the money they had created out of thin air and loaned to the government."

W.K.

The Multi-frauds of Risk Managment have Begun Unravelling

MUCH OF THIS ISSUE of *ER* is devoted to the frauds of risk-management that in several areas of the economy have begun coming apart. One of these is the Canadian federal budget process that has been based on the belief that the government hiding assets – a criminal matter in the private sector – is an aid to virtue and, at the end of the year, some of these can then be trotted out as proof of the finance minister's "fiscal responsibility."

Private corporations have used unregulated derivatives – trades in an abstract feature of a security which is unregulated and can be kept off the books – to create the illusion of more demand for the security itself. These derivatives may deal in interest earned, or the exchange value of the currency in which the underlying security is denominated, in calls or call options or swaps in trades of these abstractions ("swaptions" is only a simpler sample of what is becoming the best rewarded high technology of our period).

Another such – the hedge funds that originally were the happy hunting ground of billionaires – are now being used by more modest investors who have cashed in their profits during the aging boom market. They have also become a favorite haunt of overextended banks that by their own admission are unloading much of their bad debt on unwary modestly wealthy folk who don't know what to do with their winnings. Bankers are coming clean on such matters, since their consciences have been sensitivitized by the revelations of New York state prosecutor Eliot Spitzer. His subpoenas have achieved costly settlements by some of the greatest names of insurance for using derivatives "to aid their own results with the complex techniques that they pioneered and marketed over the past 20 years. Insurance has moved beyond its core business of insuring against fires and earthquakes" to the damage by artificial overheating and tremors of their own making.

As a result, leading Canadian bankers have moved in closed rank from opponents of regulating derivatives to supporters of the idea. Canada's banks have reached humiliating settlements running into several hundred millions of dollars. for having participated in the off-balance sheet partnerships of Enron.

The Risks of Risk Management

The change of heart of our bankers on the subject of derivative regulation has not come inexpensively for the Canadian taxpayer.

We should make clear that we are not against risk management as such. Like personal virtue it is much to be commended but devilishly difficult to achieve. Partial success towards the goal can certainly be reached by such policies as deficit budgeting by government so that during a recession a heightened degree of government spending for necessary capital purposes will help keep employment and economic activity higher. However, the risk management encouraged by hedge funds and other large financial corporations has precisely the opposite effect. It adds wind and bluster to the financial bubbles and increases the violence of the busts.

The Wall Street Journal (15/02, "Spitzer, SEC subpoena AIG over complex deal accounting" by Theo Francis) wrote: "American International Group Inc. is fresh off settlements with the US Justice Department and the Securities and Exchange Commission for its role in allegedly helping their earnings with complicated financial products for its own possible illegitimate purposes.

"The New York insurance giant yesterday disclosed new subpoenas from New York Attorney General Eliot Spitzer's office and the SEC. They seek information related to certain types of insurance arrangements 'and AIG's accounting for such transactions,' the company said.

"AIG added that it received the inquiries just after it reported its fourth-quarter earnings last Wednesday and seemingly closed the book on two regulatory inquiries that have lingered over it for months.

"The new subpoenas show regulators' mounting interest in a line of insurance products that was obscure just 16 months ago. But since regulators were caught off guard by the billions of dollars of loans that have targeted financial services firms that allegedly aid corporations in financial machinations, Enron filed for bankruptcy court protection in December 2001.

"Specifically, the subpoenas relate 'to investigations of non-traditional insurance products and certain assumed reinsurance transactions and AIG's accounting for such transactions,' AIG said. Many non-traditional insurance products blend insurance with financing. Regulators believe the products can allow users to inappropriately shift losses from the buyer's balance sheet, aiding the bottom line in the short run while misleading shareholders and regulators.

"Last fall, AIG settled allegations that it had helped PNC Financial Services Group Inc., a Pittsburgh banking company, improperly shift liabilities off its books, and that it helped Brightpoint Inc., a Plainfield, Ind. cell phone distributor, cover up losses using a bogus insurance policy. AIG agreed to pay $128 million in penalties and other costs but neither admitted nor denied wrongdoing.

"Separately, Mr. Spitzer's office has named the company as a participant in a bid-rigging scheme with other major insurers and insurance broker Marsh & McLennan Cos.; two former AIG employees have pleaded guilty in that scheme, but AIG said last Wednesday that it had found no indication of wrongdoing outside the single unit in which those individuals worked.

"Some of the complex 'alternative risk' transactions that regulators are looking into across the industry allow insurers to compensate for reserve shortfalls in the short run by seemingly transferring risk for these reserves from one insurer to another.

"AIG has long been one of Wall St.'s favourite insurance stocks, known for its steady earnings growth in an industry where results typically are banged around by everything from hurricanes to adverse developments in asbestos litigation."

The classic insurance worries may be put in the shadows by the risks of being too successful in the new jungle of derivatives technology.

William Krehm

As Though We were Hit by an Astral Body

BUDGET-TIME is the time of the Big Lie that needs ever more mendacity as cover-up. To celebrate the strange harvest brought in by Canada's new minority government, *The Globe and Mail* (24/02) carried a "Fiscal Health Report: the Past 20 Years on Canada's ever-changing bottom line" by Heather Scoffield. It began by citing the importance of the year 1995 in the lives of two prominent politicians – one on the right and the other on the left. A charming journalistic conceit, but hardly enough to make up for Ms. Scoffield not mentioning the root cause for 1995 becoming the slaughter-year for social programs.

"Feb. 27, 1995 was a fateful day for both Alexa McDonough and John Manley. The two politicians sat on opposite sides of the political spectrum, but the federal budget delivered was a thunderclap for them both. The 1995 budget would go on to define not only the careers of two politicians, but also a decade of fiscal policy, the economy and political culture of the country, and the public persona of Prime Minister Paul Martin himself."

But how different the interpretations of this crucial chapter of our history advanced by these two politicians! For Ms. McDonough the budget of 1995 was a major disaster smashing social programs that had taken generations to put in place. Rightist Liberal Manley, however, saw as key villain the huge deficit of apparently unknown origins that made it necessary for the freshly elected Liberal government to dismantle Canada's hopeful way of life, dearly purchased with the mass martyrdom of the Great Depression and World War II. But something is missing in either version – the catastrophe that led to the extraordinary budgetary measures – heroic by Mr. Manley's telling, heartless according to Ms. McDonough. It was as though some unknown astral body had hit the earth and wiped out forests and even entire species. That hidden catastrophe changed the face of Canadian politics, the pulse and purpose of our democratic process. Some strange discomfort with the logical sequence of the story, leads to it starting with

the disastrous consequences and never returning to what might have caused them. It falls to us accordingly to make good this strange omission.

The work was done for us in a remarkable book by one of Canada's great journalists, the late Walter Stewart, once editor of *Maclean's* magazine and author of an unforgettable book, the final one of a great series: *Bank Heist, How our Financial Giants are Costing you Money*. That book is dedicated "For William Krehm, Jordan Grant, Susan Bellan, Duff Conacher and all those who devote their energies to trying to bring our banks to heel." As great and tireless a researcher as Walter Stewart was, it was in my living room that he first at considerable delay saw the documented details of the revision of the *Bank Act*. In padded stealth, with neither debate in Parliament nor press release, this had done away with the reserves that the commercial banks had to deposit with the government-owned Bank of Canada as a modest proportion of the deposits in chequing accounts that they took in from the public.

These took their place alongside the Guidelines put out three years earlier by the Bank for International Settlements in Basel, Switzerland, (BIS) that declared the government debt of developed countries risk-free and hence requiring no further capital for banks to acquire.

This rewrite of the rules of banking and fiscal policy added up to the equivalent collision of an astral body and our planet. It devastated the distribution of our national income. "In five years[our chartered banks' holdings of federal debt] jumped from $25.7 billion to $94.9 billion that required practically no capital set asides." And since our banks had lost much of their capital gambling in gas and oil, real estate, and stock market plays, it seemed an ideal way of bailing them out. Yet because of its very enormity in the redistribution of the national wealth that it entailed, it not only had to be done in stealth, but constituted a shift in political power from the electorate and the productive business world to the financial sector. Former cabinet ministers could be found who were not even aware what had been smuggled in under the table by the Mulroney government between the late 1980s and 1993.

The government deficit and the debt went wild as the government paid to the commercial banks an extra $6 billion annually for simply holding government bonds in their vaults – services that the central bank – because it was its only shareholder since 1938 was the Canadian government – had done for it at practically no cost at all. For any profit of the BoC (after paying operating costs) went to that government as dividends. It was the purpose of the *Bank Act* revision in 1991: to allow the banks to hold government bonds proclaimed "risk free" by the BIS *Risk-Based Capital Requirements* guidelines brought in 1988.

How to Fill the Huge Budgetary Hole

That is the unmentioned celestial event that commentators left right, parliamentarians or editorialists, don't dare mention. To fill that huge budgetary hole, Ottawa began down-loading social programs onto the provinces without enough revenue to fund them. The provinces passed on the treatment to the municipalities, who were left holding the bag.

During the 1980s Canada's banks, had been allowed to abandon the restraints that had been imposed on them during the Depression of the 1930s. Emergency bank legislation brought in the mid-thirties had set up fire walls that separated banking from the other three pillars of the financial system – the stock market, insurance companies, and real estate financing. Each of these divisions of the financial sector kept a pool of capital, essential for its own affairs. And, given the banks' unique ability through the check-clearing system of creating money by lending out many times the amount of their own cash reserves, those capital pools of the other "financial pillars" proved irresistible to our banks as they gambled themselves into ever more trouble. They provided an additional cash base for their powers of money creation. Hence the bank deregulation of the 1980s led to widespread bankruptcies in both the US, Canada and the world at large. And the bailout from the bankruptcies and near-bankruptcies of the 1980s took the form of still further deregulation: mammoth mergers of banks with insurance companies, with brokerages, with department stores and just about anything that had set their hearts throbbing. That resulted in the current aging stock market boom, that may temporarily appear like high prosperity to those who profit from it, but already shows unmistakable signs of major disasters ahead.

What Manley Bites his Tongue About

Mr. Manley, as a former Finance Minister, knows only too well that the federal deficit that we hear so much about is not a real deficit. Rather it is mainly the result of bad bookkeeping that would have landed the CEO of any private corporation in jail. Disregarding the advice of a long line of Auditors General, until 1999, the federal government on acquiring a building or a machine or any other capital item that would last for many years, wrote off its cost in a single year just as it does the floor wax in the lavatories of government buildings. This distorted the statistics of the government's performance in a variety of ways.

It made it necessary to impose more taxation, which deepened the layer of taxation in price beyond what was already needed for the rapid transformation of our country from a semi-rural society to a high-tech one, with its rapidly expanding population flocking into the cities. This growing factor in our price rise had been mistaken by economists for market "inflation" caused by too much demand and not enough supply. It was the ideal context for the banking clique that had taken over the world's central banks, to make hay. By doing away with the statutory reserves, higher interest rates became the "one blunt tool" for licking "inflation," and as a result interest rates to productive businesses were driven into the 20% plus range. The spread between what pittance banks paid their depositors and what they charged their borrowers became indecent – as much as 18% in the early 1990s.

The next thing that Mr. Manley knows only too well but is not talking about is this: in 1999 the then Auditor General Denis Desautels, put his foot down and refused to give Mr. Paul Martin, then the Minister of Finance, an unconditional approval of two years of government balance sheets unless he committed himself to bringing in elementary accountancy that distin-

guishes between spending for capital goods and current spending for goods and services used up in the current year. During weeks of strained argument – reported only in a trade paper for accountants – the Auditor General actually used the expression "cooking the books" to describe the non-accountancy by which the government arrived at a "deficit" to justify the continued bleeding of the national treasury on behalf of the banks.

To handle a similar problem, the US, starting with calendar 1996, had brought in accrual accountancy (also known as "capital budgeting") because it recognized government capital investment as private corporations always have. This it did for 1996 and made adjustments for 37 previous years. The result was that it was able to recoup for its books $1.3 trillion of neglected capital assets. This produced a substantial surplus. But to avoid arousing the sleeping ideological dogs of the right the Clinton administration avoided calling them "investments" or "capital." Instead, it threw them into the "savings" column of its Department of Commerce accounts. But since they were not in cash which "savings" implies, but in bricks and mortar, machinery, highways and so forth, that was still a partial cover-up, but it was enough to transmit a message that bond-rating agencies have long been trained to understand with a wink and a nudge. The accountancy implied rather than correctly entered onto the books was enough to improve the government's credit standing and bring down interest rates to give Clinton a second term, and the country a period of prosperity that eventually turned into the high-tech boom and bust.

In Canada Paul Martin as Finance Minister in the Chrétien government chose an opposite course. His game was not to improve the government balance sheet. Rather he made a practice of presenting it as worse than it was, so that at the last moment he could cut social programs and only then reveal some of the reserves he had hidden and embellish his self-promotion as a prudent fiscal financier. Nevertheless in the unsavoury compromise he reached with the Auditor General in 1999, he agreed in principle to recognize federal government's capital investments and where such investments to preserve the environment, public health, or whatever, were not made, they would have to be entered on the books as a capital deficit to be addressed in the future. But above all the whole significance of "accrual accountancy" was kept secret not only from the public and the media but from Parliament itself.

Credibility by Covering Up the Facts

Of all this Mr. Manley is perfectly informed, though silent. For such details would turn to dust the great accomplishment that he claims was wrought to "regain credibility" in the great year of 1995. That could have been done by simply adjusting the books – under the proper headings, however – as the Clinton administration did in 1996. When Mr. Manley brought down the last budget under the regime of Jean Chrétien, he actually used the term "accrual accountancy," but those who followed the house session on TV could see that his fellow members did not even know what he was talking about. So within a day or two – and during the entire election campaign – that brought the minority government of Paul Martin to office – "accrual accountancy" received no further mention. Instead, the talk was about "paying down the government debt," or "paying it off completely." And Liberal and Conservative candidates discussed that to the exclusion of the too radical idea of introducing serious accountancy that would let the public know what in effect the real net deficit might be.

The concept of a "net deficit" is key. Nothing less makes the slightest sense. Otherwise you would have to give any of the homeless who sleep on our sidewalks a higher credit rating than any of our chartered banks. For the street people have no debt on their books, whereas our chartered banks carry as much debt – and more at times – than they can manage.

Are the Street People in Better Shape than our Banks?

But that is only a single storey of the skyscraper of deceit that the Conservative and Liberal positions consist of. The accrual accountancy that Mr. Manley so briefly mentioned and was the subject of the Auditor Generals' requirements covered only *physical* investments. But in the 1960s economists, largely because of the work of Theodore Schultz of the University of Chicago (in a book first published in 1961), came to recognize that the most productive of all investments that could be made was in human rather than physical capital.

That work, which won Schultz the Nobel Prize for Economics, was based on the spectacularly rapid recoveries of the war-shattered economies of Japan and Germany, which could only be explained by their highly educated and highly disciplined personnel who had come through the war substantially intact. That discovery which flourished with benign effects for a decade or two, was suppressed because it undercut the social counter-revolution that was getting underway shortly afterward. However, if you applied that you would have the books of our government in highly positive net territory, and the fateful swing-year of 1995 would finally be understood, and put behind us.

For example, that matter of paying off the debt. That "obligation" of the central bank was on every bit of paper money issued. The United Kingdom – charming homeland of archaic customs – still carries the promise "to pay the sum of" whatever its denomination is without specifying in what money. But neither the Euro, the US currency, nor the Canadian or any other major currency makes such a meaningless promise. Instead they merely entitle the paper bill "Ten Dollars," "Ten Euros," or whatever.

Surely we should eliminate such meaningless promises from our electoral rhetoric as well to make room far more significant ones that have been suppressed from official discourse for some decades.

Come to think of it, there is another British custom that is far worthier of imitating. It is the institution of a Royal Commission where the various viewpoints in handling major unsolved problems can be ventilated and put on record. It is high time that one be set up to examine the very notion of the significance of government debt and the various ideas that have been advanced to manage it in the interest of the nation.

W. Krehm

On Monetary Reform Literature in the 1930s

THE POLICY OF 1930s reformers seems to be consistent among Canadian, British and Australian writers as well as American. They were fiat money advocates or "greenbackers," which explains why Lincoln features prominently in their literature. They were indignant about the great deflationary contraction of money supply that had taken place under existing money and banking institutions. In this they were joined by many captains of industry, great merchants, and even bankers, all of whom favored some changes of policy and regulation that would assure a *stable* monetary and prices environment. (See Owen's book for the impressive membership list of the Stable Money Association.) They believed that governments had given away too much of their sovereign powers to financial tycoons and that they should assert more regulatory control in the interest of general welfare. In particular, money reformers wanted governments to issue money and spend it into circulation via important public works. Then, if the spending went a bit overboard, tax some of it back. They perceived bankers to be interested primarily in accumulating property by means of deflationary contractions of money supply. These contractions were seen to follow on expansionary periods in which bank money was created as loans by bankers out of nothing but a stroke of the pen. This bank money being quantitatively much more important than currency by the 1930s, unregulated banking was conceived to be the prime cause of business cycles and periodic panics.

The political ability of bankers to get away with this predatory scheme was perceived by the reformers to reside in the successful propaganda that money is backed by gold and that bankers lend out only the money that savers deposit with them. The reform literature is consequently heavy on debunking those two notions. Reformers were also optimistic that a campaign to educate voters in the truth about money could succeed in mounting a successful political campaign to make government take control of monetary policy. They therefore produced teaching materials and organized study clubs throughout the country. What happened to that aspiration, and is it a realistic one for our own times?

Keith Wilde

Editorial Note

There are two possible resolutions of the unresolved cadence to which Keith Wilde refers.

1. There was an immense amount of questioning by professional and amateur economists, without which the Roosevelt reform of banking, the *National Recovery Act*, and much of the rest of the New Deal would have been inconceivable. It brought about not only monetary and other reforms, but changed the alliance in power in the US by encouraging the organization of trade unions under the NRA, and bringing those unions into a broad government alliance to lift the country out of the depression. In Canada the nationalization of the Bank of Canada

in 1938 served a similar purpose. Without it, the financing of WWII would have been unthinkable, as would the postwar reconstruction. And without the efforts of McGeer and others, as regrettable as their tampering with the historical documentation was, this would simply not have happened.

2. The suppressions and tampering with the documents of history by amateur reformers is as nothing compared with the well-documented suppression of history by forces in power throughout the world. As is the lack of serious assessment of the failures of forecasts and analyses. In the case of COMER, the *Meltdown* volume (1999) summarizes what I considered essential in the forecasts of COMER and similar thinkers. I might mention the forecast of the collapse of the financial system based on the incompatibility between the deregulation of our banks that had already been bailed out by doing away with the statutory reserves and the BIS *Risk-Based Capital Requirements* guidelines that declared the debt of developed countries to be risk-free requiring no additional capital for banks to acquire on the one hand; and the simultaneous attempt of the same central banks goaded on by the same BIS to raise interest rates into the sky to lick "inflation." The deepening layer of taxation in price reflected the needs of a rapidly urbanizing society switching to a high tech economy to support a rapidly growing population. It had little to do much of the time with an excess of demand over supply. On page 96 of *Meltdown*, Volume 1, the reader will find an article of mine taken from *ER* of May 1993 – i.e., even before the phasing out of the statutory reserves had been completed, and even before we had finally dug up the text of the law that initiated it in which we clearly predicted the Mexican meltdown of the following year that almost brought down the world financial system. Only a $51 billion plus standby improvised by Washington, the IMF and Canada prevented that at the last moment, but that did not prevent the wildly idiotic combination of allowing the banks to accumulate government debt with no cash down, and pushing up interest rates that was bound to cause these bank hoards to shed value in catastrophic gobs.

Democracy – especially in so complex an economy – is unthinkable without the fullest flow of information. That, however, is what those in power have suppressed to a degree unknown in the 1930s.

W.K.

Lies Birth a Progeny of Misrepresentation

T*HE NEW YORK TIMES* (23/01, "Why Libya Gave Up On the Bomb" by Flynt Leverett) offers us a lesson of how a single misrepresentation in public policy can beget a whole further generation of distortion. Mr. Leverett, a former senior director for Middle Eastern Affairs at the National Security Council from 2002 to 2003, was in a position to know what led up to Libya's surrender of its weapons of massive destruction projects.

"Washington – As President Bush made clear in his State of the Union address, he sees the striking development in relations with Libya as the fruit of his strategy in the war on terrorism. The idea is that Col. Muammar el Quaddafi's apparent decision to renounce weapons of mass destruction was largely a result of the overthrow of Saddam Hussein, which thus retroactively justifies the war in Iraq and holds out the prospect of similar progress with other states that support terrorists, seek weapons of mass destruction, and brutalize their people.

"However, the president misrepresents the real lesson of the Libyan case. The roots of the recent progress with Libya go back not to the eve of the Iraq war, but to the Bush administration's first year in office. Indeed, some credit should even be given to the second Clinton administration. Tired of international isolation and economic sanctions, the Libyans decided in the late 1990s to seek normalized relations with the US, and held secret discussions with Clinton administration officials to convey that message. The Clinton White House made clear that no movement toward better relations was possible until Libya met its responsibilities from the downing of Pan Am Flight 103 over Lockerbie, Scotland in 1988.

"These discussions, along with mediation by the Saudi ambassador to the US, Prince Bandar bin Sultan, produced a breakthrough. Libya turned over two intelligence officers implicated in the Pan Am 103 attack to the Netherlands for trial by a Scottish court, and in 1999 Washington acquiesced to the suspension of United Nations sanctions against Libya.

"Then in the spring of 2001, when I was a member of the State Department's policy planning staff, the Bush administration picked up on those discussions and induced the Libyans to meet their remaining Lockerbie obligations. With our British colleagues, we presented the Libyans with a 'script' indicating what they needed to do and say to satisfy our requirements on compensating the families of the Pan Am 103 victims.

"By early 2003, after a Scottish appeals court upheld the conviction of one of the Libyan intelligence officers, it was evident that our approach would bear fruit. But during these two years of talks, American negotiators consistently told the Libyans that resolving the Lockerbie situation would lead to no more than elimination of the United Nations sanctions. To get out from under the separate US sanctions, Libya would have to address concerns regarding its programs in weapons of mass destruction.

"This is the context in which the Libyan officials approached the US and Britain last spring to discuss dismantling Libya's nuclear weapons program. The Iraq war, which had not yet started, was not the driving force behind Libya's move. Rather, Libya was willing to deal because of credible diplomatic representations by the United States over the years, which convinced the Libyans that doing so was critical to achieving their goals.

"The lesson is incontrovertible: to persuade a rogue regime to get out of the terrorism business, we must not only apply pressure but also make clear the potential benefits of cooperation. Unfortunately, the Bush administration has refused to take this approach with other rogue regimes. Until the president is willing to employ carrots as well as sticks, he will make little headway in changing Iranian and Syrian behavior.

"As President Assad of Syria told me, Syria is 'a state, not a charity' – it gives up something, it must know what it will gain in return."

Such a whopper on what happened when and because of what in the Libya's peaceful surrender of its nuclear armament may have helped deliver a second term to President Bush by means as flawed as what placed him in the White House in the first place.

William Krehm

The Coming Gale of Currency Adjustments

OIL IS BY FAR the most widely traded commodity of the modern era. Taking that into account, the breakdown of fixed exchange rates and the two oil crises of the 1970s in a practical sense combined to move the international economic system from being anchored to a dollar-gold link, to a dollar-oil link. For the US this meant that the dollar's role is the primary international reserve currency emerged intact from the crisis years.

The period was, despite the economic crises, also marked by a rise in trading volumes, of which the new regime of floating currencies and deregulation was not the only reason. The development of container shipping that had begun in the 1960s had by the mid-seventies fundamentally changed the patterns of intercontinental trade. Suddenly sourcing from overseas producers lost not only much of the cost barriers that earlier transport modes imposed, but transport times were also dramatically cut ensuring that delivery dates became much more predictable.

A Vortex of Change

At first the subsequent export boom out of East Asia was fuelled by local producers that penetrated the Western markets with light industrial products, which they, because of their lower labour costs, could market at much lower prices than existing Western manufacturers. But it didn't take long for the sell-everything-low-cost warehouses that at the time also were an emerging business phenomenon to realize the new possibilities the changing international trading picture opened for them. They started to set up their own sourcing offices in the low-cost manufacturing regions, thus further reducing input costs by dealing directly with the offshore manufacturers.

Costs for a wide array of products for the Western markets were thus lowered dramatically. However, because of the corporations' ability to create not only horizontal but also vertical monopolistic conditions, they were in a position to avoid passing all of the cost reductions on to consumers. Instead a substantial part of the cost reductions were turned into extra surpluses distributed partly as traditional shareholder profits and partly as skyrocketing executive pay packages.

In this vortex of change the workers of the high-cost Western industrial countries lost out, mainly because of two charac-

teristics of labour as an economic factor. Firstly, labour in this setting is very dispersed with a correspondingly low bargaining leverage. Union bargaining can to some extent offset this, but the period in question was also one of diminishing union strength. Secondly, labour is a relatively static factor that cannot respond to changes by relocating and restructuring as corporations can.

Another problem that faced the workers in the developed countries when competing with offshore labour costs is that exchange rates of the new low-cost export nations' currencies are not simply a result of cost-of-living differentials that will adjust to the higher economic growth rates, which their export industries will produce. Purchasing power parities – developed by the World Bank as an international comparative statistical device – indicate that the currencies of the developing nations typically are undervalued in a range of three to five times the official rates. In other words, the labour costs embedded in import goods are three to five times less than they would be if they simply reflected differences in living standards.

This contravenes the principle of one price to such a degree that there must be other aspects than living standards and trade balances influencing international currency alignments. One such is the concentration of the world's liquid assets in the high-income countries in the West – a heritage of European colonialism. During the early phase of Western expansionism, gold and silver, the two precious metals upon which traditional European bimetallism were based, flowed to the West in a steady one-way stream as a result of colonialism's unequal trading patterns.

After the second, or metropolitan, industrial revolution took off around the mid-nineteenth century (by 1850 Manchester had metamorphosed into the worlds first industrialized metropolitan hub) the Western states gravitated away from bimetallism and toward a true gold standard as the base for their monetary systems. Industrialism also led to the development of modern banking and a rising role of government institutions in the management of society, including the issue of fiat paper monies. Connected to these developments, new types of money forms and financial assets sprang up. Bank deposits, government bonds, stocks, equity-derived debt securities, etc., all were assets types that while not totally unknown in preindustrial Europe (and occasionally also found in proto-forms in other advanced cultures) their emergence as economic mass phenomena was unique to industrialism. Importantly, the value of these new monies and financial asset classes were no longer primarily based on convertiblity into commodities, but instead on the productive capacities of the industrial complex and governments' ability to raise taxes on that basis.

A Dearth of Liquid Assets

Since the countries on the periphery of Western industrialism – today's developing world – only had very limited abilities to participate in the processes of liquid asset creation, the divisions begun during the colonial period intensified. When the financial markets determine currency parities they consistently put more importance on holdings and ability to attract international liquidity instruments than for instance cost of living indices and trade flows. Because of that, after a number of the developing countries entered the global trading system as sourcing and offshoring destinations and began to run substantial trade surpluses, markets have been very slow to reflect this by readjusting currency parities. In fact, the markets have apparently been quite indifferent to the fact that governments in the new export countries often maintain their currencies at artificially low exchange rates in order to speed up their export-led growth strategies.

Western workers in the industries competing with low priced imports and offshoring are thus in a position where the cost levels they are up against are not only a result of the low living standards in the offshoring countries, but also an outgrowth of a historical process that concentrated the world's liquid assets in the West. In this situation, the likelihood currency alignments reflecting the new patterns of trade surpluses diminishing the cost pricing disadvantage of their wage levels is at best a long shot.

Of course, persistent trade deficits will eventually also impact asset ownership and in particular balances of assets with high liquidity in international financial markets. But while smaller nations running persistent trade deficits quickly succumb to such pressures, the position of the US is much stronger.

A combination of factors, including its economic size, its role as the world's only military superpower, and the dollar's position as the primary reserve currency, has made dollar instruments the preferred vehicle for investors seeking safety and liquidity. Such holdings of dollar assets do not necessarily have to be placed in the US itself, but can be accommodated in the tax haven banking centers that have popped up in many of the world's mini-states.

Outsourcing US Dollars

When the US started to move into a position of persistent trade deficits around 1980, economic orthodoxy would expect its government to allow markets to follow their normal course and depreciate the dollar. But with Reagan in the White House, political considerations caused the administration to follow a high dollar policy pulling in the exact opposite direction. With private savings falling and the government ready to embark on its ideologically motivated policy of tax reductions, running trade deficits was seen as a mean of financing the projected domestic deficits.

The high dollar years speeded up the dislocating of the old American manufacturing industries and the subsequent reliance on offshore imports as substitutes. This process also pushed the economy further down a path where the bulk of its value added was created in the service sectors, many of them requiring few skills and thus offering low wages. Nevertheless, during the Clinton years the economy experienced a run of a new high growth period that coupled with some modest tax hikes managed to turn the domestic deficit around. However, there was a price to pay: the trade deficits that had shrunk somewhat during the early nineties ballooned again.

The growing trade deficit meant that foreign trade partners were accumulating excess dollar receipts again, which they wanted to convert into instruments offering interest or capital gains. But after the domestic deficit had turned into a surplus by the late nineties the government's net issue of interest-bearing securities shrank accordingly. Therefore, the excess dollars in the currency markets increasingly had to be sopped up by the stock market, where they however only further fueled a bout of asset inflation already underway.

When the stock market bubble burst in 2000 this presented the incoming president Bush with a dilemma. The American corporations had by then all learned how to use the new international division of labour based on offshoring manufacturing to maximize their surpluses. Furthermore, the impact of the internet was beginning to move offshoring into white-collar industries, even including government services (calls to local government offices with questions about, for instance, tax matters or zoning statutes are in fact increasingly answered by call centers in Bangalore, India, where English speaking is widespread, has emerged as the preferred location for these new developments).

Such tendencies are speeding up, as is evidenced by the continued deterioration of the American trade deficit. And the corporate leaders crowding the Republican Party behind Bush are in no mood to see restrictive policy changes that might slow down the unfettered growth of offshoring. Once again, the interests of the American workers, who for 30 years have seen no growth in real wages, were not part of the policy equation.

The Stock Market Sops Up the Dollar Excess

Instead, the Bush administration embarked on a policy of massive, top-heavy tax reductions, a policy course that killed two birds with one stone. Firstly, it sent a lot of the money that previously had flowed into the government's coffers back into the pockets of its backers among the wealthy elite. Secondly, it necessitated a new wave of issues of government debt instruments that could serve as interest-bearing near-monies with the ability to sop up the excess dollars that the foreign currency markets otherwise would drown in.

Reagan firstly decided on the tax reduction policies and then pushed the trade deficit as a financing means. Bush, on the other hand, was confronted with a growing trade deficit that his corporate backers, all in their own self-interests, didn't want restricted. In the wake of the stock market's bubble-and-bust, that naturally had created some apprehension among foreign investors for a repeat performance, he had to recreate the domestic budget deficits to pump a new flood of near-monies back into the system.

So, as the old adage goes, things that can't go on forever, won't. When a Chinese official – who are not known to speak at their whim – during the Davos meeting in February remarked that "the US dollar is no longer (seen) as a stable currency," strong alarm bells should have gone off in Washington.

Dix Sandbeck

Condoleezza or Rumsfeld — Whom to Believe?

O N THE FRONT PAGE of *The Wall Street Journal* (11/03), symmetrically placed in extreme right-and left-hand columns are the gospels of Bush II according to his leading prophets. The Condoleezza doctrine shines through the first narrative – kiss and make up with our major European neighbours, at least if the cameras are around ("South Korean Aid to North Increases Tensions with US" by Gordon Fairclough): "Ma Jeong, South Korea – Near the barb-wired fences of the demilitarized zone that slices across this divided peninsula, a widening split between Washington and Seoul over how best to deal with North Korea's nuclear threat is on vivid display. Trucks laden with tons of construction supplies and machinery from the south start lining up here early most mornings. They are bound for a giant industrial park under construction across the border designed to help the North shore up its tottering economy.

"One snowy day last month, a South Korean soldier in green camouflage waved the convoy through a military checkpoint. The trucks then snaked under an archway marked 'Unification Gate,' headed north.

"The US, focused on preventing nuclear proliferation and disarming North Korea, is looking for ways to ratchet up the pressure on Pyongyang. But the South Korean government is busy working to help keep its former enemy in the North afloat with aid and economic-cooperation. After a fratricidal war in the early 1950s, followed by decades of Cold War, South Korea made a sharp turn in the late 1990s, moving to subsidize its erstwhile rival. Now landmines have been pulled from two parts of the demilitarized zone to allow the reconnection of roads to move goods and even tourists to the North.

"Behind Seoul's decision is a basic calculation: a collapse of North Korea, deeply militarized and impoverished after nearly 50 years of Stalinist rule, would simply be too expensive. So officials here largely oppose steps that could destabilize Kim Jong II's regime, which many US policymakers would just as soon see disappear. 'Some people seem to look for the North to collapse,' said South Korea's president Roh Moo Hyun, in an apparent reference to US hard-liners during a speech in Los Angeles last year. But that 'would cause an enormous disaster for the people of the South.' [The population of North Korea is some 22 and one half million; that of the south is just under 50 million.]

"The rift between Washington and Seoul has been in the spotlight in two developments last month. Pyongyang declared that it has nuclear weapons and is withdrawing 'indefinitely' from multilateral disarmament talks. And the US made a case to allies that North Korea shipped sensitive nuclear material to Libya several years ago. After the announcement Vice President Dick Cheney met with South Korea's Foreign Minister, Han Ki Moon, and asked whether, given the North's actions, Seoul should reconsider moving forward with aid plans." South Korean leaders retorted that it was too soon to say whether the North has nuclear weapons, and suggested "carrots" or "a cube of sugar" to entice Pyongyang back to the bargaining table and persuade it to abandon its atomic ambitions.

"For some American officials that stance is frustrating: Seoul is providing a lifeline to the government in the North. The talks, which involve China, Russia and Japan in addition to the US and the two Koreas, had been stalled since June."

Another Iraq on the Doormats of the US's Major Rivals?

"Experts in the US and South Korea were disappointed in their expectations of a collapse of the North Korean economy after the disappearance of the Soviet Union and the death of Kim Il Sung, the country's founder. But the regime proved surprisingly resilient, surviving even a massive famine." That and the reluctance of its European allies to be dragged into another Asian adventure, but this time one disconcertingly located on the very door mats of major competitive powers of the US – China, Russia, and Japan – provides compelling reason for bringing the Condoleezza doctrine to the fore.

Moreover, not only has the economy of the North turned out to have more staying power, but the South Korean economy has been less sturdy than was believed. It had been badly hit by the East Asian financial crisis brought on largely by US and the IMF's monetary policies. Nor did Seoul's growing consciousness of the vulnerability of the Western powers end there. After studying the difficulties that Germany ran into so unexpectedly when it came to the reunification with East Germany – the Seoul government has come to distrust the heroic bulletins of the Cold War period that linger on in Washington. In 1998, in response to its own financial crisis, Seoul under the previous regime embarked on a policy of cooperation and collaboration with the North.

President Clinton, along with his Treasury Secretary, Robert Rubin, had spent sleepless nights staving off an international financial meltdown brought on by the Fed's high interest rate policy and the deregulation of world banking. The main body of Bush warriors have been less open to such concerns. Putting Condoleezza to the fore, they have come to accept cooperation already under way between the two Koreas, but oppose any extension of that program unless the North abandons its nuclear weapon projects.

Seoul has been too close to an almost half-century military stalemate as well as to the weaknesses of the Western economy – from the overproduction of its automobile industry to its over-dependence on consumer debt – to share the economic orthodoxies of Republican conventions. It has a first-hand sense of the immense risks for its economy – the 10th largest in the world – in a likely influx of an estimated two million refugees from the North, if it were brought to a collapse. "Marcus Noland, a Korea expert at the Institute for International Economics in Washington, calls North Korea 'the world's largest contingent liability' and sets a price tag of some $600 billion as the costs to be faced during the first 10 years after a North Korean collapse."

Nor might the hazards of a preemptive strike on North Korea just bring in the East Asian equivalents of Syria or Iran into the fray. This time it would in one way or another be major powers operating close to their home bases. With so much hand-wringing under way about Washington's unfavorable payment position, imagine what the picture would be in the event of a preemptive strike on North Korea, should one or more of the unhappy big-powers even covertly support North Korean resistance.

"A 2004 poll conducted for the Chicago Council on Foreign Relations found that 81% of South Koreans wanted to stick with the current level of engagement or increase it. Only 9% supported a harder line toward the North.

"South Koreans view the North as less of a threat now that contacts between the two countries have increased. North Koreans look so poor. It's like South Korea in the 1960s. 'We have to help them a lot,' says 56-year-old Paek Jae Hyun, CEO of a chemical company in the South returning from a recent visit.

"But the Northerners are also seen as alien. In 2003, a group of visiting North Korean cheerleaders caused a stir when they leapt from their bus to rescue the picture of Kim Jong II getting soaked in the rain. North Koreans are taught to revere likenesses of Mr. Kim and his father, and can be punished for disrespecting their pictures. The incident prompted one weekly magazine in Seoul to ask: 'Are we really one people?'

"Park Dae Hee has been traveling back and forth to the North several times a month, delivering supplies and supervising construction of a shoe factory at the industrial park being built on the outskirts of the North Korean city of Kaesong. At first he was scared to go. Now he sees the northerners more as rather prickly little brothers.

"'They don't want to feel inferior,' says Mr. Park. But it takes three North Koreans to do the work of one South Korean. Unification would be very hard. There's such a huge economic gap between the two countries, and big differences in political views.'

"The project Mr. Park is working on is South Korea's most ambitious effort to gradually narrow these disparities. The industrial park is being developed by the South government-owned Korea Land Corp. and the private Hyundai Asan Corp. Two factories are already operating, one of which makes cookware that is on sale in Seoul department stores. An additional 13 are soon to come online in the pilot phase of the project.

"The first phase of the development is expected to include 300 factories and employ 75,000 North Koreans. Later stages will add many more plants, a golf course and apartments. About 1,800 South Korean companies have applied for spots. During the project's first nine years, it will inject $9.6 billion into the North economy. Coupled with international trade and aid, that could significantly ease the pressure on Kim John II's regime. Mr. Noland of the Institute for International Economics figures that $1 billion to $2 billion a year is enough to keep the North on 'survival rations.'"

For some people in Washington that might be less desirable, since it will certainly give them an alternative to playing Russian roulette with an existing or non-existent nuclear toy. For others it would be "the cube of sugar" that the Southern Korean diplomat spoke of. However, it could lead to the scrapping of the doctrine of preemptive strikes that is the gospel of Bush II according to prophet Rumsfeld. South Korean officials say the project shows the strategic benefits of economic cooperation. Construction has forced the relocation of some North Korean military forces away from the border. The project also sits astride one of the main invasion routes troops would have to traverse to get to South Korea.

William Krehm

Financial Fantasy

DURING A RECENT two week visit to Arizona I was exposed to the debate over the future of Social Security. The system is seriously in the red, and President Bush's solution is to privatize – permitting citizens under 55 to use up to two thirds of their tax free contribution to invest in private accounts. To make up the shortfall during the transition, the US government will have to borrow some $2 trillion – this on top of the current, and rapidly growing national debt of $7.62 trillion. Even Bush admits that his proposal doesn't fully solve the problem, but it would greatly reduce the government's obligations. So far the public reaction is highly skeptical.

Paul O'Neill, Bush's first Secretary of the Treasury (dismissed over policy differences) has a better idea (Arizona *Daily Star* – Feb 27/05). He would set up an investment account for every American at birth. The government would deposit $2000 in that account every year until the child is 18. (He does not tell us where the government would get the $144 billion annual cost – presumably it would be borrowed!) The money would remain in the account until the owner reached 65, by which time it would be worth $1,013,326 in inflation adjusted dollars, and would pay $82,000 a year for 20 years. His projections are based on a "conservative index of stocks and bonds" and a real return of 6% annually.

At first glance, O'Neill's proposal sounds wonderful, and, according to the article, it has attracted some interest from US legislators. They would be well advised to probe a little deeper. Like most financial fantasies, this one never deals with the real economy. He never tells us how the production of goods and services could be increased to validate such a huge increase in purchasing power. Perhaps in this brave new world, consumption would be restricted to the elderly. There might be enough bonds for all those accounts, as the US takes on an ever greater debt, but who will pay all the interest? There is no mention of raising taxes. Where will the needed additional shares come from and how will companies generate the wealth to pay the dividends? With the real economy, after inflation, growing at 2-3% annually, how can the stock markets grow at 6%? How many more public assets can be privatized?

This kind of fantasy stems from the delusion promoted by the financial community, that the stock market is an inexhaustible fount of wealth. The knowledgeable capitalist understands that stock ownership must be restricted to a minority. A society wherein all citizens own huge amounts of shares would vastly dilute the pool of wealth to validate those shares.

Real wealth comes from the real economy – from real resources extracted, processed, and manufactured by real machinery and real workers. Any retirement scheme ultimately depends on the ability of the productive forces in society to create enough surplus goods and services to sustain the non-working retirees. When the Canadian government increased the CPP premium recently, they recognized (not publicly of course), that maintaining consumption for seniors means reducing consumption for workers.

In the US these days, the financial fallacy is well established. Government corporations and consumers are amassing debt at a feverish pace. Because the real economy cannot sustain so much consumption, the US has to import heavily and has run up a huge and growing trade deficit. To pay for the trade deficit, it has to borrow some $2 billion a day from abroad. This can continue only as long as other societies are willing to purchase US debt (i.e., transfer some of the wealth produced in their economies to the US). This may be fine while it lasts, but sooner or later the party will end.

David Gracey

Bribing the Already Suborned

NOT THE LEAST MERIT of Stephen Zarlenga's book *The Lost Science of Money* is that it documents the repeated resurfacing of the truth about token money as opposed to commodity money. In monetary thinking over the past three millennia there has been a basic continuum of understanding of token money that does not depend on its metallic content, but on the credit of a state sufficiently well organized and concerned about the welfare of its society to make its commitment creditable without the vast expenditure in even trying to mirror the real economy with a monetary medium of an intrinsic value equal to that of the goods traded.

The champions of token money over the centuries have been of sufficient distinction, to have required massive inputs of bribery, and repression to hide the elemental facts of money creation. They can be traced as far back as Aristotle in Ancient Greece. The suppression of these traditions has in our day involved the relegation to the status of unmentionable any reference to key sections of laws still on our law books, the early retirement of academics who dare continue teaching the basic facts of central banking as could be found in textbooks little more than a decade ago – right until the our deregulated banks were massively bailed out from their losses in speculations incompatible with banking. It is over a decade since the historic purposes of central banks could be referred to in our media.

And now, as though to gild the lily, those who defend the official line are not only virtually assured lucrative careers in their chosen field – academic, journalistic, or the world of high finance, but apparently directly bribed by the government.

Thus *The Globe and Mail* (27/01, "Won't pay columnists to promote policies, Bush vows" by Alan Freeman): "'US President George W. Bush vowed yesterday that his administration will stop paying columnists and pundits to back its policies after the second right-wing commentator in a month acknowledged receiving a contract from a government agency to advance our agenda,' Mr. Bush told reporters. 'Our agenda ought to be able to stand on its own two feet.'

"The President spoke a day after Maggie Gallagher, a conservative columnist and president of her own marriage institute, divulged that she had been paid $21,500 (US) by the Health and Human Services Administration to promote Mr. Bush's $300-million marriage initiative.

"Her work included writing an essay promoting marriage that was published in a Roman Catholic publication under the byline of Wade Horn, the government's assistant secretary for children and families. At the same time. Ms. Gallagher was writing newspaper columns and appearing on television talk shows, lauding the marriage initiative.

"When confronted by *The Washington Post* about her contract, Ms. Gallagher initially seemed uncertain whether she had violated journalistic ethics by not advising her readers she was on the government's payroll. But she apologized later in the day, saying in a column that 'it never occurred to me to disclose the contract.'

"Separately yesterday, a report made public by Democratic members of the committee on government reform said Mr. Bush's administration spent $88 million last year on contracts with public-relations agencies, more than double the amount spent in 2000, the final year of Bill Clinton's administration."

Actual bribery occurs of those who have already been suborned.

This is at a time when even *The Washington Post* and other leading papers, though openly critical of official policy on other matters have not for years published anything that questions the official views on money creation. The holding of central government debt by central banks in leading countries has been shifted from a high approaching 25% of the central government's debt in the mid-1960s to around 5% today. The important point is that in most advanced countries even where the central bank is owned not by the government, but by private banks, almost all the interest paid by the government on the debt that the central bank holds is returned to the government in recognition of it having assigned to the private banks the creation of money which today is not coined gold or silver, but the credit of the central government. The result is a virtual interest-free loan, by virtue of what for centuries had been known to economists as "seigniorage."

To put matters in perspective we are going to run quotations from a book published in 1999 by COMER consisting of selections from the first decade of the existence of *Economic Reform*.

What is revealed is the very considerable elements of freedom of debate that still existed on the most sensitive areas of economic and financial policy. Even though the references will be largely Canadian, the main inspiration for the suppression of the freedom of information that spread across the world originated in the United States.

What is most alarming is that the more the official economic policy were proved misconceived and based on a massive shift of the national wealth from the productive classes to speculative finance, the more thoroughly was the freedom of discussions of these issues curbed. In 1999 COMER published a selection from the first ten years of *Economic Reform*, and from it two striking conclusions emerge. The first is the degree of open debate in the press, the universities, and at the various levels of government. The second is how dead-on our warnings were not only about the counterproductive policies that were being imposed by our central banks, but in our prediction of an abrupt ending of Prime Minister Brian Mulroney's political career, unless he reconsidered the "zero inflation" course that he had adopted.

I will reproduce a single letter of COMER to Prime Minister Mulroney that brings back that unusual age of democratic exchange of ideas, and the readiness with which Canadians in and out of office were ready to consider alternatives.

From *ER* of September 1988.

To the Right Honourable Brian Mulroney
Ottawa, Ontario

Dear Mr. Prime Minister:

Canadian Press (14/10) carries a report of a speech by Governor John Crow of the Bank of Canada in Tokyo which in part reads as follows "Some Canadian monetary specialists have suggested that the Bank of Canada could make interest rates reflect regional economic disparities in Canada 'as the Japanese do.'"

A year ago at Saskatoon the provincial premiers protested against the high interest rate policy of the BoC that was penalizing the depressed regions of the country to fight inflation in Southern Ontario. At the request of one of the premiers, the Committee on Monetary and Economic Reform (COMER) outlined a policy by which our central bank, while keeping interest rates relatively low, might apportion credit differentially among the various regions of the country according to the real productive bottlenecks.

We were told that this was not only impossible, but that it had in fact never happened in Japan as COMER claimed. In your own public utterances you seemed to identify high interest rates with "fighting inflation." More effective techniques for managing market inflation outlined by COMER and others have been systematically ignored.

We are comforted then to learn that Governor Crow in his recent trip to Japan has not tried telling the Japanese that monetary policy differentiating between industries and regions has been unknown in Japan. Much of the Japanese performance in fact can be traced to the inexpensive credit made available to strategic industries.

We would also draw to your attention that in its preamble the *Bank of Canada Act* provides that our central bank shall "regulate credit and currency to mitigate...fluctuations in the general level of production, trade, prices and employment." It does not authorize the Governor to plot violent fluctuations in the general level of production, trade and employment in pursuit of "zero inflation." That could be obtained only by achieving a "zero economy." For that the BoC studiously avoids

analyzing price movement into its very different components, some of which have nothing to do with an overheated market.

With Friday's stock market crash, you must certainly understand the urgency of such a measure. It is common knowledge among economists that it takes about 18 months for a central bank to produce a depression – twice the time that it takes a woman to produce a child. That in itself underlines the irresponsible brinkmanship of our central bank in throttling the economy until the Governor's pipe-dream of "zero inflation" has shown up in our highly defective statistics.

Depressions, Mr. Prime Minister, are easier to bring on than to undo. The one that threatens the country today is imposing severe strains on the very fabric of Confederation, and is visiting hardship on millions of Canadians. The realities of a depression would leave in tatters these buzzwords of over-orchestrated PR – "short-term pain for long-term gain" and "soft landing." The electorate is likely to prove unforgetting and unforgiving.

Yours respectfully,
John H. Hotson, Executive Director
William Krehm, Board Chairman
Committee for Monetary and Economic Reform

Australian Central Bank Insists on Reliving the Worthy Stretches of Financial History

AUSTRALIA, in the present WORLD commodity boom, occupies an increasingly key position. Immensely endowed with natural resources, it has been playing an ever more prominent part in feeding the world's hunger for raw materials, notably base metals and uranium. Naturally that is showing up in a rising price level. And the Australian central bank, obviously flaunting its "independence" from its elected government seems compelled to repeat ghastly disastrous experiments to "lick inflation once and for all."

So rising prices are once again being attacked with boots and fists rather than with analysis, even though earlier efforts towards such a "final solution" contributed to many disasters, the Iraq mess not excepted. For without such mindless provocation to a faith that sees all interest rather than just usury as a mortal sin, the present cleft between Islam and the West could hardly have attained its current savagery.

The Wall Street Journal (3/03, "Australia Raises Rates Despite Slowed Economy," Dow Jones Newswires) clues us in: "Sydney, Australia – Putting aside concerns that the economy is slowing, Australia's central bank raised interest rates to the highest level in four years because of concerns about capacity constraints and rising inflation. With the official cash rate increased to 5.5% from 5.25%, Australia now has the second highest rates in the developed world – behind New Zealand – and one of the slowest growing economies.

"Two hours after the move by the Reserve Bank of Australia, official data confirmed the economy slumped to an annual growth rate of 1.5% in the fourth quarter of 2004. That was half the third-quarter growth rate.

"Australia is a victim of its own success as it becomes harder to squeeze further growth after 14 years of expansion, economists said. 'Over recent months, it has become increasingly clear that remaining spare capacity in the labour and goods markets is becoming rather limited,' the central bank said in a statement accompanying the rate increase, the first since December 2003. 'This is starting to result in strongly inflationary pressures.'"

The logical thing then would have been to bring back the statutory reserves and raise them high enough to cut down the multiplier of credit that the banks create out of thin air as they exploit the capital pools of the non-banking financial sectors they have been able to take over under their deregulation.

But, along with the disasters brought on by Paul Volcker during his chairmanship of the US Fed when he tried wiping out "inflation" with interest rates that for productive borrowers reached into the 20% range, that is mere history, and the place for that is the waste-paper basket.

"The central bank bases its deliberations on an inflation target range of 2% to 3%. In its statement, the bank said inflation will probably reach 3% by the end of 2006, and there is a chance the forecast might be too low. With Australia's unemployment rate at 5.1% in January – its lowest in a generation – many economists had predicted the central bank the central bank would raise rates this month as skills shortages and wage spikes emerge in overstretched pockets of the economy. Complicating matters further, domestic demand remains robust and has pushed Australia's trade deficit to a record."

Higher rates, of course, will strengthen the Australian currency further and increase the unfavourable international payments balance, which by the central bank's logic will serve as further reason for shimmying up the greased interest rate pole. The only thing apparently that we learn from history would seem to be that we learn nothing from history.

"'I don't see any evidence of inflationary pressures,' said Treasurer Peter Costello, noting the lower growth rate increase meant the economy isn't presenting a 'totally consistent story,' Rory Robertson, senior strategist at Macquarte Bank, said."

The story, however, is plotted and told without contradiction by the central bank bureaucracy, while we are left wondering about the responsibility of democratic governments to look after the welfare of their citizens.

W.K.

Review of an Important Incomplete Document

Submission to Tim O'Neill, Special Advisor to Finance Minister Ralph Goodale, Review of "Federal Fiscal Forecasts and Budget Planning Procedures," by Jim Stanford, Economist, Canadian Auto Workers, stanford@caw.ca, February, 2005.

THOUGH THERE ARE MANY crucial matters still omitted, much of importance ignored by our government budgeteers is dealt with in this document. Jim Stanford had been "associated with the Alternative Federal Budget project premised on meeting the government's own deficit-reduction targets, but in what we held to be a more socially sustainable manner."

That specification calls for a high-wire act worthy of Cirque du Soleil, risky not only for broken limbs, but because it allows the government to impose the agenda. Yet it does give us the occasion to mix some sincere applause for what is included with criticism for key lessons of our history left out.

"The current methodology incorporates basic practices that skew the budget-making process in a fiscally conservative direction. This process is inherited from an earlier era in which the federal government faced the challenge of reducing its deficit, slowing an unsustainable rate of increase in its net debt and repairing its fiscal credibility in light of past missed targets.

"Today, however, the situation is radically different. Counting the 2004-5 fiscal year, Ottawa has generated fiscal surpluses in 8 consecutive years (the longest stretch since Confederation). The ratio of net debt to GDP has declined by 40% or 27 full percentage points, in the past decade, and continues to decline rapidly (thanks mostly to ongoing economic growth). Canada is now the least indebted of the major industrialized economies, and the federal debt (now below 40% of GDP) is low by both historical and international comparison.

"It may have been the case a decade ago that our budgetary forecasts had to err on the side of caution, at all costs – to restore credibility in the budgeting process, and ensure that the urgent problems of deficit and debt were addressed faster rather than slower. That is not the case today, however."

Right there, unfortunately, we must take issue with Mr. Stanford. To be accepted, as it were, as a member of the flock and to be allowed to participate in a democratic discussion of some important issues, he has chosen to pay a weighty admission fee-not to raise crucial episodes of our history that have long since been declared unmentionable. Unfortunately that means excluding the direct causes of the budget-problems of the past decade. To limit the interchange to surpluses and deficits without raising the question of what produced those catastrophic deficits that led to the *annus horribilis* of 1995, is to forgo relating our budgetary troubles to the clash of social interests, but instead treating them as a matter of solving a few mental arithmetical problems. What was involved was in fact a shift of power and accessibility to key information. Unless corrected, that threatens our democratic system.

To treat this rerouting of society's command chain and revenue so that it can be discussed in strictly arithmetical terms is like trying to understand the Great Depression of the 1930s and its eventual consequence in World War II as purely mathematical problems. Or the French Revolution. Such false solutions were prompted far less by misguided handling of quantities than by an unsustainable reshuffling of social relationships.

More than a Problem in Arithmetic

The literature on the subject is rich, if largely suppressed. I need only mention Arthur Johnson *Breaking the Banks*, Lester & Orpen Dennys, 1986, or the late Walter Stewart's, *Bank Heist – How our Financial Giants are Costing You Money*, Harper Collin, 1997. Walter Stewart, a former editor of *Maclean's*, summed it all up when he told his staff they must research every story as though they had just come to town, and write it as though they were going to leave town that night. Our criticism of Jim Stanford's in some respects laudable essay could be summed up as follows, "It is researched as though the author had come to town a generation or two ago, and intended to stay on a further generation at least."

What is missing from the tale is precisely the bailout of the banks on a world scale from their deregulated gambols of the 1980s. That is like telling the biblical tale of our forefathers' expulsion from Paradise as a misfired apple-marketing episode, with no mention of the serpent. But even without taking theological counsel, I am left with the impression that the tale of the lady with the forbidden apple and the dubious adviser keeps on repeating itself, generation after generation. Currently, it is hogging our financial pages. Leave it out, and you miss the next apple cum serpent episode that is closing in on us, and is likely to queer the budget forecasts both of our Government and of Jim Stanford.

Specifically I refer to the bailout of our banks from their huge speculative losses in gas and oil and real estate during the 1980s These were made good by allowing our banks to quadruple their holdings of Canadian federal debt without putting up any of their own money. This was achieved as part of a plan devised through the Bank for International Settlements (BIS), a non-elected institution of banking technocrats located in Basel, Switzerland. This applied to the entire market-driven part of the world, for the speculative excesses of the banks had taken place on all continents. The remedy applied was double-pronged. In 1988, the *Risk-Based Capital Requirements* were brought in by BIS – after consultations in which no elected representative of the government took part. This and other measures had been preceded by an elaborate campaign to assert the independence of the central banks throughout the world from their elected governments – even in cases where the charter of the central bank says the contrary ("the *Bank of Canada Act* clearly establishes the power of the minister of Finance the dismiss the Governor of the Bank of Canada if he failed to follow the explicit instruction of the Government in a matter of basic monetary policy). The *Risk-Based Capital Requirements* shifted the criterion for bank solvency from *cash* reserves to *capital* reserves. A bank's capital is rarely held in cash; for cash by its mere existence breeds no interest. It usually exists in the form

of bricks or mortar, machinery, or in securities of all maturities. Even more disturbing, it is usually kept on the banks' books at its original cost to the banks (its "historic" value) – rather than its current market value. Indeed, in Canada until 1991, it was completely written off in a single year.

Moreover, the debt of developed (OECD) countries was declared risk-free by the BIS Guidelines, requiring no additional capital reserves for banks to acquire.

At this very time, however, and during the early 1990s, BIS and most central banks throughout the world were conducting a no-holds-barred campaign to wipe out what they considered "inflation," i.e., any increase in price indexes whether it could be traced to a real excess of demand over available supply, or to structural factors not originating in the market economy and thus dismissed by economists as "externalities." Such factors call for more government spending to cope with the educational needs created by new technologies, a growing population, the despoliation of the environment, and the racing pace of urbanization throughout the world. For these are funded largely by the state out of taxation. This inevitably results in a deepening layer of taxes in price which is *structural* rather than *market-determined*. It cannot be made to disappear by raising interest rates or manipulating the market. It must be recognized as "structural price rise" and analyzed as such.[1] There are, moreover, many ways in which the structural price gradient, once recognized for what it is, can be harnessed for social advantage.[2]

BIS representing the ambitious of the speculative financial sector followed precisely the contrary course.

Cooking the Books in a Big Cauldron

In the early 1990s few governments distinguished between a current expense and capital investments that will remain useful and productive for decades, Most governments still do not. Spending to build a bridge or to buy a building was treated exactly the same as the purchase of soap for the government's wash-rooms. Up to 1991 in Canada there had been two main tools for combatting perceived inflation – real or imagined. Usually 8% to 10% of the deposits made by the public in banks' chequing accounts (and considerably less in the case of longer term deposits) were required to be redeposited by the banks with the Bank of Canada which paid no interest. This gave the central bank a way of combatting a rise in the price indexes other than raising interest rates. But when the reserves were abolished as a means of helping the banks cope with their immense capital losses during the 1980s, only a single "blunt tool" remained for dealing with their pet obsession with "inflation."

But in their haste to rescue the banks, BIS and the technicians they assembled in Basel to consider the new *Risk-Based Capital Requirements* guidelines, overlooked an important detail. Whenever the benchmark interest rate is pushed up, the market value of preexistent bonds falls like a rock – for their coupons will be less than what is being paid on current bonds issues. COMER grasped the point at once and through its monthly newsletter and other more personal channels sent word warning the finance minister that it had designed a bailout that was bound to undermine the solvency of our banks as much as their speculative losses in the 1980s. To no effect. In 1994, however, the Mexican banks – loaded up as they were with government bonds – declared risk-free and denominated in US dollars on the advice of an American mega-bank advisor – almost brought down the international banking system. That was staved off only by the largest standby loan on record organized by President Clinton without the backing of Congress. That fund, provided by the US, the IMF and Canada, saved the situation. As a result of that crisis, 85% of the banking system of Mexico ended up in foreign hands. That has not gone down well with a country of strongly nationalist traditions like Mexico.

By trying to flatten prices where the physical investments of all levels of government were written off in a single year, it became necessary to raise enough taxes to balance what was essentially an unbalanceable budget. Even the attempt to achieve such a feat meant that an unnecessary amount of taxation was raised, and thus the structural price gradient was exaggerated. The submission of Jim Stanford cites the raw numbers, but he does not enter into the mistaken accountancy that contributed to this. Nevertheless a series of Auditors General and at least three royal commissions recommended the introduction of accrual accountancy into the federal books in vain. (The same, of course, should be done in the bookkeeping of the provincial governments and the municipalities.)

But instead, physical capital assets – buildings, highways, power generation plants carried on the government books at a token dollar since they had been wholly depreciated in a single year – were often sold off at a fraction of their value, and the proceeds applied to "pay down the debt." Then, organized as private corporations and listed on the stock exchange these were able to exact inflated user-fees from the public for what it had already paid for in taxation. Not only were our banks bailed out from their speculative losses, but since this had to be done in secrecy, it involved a transfer of power as well as of money. Until the mid-1970s, the Bank of Canada held well over 22% of the total federal debt. And since the government of Canada was privatized by the Liberal government of Mackenzie King in 1938, the interest paid on that portion of the federal debt (less overhead costs) found its way back to the federal government as dividends. Once the statutory reserves had been abolished, and the chartered banks quadrupled their holdings of federal debt without putting up a penny *in cash or capital* of their own money, that interest stayed with them.

The Most Productive Investment Ignored

In the 1960s, on pondering the amazingly rapid reconstruction of Japan and Germany after the mass physical destruction they had suffered in World War II, economists arrived at an important conclusion. Theodore Schultz received a Nobel Prize for Economics prize for reasoning that investment in human capital was the most productive that a government could make. It mattered little that such investment was lodged in private brains and bodies: they contributed to the tax base which was the source of governmental income when needed. It had, too, the longest depreciation periods of any investments.

The education and good health of parents passes on to future generations.

Yet not even in theory is this vast investment in human capital mentioned in the endless discussions about the urgency of balancing budgets. Surely we cannot wait for the permission of the government to raise the point.

Stanford does argue with telling effect against the policy of "virtue by cooking the books" practised by Paul Martin during his years as Finance Minister. "Many advocates of debt reduction have not been displeased with the consistent 'upside' errors of recent federal budgets, since the outcome of those errors has been a significant reduction in the nominal federal debt (repayment which will total almost $70 billion by the end of the current fiscal year). In some cases, debt reduction advocates even seem to accept that Canadians need to be 'tricked' into this debt reduction (through budgetary planning practices which deliberately understate the true strength of federal finances). Apart from the distressing anti-democratic and paternalistic overtones of this approach, I also take issue with the assumption that debt reduction (especially in the form of nominal debt repayment) is indeed a positive economic goal, for a modestly-indebted country like Canada. Obviously, there are limits to indebtedness, and the costs of carrying debt increase at an increasing rate as debt burdens grow. That is why I fully accepted that Canada's debt was on an unsustainable path in the early 1990s, indeed, the Alternative Federal Budget in which I participated was premised on meeting the government's own deficit-reduction targets, but in what we held to be a more socially sustainable manner.

"But what benefit is now served by reducing Canada's debt even faster (through nominal debt repayment) than it is already declining at? Debt repayment reduces future interest charges on debt, freeing perhaps $50 million in future revenues for each $1 billion paid back. We insulate ourselves somewhat from the impacts of future financial market turbulence, although we are still very much subject to the ups and downs of those financial tides."

Amazingly, Jim Stanford, does not utter what he must certainly know: Since the early 1970s Canadian federal government debt has been the only legal tender – money that must be accepted in payment of debt, including notably by the federal government in payment of its taxes. Pay off the debt, and you will have no money. Pay off more of it than is required for circulation and money becomes scarce and increases in value.

William Krehm

1. Krehm, William (1975). *Price in a Mixed Economy – Our Record of Disaster*. Toronto.
2. Krehm, William (1977). *Babel's Tower: The Dynamics of Economic Breakdown*. Toronto.

Embedding Rumfeld's Heritage in the Military Structures

NOTHING really of importance gets wholly decided by mere debate. Such decisions more often than not are settled in large part by political and bureaucratic string-pulling behind the scenes. You reorganize the armed forces to suit your plans and they are likely to be unsuited for applying your opponent's very different ideas even if he takes over office. And that seems to be just what Rumsfeld is up to. At the other side of the first page of the same *WSJ* to offset Condoleezza's more feminine open-mindedness for setting the world aright, Greg Jaffe ("Rumsfeld Pushes Major Revamping of UD Military") informs us: "Defence Secretary Donald Rumsfeld outlines in a new, classified planning document a vision for remaking the military to be far more engaged in heading off threats prior to hostilities and serve a larger purpose of enhancing US influence around the world.

"The document sets out Mr. Rumsfeld's agenda for a recently begun massive review of defense spending and strategy. The process is conducted only once every four years. Compiled by senior members of Mr. Rumsfeld's staff along with senior officers from each of the four military services, it represents the Bush administration's best chance to refashion the military into a force capable of delivering on its ambitious foreign-policy goals."

Shifting Weapons Systems

"Indeed, the document marks a significant departure from recent reviews. Deeply informed by both the terrorist attacks of September 11, 2001, and by the military's bloody struggle in Iraq, it emphasizes newer problems, such as fighting terrorism, over conventional military issues. Mr. Rumsfeld's approach is likely to trigger major shifts in the weapons systems that the Pentagon buys, and even more fundamental changes in the training and employment of US troops throughout the world, said defense officials who have played a role in crafting the document or are involved in the review. In the document, Mr. Rumsfeld tells the military to focus on four 'core problems,' none of them involving traditional military confrontations.

"The services are told to develop forces that can: build partnerships with failing states to defeat internal terrorist threats; defend the homeland, including offensive strikes against terrorist groups planning attacks; influence the choice of countries at a strategic crossroads, such as China and Russia; and prevent the acquisition of weapons of mass destruction by hostile states and terrorist groups.

"At its heart the document is driven by the belief that the US is engaged in a continuous global struggle extending far beyond specific battlegrounds. The vision is for a military that is much more proactive, focused on changing to conflicts such as a North Korean attack in South Korea, and assuming greater prominence in countries in which the US isn't at war." Surely this implies an extension into the future of the preemptive pattern adopted in Afghanistan and Iraq. It is said that generals are always engaged in fighting the last wars. Civilian politicians taking over military strategist's role are no less dedicated to that sport. And since the end of the Iraq adventure is still not in sight, the implications of Rumsfeld's striving to leave a heritage are disturbing. The least it can mean is to pursue Bin Laden wherever he may roam in search of mass weapons of destruction. But that could open up not only a new Iraq or two, but possibly a half dozen.

Meanwhile, the very process of preemptive "democratization" is ruffling some imperial feathers especially if there is a sniff of oil in the mix. That could escalate the scale of such conflicts, but there is no indication that keeps Mr. Rumsfeld awake at nights.

The Jaffe article alludes to budget cutting in the acquisition of weapons essential for more conventional military conflicts to make room for Mr. Rumsfeld's vision.

"Already, the review is prodding the services to question the need for expensive weapons systems, like short-range fighter jets and naval destroyers and tanks that are used primarily in conventional conflicts. 'A big question is exactly how much is enough to win the conventional fights of the future, and where can we shift resources to some of these less traditional problems,' said one person involved in drafting the guidance.

"The core problems outlined in Mr. Rumsfeld's review, for example, don't seem to favor the F/A-22 jet, which is the Air Force's top priority. Unfortunately you cannot find a lot of justification for more F/A-22s in the problem sets the services are being asked to address.

"Mr. Rumsfeld has made transforming the military a priority since the Bush administration took power. But in recent years that push took a back seat to the wars in Afghanistan and Iraq. Inside the Pentagon, the review is widely seen as Mr. Rumsfeld's last big push to instill his views on changing the military. Many insiders speculate that he will leave early next year when the review is completed; he has repeatedly dismissed all such speculation.

"Mr. Rumsfeld's guidance pushes the services to rethink the way they fight guerrilla wars and insurgencies. Instead of trying to stamp out an insurgency with large conventional ground formations, the classified guidance urges the military to come up with less doctrinaire solutions that include sending in smaller teams of culturally savvy soldiers to train and mentor indigenous forces."

Helping Tottering Governments Cross the Street to Democracy

"The US would seek to deploy these troops far earlier in a conflict than they traditionally have been, *for instance to help a tottering government's armed forces confront guerrillas before an insurgency is able to take root and build popular support*. Officials said the plan envisions many such teams operating around the world." The emphasis and the amazement are ours – for surely this exposes the real essence of President Bush's sudden concern about bringing democracy and freedom to the world at large – the only justification for the preemptive interventions. For surely the US has been intervening to prop up tottering dictatorships in Latin America and elsewhere since the beginning of the 1900s, during WWII and during the cold war that followed. The US army even ran a special torture school in Panama to teach Latin American officers the less subtle arts of propping up tottering dictatorships.

"The new plan [however] envisions [still] more active US involvement, where the US is dispatching teams of ground troops to train local forces in anti-insurgency tactics. Future training missions, however would likely be conducted on a much broader scale, one defense official said."

But the US teams will not have to go far to come up against major powers – notably China and Russia, with whom the US cannot even negotiate effectively without having a clear superiority in conventional arms. That is what President Bush's "star wars" is about. That means a double increase in spending.

The economic implications of the new Rumsfeld program which may be his heritage to US military doctrine for years to come are grimly unlimited. Not the least disturbing of these is this could come at a time when the civilian economy is tanking and the only government spending that Congress may smile on is military expansion.

William Krehm

What's Good for the Goose is Not Good for the Gander

IN OUR SEPTEMBER ISSUE we recounted – courtesy of *The Wall Street Journal* – how Motorola, against its better judgement, bequeathed a modern broadband communication infrastructure to China, that currently is beginning to compete advantageously with the American communications industry. The episode is so revealing of the conditions of our world economy, that we will cite it once more.

"This mobile phone market in China is one that Motorola invented. For Robert Gavin, the company's former CEO, China in the early to mid-1980s it promised to more than make-up for Motorola having been foiled in Japan for years. But first the company had to develop a top-drawer telecommunications infrastructure. At a dreary state ceremony during a tour of the country, Galvin turned to the minister of railroads and asked whether he wanted to do a good job as minister and be done with it, or to create a world-class society. In doing so, he tapped a thick vein of economic patriotism.

"Motorola's deep and open archives show that Galvin knew that eventually the transfer of technology would create a formidable Chinese competition. Nevertheless, Motorola decided that the best strategy was to get into China early."

We commented: "In this way the curtain rose over the most incredible theater of the absurd – the one-sided duel between David and Goliath with 'little' David the heavier and by far the brighter of the two." Back to the *WSJ:* "As a result China's mobile communications network calls get through to phones on high-rises subway cars and distant hamlets – connections that would stymie mobile phones in the US.

"What no one foresaw at Motorola was that the Chinese market would become the most competitive of all. Nokia and Motorola now battle for market share in the Chinese handset business. German, Korean and Taiwanese makers figure strongly enough. And all these foreign brands are now facing intense competition from indigenous Chinese new phone makers."

At this point we bring in *The Wall Street Journal* once more (23/11, "Telecom Giants Oppose Cities on Web Access" by Jesse Drucker): "Dozens of cities and towns across the country are rushing to offer low or no-cost wireless internet access to their residents, but the large phone and cable companies, fearful of losing a lucrative market, are fighting back by pushing states to pass legislation that could make it illegal for municipalities to offer the service.

"Over the past few months, several big cities – including Philadelphia and San Francisco – have announced plans to cover every square block with wireless internet access via the popular technology known as Wi-Fi, short for wireless fidelity. Cities say these plans will spur economic development and help bridge the digital divide, making Web access nearly ubiquitous.

"But that's bad new for the large Bell telephone companies and cable operators, who are looking to their digital subscriber line (DSL) and cable modem businesses for growth. Wi-Fi, technically known as 802.11, takes existing high-speed internet connections and wirelessly extends them by several hundred feet, allowing dozens or even hundreds of people to share one subscription."

Municipalities Caught Up in Internet Wars

"Philadelphia during the summer announced that it would hook up the entire city with W1-Fi. Its current Wi-Fi service is free, but it hasn't decided whether that would continue with wider deployment. 'There are some very specific goals that the city has that are not met by the private sector: affordable, universal access and the digital divide,' says Dianah Neff, the city's chief information officer. Less than 60% of the city's neighborhoods have broadband access.

"However, last week, after intensive lobbying by Verizon Communications Inc., the Pennsylvania General Assembly passed a bill that would make it illegal for any 'political subdivision' to provide to the public 'for any composition any telecommunications services, including advanced and broadband services within the service territory of a local exchange telecommunications company operating under a network-modernization plan.' Verizon is the local exchange telecommunications company for most of Pennsylvania, and it is planning to modernize the region using high-speed, fiber-optic cable. The bill has 10 days for the governor to sign it or veto it.

"The Pennsylvania bill follows similar legislative efforts earlier this year by telephone companies in Utah, Louisiana and Florida to prevent municipalities from offering telecommunications services which could include fiber and Wi-Fi.

"Critics denounced this legislative tactic, arguing that the US lags other countries in broadband internet access because the phone and cable companies have been slow to roll out the service in some areas.

"'We should be encouraging our municipalities to take a major role in broadband, the way other countries are doing,' says James Baller, an attorney in Washington, DC, who represents local governments on telecommunications issues.

"The telecom companies argue that it is unfair for them to have to compete against the government."

However, that raises a serious problem with the moral principles quoted when millions of jobs and livelihoods are wiped out through Globalization and Deregulation. On such occasions the wisdom of Joseph Schumpeter is cited like holy scripture arguing the "destructive development" of capitalism. Capitalism destroys economic patterns to make way for greater efficiencies that – like the Road to Tipperary – can be very long and winding. Why does the Schumpeter principle of destructive progress disappear when very influential forces stand to suffer?

"What is good for the goose, is good for the gander" should be the first test of good faith, let alone of good legislation.

William Krehm

Washington Discovers the Evils of "Oligopsony"

THERE WAS SOMETHING PORTENTOUS when Columbus, having discovered America, honestly believed that he had come to India. Ever since, US governments have been prone to confusion where continents are concerned. The are too ready to impose as benefactions overseas what they would see as evil back home.

The Wall Street Journal (27/01, "Bully Buyers – How Driving Prices Lower Can Violate Antitrust Statues" by John R. Wilke) informs us: "As more of the world's markets become dominated by a few big companies, a rare form of antitrust abuse is raising new concern: when corporations illegally drive *down* the prices of their suppliers.

"On the coast of Maine, blueberry growers alleged last year that four big processors conspired to push down the price they would pay for fresh wild berries. A state-court jury last year awarded millions in damages. In South Carolina, International Paper Co. faces a lawsuit that it conspired with its timber buyers to depress softwood prices in several states. In Alabama and Pennsylvania, federal antitrust enforcers last year targeted insurance companies that imposed contracts forcing down fees charged by doctors and hospitals. The insurers abandoned the practice."

Super-inflation on the Top — Deflation Below

However, the same government has pushed through globalization that seeks to level all barriers that prevent the ever fewer large corporations from organizing to keep prices low. It has also mobilized the international monetary bureaucracy – the International Monetary Fund and the World Bank – to increase Third World companies' exports of staples – no matter at what prices to service their debt. It is servicing debt rather than the interplay of supply and demand that increasingly determines the prices of staples on the world market. At the same time other features of the Globalization and Deregulation program make local governments liable for damages if they outlaw advantages already enjoyed by foreign corporations that have proved ruinous to the environment or society.

And it is equally clear the rejigging of the international system so that interest rates are the sole "tool" for "fighting inflation" hit the Third world between the eyes. As did the removal of the firewalls between banking and stock market gambles financed at wild leverages by "derivatives" that put them under the wheels of the financial juggernauts. That. too. can be seen as a means of "fighting inflation" since it allows the US to import at bankruptcy prices – largely denominated in US currency that the US financial system can produce at practically no cost. That provides more elbow-room for the financial hyperinflation that has taken over both in the US and abroad.

But let's return to the tardy but yet very different reactions to Monopsony on the home front.

"The power to drive down prices is an issue as well in a Federal Trade Commission investigation of R.J. Reynolds Tobacco Co.'s pending $2.6 acquisition of BAT PLC's Brown & Williamson unit, lawyers close to the case say. The FTC is looking at whether the combined company could force tobacco-leaf growers to accept lower prices. Other major US cigarette makers recently agreed to pay tobacco farmers $1.2 billion to settle a private lawsuit accusing them of secretly agreeing to avoid competitive bidding at tobacco auctions.

"'Price fixing and other forms of collusion are just as unlawful when the victims are sellers rather than buyers.' R. Hewitt Pate, the Justice Department's antitrust chief, told a Senate Judiciary Committee hearing late last year. The hearing aired farmers' concerns that a few giant agribusinesses now control commodity prices in many markets.

"Usually relegated to the back pages of law books, this mirror image of monopoly is known as 'monopsony,' or when more than one company is involved, 'oligopsony.' It arises when one or more companies gain enough buying power to push their suppliers' prices down.

"It isn't a new legal theory, but it is getting more attention now because of the rise of giant companies in a global marketplace. Buyer muscle has become more visible in recent years as markets become more concentrated through mergers and joint ventures. In meat-packing, the business of slaughtering cattle and pigs, four companies control 80% of the market. In four out of 10 US cities, a single health insurer has at least a 50% market share. Concentration is also rising in markets from aluminum refining to baby food.

"Most of the time, there is nothing wrong when big companies squeeze suppliers for lower prices. Hard bargaining by profit-minded business buyers can help drive down prices for consumers.

"But if dominant buyers use their clout to distort the market and push prices down, the legal theory goes, consumers ultimately can lose. That's based on the assumption that producers will stop innovating, or producing at all, if they can't get a fair price. Monopsony, which has been found to violate federal antitrust statutes, can be alleged in either government or private suits.

"Finding the fine line between healthy, price-cutting competition and harmful price-reducing monopsony has historically made government antitrust enforcers cautious about taking action in this area. The world's largest retailer has enormous power to squeeze suppliers, who have repeatedly asked regulators to rein it in. But many economists see Wal-Mart as an example of how buyer power can benefit consumers."

What is odd is that the learned legal experts, undoubtedly advised by learned economists, overlook that before a mortal can become a consumer, he must be a producer. And by ruining producers and Third World countries, they are doing nothing for the mass of consumers at home, many of whom will find themselves without a job, or working at ever lower wages.

And meanwhile the rate of growth achieved in the stock market prices of the shares of the aforesaid large corporations is extrapolated into the remotest future and incorporated into their current price. As is the rate of growth of the rate of growth of that price, and the past acceleration of that growth rate, and all higher growth rates to infinity.

For all these "higher derivatives of growth" are driven to keep pace with the increase of the rate of growth of the stock price. And the slightest failure to keep up those growth rates will bring the stock price crashing. And those stocks serve as collateral for further financings, and the slightest failure to maintain the pattern and justify what has already been embedded in the stock price, leads to its collapse. This happens to be the mathematics of the atomic bomb – exponential growth. So the blood squeezed out of Third World producers is never enough since the rate of increase of that process has to be maintained. And before the CEOs can admit to failure at this, they are likely put everything they learned at Sunday school on hold and cook their books and bribe their accountants. That is why the high courts of the superpower will have to learn something about the pitfalls of official economics.

William Krehm

The Crumbling of our Auto Titans

LIKE THE HAPSBURGS at the pinnacle of their glory, imperially overexpanded and incestuously over-married, our world-wide auto industry is faced with survival problems.

The Wall Street Journal (24/01, "For GM and Fiat, A Messy Breakup Could be in the Works" by Gabriel Kahn, Stephen Power and Alessandra Gallani) provides the latest development in the epic: "Turin, Italy – Nearly five years into a partnership, once touted as made in heaven, General Motors Corp. and Fiat SpA were in tense talks about a possible breakup that could further batter their finances and reverberate across the auto industry.

"Despite months of negotiations, the two sides seem miles apart on the major sticking point: a 'put' option that could force GM to buy 90% of Fiat's ailing, debt-laden auto unit that GM doesn't already own. Fiat's CEO, Sergio Marchionne, has stated repeatedly that he has the right to exercise the put beginning today, when a so-far unsuccessful mediation process expires. GM CEO Richard Wagoner Jr. insists the option is invalid."

That showed that the regal auto industry has also been sucked into this derivative age that brings no free solutions, but inflates greed like soap bubbles.

"GM, which paid $2.4 billion for a since-diluted 20% stake in Fiat's car unit in 2000, faces a possible cut in its credit rating. In its core market of North America, it has been losing market share and been forced to cut production amid increased competition from Asian rivals such as Toyota Motor Corp. and Nissan Motor Co. If GM is forced to pay a hefty settlement to wriggle out of the put option – or worse, has to acquire the Italian auto maker and its $10 billion in debt – it could weigh heavily on an already burdened balance sheet.

"The situation is even more dire for Fiat, an Italian industrial icon that also owns businesses such as Iveco trucks, CNH farm equipment and Ferrari sports cars. Fiat Auto's operating losses for 2004 are expected to total around $1.3 billion. With Fiat Auto burning through cash, the put option has emerged as a potential lifesaver for Mr. Marchionne, a turn-around specialist who arrived at the Italian auto-maker in June following a management shakeup. People say he hopes to force GM to pay handsomely to get out of the obligation, thus buying Fiat some time. [A put gives its owner the right but not the obligation to force his counterparty to buy what it covers at a specified price.] But the price would have to be in excess of nearly $2 billion – to provide the car unit the 18 months of extra time to tide it over as it tries to bring important new models to the market.

"Fiat Auto is running on fumes. In a rapidly consolidating industry of global giants, it is caught in a trap of high fixed costs and shrinking market share. In a document presented to one of Fiat's creditor banks earlier this month, Fiat SpA, reports that without a payment from GM, the conglomerate's current cash and cash equivalents will last only between 13 and 20 months. But while Fiat needs a quick resolution, GM stands to gain by postponing the matter."

No Brakes on the Overexpansion of the World Auto Industry

"The showdown over the hobbled Italian auto maker comes as the global auto industry is grappling with an immense overcapacity. Auto companies have the ability to make an estimated 24 million more cars than they can sell each year. The glut is prompting price wars that are dragging down profits.

"The big players' strategy of making alliances with small and often weak manufacturers has contributed to the glut in recent years, with Ford Motor Co. pumping money into Japan's Mazda Motor Co. and GM acquiring Daewoo and investing in Fiat Auto. Just last week, some of Japan's biggest companies were preparing a $3 billion bailout of Mitsubishi Motors Corp. They reasoned that partnerships could yield cost savings by achieving economies of scale without the hassles of a full merger. But the Fiat deal, which included the Italian company taking a 5.1% stake in GM, has sorely tested that strategy."

The trouble is that Deregulation and Globalization has put so many balls in the air, that it is next to impossible to keep track of them. Besides, there is always the consoling credo that a completely deregulated market will be self-balancing and thus take care of all tough questions, provided that you keep growing big enough to wipe out your competitors. Add to that the environmental, cultural and countless other issues brushed aside as "externalities," and the stage is set for major troubles.

"When Mr. Wagoner negotiated the Fiat tie-up, he agreed to another clause – a put that gives Fiat the right to force GM to buy out all of the Italian company's car unit at a price to be negotiated. Now, five consecutive years of losses in Europe are forcing GM to hack at its overcapacity. It is shedding roughly 12,000 jobs, mostly in Germany. In the US, GM is closing plants in Maryland and New Jersey.

"Rivals would benefit greatly if weaklings such as Fiat Auto – whose capacity of around 2.3 million cars a year outstrips its annual sales by more than 400,000 vehicles – went out of business. But shutting Fiat Auto would spark a political firestorm in Italy, where the company remains a linchpin of the industrial base and its controlling shareholders, the illustrious Agnelli family, enjoy a status close to royalty.

"As part of the 2000 agreement, GM and Fiat formed two joint ventures in Europe and Latin America. One venture pooled purchasing operations to save money. Another called Fiat-GM Powertrain BV, developed engines and transmissions. They are now yielding significant economies. At the same time, the uncertainties of the alliance are threatening the health of the joint ventures. Major decisions have been frozen for six months because neither side is willing to invest in a product as long as the two are threatening to sue each other.

"GM has enlisted an armada of investment bankers and lawyers to argue the case: that financial moves by Fiat have rendered the put option invalid, including the sale of a chunk of Fiat Auto's financing arm. Mr. Marchionne, by contrast, is conducting the negotiations with little help from the outside. A lawyer by training, he has argued repeatedly that he believes GM's claims to be groundless.

"In a filing with the Securities and Exchange Commission in the US last year, GM indicated that if it were forced to take over Fiat Auto it would be reluctant to contribute any additional capital to the Italian company. GM also indicated that if Fiat Auto was insolvent at the time of acquisition, GM wouldn't have to assume the Italian unit's debt. Without fresh funds, Fiat Auto could quickly turn insolvent, possibly leading to massive factory closings and the loss of tens of thousands of jobs in Italy. The threat of such action, say industry analysts, could prompt Prime Minister Silvio Berlusconi to intervene with a government bailout. Ministers in Mr. Berlusconi's government insist that no state aid will be forthcoming. Last week, GM wrote down its remaining stake in Fiat Auto to zero...."

Obviously the mega-corporate tussle is taking place on the lip of a precipice.

"According to a person close to the negotiations, GM is trying to argue that Fiat Auto has a negative value. Fiat SpA, the parent company, has an overall market cap of about $7.5 billion. The Fiat Auto unit alone carries debt on its book totalling around $10 billion. This person argues that if Fiat tries to exercise this put option, the Italians may have to compensate GM. The original deal between the companies stipulates advisers to each side must propose a value of Fiat Auto before the put is exercised.

"Fiat rose to prominence in the '50s and '60s, when it could claim the dominance of the Italian market. Its owners, the Agnellis, were powerful and fashionable figures hobnobbing with the likes of the Kennedys. As the market liberalized in the '90s, Fiat's chunky sales network and laggard technology left it unprepared to handle the flood of competition. When Fiat linked up with GM in the boom year of 2000, neither believed things would ever get so ugly.

"Other members of the family, including Mr. Agnelli 's younger brother, Umberto, disagreed. They no longer felt duty-bound to keep Fiat in Italian hands, especially if that risked the family's own money. Still both companies acted as though they had just sealed a love match."

A Peek under the Hood of the Compulsion to Grow

"General Motors never grasped the complexity of Fiat Auto, and the tactics it used to prop up sales in its most important market of Italy. According to Mario Rosso, a former Fiat executive who handled the government liaison office in Rome, Fiat Auto relied on the government to offer tax breaks for trading in used cars for new ones. This helped pump up sales, but foreign competitors were barrelling into Italy with cheaper cars and stronger sales networks. And the Italian government no longer doled out favors as it once had.

"By the end of 2/2002, Fiat Autos was out of gas and sucking cash from the group's truck and tractor units. Desperate, the group put many of the group's best assets up for sale. It sold off its stake in GM. The government lined up banks to extend the group nearly $4 billion in new loans, convertible into equity. The Agnellis eventually agreed to open the family treasure chest and kick in about $325 million. GM, asked to pitch in, stayed out, and its 20% stake in Fiat Auto was diluted to 10%.

"As Fiat Auto skidded, the put option swelled in importance. Fiat's calculation: With the put, it could force GM to pay up to free itself from the obligation to buy the Italian auto unit. But negotiations went nowhere because of the disarray in Fiat's senior ranks. The Agnellis ran through five CEOs in less than two years. The chairmen changed as well as Umberto Agnelli took over and then died a little more than a year later.

"The music changed abruptly when Mr. Marchionne arrived. An Italian who grew up in Canada, he was an outsider to the insular world of Fiat. He quickly seized on the option as the best solution for tackling the auto unit. Alexis Boyer, analyst at Deutsche Bank, says when he met with Mr. Marchionne, the Fiat chief didn't even try to argue that the company's auto unit could be fixed."

The Globe and Mail (21/02, "Fiat plays the Italian heritage card" by Jane Barrett, Milan) reports the resolution of the stand-off: "Last week, GM gave Fiat back its stake in Fiat Auto and $2 billion (US) for Fiat to cancel the put option that allowed it to sell." That is, it paid them $2 billion and surrendered its 10% interest in Fiat Auto for releasing it from buying the balance of the auto firm at what had seemed an attractive price a few years ago!

The Fiat-GM wrestling match has implications far beyond Italy or Detroit. Globalization and Deregulation, that so readily trips off wagging tongues, may mean many contradictory things. The industry has an immense need for capital investment to meet environmental obligations that are just coming to be recognized. That will not only require reworking the fuelling systems of cars, but probably public investment to make the new fuels available to motorists. And of course the additional highway systems to accommodate the growth that is at the core of the industry's plans for survival. Standing still or even downgrading the growth compulsion is simply not an option. But the G&D of the European Union in monetary matters is constitutionally stuck in views that were completely discredited in the 1980s and 1990s. That makes both capital and other costs dear and uncompetitive. The result is an increasingly aggressive competitive warfare that cuts across cultural boundaries at the very time that political mergers are expanding and imposing bruising ideological hangups. Military spending has always been a tempting exit for dead-ended civilian economies. And that is why the second term of the second Bush is sending shivers down the world's spine. Solutions will be sought in outer space that are so clearly unavailable in the rigged realities of this planet.

W.K.

Open Letter to Jack Layton, Leader of the NDP

OUR CONGRATULATIONS for a unique opportunity that has arisen for bringing both this country and your party out of the brambles in which they have both been for at least a quarter of a century. You have certainly helped bring that opportunity about, and for that we offer you our congratulations and best wishes in making full use of it. That would bring to life again Tommy Douglas's great heritage in contributing to the nationalization of the Bank of Canada in 1938.

That nationalization made possible the financing of a major part of the federal government's capital projects with the Bank of Canada on a virtual interest-free basis. The money paid to the BoC as interest on such loans came back to the federal government as dividends. An essential part of the mechanism that made this possible were the statutory reserves that required the banks to redeposit with the BoC some 8% to 12% of the deposits received by banks from the public in chequing accounts.

These statutory reserves served two vital purposes: (1) they provided more elbow-room for the federal government to finance its capital projects from the BoC within the constraints in force on an interest-free basis; (2) they offered an alternative to raising the benchmark rate of interest set by the BoC for overnight-loans between chartered banks to help them meet their cheque clearing obligations. Once these reserves were phased out over a two-year period in the 1991 revision of the Bank Act, higher interest rates became "the one blunt tool" for "controlling inflation." The result: in the mid-1970s the Bank of Canada had held well over 20% of the federal debt. Within a few years it was down to almost 5%.

We note that the NDP did include bringing back the statutory reserves among its policy *options*. More than that, it is an absolute necessity to reverse the trend of Canadian politics towards disaster bred by greedy privilege.

The NDP could reclaim the traditions of Tommy Douglas, by proposing a gradual reintroduction of the statutory reserves, say over a 3-year period. Neither the UK nor the US ended reserves as Canada and New Zealand did. In Britain they were simply reduced to 0.35 of one percent but are still on the books; in the US they also remain but have been reduced to irrelevance by the shifting of deposits from reservable accounts to non-reservable accounts at the close of bank hours, and back to reservable accounts when the banks open their doors again. Bringing the reserves back in Canada to their former levels over a two or three-year period would give the banks an ample opportunity to readjust to the return to a statutory reserve regime. This is of particular importance since the Bank of Canada is in the process of pushing up interest rates again despite the limp state of the economy.

I would be happy to meet with you to elaborate on our proposal.
William Krehm, Chairman, Committee on Monetary and Monetary Reform (COMER)

Afloat on Two Seas?

THE WALL STREET JOURNAL (3/02, "President Provides New Detail of Plan for Private Accounts" by John H. McKinnon and Cristopher Cooper) informs us: "President Bush planned to use the State of the Union address to give the first broad details of his Social Security overhaul, which would divert up to one-third of the system's payroll-tax revenue to individual accounts beginning in 2009. [He] disclosed that his plan would leave benefits untouched for Americans age 55 or older – roughly one-fourth of the country's population, but a higher share of the electorate because older voters turn out [to vote] at higher rates. That concession is designed to damp the political fears of Republicans and the ammunition of Democrats in Congressional battles ahead.

"Missing from Mr. Bush's address were important details of his plan, including covering the costs for the transition to private accounts and scaling back growth in Social Security's guaranteed benefits for millions of middle-age and younger workers. Those difficult decisions will be made in negotiations with Congressional leaders in coming weeks."

The risks to which this will expose a substantial amount of the social security of the retired is evident from almost any issue of the Journal quoted. Thus the "Money & Investing" section of its 17/02 issue on its very first page contains the following:

"[Wall] Street's Top Dogs get Top Dollar" by Ann Davis reports: 'In a year when stocks of US brokerage companies sported modest gains and in one case a big decline, chief executives at four of the largest brokerage houses pulled in $110.1 million among them, a sharp rise from a year ago. The four major firms that have released CEO pay so far – Merrill Lynch & Co., Morgan Stanley, Goldman Sachs Group Inc., and Lehman Brothers Holdings Inc. – gave top dogs an average raise of 33%, while those firms' stocks rose an average of 4.7%. Even in the case of stronger performers such as Lehman, CEO pay rose by a far higher percentage than stock returns. Lehman's shares rose 16% in its fiscal year that ended Nov. 30, compared with the S&P's return of 11% over the same period. CEO Richard Fuld received a 22% raise.'

That strongly suggests that it is the distribution of power – within the company and within society – that determines the division of income between shareholders and the high executives. Certainly not anything that could pass even in the dark for economic logic. And it is to this rigged crap game that President

Bush is determined to entrust pensioners' retirement funds!

But supporters of such privatization will say the results are more favourable over the long term. Well-heeled and especially well-connected players who can sit out the busts of the stock markets, may come up winning at the expense of those less well equipped. Ordinary retirees, however, supporting a many-levelled investment bureaucracy paid off the top from the skimpy retirement savings of the ordinary Joe, would hardly stand a chance of not getting flayed.

Alongside the article from the one just quoted is another article, "Ebbers Lawyers Paint Sullivan as Chronic Liar." The CEO of WorldCom, Bernard Ebbers, is on trial for fraud in the greatest such case on record, and Mr. Scott D. Sullivan, the corporation's former chief Financial Officer has turned witness for the prosecution. Mr. Ebbers is on trial on charges of WorldCom's $11billion fraud, and if convicted faces 30 years in prison. Mr. Sullivan has pled guilty to fraud and is a cooperating government witness.

This is only one in an unbroken chain of such trials. On the same page of the same issue of the *WSJ* is yet another article, "Hedge-Fund Partners Face Fraud Charges Over Missing Money."

Hedge funds were once the private reserve of investors or speculators who could afford to gamble in dizzily leveraged derivatives with hundreds of millions of dollars. Today, with excess speculative money sloshing around from big killings, such funds have become a favourite decoy for the unwary. Since money creation was shifted to private banks from direct control by central banks, it is the stock market and other bank-controlled institutions that have taken over. On the same page of the *WSJ* ("Hedge-Fund Partners Face Fraud Charges Over Missing Money" by Ianthea Jeanne Dugan) sets the scene: "The Securities and Exchange Commission accused three partners of North Shore Asset Management LLC, a Chicago-based hedge fund, of fraudulently sinking $37 million of investor money into hard-to-trade stocks.

"The SEC lawsuit, filed in a federal court in New York City, represents an effort to corral allegedly fraudulent activity by hedge funds – private investment partnerships mainly for rich and institutional investors, that make high-stake bets on stocks, currencies and other global markets, often borrowing money to boost returns."

With so much money from market gambles seeking investment opportunities, more and more money managers are driven to produce escalating results in an ailing real economy. The risk factor climbs, as do the number of corners cut. There has thus been a deepening detachment of our financial institutions from the producing economy, with results that are clogging the American law courts. The increase of speculative profits, real or fictitious, are projected into the indefinite future and incorporated into the present market price of securities, or detached derivatives of securities such as the *increase* of its annual profit, which can be exchanged against an unrelated derivative of a quite different security (swops). Or against the mere option to make such an exchange. The fact that leading accountancy firms have been caught and fined for devising such scams indicates that it is

becoming something like the survival norm in privileged financial circles. The rewards of CEOs – unrelated to anything earned in the productive economy – points to a power mal-distribution that leaves no room for morality. For the failure to maintain a rate of growth already imbedded in stock prices will bring down the house of cards To prevent that the speculative financial sector must appropriate every capital pool in sight. That explained the banks taking over the brokerage firms, then the insurance companies, and now part of the retirement pensions. Without that the big game could simply not go on.

The Record of Privatized Social Security in Other Lands

The bailout of the distressed banks in the late 1980s and early ninety nineties did away with the firewalls between banking and the stock market, insurance, and real estate mortgages. This gave the banks access to the capital pools and multipliers with which to compound their own powers of money-creation. It also added up to a an immense shift in the distribution of political power. This is what is fuelling the current push across the world for the privatization of social security funds, as has already been done with government capital assets.

The Wall Street Journal (identical issue, 'Some Bush-Style Social Security Scenarios" by David Wessel) examines the record of such privatized social insurance elsewhere. "The White House is being stingy with specifics about far-reaching changes to Social Security that President Bush is seeking, reflecting an apparently tactical choice: more details could doom the proposal. But the president and his aides have said enough to allow outsiders to plug numbers into spreadsheets to illustrate how Bush-style Social Security might work. The examples – which the White House says are 'premature' – underscore how far Mr. Bush would move Social Security away from a system that offers monthly payments regardless of the financial market's ups and downs to one in which retiree benefits depend heavily on stock and bond performance."

In Mr. Bush's plan, "retirement benefits wouldn't change at all for workers or retirees 55 or older, and wouldn't change very much for workers now in their 40s or early 50s. But for younger workers, particularly today's teenagers or those in their 20s who would spend their entire working lives under the new system, Social Security would be very different.

"They would continue to pay 12.4% of their wages into Social Security, split evenly between employer and employee, but they could divert up to 4% into a private account. When upper-wage workers in this younger cohort retire in mid-century, 85% more of their total Social Security benefits – the traditional program plus what they draw from their private accounts – would come from that private account.

"A young man born in 1990, at retirement, would draw both from his private account and from traditional Social Security. But that traditional benefit would be reduced twice from levels under current law: once because he diverted some of his payroll taxes into a private account and a second time because Mr. Bush proposes to reduce promised benefits across the board to make Social Security solvent for the long haul.

"If the law remained unchanged, such a worker is scheduled to get $22,863 a year in Social Security retirement benefits. But benefits were reduced to make Social Security stable, using an approach that a Bush-appointed commission favored, he'd get $18,406 a year. All that's before any private account [drew its share].

"Under a Bush-type plan, if the worker opted for a private account, his traditional retirement benefit would be reduced sharply. He'd just get $2,191 a year from traditional Social Security. If his stock and bond mutual funds earned 3% a year after inflation, he'd have a $234,012 nest egg at age 65. If he turned that into an annuity at retirement, he could get another $16,215 a year for life from his private account for a total annual benefit of $18,406. If stocks and bonds earned $4.6% a year after inflation, he'd get $29,396 a year. If they earned less, he'd do worse. But he'd get that same $2,191 traditional Social Security check no matter what the markets do.

"*The Wall Street Journal's* examples rely on a spreadsheet built by Jason Furman, a New York University economist, who opposes Mr. Bush's proposal.... The White House takes issue with Mr. Furman's estimates. 'Any numbers are premature,' said White House spokesman Trent Duffy. We can't verify Mr. Furman's numbers, and we have concerns about their accuracy.'

"The White House won't say when, or even if, Mr. Bush will make public a detailed plan."

An Example of What the Private Nest Egg will be Exposed To

Citigroup is no fly-by-night operator. It is the largest financial conglomerate in the world Hence the report of *The Wall Street Journal* (3/02, "Bond Strategy Haunts Citigroup" by Silvia Ascaraelli) acts out what we said earlier about the blind drive for profit growth by just about any means in the deregulated financial sector.

"On July 16, a senior Citigroup Inc. executive in London told traders [of his firm] on the European government bond desk they weren't making enough money and ordered them to come up with new trading strategies.

"About six weeks later, six bond traders pushed the button on a huge bond-trading strategy dubbed 'Dr. Evil,' according to a report by a German financial regulator.

"The frantic trading roiled the massive markets for European government bonds and futures contracts, and netted Citigroup an estimated 15 million euros or about US $20 million, in just two hours on August 2. It also embroiled Citigroup in months of controversy just as Chief Executive Charles O. Prince was seeking to clean up the Bank's reputation after it was tarnished by the scandals at WorldCom and Enron Corp.

"Citigroup in a statement yesterday reiterated its remorse over the trading.

"Financial regulators in the UK, Italy and France are examining whether the trades violated their rules. German prosecutors are investigating the six traders for possible criminal violations after German securities regulators found indications of market manipulation. Citigroup and the traders could face administrative sanctions from Eurex, the derivatives exchange, where the futures trades took place.

"One of the Citigroup bond traders that day wasn't even licensed to trade for Citigroup on Eurex, a unit of the German stock exchange operator Deutsche Boerse. Instead he executed his trades using the name of a licensed Citigroup trader. A Citigroup spokesman declined to comment.

"The regulators' report said the trading strategy was approved by at least two managers of Citigroup, including Stephen Compton, the bank's London-based head of European inter-rate trading, who oversees trading in all government bonds and bond-based derivatives in Europe.

"Citigroup is a big player in trading European government bonds and in futures trading on Eurex. The European government bond markets have become increasingly liquid since the advent of Europe's common currency in 1999, when bond markets from Spain to Finland were redenominated into Euros. The 12-country euro-zone market is valued at about $4.9 trillion, according to the Bank for International Settlements, slightly shy of the $5.3 trillion US bond market The benchmark futures contract is the German government's 10-year bond future, traded on Eurex.

"Citigroup's regulatory problems in Europe are in addition to an unrelated scandal last year at Citigroup's private bank in Japan, after which the private banking unit lost its license to operate in Japan over mishandling the accounts of some wealthy customers.

"In the wake of the Japanese scandal, Mr. Prince apologized profusely to Japanese officials, taking the unusual step of a long, deep bow. He also dismissed or sought the resignation of a number of employees in Japan, and asked three of the most senior New York-based executives, including Vice Chairman Deyck Maugham to leave the bank."

However, despite the dismissals, and the depth of Mr. Prince's bow, it is hard dismissing the impression that the real sin of those punished was getting caught. The dominating compulsion is to grow and expand. Ablution will come with success at the game. Hardly a setting for the retirement savings of hard-working citizens.

William Krehm

Relating the Public and Private Sectors

THE DEVELOPMENT of human societies has followed a long-term trend of moving from simple to complex forms. This has manifested itself both by the increasing private economic activities as well as by expanding public superstructures. We must assume a strong correlation between these two phenomena. With the emergence of metropolitan industrialism around 1850 both trends took a sharp tick upwards.

The social structures that emerged after industrialism turned the majority of society's population into metropolitan dwellers were based on the new high intensity economic activities. The bulk of activities in the metropolitan cities were monetized, or in other words, intermediated by cash transactions – another significant departure from the pre-industrial economy that still had a high degree of non-cash transactions.

The concentration of the population in large cities created a need for much more complex social networks. This was reflected in a sharp rise in the level and types of government institutions, many of them in areas that either were totally new or at best previously had existed only in very rudimentary forms. Prominent was the need for a literate workforce. Life in metropolitan cities is almost unmanageable for citizens without literacy.

As a consequence, the early industrializing countries in Western Europe and North America all implemented far-reaching reforms that made basic education a publicly delivered free social good. Literacy became a social skill extending to all classes of society and not only, as it had been earlier, restricted to noble families, and minor groups of professionals and bureaucrats in the market towns and administrative centers.

During the market town phase of economic development, manufactured goods were produced in local workshops, and the bulk of their products were consumed locally. Industrialization changed this radically as few of the manufactured goods were consumed where they were produced. Mass production made it possible to market goods more cheaply and over much larger areas.

This, in turn, necessitated the establishment of large-scale transportation networks, which at first relied on massive expansion of canal systems and the new invention of railroads. The large population concentration in the metropolitan cities also gave rise to other infrastructural needs, including local transit, water supply, sanitation, street lightning, gas works, etc.

Industrialization not only changed the material aspects of life. Society's structures also underwent major changes as a consequence. In settlement patterns dominated by villages and small towns, the extended family traditionally is the primary social unit. Health and old age care had generally been taken care of within these larger family units.

With the population concentrated in the metropolitan cities, the extended family broke up and lost its role as a significant factor in the provision of society's social safety net. Accordingly, new institutions were called for. The change was also spurred by the development of modern scientific medicine that turned health care into a highly specialized field and, as such, necessitated the establishment of hospitals and medical universities.

Another important development that took place during the formative period of metropolitan industrialism was separating science from the dogma of Christianity. The spirit of the times was positivism; what mattered in science was rational observation of facts and things that could be measured. This was the basis for the great strides in the technical sciences from which industrialism had sprung, and it seemed to some that social sciences would do well to take their cues from the new methods of the exact sciences.

In this spirit, the science of economics also underwent a major revision that resulted in the establishment of neoclas-sical economics. But in what must be considered a historical oddity, the leading economists of the day chose to promote a version of economics that almost totally ignored the obvious correlation between the rise in industrialism and the vastly expanded government involvement in providing and managing the distribution of social goods. Instead the neoclassical econo-mists focused on developing a new theory of market value. Classical economics had principally revolved around the labour theory of value. However, this theory ignored other factors of production, and furthermore had to assume that economic actions included an explicit "memory" of previous states. This, as increasingly apparent, was not defensible since all individual economic agents only consider their own profit-loss relations when transacting in markets

The main discovery that led to the establishment of neoclas-sical economics was the marginality principle. It worked much better in explaining how value formed for a marginal unit ex-changed at any point along the exchange chains that transformed resources and factors into final consumers products. And what was seen as a strong bonus, marginal value relations could be expressed in mathematical formulas. With this change, it seemed that economics moved much closer to the exact sciences.

The Incompleteness of Social Choices

The logic of defining value at the point of exchange by the marginal principle at first swept all before it, leaving the labour theory of value behind as an interesting but strictly historical phenomenon. But soon it became apparent that neoclassical economics, despite all of its systemic rigor, had left two major problems untackled.

Essentially, neoclassical economics is only a theory about private individuals transacting in markets and leaves out all the activities in the vastly expanded public domain. Furthermore, it provides no mechanism for adjusting value for the influence of such "externalities." Both these problems have received ex-tensive scrutiny by various theorists from the 1930s onwards, but the defenders of neoclassicism have argued that both arise as results of market failures. The problems are therefore, in their opinion, not theoretical but political ones. Society must show the political will to pursue and fully implement market-based solutions in all areas and the problems will recede into insignificance.

The postulate that all public activities and externalities are caused by market failures is, by its very nature, not subject to testing – requiring a total market to prove it true or false. However, any study of society's historical development as well as of conditions in all modern societies doesn't make this a very plausible method. Just to mention one thing, we saw above that metropolitan industrialism was dependent on a policy of extending basic education to the population at large – a major social project that could not have been achieved by any conceiv-able private means as they existed at the time.

Similarly, the claim that the effects of negative externalities is simply a product of market failures and thus can be solved by extending property rights is not a credible one in view of human behavioral patterns. The self-interests of opportunistic individuals will whenever possible try to push costs into the social commons. Likewise, big corporations will always have many ways to hide adverse information and have highly specialized legal counsel at their disposal whenever need be. Thus, the claim that sufficient information will be voluntarily disclosed and that a fair playing field exists when interest conflicts related to externalities are before the courts is a spurious one.

The fact is that neoclassical economics by its narrow focus on the private market sector never has made a convincing case against public engagement in creating and distributing social goods, nor its involvement in curbing negative externalities. Thus, the current political vogue of postulating that markets and private property must be expanded at all costs is ignoring the other possible conclusion – that there from the outset has been something fundamentally incomplete in the neoclassical framework.

Often, the attack on public institutions has been framed as attacks on what in reality is a bureaucratic problem. However, that is not a problem specific to public bodies but is shared with large privately owned corporations.

One course of action is to make more room for inputs at the grass-root level in both sectors.

It is high time to discard the neoclassical paradigm, or, at the very least, reformulate it as a theory only valid for restricted and closed conditions.

Dix Sandbeck

REVIEW OF A BOOK BY PAUL KRUGMAN,
W.W. NORTON & COMPANY, 2003

"The Great Unraveling: Losing Our Way in the New Century"

PAUL KRUGMAN was once selected as "best American economist under 40." What they couldn't quite bring themselves to say, snorted a friendly colleague of mine, is that he is the best of the current crop, no matter what their age. (My friend is himself a well-trained and self-confident economist who retired early as a senior policy adviser in Ottawa – in disgust.) Acting on his advice several years ago, I began to pay attention when Krugman bylines caught my eye. Since spotting his column in *The New York Times* shortly after it started, I have rarely missed one of them. The just-released *Great Unraveling* was therefore a welcome stuffer in my Xmas stocking at the end of 2003, but I put it on the shelf in the belief that most of the content was still fairly fresh in my memory. It was a year later, after the re-election of the Bush team and Republican majorities in both House and Senate, that an urge to refresh one or more of those memories caused me to open the book and to then recognize that I had been denying myself the most important and electrifying part.

It is no longer news that G.W. Bush is making good on his triumphant post-election declaration that "I have political capital and I intend to spend it!" His high-profile attack on Social Security is the symbol and substance of those intentions. As you read the following excerpts and paraphrases from Krugman's Preface and Introduction, keep in mind that he wrote them a full year before the election of 2004.

Krugman begins by explaining that as an economics professor, one of his main specialties has been international *financial* crises. He therefore did not expect that as a columnist he would be spending a lot of time on domestic politics, since everyone assumed that American policy would remain sensible and responsible. "But as events unfolded, politics inevitably intruded…. It gradually became clear that something deeper than mere bad economic ideology was at work. The bigger story was America's political sea change…. More and more, I found myself speaking very uncomfortable truth to power…. If I have ended up more often than not writing pieces that attack the right wing, it's because the right wing now rules – and rules badly. It's not just that the policies are bad and irresponsible; our leaders lie about what they are up to. I began pointing out the outrageous dishonesty of the Bush administration long before most of the rest of the punditocracy."

In explaining why he saw what others failed to see, Krugman points to his training as an economist in contrast to the political reporters whose style is to give equal credence to the opposing claims of politicians regardless of the facts. "I did my own arithmetic – or, where necessary, got hold of real economists who could educate me on the subjects I wrote about – and quickly realized that we were dealing with world-class mendacity, right here in the USA." In pointing up this contrast, Krugman also recognized that business reporters know a bogus number when they see it and have often accused top officials of outrageous mendacity at the same time as political pundits are still dripping phrases about their sterling character. "But the writings of business reporters necessarily have a narrow focus, and rarely affect political commentary. With a wider brief, and a spot on the Op-Ed page, I attracted a lot more attention."

What the Militant Right Throws Overboard with a Rock Attached

At least as important as his ability to see the lies is his willingness to call them that. This he explains in part as his distance from the groupthink that dominates the perception of Washington journalists who go to the same dinner parties. As a professor in New Jersey (Princeton) he never bought into the shared assumptions and story line (e.g., before 9/11 George W. Bush was dumb but honest; after September 11 the new story was "Texas Ranger to the world"). Furthermore, as Krugman acknowledges, he "couldn't be bullied in the usual ways. The stock in trade of most journalists is inside information – leaks from highly placed sources, up-close-and-personal interviews with the powerful. This leaves them vulnerable: they can be seduced with offers of special access, threatened with the career-destroying prospect that they will be frozen out. But I rely almost entirely on numbers and analyses that are in the public domain; I don't need to be in the good graces of top officials, so I also have no need to display the deference that characterizes many journalists…."

That explains why Krugman is able to spot the lies and the hidden agenda, and why he is fearless in exposing them. Most of that I could have figured out for myself, if challenged. The really electrifying part of his Introduction is his explanation of what it all means and why we should not have been surprised at events and statements that have dominated news out of Washington over the past few months. Krugman says he discovered it himself only just before completing *The Great Unraveling*. And he found it in the doctoral dissertation of the young Henry Kissinger, published in 1957. That book was about diplomatic efforts to reconstruct Europe after the battle of Waterloo. "But the first three pages...sent chills down my spine, because they seem all too relevant to current events. In those first few pages, Kissinger describes the problems confronting a heretofore stable diplomatic system when it is faced with a revolutionary power – a power that does not accept that system's legitimacy.... It seems clear to me that one should regard America's right-wing movement – which now in effect controls the administration, both houses of Congress, much of the judiciary, and a good slice of the media – as a revolutionary power in Kissinger's sense. That is, it is a movement whose leaders do not accept the legitimacy of our current political system."

As of mid-spring in 2005, that information is no longer news, but keep in mind that Krugman wrote the lines in the summer or fall of 2003. He then felt it necessary to put a substantial quantity of evidence in front of his readers to persuade them that he was not overstating his case. In the light of what we have seen and heard since Bush's second inaugural, we no longer need to rely on clues and inferences to be convinced that "...there's ample evidence that key elements of the coalition that now runs the country believe that some long-established American political and social institutions should not, in principle, exist – and do not accept the rules that the rest of us have taken for granted."

The important instances Krugman provides in support of this rule include:

1. New Deal programs like Social Security and unemployment insurance, Great Society programs like Medicare. "The Bush administration's economic ideology...regards the very existence of those programs as a violation of basic principles."

2. Foreign policy: "Since World War II the United States has built its foreign policy around international institutions, and has tried to make it clear that it is not an old fashioned imperialist power, which uses military force as it sees fit. But... the neoconservative intellectuals who fomented the war with Iraq...have contempt for all that.... They aren't hesitant about the use of force; one [of them] declared that 'we are a warlike people and we love war....' [A] senior State Department official, John Bolton, told Israeli officials that after Iraq the United States would 'deal with' Syria, Iran, and North Korea." (As I write this on April 19, the Senate Foreign Relations Committee has been unable to agree on sending Bolton's nomination as Ambassador to the UN to the full Senate.)

3. The separation of church and state: It is one of the fundamental principles of the US Constitution, but House majority leader Tom DeLay has said that he is in office to pro-mote a "biblical worldview." Consistent with that, DeLay has denounced the teaching of evolution in schools. (News of early 2005 is that biology teachers in U.S. schools are now reluctant to mention evolution at all, in fear of troubles from being politically incorrect.)

4. Legitimacy of the democratic process:

"Paul Gigot of *The Wall Street Journal* famously praised the 'bourgeois riot' in which violent protestors shut down a vote recount in Miami. (The rioters, it was later revealed, weren't angry citizens; they were paid political operatives.) Meanwhile, according to his close friend Don Evans, now the secretary of commerce, George W. Bush believes that he was called by God to lead the nation. Perhaps this explains why the disputed election of 2000 didn't seem to inspire any caution or humility on the part of the victors. Consider Justice Antonin Scalia's response to a student who asked how he felt making the Supreme Court decision that threw the election to Bush. Was it agonizing? Did Scalia worry about the consequences? No: 'It was a wonderful feeling,' he declared." In several of his *NYT* columns of 2004, Krugman worried about inadequate preparations to assure an honest vote in the elections of last year, and as we now know, there were widespread and bitter denunciations of interference with voters who were expected to favor nominees of the Democratic Party.

The Ensconced don't Like "America as It Is"

In this 2003 book, Krugman challenges his readers to face the clear implication "that the people now in charge really don't like America as it is. If you combine their apparent agendas, the goal would seem to be something like this: a country that basically has no social safety net at home, which relies mainly on military force to enforce its will abroad, in which schools don't teach evolution but do teach religion and – possibly – in which elections are only a formality. Yet those who take the hard-line rightists now in power at their word, and suggest that they may really attempt to realize such a radical goal, are usually accused of being 'shrill,' of going over the top. Surely, says the conventional wisdom, we should discount the rhetoric: the goals of the right are more limited than this picture suggests. Or are they?"

Therein lies danger, Krugman argues, backed up the following passage that he quotes from Kissinger:

"Lulled by a period of stability which had seemed permanent, they find it nearly impossible to take at face value the assertion of the revolutionary power that it means to smash the existing framework. The defenders of the status quo therefore tend to begin by treating the revolutionary power as if its protestations were merely tactical; as if it really accepted the existing legitimacy but overstated its case for bargaining purposes; as if it were motivated by specific grievances to be assuaged by limited concessions. Those who warn against the danger in time are considered alarmists; those who counsel adaptation to circumstance are considered balanced and sane.... But it is the essence of a revolutionary power that it possesses the courage of its convictions, that it is willing, indeed eager, to push its principles to their ultimate conclusion."

That "sent chills down my spine", says Krugman, "because

it explains so well the otherwise baffling process by which the [Bush] administration has been able to push radical policies through, with remarkably little scrutiny or effective opposition...from the American political and media establishment... over the past two years."

A year and a half later, these words sound almost stale as the Bush agenda unrolls before our eyes. And to the list of fundamental institutions that the revolutionary force intends to overthrow we can now add the system of checks and balances that is a central feature of the U.S. political system. For in the aftermath of the orgiastic Terry Schiavo feeding tube incident, Tom DeLay is campaigning to make the judiciary subject to the legislative branch.

The policy agenda that Krugman inferred from what he saw and heard in application has been explored and explained by political historians as a deliberate, well-orchestrated and abundantly funded campaign that got underway with the nomination of Barry Goldwater as Republican presidential candidate in 1964. Several analyses of this kind have appeared since the November 2004 election, but one of the best preceded it by a few weeks. It is an essay by Lewis Lapham in *Harper's Magazine* of September 2004, titled "Tentacles of Rage: The Republican propaganda mill, a brief history."

Keith Wilde

The Perils of Symptom Intersections

A T THE BEGINNING of our search towards an understanding of any crucial problem, we must check the language used to discuss it. Are we preempting our research with an answer locked into accepted terminology such as "inflation"? Does it allow us to sort out the strands of different causes that may contribute to apparently similar results? Some of these may be providing socially indispensable returns for the higher prices they contribute to, while others may simply reflect the appetites of a particular social group. Should we not try sorting out the final effects from similar symptoms thrown up en route?

What we need is a map that will track two alternate policies not to "a crossroads of symptoms," easily mistaken for an equilibrium point, but which may just be an intersection of independent causes en route to their ultimate effects. We must consult our map to see whether those paths, after intersecting, simply pursue each its different course to its own goal, perhaps leading us where we had no intention of going. Price stability is usually defined as a condition where changes in the prices of individual commodities average out to zero, so that the index is flat. Simplified to two commodities they may vary but meet – that is, their changes average out at a certain point of their trajectory to zero, which is taken to be price stability. But since many different factors are at work the two lines may continue their independent course, with causal factors for which the supposed equilibrium point has no special significance. One

of these lines may be the price effects of new taxation imposed for essential measures for our health or educational systems or for environmental conservation, but which economists dismiss as externalities. Or to bail out our gambolling banks, which for reasons carefully hidden, give it top priority.

To get our important point across, let us try another simile, and deal with the trajectories of common physical symptoms of two very different causes at their intersection. A flushed face may be the result of strenuous sport, or of a serious infection. Not to make the distinction, but instead employ a drastic means to bring down the subject's temperature, would not be wise.

We must avoid preempting the search by referring to a super-historical ideal like "the pure and perfect market" on which all actors are of such infinitesimal size that anything they do or leave undone cannot affect the price level. Such a world never existed, and least of all exists in this day of international conglomerates.

Use History, Not an Imagined World of Self-balancing Markets

On May 23, 1991, in his annual report the General Manager of the Bank for International Settlements, Alexandre Lamfalussy, laid down the goal of "zero inflation" in these terms: "It has been argued that a quality bias in price level calculations implies that inflation in the range of $1/2\%$ may be considered price stability for all practical purposes. Nonetheless, the move from an environment of low or moderate inflation to one of no inflation implies an important psychological shift. It has proved very difficult in recent decades to do better than achieve merely low inflation and to move to actual price stability, even in those countries with the best price performance." BIS is a sort of central bankers' club that argues for the independence of central banks from their governments even if their charters – as is the case of the Bank of Canada – openly gives the Finance Minister of the government the power to fire the head of the Bank of Canada – if he fails to comply with the government's written directives on general policy. At the Bretton Woods Conference that planned the postwar economic organizations in 1943, Resolution Five was adopted on the initiative of certain governments-in-exile because of the speed with which BIS had delivered to the Nazis the moment they occupied Prague in 1938 the gold reserve entrusted to them by the government of Czechoslovakia. That Resolution called for the liquidation of BIS at the earliest possible moment. That caused BIS to cultivate a low profile, and that low profile in turn commended it as an ideal bunker for plotting the deregulation of the banks throughout the world from the severe restraint that had been imposed on them in the depth of the Great Depression. The reason: the Depression had been brought on to a considerable extent by the speculative activities of the banking systems.

From the BIS emerged the gush of propaganda that predicted that hyperinflation similar that destroyed the German currency in 1923 would ensue if the slightest price inflation were tolerated. But that German hyperinflation was the result of a lost world war, of the reparations imposed on Germany in strong foreign currency that it was not allowed to earn, of the occupation of the industrial heartland by the French and Belgian armies when Germany suspended its reparation payments, of a general strike supported by the entire political spectrum. What the BIS implied was that had interest rates been pushed up sufficiently to fight inflation, there would in retrospect have been no lost World War, no reparations, no occupation of the Ruhr by the French, no general strike.

Economic historians like Fernand Braudel have emphasized what official economists are blind to: life in cities requires increasingly more services than life in the countryside.

The Gush of Propaganda that has Replaced Analysis

During the Depression of the 1930s, governments eventually came to play a greater part in their economies. The war and the reconstruction, the vast post-war migration, and the population shift from countryside to cities, the post-war baby-boom that skewed age patterns to require more hospitals, schools, and other public services than in the past. All this is ignored in most discussions of "inflation." Yet all these factors and many more drove up the share of public investment within the economy. And it was paid for by taxation, that became a deepening layer of price.

The rise of the price indexes thus came to reflect two distinct processes. There may have been too much demand to be supplied by available production. That could be termed "market inflation." But on top of that was a deepening stratum of taxation unrelated to the supply-demand imbalance. That reflected the growing importance of government investment in physical and human capital within the economy. This was paid for out of taxation that thus showed up in the entire national product and thus in the price index. It must be given a distinct name to avoid sowing confusion. In a paper published in *Revue Économique* in Paris (May 1970) I chose to call it the "social lien," since it had to be paid for out of the prices of other goods and services.

Price had become pluralistic, reflecting the what had happened to the society it served.

On the other hand, if we recognize it for what it is and adopt the corresponding accountancy, governments would not try to pay for public investment, whether in physical or human capital, in a single year. For the benefits of such investment will last for years, and the pattern in the private sector is to depreciate the capital investment over a similar period. More taxation collected than strictly needed will add to the social lien and to the upward price gradient. That is coming to be recognized tacitly by many governments, but has still not done away with the alarms about budgetary deficits of governments that apply no such depreciation for government investments.

Human capital – public expenditure for education, health, social welfare, is never treated as a public investment on the government's books. However, in the 1960s careful research on the astoundingly rapid recovery of Japan and Germany from the devastation of WWII, had led economists to recognize that investment in human capital was the most productive that can be made. It matters little that physically that asset is lodged in private bodies and brains. Its contribution is made to the tax base, which is the source of government revenue and credit.

Theodore Schultz of the University of Chicago was awarded the Nobel Prize for Economics for having developed the point. Today he and his great work are significantly forgotten.

Since 1996, the US has introduced into its books the depreciation of its physical investment over its useful life, rather than a one-year write-off in the year in which it was made. Canada under the pressure of the previous Auditor General finally prevailed on Mr. Martin the then Finance Minister, to do likewise, but the revision of our government books is apparently proceeding at a leisurely pace. In neither country has the public been informed of what was being done. In neither country, too, has there even been mention of extending such accrual accountancy to investments in human capital, though almost a half century ago economists were forced to realize that investment in education, health and social welfare is the most rewarding investment a government can make.

Such "accrual accountancy" or "capital budgetting" will, to be sure, show a greater debt, but the portion of that debt incurred for capital purposes will be shown separately from spending for current purposes. Robert Eisner of North Western University a quarter of a century ago did detailed studies that showed that government investment if not paid off in a single year would lose part of its real value by the very upward price gradient due to the increase in this not-recognized layer of taxation. That in turn would attenuate the steepness of the climb of the price index. However, the brilliant work of Eisner, like so much else that clashes with the dominant ideology, has been buried without a marker on its grave.

Over two years ago BIS, the Fed and other central banks started talking about "good inflation" and "bad inflation". Up to 2% – occasionally even to 3% – "inflation" was good. Beyond that it became bad once more. However, like other insights that fleetingly reverse economic orthodoxy, "good inflation" has disappeared once again even before it was properly introduced.

Currently interest rates are being pushed upward once more to "lick inflation."

That gives you the measure of the trouble for economists arising from the very language they speak.

Today the recent talk about "good inflation," a "necessary lubricant of our economy," has already vanished. The talk on all continents is once against the dangers of inflation and the need to "pay down" the debt. What, however, are they going to "pay off" the debt with? The only legal tender in existence throughout the world is government credit. Such nonsense issues monopolize our think-space and our political discussion space. Unless we address that issue our democracy will go on crumbling.

William Krehm

REVIEW OF A BOOK BY A. CHOMSKY, B. CARR AND P.M. SMORLAKOFF (EDS), DURHAM AND LONDON, DUKE UNIVERSITY PRESS, 2005

"The Cuba Reader: History, Culture, Politics"

THIS COMPENDIUM, mostly translated from the Spanish, offers a wealth of nuance from a generally left of centre viewpoint. Its great merit as it ranges over hill, dale and mountain is that it focusses on what has made of Cuba a special gem of Latin America. Neither the epics of Latin America as a whole or of Cuba in particular could have arisen without their mountainous settings. Fidel Castro retreated with two or three dozen revolutionaries into the Sierra Maestra of the eastern part of the island under very noses of the US secret service and their pet dictator Fulgencio Batista. And the very heroism involved was too out-sized, once victorious, to endure completely uncorrupted. In his book on the early Castro Revolution, Hugh Thomas described the typical white Cuban male excelling at only two things – managing a sugar estate and facing a firing squad. But Castro was to change that equation. Like him or hate him, he stood up to the United States that so repeatedly had frustrated Latin American freedoms.

After the work of the great Liberators of South America came the US proclamation of its Monroe Doctrine, declaring Latin America its private preserve. But that was as nothing compared with the Platt Amendment passed by the US Congress in 1901. You may have heard of that amendment vaguely as the big bully on the block meddling in the affairs of a neighbouring small nation after it had practically won its independence from Spain after almost a half century of bloody warfare, but to appreciate it fully you must read a summary of the Amendment. It provides: (1) "The government of Cuba shall never enter into any treaty or other compact with any foreign power which will impair or tend to impair the independence of Cuba, or in any manner authorize or permit any foreign power or powers to obtain by colonization or, for military or naval purposes or otherwise, lodgment in or control over any portion of said island; (2) The said government shall not assume or contract any public debt or pay interest upon which, and to make reasonable sinking fund provisions for the ultimate discharge of which, the ordinary revenues of the island after defraying the current expenses of government shall be inadequate. (3) The government of Cuba consents that the US may exercise the right to intervene for the preservation of Cuban independence, the maintenance of a government adequate for the protection of life, property and individual liberty and for discharging the obligations with respect to Cuba imposed by the Treaty of Paris on the US.... (5) That the government of Cuba will execute and as far as necessary extend, the plans already devised or other plans to be mutually agreed upon, for the sanitation of the cities of the island, to the end that a recurrence of epidemic and infectious diseases may be prevented, thereby assuming the protection to the people and commerce of Cuba, as well as to the commerce of the southern ports of the US.... (7) That to enable the US to maintain the independence of Cuba, and to protect the people thereof, as well as for its own defense, the government of Cuba will sell or lease to the US land necessary for coaling and naval stations at certain specified points to be agreed upon with the president of the US."

The Tale of the Conquest of Yellow Fever

The book carries cartoons in the US press of the period advocating the intervention of Uncle Sam in Cuba. The Cubans are shown as positively simian in appearance and manner, and invariably black. Puerto Rico, already in Washington's colonial stable is presented as a demure, white, well-dressed youngster holding Uncle Sam's benign hand. But the real payoff was yet to come.

"The US military occupation of Cuba (1898-1900), which followed the defeat of the Spanish army, [had as one of its purposes] built into the Platt Amendment that the Americans would make it sanitary enough for commerce and immigration. About that Nancy Stepan (p. 150) recounts a burlesque tale. When the Yellow Fever Commission triumphed over yellow fever in Havana in 1900, by confirming that it is transmitted by the Aedes Aegypti mosquito, the matter was of immense satisfaction in the US. Yet the mosquito theory [of its origins] had been in existence for nearly twenty years. In 1881 the Cuban physician Carlos J. Finlay proposed that the Aedes mosquito transmitted yellow fever from person to person through its bite. One may well ask why there was a 20-year delay in confirming his work.

"To a large extent, indeed, North America's entry into the Cuban war against Spain and the occupation of the island was justified by the belief that the US brought to Cuba a moral, political and technological superiority not to be found in Spain or Cuba. But between January, 1900, and December of that year the cases of yellow fever in Havana had risen from a handful to 485. Only then did the American scientists turn to the work and collaboration of the Cuban Finlay and within months yellow fever was conquered. Shortly afterwards that control of yellow fever made possible the construction of the Panama canal."

In all his contradictions, Fidel Castro reflects the very different social implications of Cuba's two main crops: tobacco, of native origin, requiring great skills and little equipment but the dedication of small growers; and sugar, a foreign crop requiring much capital for mechanical equipment of the mills. You catch a glimpse of what may have influenced the otherwise highly disciplined Fidel Castro, particularly proud of his government's health record, until his recently obvious throat troubles, rarely photographed without his big Cuban cigar. Sugar, on the other hand, was a feudal crop, with Haitian field workers smuggled into Cuba by contractors who recruited them with much misrepresentation and liquor. Local Cuban field workers during off-season, having neither jobs nor savings, fed themselves by growing food crops between the cane rows.

"In economic life, too, Cuban sovereignty was quickly weakened. The Reciprocity Treat signed with the US in 1903 privileged Cuban access to the US sugar market but at a substantial cost. US manufactured goods and other products could enter Cuba, establishing an informal economic protectorate and consolidating Cuba's role as producer of a single crop (sugar). For the next fifty years, Cuba's economic prosperity would depend on the outcome of Byzantine struggles over the fate of Cuba's tariff privileges in the US Congress. Economic dependency and US military intervention and hegemony did not promote good government. Cuban politicians viewed a bloated, corrupt state as the only opportunity for acquiring wealth.

The arrival of F.D. Roosevelt in the presidency, reduced US backing for a particularly bloody regime of Gerardo Machado (1925-33). While mobs, looted, burned and killed. Machado resigned and fled." The entire procedure was supposed to have been carried out in "legal form" according to the Constitution, that is under the influence of [US] Ambassador, Sumner Welles (p. 274). And the 1930s, in Cuba as throughout the world, were a time of economic collapse and widespread rethinking of economic and political orthodoxies, not least in the US itself. The numerous young exiles who had fled the country during the Machado years now came back home from the capitals of the world with heads full of exciting new ideas.

The Return of the Exiles with Heads Full of New Ideas

"The neo-colonial 'politics of disappointment' facilitated the coup d'état launched by Fulgencio Batista in March 1952, which inaugurated seven years of increasingly repressive government.

"The Cuban Revolution of 1959 was one of the most profound revolutions in Latin American history – in many ways more than the 19th century wars of independence that left unchanged the basic structures of Latin American society. The post-Stalinist, Third World revolutionary Marxism that it helped define was also a factor in the emergence of a youthful New Left in Europe and the US.

"In the US, this dynamic tended to be perceived in Cold War terms – and indeed, the Soviet Union sought to present itself as a defender of colonial peoples (at least those outside its own sphere of influence). The locus of the Cuban revolution shifted towards the Left in the first two years. This happened because of the pressure from workers, agricultural laborers, and peasants anxious to broaden and deepen the initial cautious policies of the new government and as US resistance to economic nationalism and social reform led to the breaking of diplomatic relations. Along with these factors came a growing reliance on the Soviet Union.

"The agrarian reform, enacted in the summer of 1959, set the stage for an aggressive commitment to redistribution of the country's wealth for the good of the nation as a whole. 'Great landowners must understand that their duty is to adapt themselves to the new circumstances.... Not a single Cuban must suffer from hunger,' declared Fidel Castro. Nationalization as a policy gained strength until 1968, when the last remnants of the private economy were essentially abolished.

"In the economic sphere, Cuba's growing dependence on the Soviet Union reproduced the old colonial pattern of reliance on exportation of a single crop – sugar – with the important differ-ence that the USSR chose, for political reasons, to subsidize Cuba's economy, instead of profiting from it as had previous colonial powers. In the political sphere, Cuban leaders found themselves obligated to support the USSR when it might have been more in their interest not to, though they sometimes continued to challenge Soviet policies on the international level." The shipping of Soviet nuclear missiles to Cuba, would never have happened had it not been for Washington's dunderheaded nostalgia.

The Argentinian "Che Guevara" tells the story how he joined Fidel Castro and eighty other conspirators in Mexico and set off in the motorboat Granma in late November 1956. Their initial experiences were disastrous, but hardened the 21 who survived after the first weeks on Cuban soil. Taking refuge in the mountainous terrain of the Sierra Maestra the guerrillas managed to win the support of the local peasantry, who had suffered from the land-grabbing of speculators and local army chieftains. Become seasoned warriors from the defeats suffered, the band soon emerged as victors. The government responded by resettling thousands of peasants in the cities. Children died for lack of food and medical attention. The scandal of this cruelty not only rocked Cuban public opinion but echoed abroad. The government reversed itself. That brought the Castro band recruits and soon they established links with the cities below.

21 Survivors of the Granma Make a Revolution

Oddly enough, the US State Department, though it held Batista in low regard, was determined to keep the Castro group with its aggressive nationalism and social reform ideas out of power. One CIA group, however, viewing the problem in its geopolitical context, saw an early approach to Castro "in a context of checks and balances" to be in Washington's interest. Castro, however, was not a leader to be checked or balanced.

That soon appeared in his social programs. When we try to assess the justice or injustice of Washington's tightening boycott against Cuba, we need a sense of what the Castro regime brought to Cuba. Nutritionist Medea Benjamin lived in Cuba from 1979 to 1983 – well before the collapse of the Soviet Union and long enough for Castro's redistribution of the national income to have taken effect. She was there working for a project for the Institute for Food and Development Policy about food and hunger in Cuba. "'Landing in Havana, the head of the Nutrition Institute laughed when I told her I wanted to work with malnourished children.' What an immense pleasure to live in a society that had abolished hunger! The revolution's leadership viewed inadequate income as the reason why people were undernourished, so it put into motion policies to boost the earnings of the poorer half of society and to enlarge the share of their earnings they could spend on food. But once people had more money to spend on food it became clear that there was not enough food to go around. One simple solution to that would have been to let prices rise, and reduce the number of Cubans able to buy food. That would have dealt with the shortages but not with people's hunger. As Castro recalled years later, 'A price policy to compensate for this imbalance [between supply and demand] would have been a ruthless sacrifice of the population with the lowest income. Such a policy was acceptable for luxury goods, 'but never for necessities.' The government chose a more equitable distribution – by need rather than by income – rationing. At the same time it generated fuller employment. With the large estates converted into 'people's farms' by the first agrarian reform, there were 150,000 year-around jobs on these lands in August 1962 compared to fewer than fifty thousand in 1959. During the 'dead season' on sugar plantations workers now found steady work on the construction projects that sprang up everywhere – roads, schools, clinics, government offices, housing, etc. While only 29 percent of rural workers earned more than 75 pesos a month as of April 1958, two years later 44% did.

"What did people do with so much extra money? Among the most pressing desires for the poor was to eat more and better. Nationwide consumption of such coveted foods as pork and milk soared, beef consumption shot up by 50% in just two years, But supply failed to keep pace with the growing demand. The Eisenhower administration's 1960 embargo on most exports to Cuba seriously disrupted the island's agriculture, which had become dependent on the US for farm machinery, fertilizers, pesticides, seeds. Repeated military attacks culminating in the Bay of Pigs invasion of April 1960 exacted a toll on production. Finding fewer consumer goods to buy, especially imports from the US, tenants and sharecroppers had little need for cash and produced less for the market. In an attempt to stem speculation, the wholesale food business was nationalized and those retail stores accused of hoarding and profiteering were taken over by the government. And in August 1961 a law was passed prohibiting the resale of certain goods. A rationing system was introduced for all Cubans covering the most important food items."

Cuba's Medical Diplomacy a Model for the Big Powers

"Medical diplomacy has been overlooked in analyses of Cuban foreign policy. Dozens of countries have received long-term and emergency Cuban medical assistance, medical education and in the donation of equipment, medicines and supplies. This was done despite the fact that half of Cuba's physicians emigrated shortly after the revolution, reducing the number of Cuban physicians from about six to three thousand. The program involves some 16,000 doctors, teachers, construction engineers, agronomists, economists and other specialists serving in twenty-two Third World countries."

On the other hand, on a recent visit in Cuba, I was struck by the fact that it was practically impossible to purchase any aspirin. In view of this tremendous altruistic achievement, of a country itself beggared by an economic boycott, might we not expect that President Bush's democratic heart might not be moved to exempt trade in aspirin with Cuba?

With the collapse of the Soviet Union, in the early 1990s, new draconian austerity measures were introduced because of the disappearance of the Soviet subsidy. A "Special Period" for belt-tightening was introduced. The government gave hard currency exports priority over islanders' needs and wants as its deficit rose. Cutbacks in Soviet grain deliveries meant less feed for chicken and cattle, and less wheat for bread. And people were now obliged to make numerous trips to stores, since not every item was available on a particular day.

The Ghastly Effects of the US Embargo

Unemployment spread. Workers who lost their jobs were given the right, under the new policy, to select from three alternative jobs. If they refused the options, they were entitled to unemployment insurance, first for three and later for one month. Previously there had been no limits on unemployment compensation. Susan Eckstein (p. 610) writes "One university professor informed me that about half the labor force in the light industry sector and in many ministries had been let go when the "Special Period" was proclaimed, Castro began courting foreign investment as never before. He publicly defended the 'creeping privatization' and economic 'denationalization' involved. 'Capital yes, Capitalism no,' became the slogan of the day. In the main, plants built with Soviet-bloc assistance ran the risk of becoming tombstones of bygone 'Communist solidarity.' To offset such obstacles, the government exempted investors from compliance with labour laws and it allowed unlimited profit repatriation for up to ten years. The government also agreed to bear construction and infrastructural costs." Many of the impressive restoration of old buildings on Havana's Prado were done with foreign financing under such plans.

But the greatest expectations for coping with the "Special Period" were placed on the tourist industry. That sector had grossed $200 million in 1989, and by 1992 that had risen to $700 mllions. Despite the US embargo 424,000 tourists came, but since the sector is import-intensive, only half that amount was netted in foreign currency. To the shame of most Cubans even the Ministry of Tourism began running tourist advertisements abroad featuring bikini-clad sexy Cuban girls. The government's interest in hard currency led it to play on its pre-revolutionary reputation and to reverse its earlier puritanical stance on such matters. Cuba threatens to become a major bordello of the world once more.

William Krehm

A WAY OUT — FREEDOM OF DISCUSSION

With difficult problems for survival and caught in the gunsights of its powerful northern neighbour, a lot of consideration must be given to the best course to follow. An important contribution to the book reviewed is the essay on Civil Society by Haroldo Dilla, who had been an investigator attached to the government think tank, the Center for the Study of the Americas. "In the mid-1990s CEA became the target of hard-line criticism, leading to the dispersion of some of Cuba's most creative intellectuals. Dilla is currently living in the Dominican Republic, where he is Research Coordinator at Latin America Faculty for Social Sciences. He writes, "The first time that I heard someone argue about the importance of civil society in Cuba was in 1984, during a talk by the well-known political scientist Rafael Hernandez at the then-vigorous Center for the Study of the Americas. At the time Cuban society was still not very differentiated socially and had been shaped by the intense process of social mobility led by a government that had had relatively plentiful resources and considerable social autonomy. Thus, ideas like those of Hernandez were viewed at best as needless intellectual subtleties. The situation changed in the late 1980s when Cuban society began to undergo a profound transformation as a result of the acute economic crisis and the gradual dismantling of prevailing forms of social and political control. The economic reforms implemented by the government to address the crisis opened considerable space for the market and the circulation of dollars, while undermining the average citizen's purchasing power. One of the significant signs of this change has been the decline in the state's previously unchallenged capacity to control the distribution of resources, social and political discourse, and ideological production.

"The partial withdrawal of the state opened spaces that were filled by associations, communication networks, or simply aggregates of people. Independent spaces for activities and debates appeared that were unthinkable only a few years earlier, whether as a result of the opening of the market or as result of the inability of the old ideological apparatuses to control the whims of thought. A civil society demanding its own space began to emerge in Cuba.

"In the early 1990s, pronouncements about civil society were very cautious, given the reticence of the people involved to discuss a subject that had been proscribed by Soviet Marxism. To make matters worse, it was also a topic that appeared in the US agenda aimed at subverting the Cuban Revolution. Fortunately, this reticence vanished in 1992 when Fidel Castro made a positive allusion to the role of civil society in Latin America in a speech at the Rio Summit. Cuban intellectuals interpreted that speech as a signal that the subject was now safe to talk about. Everyone simply wanted to know whether the role of civil society would be positive or negative in rebuilding Cuba's consensus. The new debate was constrained by hostility from two fronts. On the one side, there was the hostile meddling of the US government interested in using Cuban civil society for subversive and counter-revolutionary ends. On the other, there was the Cuban political class, which was not inclined to allow competition in the control of resources and values."

W.K.

STEPWISE TRADING AWAY THE EMBARGO FOR MORE DEMOCRATIC LIBERTIES

Having from *The Cuban Reader* an objective account of the suffering inflicted on the Cuban people by the US embargo, we will attempt a purely apolitical program for removing some of the worst features of that 45-year policy misstep of Washington that would be to the eventual advantage of both parties. Before clipping the claws of this beast unknown in international legal lore, a few observations are in place. There is no use seeking a solution in the laws of war, for there has been no official war between these two nations. And to suggest that Cuba, even were it not impoverished to a state approaching beggary, is in any way a military threat to the US is ridiculous. The aggressor on all previous military encounters between the two nations was the United States. The success of a tiny nation in repelling at-

tacks planned and backed by the US, the attempts as assassinating the Cuban head of state have no justification in the law of nations. Nor has it earned the US esteem in Latin America and throughout the world. The lack of support of the US embargo is indicated by the fact that the rest of the world is engaged in trading with Cuba, even though its demeaned condition due to the US embargo restricts the scope of possible trade and investment by other countries.

We would propose that the United States and Cuba, brought together by some peace-loving powers, join in a staged plan for Cuba to start making carefully defined criticism of Cuban government policy within that country in return for specific successive reductions in the scope of the US embargo against trade and investment by US citizens with that republic.

Since each stage would be preceded by friendly negotiations, the two countries could take equal credit and responsibility for the steps in such a plan. The choice of the successive relaxations of the embargo, and the greater freedom of expression in matters not affecting the basic communist regime would lie entirely the hands of the two countries affected, so that they would not surrender control of the timing and the nature of the mutual concessions.

After all, the Soviet Republic in its early days went through its New Economic Policy and came out of it stronger. The Castro regime, due to the disappearance of the Soviet subsidy, has already had to make far greater concessions to the a free market economy than would probably be necessary by allowing a greater degree of criticism by a loyal opposition in its administration of the mixed capitalist-economic economy of the country as it exists today. Starved of resources, it is also beset with serious inefficiencies some of which can be traced to the absence of an independent loyal opposition. What the proposed plan would offer would be freedom in the press and forums to express views critical of government administrative policies, without even increasing the amount of private investment that exists today. It is even conceivable that the proposed plan would make it possible to do away with undesirable private sector innovations that have already been granted – for example, the notorious expansion of the sex trade.

Given the degree of this indignity that the embargo has visited on an innocent nation, it is certainly worth the effort. If either side refuses to join the other in even exploring the possibility of embarking on such a plan, it would certainly forfeit credit in the eyes of the world.

Progress on the scheme just outlined, might pave the way for a far more ambitious project: the organization of a Latin American central bank that would not replace, but rather would supplement the present central banks of the individual Latin American countries. The readers of *Economic Reform* will have noted the disastrous effects in countries like Mexico, Ecuador, and the Argentine of having in one way or another adopted the US dollar either for their currency or required as backing for their own. Great effort was made by rightist think tanks and individual economists for a similar arrangement in Canada, which fortunately our government had the good sense to resist.

A Latin American Central Bank

When the central bank of any country adopts the currency of another as its monetary base or the backing for its monetary reserves that is tantamount to a free loan of the amount of the foreign currency used for such. About 60 percent of the world's central bank reserve are in US dollars and that is one of the things that still allow the US to live with its enormous debt.

A Latin American bank such as we propose would have its reserves made up almost entirely of currencies of the Latin American countries (say in the proportion to their Gross Domestic Products), with just marginal amounts of dollars, pounds, euros, yen and yuan. With its reserves thus constituted, the L.A. Central Bank could concentrate its finance on trade and investments amongst the Latin American countries. This would provide a tremendous help to them in overcoming their inherited role as borrowers, with endless frustrations barring the way to financial independence. Since the Mexican banking crisis begun in 1994, that country's huge foreign debt contracted in US dollars on the advice of foreign banking consultants, resulted in 85% of the Mexican banking system ending up in foreign hands. A big pill for a country as nationalist as Mexico to swallow!

A further word of explanation is in place here. When a private bank makes a loan it creates a multiple of the money base actually in its vaults. The rest is essentially float and fiction. What ultimately backs it all up in addition to the bank's own capital, and the deposits made by the public, is the creditworthiness of the government, through its central bank as "lender of the last resort." The government actually *invests* the money it creates into existence. What banks must keep their eye on is making sure that they will always have the legal tender in their vaults to honour a cheque drawn on them. In recent years, the statutory reserves required to back the money it created were done away with altogether, or almost so in the case of the US, so that the leverage that banks operate with is greater than ever. Today the credit of the financially powerful states plays the role that was once assigned – at least in theory – to gold and silver. That has made it more difficult for a borrowing nation to meet its own financial needs, let alone developing into a lender. That is why our proposal for a Latin American Central Bank is all the more timely for dealing with situations like those of Mexico, Cuba, Ecuador, the Argentine and Brazil, and Latin America as a whole.

The very mention of a Latin American central bank owned by governments and financing essential public investments at near-zero interest rates is certain to elicit objections that Latin America is far too corrupt to indulge in such plans. Perhaps because He on High had foreknowledge that somebody was going to propose this plan for a central Latin American bank that would invest money into existence rather than borrow it into existence, that the Attorney General of New York State, Eliot Spitzer was inspired to continue and even intensify his investigations of corruption on Wall St. Currently he has disclosed such "cooking of the books" in the very re-insurance industry – the ultimate guardian at the gates. No matter how great the corruption in some Latin American circles might be, what Mr.

Spitzer has disclosed would be hard to match.

And one of the purposes of both our proposals is to come to the help of Washington to step down with some grace from its dangerously tempting role as lone economic superpower that no longer is based on reality. Moreover, international interest rates are rising ominously once again as the one "blunt tool" to fight rising oil prices. But higher interest rates happen to favour money-lenders and penalize productive effort. If it is true that it would be wise for Cuba to tolerate some loyal criticism within its chosen system, it is no less a fact that Washington could also profit from a coordinated abandonment of its Big Bully – Bad Loser role.

W.K.

The CBC National Invites Us to Send in Questions about the Sponsorship Scandal

AW C'MON GUYS, what's a hundred million between friends?

Why are we getting so much coverage about a mere $100 million while ignoring the really big scandal – the Mother of all scandals – the one which doesn't involve millions of dollars, or even hundreds of millions of dollars, but hundreds of BILLIONS of dollars?

And why focus on the Liberals when the Conservatives are just as guilty for this bigger boondoggle – the one which saw our national debt grow from $30 billion to almost $600 billion in just 20 years – 1977 to 1997?

Why isn't this massive mishandling of our money getting the attention it deserves?

Richard Priestman

Coexisting with Mother Nature

A review of The Natural Step – From Consensus to Sustainable Development.

THIS REMARKABLE DOCUMENT was reprinted by Ontario Hydro in 1996. That, of course, is sadly ironical, because long since Ontario Hydro has been broken up and mostly privatized in an atmosphere of scandal.

"The Natural Step is a movement started in Sweden by Dr. Karl-Henrik Robert. It is based on the belief that only by working within the natural cycles of the earth can we survive and prosper. It came into being as a dialogue and consensus beginning with scientists and spreading into the community at large. It has identified four basic and non-negotiable 'systems conditions.' Swedish businesses such as IKEA, Electrolux and Scandic Hotels, among others, have adopted these systems conditions as part of their planning and operations:

1. *Nature cannot withstand a systematic build-up of dispersed matter mined from the Earth's crust.* This ultimately means that fossil fuels, metals and other minerals must not be extracted at a rate faster than they can be redeposited into the earth's crust. This requires a radically reduced dependency on mined minerals and fossil fuels.

2. *Nature cannot withstand a systematic build-up of substances produced by humans.* This means that substances must not be produced and released into the ecosphere at a rate faster than they can be broken down and integrated into the cycles of nature or deposited into the earth's crust. This requires a greatly decreased production of naturally occurring substances that are systematically accumulating beyond natural levels.

3. *Nature cannot withstand a systematic deterioration of its capacity for renewal.* This means that we cannot harvest or manipulate ecosystems in such a way as to diminish their productive capacity, or threaten the natural diversity of life forms (biodiversity). This requires that we critically adjust our consumption and land use practices to be well within the regenerative capacities of our ecosystems.

Therefore, if we want life to go on, there must be fair and efficient use of resources.

Basic human needs therefore must take precedence over the provision of luxuries for the select few. Social sustainability must occur with a resource metabolism meeting system conditions 1–3.

The Natural Step is now spreading throughout the world and is active in the UK, New Zealand, Australia and the Netherlands, and the US and is about to be introduced into Canada.

The Natural Step is based on the laws of natural science, including the laws of thermodynamics and matter conservation, and the cyclic principles of ecology.

It is based on systems thinking, focusing on first-order principles at the very beginning of cause-effect relationships, which promote simplicity without reduction. It recognizes that what happens in one part of the system affects every other part of the system, often in unexpected ways.

A Compass for Sustainable Development

Karl-Henrik Robert, Herman Daly, Paul Hawken and John Homberg – Methodology

Environmental problems have multiplied and changed character during the past decades: from local to global, from distinct to diffuse, from short time delay between cause and effect to long time delay, and from relatively low complexity to high complexity. This has increased the need for a compass to point us in the direction of sustainability.

A compass uses a sensitized needle which responds to the lure of magnetic north. The model we develop below is a means of sensitizing our society – but what is the lure, the magnetic north? It is the ethical insight that destroying the future capacity of the earth to support life is wrong.

To successfully implement sustainable development, professions, experts and the general public all need to be engaged. There must be a re-balancing in society between the sharing of existing scientific knowledge and the further expansion of that knowledge. The scientific background to our model is not new – indeed it derives much value from being based on the most basic laws of science. All physicists know and accept these laws (first and second laws of thermodynamics and the principle of matter-conservation). But the voting public does not understand them and often scientists themselves fail to see how these laws set the context for sustainable development. In a democracy, public policy cannot rise above the understanding of the average voter. Consequently, the sharing of knowledge is at least as critical for democracy as the distribution of income. [And we would add – likewise the contrary. Everything in square brackets is our comment.]

Among the "critical requirements for a theoretical model of sustainability," there are listed:

• The model must be based on a scientifically acceptable concept of the world.

• The model must contain a scientifically supportable definition of sustainability.

• The overall perspective must see the economy as a subsystem of the ecosystem.

• It would be an advantage if the model could also be used as a starting point for developing "new economics" – as a way to recognize new and wider patterns of values within old and basic economic principles." [Had the authors devoted as much study and attention to what is sustainable in official economic doctrines, they would find some of their comments far out on a limb. No economic doctrine based on exponential growth such as is assumed by conventional economic doctrine can be compatible with a sustainable treatment of the environment. We reproduce the essence of this impressive study for its handling of the physical and general social aspects of ecological conservation, not for its few feeble references to economic theory.]

"It is difficult to fully account for the costs of pollution and depletion of finite resources. Such costs tend not to escalate until something dramatic occurs., which means that the feedback comes too late. For example, a gallon of water is worth little today, but what will the last gallon of drinkable water be worth? This is a serious draw-back for margin-based valuations." [However, for a century and more economics has been taken over by marginal utility theory – e.g., the amount of increase in satisfaction resulting from the next infinitesimal increase in the consumption of whatever resource or product. And in such an operation the amount of satisfaction or destruction of the resource before the value of a current added increment of either process is disregarded. In calculating the rate of increase of the satisfaction or the amount of pollution, the constant in the expression for the current state simply disappears by the very procedure of differentialtion. And if the process is extended into the future through the integration process of calculus, the constant added is arbitrary – i.e., it does not have to be specifically evaluated.... Anyone with an elementary knowledge of maths will see at once that marginal value theory is the dead opposite of what the authors of the paper are proposing in their excellent program for a sustainable ecology.]

"This dilemma can be solved by proceeding from the overall physical conditions for sustainability, since nature must survive independently of how it is economically evaluated. Therefore, there is no guarantee that all environmental costs can ever be internalized in a way that prices alone will provide enough information to foster development towards sustainability." What the authors referred to as "basic and old economic principles" cannot begin to deal with the deterioration of the ecology. The ecology, as also public health, education, and much have simply been declared "externalities" – i.e., literally shown the back door.

One Dimensional Physical Models —
Matter Matters Too

Many scientists have realized the difficulty in trying to evaluate the stock of natural capital in monetary terms. This has led to attempts to change the unit of value from monetary terms to something "closer to nature." The most common attempts build on various units or "currencies' related to energy flows in both society and nature.

First of all, these scientists have generally observed the difficulty of auditing the complex interrelationships in nature with one single currency. For instance, accounting for pollution of mercury in a lake in energy or exergy (i.e., the degree of order within energy and matter) terms, would lead to an inappropriate and highly coloured description of reality. The world functions on the basis of many qualitative properties of matter that are simply not reducible to differing quantities of energy or exergy. As N. Georgescu-Roegen noted in reply to the modern versions of an energy theory of value: "matter matters too."

Furthermore, efforts to apply various energy terms as an appropriate currency are based on the assumption that the lack of energy provides the overall restrictions for societal metabolism of resources. But the global use of energy only correspond to around 1/13000 of the incoming energy from the sun. Thus, the bottle-neck for sustainable development is the complex pattern of all the material flows in society includes the resource sinks for society's metabolic wastes. These flows are generated not only by the energy sources (for instance fossil coal leading to flows of carbon dioxide and polluting metals), but also by the other material flows that are linked to the energy flows (mining, production, packaging, distribution and disposal). Besides the material flows, surface area provides another limiting factor; both as space for human activity and as the basic "net" for capturing solar energy that drives the material cycles by which dissipated quality of materials is reconstituted.

"Due to ecological complexity and delay-mechanisms, indicators late in the cause and effect chain have generally led to such complicated and incomprehensible results that the experts applying them have lost overview and control. If we, for instance, apply emissions of CO_2 as an indicator for the impact of fossil fuels, we end up with two major problems. Firstly, the complexity of negative and positive feed-back loops that are related to the accumulation of CO_2 in the atmosphere leads to such complicated calculations that we lose control. This in turn may lead to complicated disputes regarding the allowed threshold for accumulation of CO_2 in the atmosphere, where we tend to forget that any systematic accumulation is definitely non-sustainable. Secondly, the accumulation of CO_2 is but one of many molecules or elements that accumulate in nature due to the transformation of fossil fuels to dispersed waste. In this respect, the accumulation of CO_2 could be regarded as an indicator for a net increase of other types of waste such as metals like cadmium or lead, or sulphurous acid rain.

Society is influencing nature through an exchange of energy and matter. Matter is mined or drilled from the earth's crust and is delivered to the ecosphere. Molecules and compounds are produced in society – intentionally in production, as well as unintentionally in for instance sewage water or smoke from incineration processes – and delivered to the ecosphere. We are also physically *manipulating* natural systems through expansion of the technosphere and other interventions.

For example, natural ecosystems are replaced with monocultures to increase yield, but at a cost to resilience and biodiversity. Another example is the flows of copper from the earth's crust to the ecosphere from mining. It has increase five times since 1945, and is today 24 times larger than the corresponding natural flows. Production of new compounds has literally exploded In the present industrial society tens of thousands of chemicals are used regularly. There, for example, over 70,000 on the *US Toxic Substances Control Act* inventory. Many are produced in such volume that the limits of natural mechanisms by which they are turned into resources or stored away – are exceeded. This means that sedimentation processes, as well as biodegradation followed by re-entry into the cycles of nature, are exceeded leading to accumulation in the ecosphere.

Some of the substances accumulate directly in nature, some accumulate in society until they eventually leak out into nature. For example, heavy metals are leaking from the stockpiles of society. And they will continue to accumulate in nature even if we cease completely to mine them. The rate of manipulation and harvesting from ecosystems is also excessive. The global fish catch has for instance increased 4.5 times since 1950 while all 17 major fishing areas in the world have either reached or exceeded their natural limits.

Basic Science

Matter and energy cannot be created or destroyed (according to the first law of thermodynamics and the principle of matter conservation).

Matter and energy tend to disperse (according to the second law of thermodynamics). This means that sooner or later, all matter that is introduced into society will be released out into natural systems.

Material quality can be characterized by the concentration and structure of matter. We never consume matter – only its exergy, purity and structure.

Net increase in material quality on Earth can be produced only by sun-driven processes. According to the second law of thermodynamics, disorder increases in all closed systems. Consequently, an exergy flow from outside the ecosphere is needed to increase its order. The exergy flow from the sun is far greater than the exergy flows inherent in gravity in the solar system (creating, for instance, tidal flows) or the exergy flows from radioactive decay inside the Earth (creating geothermal heat).

Basic science and the precondition of our lives lead to the cyclic principle that waste must not systematically accumulate in nature, and that reconstitution of material quality must be at least as large as its dissipation. Consequently all matter must be processed in cycles, i.e., the societal metabolism must be integrated into the cycles of nature. From this four conditions for the maintenance of quality of the whole system can be deduced.

1. *Substances from the Earth's crust must not systematically increase in the ecosphere.* In practical terms this means, in relation to today's situation: radically decreased mining and use of fossil fuels.

2. *Substances produced by society must not systematically increase in the ecosphere.* In practical terms: Decreased production of natural substances that are systematically accumulating, and a phase-out of persistent unnatural substances.

3. *The physical basis for the productivity and diversity of nature must not be systematically diminished.* This means: our health and prosperity depend on the capacity of nature to re-concentrate and restructure wastes into resources.

4. *Fair and efficient uses of resources with respect to meeting human needs.* In a sustainable society, basic human needs must be met with the most resource-efficient methods possible, and their satisfaction must take precedence over provision of luxuries.

In practical terms this means: Increased technical and organizational efficiency throughout the whole world, including a more resource-efficient lifestyle particularly in the wealthy sectors of society. *Furthermore, it implies improved handling of population growth.* [Last emphasis is ours.]

W.K.

[SIDEBAR]
Yet the Official Prophet Drones On in Another Language

How different the Natural Step Analysis from the latest utterance of the official prophet Alan Greenspan, chairman of the US Federal Reserve (*The Globe and Mail*, 04/05, "Greenspan plays down oil 'frenzy'" by Barrie McKenna and Patrick Brethour"):

"'The Fed Chairman said he believes soaring [oil] prices have laid the foundation for their own decline, with the futures market now priced so that refiners and others have an incentive to buy oil and stockpile it. That will likely support increased inventories of crude oil,' Mr. Greenspan told the conference in San Antonio, Tex., over a satellite link. 'If sustained, these market technicals could encourage enough of an inventory buffer to damp the current price frenzy…. High prices will spur investment in new sources of supply.' Conversion of the vast Athabasca oil sands reserves in Alberta to productive capacity has been slow. But at current market prices they [and] coal bed methane gas deposits are becoming competitive as prices rise. The unconventional is increasingly becoming conventional.

"He also referred to potential energy sources in the future, 'perhaps a generation or more.' He said natural gas hydrates, which exist as ice-like structures on the sea floor, store 'immense quantities of methane.'"

These distant solutions to society's present apparent needs contradict the warning in the above document: "Matter is mined or drilled from the earth's crust and is delivered to the ecosphere. Molecules and compounds are produced in society and delivered to the ecosphere…. In a sustainable society, fossil fuels, metals and other minerals must not be extracted at a faster pace than their slow reposit and reintegration into the Earth's Crust" (page 31). In short what for Mr. Greenspan is a future solution, by scientific logic actually adds to the extent of the underlying problem.

William Krehm

Has our Finance Minister Finally Awakened to Something Important that We've Been Saying for 35 Years?

A NASTY SPAT has broken out between the federal and Ontario Liberal governments as reported in *The Globe and Mail* (26/02, "McGuinty's arithmetic doesn't add up, Goodale says" by Murray Campbell): "[Federal Finance Minister Ralph Goodale] dismissed the [Ontario] Premier's contention that there is a $23 billion gap between what Ontario taxpayers send to Ottawa and the money the province gets back in transfer payments. He said Mr. McGuinty is ignoring the benefits Ontario gets from a range of other federal schemes, such as those to the automobile industry or to encourage scientific information.

"'I find when dealing with almost all provinces…they only tend to measure what comes in a formal government-to-government transfer, the other things don't count,' Mr. Goodale told the editorial board of the *G&M*.

"Well, the other things do count when you add in the other ways the government of Canada either invests in or transfers money to people and projects in Ontario that doesn't happen to go through the Ontario budgeting system. Those other transfers are also very large and they are growing with time."

"The Finance Minister said he understands the financial pressures that Ontario and other provinces are under and why they demand more money from Ottawa. He noted, however, that federal transfers are at a historic high and that some of these transfers, particularly for health care, have built-in escalators that automatically increase the [payouts] to the provinces."

It is not very often that we have had occasion to congratulate our Finance Ministers. Mr. Goodale has earned our applause with these remarks, but only on a single condition: he must go on to generalize the shift of wealth between one level of government and another, that most definitely occurs when that government makes capital investments that indirectly benefit the production and the productivity in those other levels. But that is also what happens on an even larger scale when expenditures of all levels of government financed by taxation go to provide necessary infrastructures to the private sector itself. It matters less in which jurisdiction the physical capital assets in which such public investments are embodied end up. What is important is that they are made outside of market circuits in which there must always be a balancing of benefits received and cash payment received for them. In the case of human capital investment by governments of all levels the end result of such outlays end up in human brains and bodies. Nevertheless they are essential investment without which the private sector could not function.

Note well, our congratulation to Finance Minister Goodale have to do with his recognition of the circulation of cash-costing benefits amongst the various government levels rather than between the public and private sectors of the economy., but it is a doughty beginning, and we wish him well in pursuing it further. For some amazing revelations and rethinking of old, discredited nostrums passing for economic truths lie at the end of that rainbow.

William Krehm

Are General Motors and Ford Themselves on a Conveyor Belt?

GENERAL MOTORS is the last and greatest of the U's big auto three to have grown itself into serious financial difficulties. We are talking then of the likely bankruptcy of an industry that developed what was probably the defining feature of the US industrial age – Henry Ford's moving production lines that brought the product to the worker and thus determined the pace of his own breathing, and moving, and thus reduced him to an automaton. Today that industry is itself unable to keep up with growth dictated by another sector – speculative finance. The latter in its way is also a sort of a conveyor belt but one that speeds up at an exponential rate that is beyond the stamina of men, beasts, and the economy itself.

Nowhere is this more graphically illustrated than in the changing relations between General Motors Co. and General Electric Co. where financial growth rates have come to clash with paces possible in manufacturing and the financial sector. In their own different degrees of success, both these corporations, once great manufacturing companies, have transmuted into financial giants.

Thus *The Wall Street Journal* (23/03, "General Motors Loan Agreement with GE May Come to an Early End" by Kathryn Kranhold) sheds light on this crucial situation:

"General Motors Corp.'s recent financial troubles could bring to an early end a $2 billion loan-facility agreement with General Electric Co.'s commercial lending arm. The agreement which had been scheduled to end in December 2005, allows GM to pay its suppliers early. Under the program GE pays GM suppliers within days of the receipt of a bill. Then GM pays GE within the traditional 45-day or 60-day cycle. The supplier is typically paid at a discount.

"GE told GM in May 2004 that it would be ending the program, called 'trades payable,' in December 2005. But GE said that GM's recent setbacks triggered covenants in the contract that allow GE to accelerate the winding down of the facility before December.

"The GE spokesman, Stephen White, said, 'We've preserved these rights,' related to the loan covenant. 'We haven't made any decisions. We're still discussing.'

"GM said it would continue such a program through its own financing arm, GMAC Commercial Finance, and that it is ramping it up to do so now. Jerry Dubrowski, a GM spokesman, said the auto company has been seeking an alternative provider since GE said last year it was exiting the trade-payable business."

Teetering on the Edge of Junk Status

"The discussions follow GM's announcement last week that 2005 profits will fall short of previous expectations. The main reason is its deep losses in the North American auto business. Its credit rating is teetering on the edge of a downgrade to junk status. GM is seeking cuts from its employees as it works to shore up its auto business."

This gives us an intimate peek into the digestive organs of two originally manufacturing behemoths that have simply shifted species. One has become essentially a financial mega-corporation, and the other a still a manufacturer that has been compelled to develop a frail, financial facade.

But it was consumer credit, that helped create deceptive hopes of market expansion internationally, above all in the US. Eric Reguly, economic columnist of *The Globe and Mail* (16/04, "Is GM driving off the proverbial cliff? Don't bet against it"): "Could General Motors, the biggest auto maker, go bankrupt? Not readily, but not inconceivably either. This week as GM shares hit new lows, and GM debt faced a trip to the junk yard, another mighty motoring name, MG Rover Group went to the great rust yard in the sky. Rover, a century old, was once the third biggest car maker on the planet (when it was known as British Leyland). At its peak in the 1960s, it had 250,000 employees and produced 40% of the cars sold in the UK. Its marques included Triumph, Austin, Land Rover and Morris.

"It's been a slow motion car crash ever since. But as late as the 1960s, Rover's demise was unthinkable. That was because Rover had then come under the ownership of BMW which had ambitious plans to turn Rover into a mass-market non-luxury brand. Instead, the 'English patient' delivered $6 billion losses to BMW. The Germans gave up, although they kept the hot-selling Mini Cooper and sold the carcass for $15 to a venture capital group. Rover's UK market share promptly slipped to 3%. Now it's nil.

"GM's North American market share loss has been nearly as dramatic. It was about 44% in the early 1980s. By the late 1980s, as imports came on strong, it was about 35% (although still high enough to put the GM label on 1 in 5 cars made globally). Today its less than 25%. But that's not the main problem.

"GM pays more for health care – the equivalent of $1,525 per vehicle produced – than it does for steel. GM is the country's largest single private health care buyer. Don't think of it as a car maker; think of it as a life-support network for 1.1 million employees, retirees and their dependents. Last year, GM's health care bill was about $4.6 billion. It will be $1 billion higher this year. Now you know why GM, Ford and Daimler-Chrysler like building cars in Canada, where the taxpayer funds most of the health care costs."

Why Car Companies Love Building Cars in Canada

This is a detail that is hardly mentioned in the rasping political debates on our health care. They include part of the cost of keeping our industry at home and in reasonable shape.

"It gets worse. GM's contracts with the United Auto Workers give laid-off workers 95% of their base pay, plus benefits, for up to five years. The American investment strategist Gary Shilling says the combination of the extraordinarily high labour and health care costs, combined with an aggressive price strategy (rebates, zero money down, zero interest on auto loans) conspired to give GM a profit of only $290 per auto sold in North America last year. Toyota earned $2,000."

At this point the predictable comment of many would be "those greedy unions." But it is not so simple as that. Under Eisenhower the essence of managerial acumen was to settle with unionized labour by offering them a cut of the future in pension obligations instead of greater current wages. Current profits and executive options were determined by the current profits not by the long-term solvency of the firm. In short the whole economy was developing that forward list that extrapolated past rates of growth into the indefinite future, by courtesy of the self-balancing market. A more realistic appreciation of health and population trends would have identified what was unknown and unknowable in the future, while current wage increases provided current costs to the firm. *It would have provided a relationship between more eventual costs and the production cycle for which they were incurred.* Now not only the pensioners but the firms themselves are faced with the consequences of that executive irresponsibility. The government which is the lender of the last resort for distressed banks too big to be allowed to fail should have been the insurer of the first and last resort for the welfare of the population as a whole. Anything less is a gamble.

Reguly in fact terminates on this solemn note: "Chrysler almost went axles-up in 1980. It would have gone bankrupt were it not for emergency loan guarantees from the US government. GM's continued erosion is all but certain and a massive restructuring that may land it in the bankruptcy courts is not out of the question. GM's present plight is a crisis of the American financial system."

William Krehm

Let Us not See Ourselves Lapsing into Sainthood

LET US NOT LAPSE into the flattering belief that good advice and helpful examples flow only southward across our overburdened bridges to the United States. Much of what we have learned about the transgressions we have even encouraged our banks to undertake has come from regulators south of the border. Our own authorities seem to have been in utter somnolence, occasionally emitting nothing but a snore. It was from US authorities that we learned about the involvement of three of our major banks in the Enron trading partnership mess to the extent of being fined hundreds of millions of dollars, and this was a decade after our government had bailed them from their losses in the 1980s with an annual subsidy and then deregulated them to gamble with ever greater leverage at the expense of their clients and the government. That happened for no better reason than because it was argued that our government was not to be trusted to create the country's legal tender, but only the banks who had just been bailed out by that same government.

In the United States, in contrast, careers have been made by prosecutors exposing banking conglomerates' illegal activities. Indeed, the US has been described as the greatest laboratory on money creation in the world since colonial times. Only now when the involvement of most of our largest banks in some of the most malodorous scandals in the US has been disclosed by US investigators, has there been minute effort of the Canadian authorities to close the gap between the curiosity of investigative authorities in the US and those north of the border.

G.W. Bush, having pick-pocketed a second term, is not likely to encourage further zeal on the part of the Security and Exchange Commission. Thus *The Wall Street Journal* (20/12, "Bush's Donaldson Dilemma" by Deborah Solomon and John D. McKimmon) had this to say: "Now that President Bush has replaced most of his cabinet, he is expected to turn his attention to the chiefs of the various government agencies. Few decisions will be as tricky as deciding whether to keep William Donaldson as chairman of the Securities and Exchange Commission.

"Mr. Donaldson, a 73-year-old former Wall St. executive and long-time friend of the Bush family, has quietly let it be known in the White House that he would like to remain as the nation's top security cop. But the business lobby, fed up with what it believes is an overzealous SEC and a chairman that has been a tougher regulator than expected, has made it equally clear that it would like nothing better than to see Mr. Donaldson gone. Business believes its complaints about burdensome regulations are going unheeded. They are being forced to spend too much time and money trying to comply with a slew of new regulations under the 2002 *Sarbanes-Oxley Act*. They have also aimed at other SEC initiatives, including plans to give shareholders more power to nominate directors, register hedge fund advisers and require independent chairmen for mutual fund boards."

Mr. Donaldson, no matter what his private inclinations, has been feeling the hot breath of Eliot Spitzer, Attorney General of New York State. In contrast, it is only now that Canadian authorities seem to be stirring themselves to rain a bit on what has up to now been Bay Street's private party.

Angering some members of his own party, Mr. Donaldson has clashed repeatedly with his two fellow Republican commissioners and instead sided with the two Democrats to win 3-2 votes on some key matters.

And with such blasts blowing in from our neighbour, Ottawa and some of our provinces have finally come around to looking into the morality in the magic realm of high finance.

Until last September, improper insider trading wasn't even a criminal offence, while south of the border, disgraced CEOs were going to jail. Here, financial crooks are used to cutting deals with regulators and putting up with small fines that could be absorbed as a business expense.

In 2003, to rejig some trust in capital markets, the RCMP and the federal Justice Department, with the cooperation of provincial securities commissions, the Investment Dealers Association set up IMFET – the Integrated Market Investment Enforcement Team. Provincial regulators turn the biggest and worst cases over to them. What brokers do with margin accounts no authority seems to have the time of day for. The good Lord created small fish, it seems, to be fried.

The maximum penalty for fraud is now 14 years – close to what they dish out for murder. Unlike Spitzer, who can seek quick penalties in civil courts before he gets nasty with criminal indictments, Canadian enforcers have to deal with a ponderous system that requires more investigation before accusations can be made. IMFET's Toronto branch can currently handle about six or seven cases at a time.

In effect IMFET is our new national regulator of the worst offenders.

Spitzer in the US depends on his own staff, making his own decisions, sends a challenge to the SEC and other local authorities not to be left too far behind, without in any way being dependent on their cooperation. Handling six or seven cases at a time in Toronto where most of the skullduggery occurs is not reassuring. It means that big cases like Nortel are likely to get more of the attention. Modest margin accounts are likely to remain fair game for bank-controlled brokerages attempting to make up for the enormous fines incurred for their involvement with Enron and other large sinners.

Referring them to their private lawyers for justice as has been the case to date, is mockery. None of these small investors can afford to talk to a lawyer. A few well publicized convictions for abuse of margin account collateral, for example, would be helpful. And what is perfect legal practice today – hiring out the margin client's security to short his shares, should be ended. Not only does it victimize the client, but destabilizes the stock market. Banks and Brokers addicted to that should buy themselves a casino and surrender their brokerage licence.

The Globe and Mail (27/12, "Lawyers brace for rise in class-action lawsuits" by Beppi Crosariol") paints the prospect: "Dramatic amendments to Ontario's *Securities Act* due early in the new year are expected to spawn a wave of shareholder class action lawsuits – and a wave of business for law firms with burgeoning corporate governance practices.

Class Action Suits will be Coming to Canada

"The changes, aimed at helping to restore investor confidence in the wake of recent accounting scandals, will make it much easier for investors in the so-called secondary market to launch class action lawsuits against officers, directors, spokesperson and other key figures of public companies for issuing false or misleading statements, or for failing to promptly disclose information that could influence stock prices.

"That is very significant because the vast majority of stock transactions take place on the secondary market, says lawyer Ava Yaskiel, a partner of Ogilvy Renault LLB. It's going to be front and centre in the Ontario courts for years to come.

"Until now securities laws in Ontario and the rest of the country have provided remedies only to those investors who bought shares of companies on the basis of comprehensive disclosure documents, such as prospectuses, memorandums and takeover-bid circulars. Typically such shareholders buy into companies through initial offerings in what's known as the primary market.

"That will change, however, with the new law, commonly referred to as Bill 198, which has been given royal assent and is expected to be enacted in the first quarter of 2005.

"Under the new legislation, investors would be able to sue for two types of misconduct: a misrepresentation made in disclosure documents, and a failure to make timely disclosure of a material change. Any company issuing a press release that's amending or revoking a prior release is going to be in the bomb sights. That means more business for lawyers.

"The legislation is notable also for the broad scope of potential defendants it will expose to liability. Not only does it pertain to the company and its directors and officers, but also to investment fund managers, spokespersons, experts (such as accountants, lawyers, financial analysts and geologists) and so-called influential persons (such as stock promoters or majority shareholders with a significant influence on the company).

"To date, the only recourse for disgruntled investors who bought shares in the secondary market has been via common law, specifically by alleging fraud. But the barrier to establishing wrongdoing under common law has been much higher under the coming securities changes, 'says Matthew Fleming, a lawyer at Fraser Milner Casgrain LLB. Under common law, plaintiffs must prove that they relied on alleged misrepresentation when they bought or sold shares.

"'Such a requirement was often fatal to plaintiffs in securities class actions because the issue of whether each member of the proposed class relied upon the alleged misrepresentation was generally deemed to give rise to too many individual issues,' Mr. Fleming explains.

"In contrast, the *Securities Act* amendments make an automatic assumption that the plaintiff relied on the information. Mr. Fleming says changes similar to Ontario's are in the works in British Columbia. Beyond that, no secondary market liability provisions exist in Canada. The Ontario amendments mirror US laws dating back to the 1930s that have made class action suits there the subject of regular newspaper headlines.

"The US laws have been criticized for spawning a 'greenmail' phenomenon in which malicious lawsuits with little merit – known as strike suits – are launched in the hopes of extracting large settlements from deep-pocketed corporations. And sometimes the publicity around one suit will breed other gold-diggers. 'It's almost like a cockroach-type theory applied to class-action lawsuits. One is filed, and before the end of the day you can bet that a slew of others will follow,' says Richard Wertheim, a corporate governance partner at Wertheim & Co. Inc.

"Lawyers generally applaud the legislation for placing a cap on penalties, thereby guarding against a company's downfall in the wake of a shareholder lawsuit, as happened in the case of the infamous Texas energy trading giant Enron Corp. A company's liability would be limited to either 5% of its market capitalization or $1 million, whichever is greater. The penalty limits for individuals, meanwhile vary with that person's responsibility in the case. A spokesperson, for example, would be liable for up to $25,000 or 50% of the aggregate of the person's compensation from the company and its affiliates over the previous 12 months. The same would apply to a director or officer."

W.K.

The Fate of American Student Debtors in an Epoch of Low Interest Rates

AT THE END OF WORLD WAR II the US government looking ahead, sent many economists to Japan and Germany to predict how long it would take for those countries to make good the devastation of the war and emerge once again as formidable competitors on the export market. One of these, Theodore E. Schultz, of the University of Chicago, years later, in 1961, wrote: "Having had a small hand in this effort, I have had a special reason for wondering why the judgements that we formed soon after the war proved to be so far from the mark. The explanation that now is clear is that we gave altogether too much weight to non-human capital. We fell into this error, because we did not have a concept of *all* capital goods and therefore failed to take account of human capital and the important part it plays in production in a modern economy.

"We were taught to believe that a country which amassed more reproducible capital relative to its land and labor would employ such capital in greater 'depth' because of its growing abundance and cheapness. But apparently, on the contrary, the estimates now available show that less of such capital tends to be employed relative to income as economic growth proceeds…. For my purpose all that needs to be said is that these estimates of capital-income ratios refer to only a part of all capital. Human capital has surely been increasing at a rate substantially greater than reproducible (non-human) capital. We cannot, therefore, infer from these estimates that the stock of *all* capital has been decreasing relative to income." The income of the US

has been increasing at a much higher rate than the combined amount of land, man-hours worked and the stock of reproducible capital used to produce the income. Moreover, the discrepancy between the two rates has become larger from one business cycle to the next in recent decades.

"To call this discrepancy a 'measure of resource productivity' gives a name to our ignorance, but does not dispel it."

In quoting these passages from Schultz in *Human Capital* (Columbia University Press, 1971, p. 51 et seq.) in my *Price in a Mixed Economy – Our Record of Disaster,* Toronto, 1975, I added: "Not only is education capital, but it is the most dynamic of all capital categories, endlessly revolutionary in its effect. The typical capital accumulation of earlier generations – railways, factories, machines – served as a repository for society's inertia; its growth gave rise to spreading ranks of bondholders, rentiers, and passive stockholders. Over long periods its increase seemed to blunt the economy's hunger for more capital – to hold back technical innovation at times. Capital placed in education has quite the opposite effect. It speeds the rhythms of change, shrinks write-off schedules, hastens obsolescence. It consigns to the scrap heap those solid tangible investments: factories and machines, which had been regarded as provident investments par excellence.

"Nor does the misrepresentation stop there. If education must be considered an investment, then health and welfare of those in whom that investment is stored cannot be less important."

What Governments Forget in their Debt Collection Fervour

All this seems to have been forgotten, from the evidence of *The Wall Street Journal* (6/01/05, "US Gets Tough on Failure to Repay Student Loans" by John Hechinger): "In dealing with material investments of the public sector, our government were so carefree that until recently (01/01, 1996 in the US), when it recognized them as 'savings' in their statistics. Yet 'savings' they certainly were not, they were not in the cash form this implied. Canada, though it has agreed under pressure from the previous Auditor General to recognize physical investments of the federal government as capital, has still done little to revise its books accordingly. Human capital is still ignored even in principle. But when it comes to a student loan not being repaid – at times for good enough reason – the state in either country would seem deaf, dumb, and unrelenting."

There is not among investments in the private sector any known guarantee against investments going sour for quite irreproachable reasons. That is why the institution of protection against bankruptcy was devised. But Mr. Hechinger writes: "Years after a political outcry over high levels of student loan defaults, the Education Department has become one of the toughest debt collectors around. A 1998 change in federal law, for instance, made it extremely difficult for people to escape student loans through personal bankruptcy. The Education Department also can now seize parts of borrowers' paychecks, tax refunds and Social Security payments without a court order, a power that only the Internal Revenue Service, among federal agencies, regularly wields. Access to a government database of the newly employed has enabled the department to make much more effective use of private collection companies. And there is no statute of limitations on student loans, unlike most consumer debts. It can go after even decades-old student loans. For current loans that go into default, the department now projects it will ultimately retrieve every dollar of principal, plus almost 20% in fees and interest, a prediction few private lenders would be bold enough to make.

"'Student-loan debt collectors have power that would make a mobster envious,' says Elizabeth Warren, a Harvard Law School professor and bankruptcy specialist." The *WSJ* cites some specific instances of how this translates into social justice or even economic sense:

"The bill collector called when Clay Stanley, gaunt and suffering from AIDS, lay bedridden in his apartment, back from the hospital after a bout with a viral infection. The call concerned a matter that Mr. Stanley had long forgotten – student loans he took out two decades before. The private collection agency, acting on behalf of the US Department of Education, said Mr. Stanley must pay $69 a month or the government would take a larger sum than that each month from his Social Security disability check. Mr. Stanley says, 'I didn't know what to do, so I said, "OK,"' he says.

"The government's toughness traces back to the 1980s, when politicians became alarmed by high levels of student-loan defaults. Some [also] waged a campaign against deadbeat doctors, lawyers, and other professionals taking advantage of the government. Today the default rate on recently made loans is way down. It was 5.2% last year, down from 22% in 1990. Graduates of four-year or graduate programs at private universities default at a 3.1% rate, while students at trade schools and community colleges default at 5.2% overall rate. Studies show that those most likely not to repay, didn't complete their studies.

"Though the US government makes some of the loans directly, most are made by private lenders such as banks, with the government guaranteeing payment. The guarantees plus federal interest-rate subsidies let lenders offer low rates despite students' scant credit history. The rate on new student loans, set annually and tied to Treasury bills, is now 3.37%. Repayment term is usually 10 years, and repayment must begin six months after graduation. If no payments are made for 270 days, loans are in default. Then the state agencies – which both administer the loans and offer lenders an initial guarantee – will try to collect. If they can't, they will they will kick the loans back to the Education Department. The department has a stable of collection firms it uses. Under federal law, the collectors are entitled to 20% of what they recover. These fees are added to borrowers' loan balances."

A National Directory for the Newly Employed as a Debt-collecting Tool

"Four years ago, the collectors started using a national directory of the newly employed compiled from employers; filings with state employment divisions. That has helped in tracking down defaulted student-loan debt, which now totals $30 billion.

"In 1998, largely unnoticed, the federal law governing the

loans was changed so borrowers could shed them in bankruptcy only by proving it was an 'undue hardship' to repay. Student loans thus joined a rarified class of obligations, such as child support and restitution in criminal cases, that can almost never be shirked. It is a very hard test to meet, as cases such as Carol Ann Race's show.

"In the 1980s, Ms. Race borrowed $20,000 to study theology and philosophy at the University of St. Thomas in St. Paul, Minn., and another school. Now 42, she has five children, aged four through 11. Two are autistic. Her husband earns $18,000 a year as nursing-home aide. The family lives in Bertha, Minn. on $28,000 a year, including government disability payments to the autistic children.... Mrs. Race says she made $300 monthly payments on her student loans for 2 $1/2$ years before she lost her job as a religious educator in a church in 1994.

"She filed for bankruptcy in hopes of getting the loans – the family's only debt – canceled. A year ago, US Bankruptcy Court Judge Dennis O'Brien ruled against her. In an interview, the judge says he wanted to let her out of the loans but was sure he would be reversed on appeal. His opinion said that because of higher court rulings, he couldn't cancel her student loans unless he found that repayment would 'strip Race or her family of all that makes life worth living.'

"The language of the higher court in this matter is in itself a subject for wonder. For example the survival of Negroes in the Americas is itself evidence that slavery did not meet such demanding specifications, otherwise there would have been mass suicides among the slaves and no progeny.

"At the end of her case, Ms. Race owed $34,000 at 7% interest. Pursued by two state agencies that made the initial guarantees, she has signed up for a repayment program with a 5.125% rate; the payments will be linked to family income. She says she will be paying the debt for decades, making it difficult to set aside money to care for her children.

"In the mid-1990s. abuses cited by lawmakers were infrequent. 'More perception than reality.'

"But not long after, in 1998, Congress tightened the bankruptcy treatment of student loans. The changes resulted from wrangling over an education bill, says Henry Sommer, editor-in-chief of *Collier on Bankruptcy*, a legal reference work. The Clinton administration was seeking a reduction in student-loan interest rates, a move lenders opposed. The administration agreed to provide a subsidy to cushion the rate cut for them. At the same time, the government changed the treatment of student loans in bankruptcy, which would mean smaller losses for the Education Department and taxpayers.

"A trouble with the politics of compromise is there rarely room or insight left for the deeper perceptions of social-minded thinkers, who may have been honored for their highly esteemed work, but have no presence when the 'political center' gets patched together by politicians and financiers.

"That leaves borrowers like Jonathan Gerhardt, 46, little choice but to pay. He is a cellist. The child of two classical musicians in Columbus, Ohio, he studied at the New England Conservatory of Music, performed with two city Orchestras and finally won a spot as principal cellist of the Louisiana Philharmonic Orchestra in New Orleans. Despite climbing this high in the field, he was earning just $20,000 a year three years ago, including pay for teaching cello at Tulane University. He buckled under his $100,000 in student loans and filed for bankruptcy.

"Lawyers for the Education Department and a guarantee agency that held some of the loans sought to make him pay. The opinion of a bankruptcy court in New Orleans says Mr. Gerhardt could trim his expenses, such as $23.90 for Internet access and $48.51 for a gym membership. They also suggested he get rid of his cat to save $20 a month."

Politics of Compromise Leave Little Room for Social Sensitivities

"Bankruptcy Judge Jerry A. Brown, however, said Mr. Gerhardt had to work out to relieve back pain from playing the cello, and needed the Internet to look for extra work. 'Expenses related to his cat are not luxuries, considering he is single and lives alone,' the judge wrote. He ruled that repaying the loans would be an 'an undue hardship' and expunged it.

"The Education Department appealed. A federal appellate court sided with the government. It suggested Mr. Gerhardt find a job as a music-store clerk!"

That sure put the muses in their places.

"Mr. Gerhardt says he is already working 60 hours a week including rehearsals for the Louisiana Philharmonic, practising and teaching. He recently moved into an apartment with a roommate, saving $50 a month in rent. He says he stopped taking annual trips to Ohio to visit his 51-year-old mother, and doesn't believe he will ever be able to support a family or afford a house. Mr. Gerhardt is now paying $200 a month towards his loan. The government wants $900."

The great insights of Theodore Schultz have been buried not by gentle shelf-dust, but by dirt and rubble loaded as though by an earth-mover. Capital budgeting even when brought in on physical investments of government under President Clinton were sedulously hidden not to upset Wall St. But even Schultz's perceptions on the unique productivity of human capital, failed to raise the importance of its cultural heritage to a society's functioning. And that, however, was very evident in the cases of Germany and Japan – the two countries whose postwar resilience Theodore Schultz studied. Hopefully our great neighbour, so intent on recasting the world in its image, will awaken to the importance of the leading members of the orchestras of a significant city passing on the genes of their talents to future generations, and even affording to keep a cat.

William Krehm

Why Canada Needs a Royal Commission on Monetary Policy

IT ALL HAPPENED so suddenly. The miracle of growth and increased efficiency was winning all hands down, when, like a clogged plumbing line, it all started backing up. The smelly stuff that has deluged our federal politics, as the crescendoing investigations headed by New York State Attorney General Eliot Spitzer move from one exalted business sphere to the next higher up, expose ever greater corruption. In these investigations several of Canada's largest banks have been convicted and fined. For the first time Canadians caught a glimpse of how our banks were using their bailout entitlement money. Scarcely the stuff that makes you want to throw out your chest and sing *O Canada!*

And closely intertwined with this – although those in the media and government make a point of missing the link – comes the down-grading to junk and near junk status of the debt of several of the largest icon corporations that had framed the American dream. *The Wall Street Journal* (13/05, "Hunting the Nearly Extinct 'AAA'" by Mark Whitehouse) remarks: "General Motors Corp. used to be one of the companies with a top rating. So did Ford Motor Co. and American International Group Inc. But over the years, the elite of American business, the triple A-rated company, has become an endangered species. Its disappearance has brought sorrow to borrowers and investors alike. Companies with lower credit ratings pay more – in the form of higher yields – to raise money in the bond market. And while bondholders surely appreciate the yield bump, they also lose principal when the price of a downgraded company's bonds fall.

"Indeed, bondholders of all stripes suffered after Standard & Poor's moved to demote General Motors and Ford to below-investment grade status, ultimately dumping about $85 billion of the auto makers' debt into the high yield or junk, market. These downgrades have caused investors to reassess their appetite for all risk. The proof: junk bonds are paying yields a percentage point higher than they were only a month ago. And the cost of insuring against corporate defaults has risen sharply in the credit derivatives market, where investors parcel and trade risk.

"Only six US non-financial companies now sport a triple-A debt rating from S&P – among them General Electric Co. and United Parcel Service Inc. – compared with 12 in 1980. In the same period, the tally of banks, utilities and industrial companies enjoying a Moody's top rating has fallen to six from 58. (Some blue-chip companies such as Microsoft Corp. – don't issue bonds and therefore have no ratings.)

"Companies appear to fall from grace faster than in the past. In addition to current concerns about credit quality, this likely reflects the tougher views the rating companies have taken since they were criticized for failing to anticipate Enron Corp.'s bankruptcy. Moody's downgraded a record 652 ratings in 2002, almost five for every upgrade. S&P's downgrades peaked in 2001 at 771, or about 5.5 for every upgrade.

"In the larger context of US economic history, the dwindling list of triple A's reflects a tectonic shift in priorities. 'As the US lost its dominant position in the world economy, competitive pressures forced companies to assume more risk,' says John Lonsky, chief economist at Moody's. You can't grow without risk.'

"For many established companies, the decision to borrow more money made sense. Because interest payments are deducted from taxable income, debt is usually the cheapest way to finance growth. But more debt means lower credit ratings.

"Coca Cola Co., for example, lost its triple-A rating from S&P in July 1986 when it took on debt to create a new bottling network. Although the move was bad for the company's rating S&P's Mr. Nicholas Riccio believes it was better for the business. 'They chose to do that to enhance value for shareholders,' yet the move weighed on bondholders. Coke is now rated single-A plus, four notches below triple A."

In the same issue of *The Wall Street Journal* ("Hedge Funds Amass Clout in Public Firms, Then Demand Management Boost Share Price" by Henry Sender) introduces another factor in this down-grading of what Americans were once most proud of.

"A Boston-based hedge fund that has a 6.2 % stake in OfficeMax Inc recently demanded that the office-products retailer improve its stock price. The $1.1 billion fund called K Capital Partners PLC, didn't stop there. It then called upon CEO George Harad to give up certain pay and pension benefits, put forth in the name of a potential board member and hired Blackstone Group to examine strategic options to boost the value of the stock. OfficeMax – one of several companies that have come under attack from hedge funds over performance issues – agreed to appoint an additional independent member of the board.

"Such calls to boost performance have become a rallying cry for hedge funds that have taken increasingly large positions in public companies and then demanded management work harder to increase shareholder value. Just this week financier Carl Icahn with a stake in Blockbuster Inc., won a seat on video-rental chain's board. And Mr. Icahn, supported by hedge funds, is now demanding that management curb spending and boost the dividend to get Blockbuster's share price up.

"'A number of hedge funds have become the corporate activists of this generation,' says Alan Jones, managing director and head of global corporate finance at Morgan Stanley. 'They are increasingly agitating for change even to the extent of putting companies into play.'"

In this way, note well, they are the complement of the Merger and Acquisition (M&A) departments of our deregulated banks. For when share prices go up, so does the value of the corporation, and then there is a large bonus to be earned by the hedge fund shooting with maximum leverage made possible by derivatives. "It is a high-stakes game and one that the hedge funds didn't play in the past." It is one of the fruits of dismantling of the firewalls that the Roosevelt administration had set up to separate the four pillars of the financial sector: banks, the stock market, mortgage lenders, and insurance. Each of these has its own liquid capital pool to meet the obligations of its particular industry. And derivatives can raise the financial multiplier especially of the banks to a higher order. With derivatives you don't waste your time and resources raising roses. Instead you deal only with the merest fragrance of the rose, and leave the hard work to the clods. You acquire not the entire security, but an abstracted feature of it – the increase – or fall – in its yield, or in the exchange value of the currency it is denominated in. You can swap these, as exchanging the dividend or interest paid by one share of stock for that of a bond, or you can acquire an option to do anything you wish with these – like acquire an option to do such a swap (a "swaption").

A Swaption to Cook your Books

Since many classes of derivatives are not regulated, they can be kept off the company books, and indeed conducted in offshore havens. The result: instead of the single bank multiplier creating money by lending out many time the cash it retains in its vaults and with the central bank, you have a many-storeyed structure with a rising composite multiplier at each successive storey. These are determined by the compounding by bank or other multipliers of the successive capital pools tapped through merger and acquisitions. That is why the banks up to very recently resisted tooth and nail the regulation of such derivatives that are still unregulated, i.e., beyond control or even the ken of any regulator. That makes them an easy way of keeping skullduggery off a firm's balance sheet – as in the notorious partnerships of Enron in which three of Canada's topmost banks were involved up to their eyebrows.

Only recently have the Canadian bank executives suddenly switched to arguing for the complete regulation of derivatives. That suggests that they are alarmed by the pyramided inflation of assets off and on their balance sheets. In the words of the CEO of the TD Bank because unregulated derivatives are a notorious way of banks unloading their bad debt syndicated for aesthetic effect onto innocent investors. It could be disastrous, he said, and potentially bad for the banks' reputation.

Meanwhile on the strength of this dynamic of M&A and G&D (Globalization and Deregulation), the pattern of growth has done wondrously well, thank you. In Canada the ratio of bank assets to the legal tender in the banks' possession that was 11 to 1 in 1946 is now not too far from 400 to 1. And all public firms are under the compulsion to extrapolate the rate of growth already attained – in fact or fiction – into the remotest future and then, discounted at a modest rate for their current value, incorporated into current share prices. It works wonders for achieving the strike price of high executives' options – the level at which executives can cash in their options at a good profit. Yet like all deals with the devil, it does have its price. For once these highly putative valuations experience a single shortfall, the whole house of cards flattens. And then adios options, princely life styles, new expensive wives! So inviting accountants and auditors into the game becomes a necessity.

It is not difficult plotting the course of M&A that weds the multipliers of banking to the consolidated pools of liquid capital of the non-banking factors that the great Roosevelt banking reform of 1935 separated with fire walls. One by one as the firewalls have been razed, those corporations have been acquired by banks and their liquid capital pools tapped – right to the mighty re-insurance companies that are very guardians of the over-advertised "risk management" at our outermost gates. We can imagine the uproar in the software design department in the afterworld where new entrants are assigned to the glowing depths or the heavenly rewards, trying to sort out who goes where.

And yet it has not occurred even to Mr. Eliot Spitzer that there is something systemic to the all-engulfing disparity between rewards to average toilers and those to high executives – something to be reckoned in digits rather than in mere unit counts. If there were so sensational a spread of petty crime in a given area, sociologists would long ago have been brought in to study the systemic causes. However, the major crime, and the corruption of corporation auditors have been treated to date as free-standing turpitude.

Surely in Canada the time has come for a Royal Commission to enquire into the state of economic theory and policy-making over the past three decades. The Globalization and Deregulation that has for too long had a virtual monopoly of the academic media and policy field. Our universities have long since been cleared of the last dissenting economic staff. Many of them hold their noses as they teach what they have long ceased to believe in. There are grades of heroism, and not every academic with a family to support dare speak his full mind at risk to his livelihood. Yet administrative muscle alone is helpless to prevent the cave-in of anti-social policy over the longer run. That point is driven home by the sudden sell-off of our booming stock market currently under way.

And into this over-stressed situation the hedge funds barge, determined to extract the quick super-profits to which they are committed and that the fatigued stock market denies them…. For the purpose they have mustered their ancestral powers of turning black into white, liabilities into assets, and back again. If we wish to get this witchery under control, we must track it to its beginnings. For from the tiny acorn comes the mighty oak. And where do we find that in finance? Why, in brokers' humble margin accounts, where the client's security is put up as collateral with the broker for the money still owed for its purchase. Not only does the broker charge the client interest for the unpaid portion – fair enough – but rents our that security for good money to a third party who wants to short the stock and has to find shares to sell. That systemic windfall – second or third profit the broker has scored from the client – the broker keeps. And the proceeding is against the client's interest. The victim-client is not even informed of its existence. Obviously that innocent sport contributes vastly to the volatility of the market in vulnerable moments.

A Talent for Picking their Clients' Pockets

So bountiful a combination of talent and opportunity for picking a client's pockets could not know not where to stop. But to complaints of the client the OSC has had a single answer – "Retain a lawyer." The fact is that most margin account clients cannot afford to talk to a lawyer let alone retain them to sue a bank. That fertilizes the acorns in the stock market to grow into oaks and they keep right on growing to get into heaven their own way.

During the Depression of the 1930s and after WWII, when there was still a far greater opportunity for dissident ideas in and out of legislatures, Royal Commissions were a staple means of assembling information on all sides of crucial problems. Similar parliamentary enquiries guaranteed an adequate availability of the various sides of important policy problems. Those in the UK are still classic sources of what money is about, and even Karl Marx dipped into them for his evidence. Never were they more than necessary than in the matter of monetary and economic policy today. The demand for such should be a key issue in the common election campaign. The commitment to call for a Royal Commission to examine the state of economic theory as it affects economic and monetary policy must be demanded of all political parties. Those that evade such a commitment clearly have far more to conceal than the sponsorship scandals that have hogged our think-space.

William Krehm

Why the EU is Striking Out

THERE IS AN INTIMACY between the political-juridical system and the currency that has always been. imperfectly recognized. And yet ignoring that relationship can only be an invitation to disaster.

There was a time when in theory money was seen as a commodity that actually embodied the value that it was chosen to represent – whether gold or silver. But even then there was not nearly enough of the favoured metal around to serve the purpose – especially in times of dynamic development it required the power and credibility of the state for what was partly fiction to prevail. But it is a long time since even the pretence of the currency containing the worth that it represented was abandoned (in the UK this happened with gold in 1931; in the US in the early 1970s). What remained to back currencies was the credibility of the state. The currency itself had become token money.

And that is why there was something basically wrong-headed about the sequence chosen by the Europeans seeking to bridge and bury the bloody historical rivalries on their continent. Unfortunately this ambitious political idealism for unifying Europe coincided with a most unidealistic suppression of all that had been learned about money and banking in recent years. The Great Depression of the 1930s and through it World War II had been ushered in by the excesses of an unbridled banking system. The Roosevelt regime had imposed severe limitations on the amount of credit banks could create, and the uses they could make of it. Banks were severely limited to banking, and specifically could not invest the credit they created in the other "financial pillars" – the stock market, insurance, and real estate financing. All these industries required their own liquid capital pools, and allowing banks to preempt them in their search for greater profit, escalated the risks that banking of any sort involved.

One by one these safeguards were removed, so that rather than the two main policy tools for avoiding inflationary excess – controlling the volume of credit banks could produce by requiring they redeposit a portion of the deposits entrusted to them by the public; and the ability of the central bank to raise or lower the benchmark interest rates at which banks lend each other overnight loans. This implied so great a redistribution of the national wealth as to represent a power shift. These statutory reserves had provided governments with access to financing by their central banks at a near-zero interest rate and the former now became dependent on financing by the commercial banks. Moreover the Bank for International Settlements, had declared the debt of developed countries risk-free and hence requiring no additional capital for banks to acquire.

But all this the European Union forgot about. Worse yet, both Germany and France had after the two world wars seen their currencies wiped out or almost wiped out. That made them particularly vulnerable to highly promoted notions that "inflation" – identified with all higher prices – was the chief, indeed, the only enemy to be held in check. What was suppressed was that in a pluralistic society prices may move up not only because of an excess of aggregate demand over supply, but because of the vast infrastructural investments by government made necessary, by the jump in inactive over active population due to the baby boom, countless technological revolutions, urbanization, mass migrations. These had to increase the layer of taxation to finance the growth of essential public investment within the total production rather than an imbalance between aggregate supply and demand. Elsewhere in this issue, we have dealt with the resistance to the introduction of accrual accountancy in the government books that would write of such investments over their useful life rather than entirely in the year in which they were made. This issue of ours, though not planned as such, might have been put together to prepare the reader for grasping the essence of the EU crisis. The extent to which the European leaders, particularly those of their central bank, seem unaware of these factors, is incredible.

The main villain of the piece is the foible of grand planners to assume that they can ride to their idealistic goal bareback on the single variable of their model in a world growing more complex in uncountable dimensions. Economists do away with all other factors by calling them "externalities," and suppressing any questioning of this orthodoxy. No better formula could be devised for nasty surprises. The plight of the EU is but one of these in store.

There is to begin with the intimate relationship between the credibility of the political system and the currency already mentioned. With the exception of the British pound, this is attested by what you can read on the US dollar, the Canadian dollar, or the Euro. You will find on these bills not the promise to pay the whatever the value of the currency note might be, but the statement of identification: "five dollars" or "five euros." It is the currency, the end of the legal tender line, acceptable for the payment of taxation by the government whose credit is its sole backing.

Government Credibility Alone Backs Currency

On the other hand a clear understanding that it is the credibility of government that is eventually the only monetary standard, might cause governments to pause in what responsibility and political gambles they undertake. Globalization and Deregulation is an enticing formula for deregulated financing concerns that have incorporated the rates of growth extrapolated into the indefinite future and then discounted for present value incorporated into today's stock price. But this entire system like an executioner, has been left with one "one blunt tool" to achieve what is taken to be its major task – "to fight inflation." But interest itself is the nuclear income of money-lenders, a sub-class of entrepreneurs that has been known to become sufficiently parasitic to be proscribed by three major religions. Obviously declaring interest the sold blunt tool for keeping the economy justly balanced could not but be a provocation to Islam, which the Lord undoubtedly for a credible enough reason, placed in charge of much of the gas and oil that the United States and Europe seem to find essential to their indispensable growth.

The countries of Europe have their specific cultures, that they and the world as a whole have valued high. The credibility of a nation – and hence of its currency – will in the long run be judged to no small extent by how it has taken care of this irreplaceable inheritance – provided by nature and that developed by its forebears. The quotation of its currency is a lesser matter of tactics related primarily to its balance of payments.

But we are not at the end of the "externalities" that have returned to haunt the EU in the loss of the French and Dutch votes on the acceptance of the European Constitution.

The European Central Bank (ECB) does have statutory reserves that banks must leave with the ECB. *But on these the ECB pays interest unlike most other central banks where statutory reserves must be deposited by the banks with the central banks to back their loans without earning interest.*

We hear a great deal about the deficits run up by the leading members of the EU – France, Germany and Italy, in excess of the 3% maximum of their budget. What we do not hear of is that if they simply discontinued the interest paid by the ECB on the statutory reserves deposited with them by the banks and gave the member government the near-free use of those reserves – as is done where such reserves exist outside Europe, those deficits would substantially disappear.

The Outspoken Militancy of the ECB

But these significant silences are matched with a particularly uncompromising outspokenness of the officialdom of the ECB. *The Wall Street Journal* (03/06, "Doubts Swirl About EU Future" by G. Thomas Sims) informs us: "ECB President Jean-Claude Trichet, a Frenchman and self-proclaimed 'militant' of a closely bound European Union, called the current turmoil over Europe's future an exceptional moment. 'I would say it does only one thing: it reinforces our sentiment of responsibility. Structural change by reluctant Europeans – such as loosening job-protection laws or decreasing non-wage labor costs – is the medicine the economy needs,' he said, 'especially to reduce unemployment that is producing unrest. In countries with structural reforms, we don't have mass unemployment.'"

There are substantial differences in the rates of unemployment and growth amongst the members of the EU. Clearly different benchmark interest rates – they are rarely used in overnight borrowing from the central bank itself but determine to a large extent the entire structure of interest rates in the given country. The point was raised in Canada by COMER in an article in its May 1989 issue by Harold Chorney, of Concordia, to deal with the diversity of unemployment figures at the time of 4.6% in Toronto and 12.8 in Saint John's, NF. It is significant that what our government and central bank did not give the time of day to 16 years ago in Canada should be cropping up as a major source of trouble in the EU 16 years later.[1]

"The ECB is trying to steer the economy of a region in which the four largest nations – Germany, France, Italy, and Spain – are growing at vastly different speeds. The ECB's key-term rate for the 12 nations that use the euro is 2%. Peter Dixon, economist at Commerzbank in London, reckons that Italy could use interest rates closer to Zero and France and Germany 1.5% or 1% Booming Spain, meanwhile, might be better off with a rate of 3%." It is important to note that these are little more than benchmarks since for a commercial bank to apply for a loan to the central bank would be a serious mark against it. The benchmark rate determines the considerable higher rates that is actually paid for overnight borrowing by one bank from another. The persistent use of the benchmark rate without further explanation of its theoretical nature is a self-dealing habit of bankers in such discussions.

It will be hard resolving the EU crisis without raising some basic questions of money creation.

In Germany, which wants lower rates to help boost economic growth, a poll published yesterday in Stern magazine said 56% of Germans wanted to ditch the euro to have their German marks back. Wolfgang Clement, the economics minister, in a speech yesterday said, "The European-wide common interest-rate level doesn't honor sufficiently Germany's contribution to Europe's stability.

"Meanwhile, some countries are rejoicing that they agreed to stay out of the euro. Britain is benefiting 'enormously' because the Bank of England still can set interest rates, said Michael Saunders, economist with Citigroup in London, point to UK's economic growth rates well above the euro-zone average.

"By late Thursday evening in Europe, the euro had recovered slightly to $1.2277; at 4 p.m. in New York it stood at $1.2277. It is still down about 10% from its high at the end of last year and is down about three cents from $1.2574 before the French and Dutch referenda."

The *WSJ* (31/05, "French 'No' Highlights EU Troubles" by Marc Champion, Dan Bilefsky, John Carreyron): "The loss of a pan-EU foreign minister also would be a serious setback. After the divisions [over] the US-led war in Iraq, the EU has been trying hard to play a more effective role in security affairs. France, Britain, and Germany, for example, have been conducting negotiations with Iran aimed at persuading the regime there to abandon a nuclear-fuel production program that could be used to make weapons.

"'This was not just about France, or about this constitutional treaty,' said Simon Serfaty, Europe specialist at the Center for Strategic and International Studies in Washington, DC. 'France is just one piece of the whole political and institutional disarray in Europe and for global security.'"

That is still underestimating the problem as the bill is being presented for several decades of suppression of the freedom of discussion on basic economic matters.

Willam Krehm

1. The Chorney article can be found on page 9 of *Meltdown: Money, Debt and the Wealth of Nations: As Documented in the First Decade of Economic Reform.*

THE WINDSOR STAR, THURSDAY, MAY 12, 2005

Opinion

GOVERNMENTS put bank profits over tax savings. Less than 4% of money supply is non-interest-bearing credit.

Letter writer André Marentette correctly referred to the *Bank of Canada Act* provisions for loans from the bank to provincial governments, which could be almost interest-free. He is also aware that municipalities, as wards of the provincial governments, could also access such loans.

In fact, when the act was originally passed, supplementary legislation provided specially for loans to municipalities.

What he does not address is why governments of all political stripes have not made use of this source of funds. When I raised this point with the leader of one of the national parties, I was told that "it would be inflationary." I refrained from pounding the table in frustration at this mindless parroting of the line given out by the chartered banks whenever Bank of Canada financing of government debt is raised.

Nor did I wait for the inevitable corollary example of Germany in the 1920s, but patiently explained that it is not who created the nation's credit, but how much is created, that determines whether the effect is inflationary or deflationary. If the government borrowed from its own bank, the Bank of Canada,

instead of from the private banking system, there would be no difference in the total credit created. Therefore, no inflation. The only significant difference would be who receives the benefit of the interest charged – bank shareholders or Canadian taxpayers.

Mr. Marentette got it right. Governments for the last 30 years have been more concerned with the profits of the banks than with the pockets of the taxpayers. Need we ask why? Today, less than four per cent of the Canadian money supply is publicly created, non-interest bearing credit.

On every other dollar, a rental fee is being paid to one of the chartered banks. When will we hear a government calling for, say, 20% in 2020? They could begin by borrowing, when needed, from our own bank. If there were two gas stations in your town and you owned one of them, which would you get your gas at?

Prof. Gordon Coggins
Brock University (retired), Windsor

REVIEW OF A BOOK BY JOHN PERKINS, SAN FRANCISCO, BERRETT AND KOEHLER PUBLISHERS

"Confessions of an Economic Hit Man"

THE AUTHOR spent most of his working life employed by MAIN (Chas T. Main Inc.), a firm which did consulting work for the World Bank and private US banks and corporations. His task was to investigate a target country, assess its potential for development, its capacity to utilize foreign investment, and to prepare a report incorporating recommendations for lending. His real task was "to convince third world countries to accept enormous loans for infrastructure development – loads much larger than necessary – and to guarantee that the development projects were contracted to US corporations like Halliburton and Bechtel. Once these countries were saddled with huge debts, the US government, and the international agencies allied with it, were able to control these economies and ensure that aid and other resources were channelled to...building a global empire" (p. 248).

Perkins' basic thesis will surprise no one who is familiar with the growing body of literature on the World Bank and the IMF, notably Stiglitz's *Globalization and Its Discontents*. However, Perkins details how the system operated on the ground. This book is the smoking gun.

The scenario is as follows. The foreign "consultants" work with the local and usually corrupt business and political elite. These individuals stand to benefit by siphoning off some of the loans – and often sending the funds offshore. They will also profit from the "development." Export firms, for example, will benefit from better roads, harbours, and power systems. These companies will cream off the gains. and the working population will be left with the unrepayable debt plus interest. and with the cuts in social spending forced by repayment. If leaders are too honest and refuse to accept this mode of development, they can be coerced or eliminated (Arbenz, Mossadegh, Torrijos – the list is long). In Indonesia, after Sukarno had been replaced by Suharto, Perkins was told to "develop this master plan...make sure that the oil industry (foreign owned) gets whatever it needs...for the duration of this plan." In Ecuador the ruling elite "saddled their country with huge debts borrowed from international banks on the promise of future oil revenues." Huge construction contracts were awarded to US firms. Oil lands were expropriated from the Indians. But resistance developed and an honest politician, Jaime Roldos, was elected president. He insisted on national control of oil to serve national interests, and expelled one of the US agencies from the country. Soon after he died (like President Torrijos of Panama) in a helicopter crash.

This is not an easy book to read. It is poorly written and poorly organized. The author is overly preoccupied with his personal story, and the book is padded with too much general material which is not well integrated with his new information. Nevertheless this is an important book. It is unfortunate that it has made so little impression to date.

David Gracey

The Crazy World that Central Banking has Become

THE TASKS OF CENTRAL BANKING have always been a bit vague and often incompatible. The Bank of England, for example, was set up by a group of English carpet-baggers who learned the tricks of the trade from the camp followers of William of Orange. Married into the English throne, he used his position to reward his Dutch cronies and their English accomplices by giving them a charter to issue paper money out of the void and then lend it once again to the monarch to finance his continental wars. And since that was a brilliant business it went far towards assuring there would be few dull spells of peace. Yet banking insolvencies spread even more rapidly than the pox, the Bank of England found itself out of sheer selfishness pushed into philanthropy as the Banker of the Last Resource.

Our Unprecocious Central Banks

As world trade resumed after Napoleon had been dispatched to St. Helena, the Bank took over the business of defending the currency when the balance of payments turned against Britain. The gold standard was in theory supposed to look after that, but in fact never really worked as automatically as was claimed and emergency gold loans took place between one central bank and another to stave off financial crises. There were learned discussions about whether the country's gold reserves should or should not be concentrated in the Bank of England, and gradually it moved in that direction. The essence of what we know about central banking was not really learned until the Great Depression of the 1930s. Central bankers were anything but precocious learners. When the financial world had gambled itself into bankruptcy it was left to non-banker economists to put central banking on a society-friendly footing. Under Roosevelt in the mid-1930s, the banks, separated by fire walls, were not allowed to invest in the other three "financial pillars" that kept their own reserves – capital pools necessary for their own business – the stock market, insurance, and real estate mortgages. And the banks had to leave as cash reserves a percentage of the loans they made, i.e., the multiple of credit they created on the base of the cash in their vaults. Such reserves earned them no interest, because cash money whether paper bills or coins do not automatically breed interest, unlike money created by being lent out by banks.

That came to be recognized as an essential feature of money, since when interest rates go up, the value money earning a lower rate of interest would drop to less than par. In banking lingo it is termed "near-money" because its market value goes up or down in the opposite direction of interest rates. Doing so, it acts a bit like a drunk and sets a bad example to the citizens at large. That is all right for a bond, but not for cash. Those interest-free reserves that banks had to redeposit with the central bank as a proportion of the deposits they took in from the public – a greater proportion if they were deposited in chequing accounts, a lesser in longer-term accounts – gave the government virtual interest-free use of the central banks for its own borrowings. For within the constraints in force, it could itself borrow from the central bank and get the interest it paid on such loans back almost wholly intact as dividends in the case of Canada after 1938 when our central banks was nationalized and the UK after the nationalization of the Bank of England after World War II.

But even where the central bank is privately owned as is the US Federal Reserve System, almost the same proportion of the net earnings returns to the government by virtue of the ancestral sovereign's monopoly in coining precious metals (known as "seigniorage" to the *cognoscenti*). The more prosaic truth is that it was found a highly sensible thing to do, because even for bankers it was a wise thing to prevent the government from being bankrupted by too much greed. For should that happen, who would be left to bail them out?

The Confusing Mysteries of Money

Such near-costless financing of government projects through the central bank was used timidly the latter thirties, except in Germany, considerably more daringly during the war and still more so to achieve the reconstruction of the world from 16 years of devastating depression and warfare. And while achieving that and settling an immense immigration, Canada managed to reduce its federal debt from well over 140% of the GDP to little more than 20%.in less than three decades. This was a striking demonstration of how the central bank could be used to finance essential government investment for the benefit of both the private industrial sector and for society as a whole.

However, the financial sector, having recovered from its collapse in 1929, was ready for a brilliantly prepared comeback. Our new pluralistic economy was rapidly urbanizing, with new technologies that required far higher inputs of government investments paid for out of taxation. The result was an ever deeper layer of taxation in the price level. Any upward movement of the price index, however, economists continued to view as "inflation" that would result in the ruin of the currency. There were at the time two main means at the disposal of central banks to check an upward push of the price level: it could raise the benchmark overnight interest rate set by it, for banks making loans to one another to meet their cheque-clearing obligations. Or it could increase the statutory reserves – the banks put up with the central bank. This decreased the leverage of the loans a bank could make as a multiplier of the cash it actually held in its till. By depending less on a higher benchmark rate – that almost automatically raised rates to a far higher extent throughout the economy, and more on adjusting the statutory reserves, the central bank was able to avoid bringing on a recession. Interest rates, moreover, are the financial equivalent of the dice shaken in a gambling den, and the staple income of banks. And the banks and other financial institutions during the 1980s profited by the deregulation of what they could do with the money they created by lending out on a sliver of cash base. In the process, they lost much of their capital in gas and oil, real estate and other gambles

They were saved from mass bankruptcy by some hasty, badly thought-out emergency measures brought in from various points on the globe. Let us take them one at a time to work our way to an understanding of the present plight of the South Korean central bank sitting on a variety of chairs at the same time.

BIS — The Bunker for the Bankers' Comeback

From the Bank for International Settlements in Basel, Switzerland, came the guidelines for the *Risk-Based Capital Requirements* of banks. In 1988 with the banks internationally reeling or worse from their non-banking excesses made possible by their deregulation, BIS rushed to their rescue with its *Risk-Based Capital Requirements*. The most important feature of this seems to have escaped the attention of critics. The main concern in keeping a bank's doors open is not its capital reserves, because these include its investments that are not cash and hence illiquid, but – if the capital is really there – its solvency. The two are very different, since a bank's liquidity depends on its always having enough cash to meet its obligations. Solvency, on the other hand, involves its net worth and includes its investments not only in real estate, but in long-term loans that cannot be readily converted into cash with which to honour claims on the bank. There is the further detail that most banks use the historic value of investments – i.e., their purchase price – rather than their current market value. There is then a considerable degree of latitude, quite apart from the fanciful accountancy that bank deregulation has encouraged.

Moreover, the disastrous effect of two of the rescue measures combined also escaped the rescue designers' scrutiny. The phasing out of the statutory reserves in Canada (1991 to 1993), added to the leverage of (credit) money creation; and the declaration of debt of the governments of developed coun-

tries to be risk-free, by the BIS *Risk-Based Capital Requirements* guidelines that made it possible for banks to quadruple their holdings of federal government debt, without putting up any of their own money. Yet at the same time the same Bank of Canada that sponsored these measures was conducting a campaign to flatten out the price index at all costs. However higher interest rates applied to hoards of government bonds bought entirely on the cuff is like applying a lit match to a gasoline tank – the pre-existent bonds with far lower coupons collapse in market price. Again COMER in great loneliness warned against that outcome. The opening disaster first took place in Mexico where most of the debt had been denominated in US dollars on the advice of foreign consultants, and well-informed money had every facility for taking flight. The US government, with the help of the IMF and Canada put together the largest standby fund ever – over $51 billion US. That prevented the disaster spreading to the entire international banking system. Nevertheless it did provide the background for the East Asiatic meltdown in the 1998, that quickly spread to Russia.

Central banking had been disarmed and disoriented. It no longer had a clear notion of what it was for and how it could achieve its contradictory goals.

With that we are able to appreciate *The Wall Street Journal's* report of the difficulties of South Korea's central bank in plotting a course over these shifting sands (19/04, "South Korea to Rejigger Reserves" by Gordon Fairclough): "Seoul, South Korea – Twenty-five years ago when Choo Heung Sik first helped manage the foreign-exchange reserves of South Korea's central bank, his choices were limited to parking money in commercial-bank accounts or buying short-term US Treasury bills and rolling them over.

South Korea Retains an Investment Counsellor

"The Bank of Korea, like other central banks around the world, is looking at a range of higher-yielding returns on a mounting piles of reserves. At the end of March, South Korea's reserves were the fourth-largest in the world – $205.5 billion.

"Among the choices under consideration: More corporate bonds and expanded holdings of mortgage-backed securities. Mr. Choo, who is a chartered financial analyst and has spent his career at the central bank, declined to be more specific, saying he didn't want to roil markets. South Korea's moves are being watched closely by currency traders. Many traders remain suspicious that the bank's decision to diversify investments is actually a smoke screen for plans to move holdings out of dollars as the US currency falls. South Korea doesn't disclose the percentage of its reserve held in dollars.

"The Bank of Korea's governor, Park Seung, this month repeated that the bank doesn't have any plan to sell dollars because that would lead to a further appreciation of the local currency, the won. The bank has long tried to slow the won's rise against the dollar to protect export industries."

That problem, however, was largely created by Globalization and Deregulations that pretended that the world, become one vast market, would gain in efficiency and that the liberated market would take care of the rest. Instead we have central bankers around the world with unavowed agendas of manipulating their currencies and the exchange value with the US dollar. That in turn is increasingly dependent not on its production of goods and services, but on its financial services and its privileged position as some 60% of the central banks throughout the world keep their reserves in US dollars that cost Washington next to nothing to print. Besides not only oil, but many other raw materials that the US imports in increasing amounts are quoted in dollars, so that when the Federal Reserve tries to keep the dollar low it is not only helping its exports but keeping the price of its imports low.

But how have central banks got so involved in manipulating the terms of trade when Globalization and Deregulation were supposed to overwhelm the world with the benefits of self-regulating markets?

The Wall Street Journal's points out yet another such clash between what central banks are supposed to be about, and what they are in fact spending their time doing: "Central banks, whose role is to safeguard macroeconomic stability, historically have shown little interest in returns, opting instead for safe, short-term investments so that money is available on short notice to intervene in currency markets or cope with a sudden shift in capital flows. That is changing as foreign exchange reserves pile up, at times exceeding the amounts experts say are needed for policy reasons. The trend has been especially pronounced in Asia, as trade and capital flows, currency-market interventions and other factors have led to sharp jumps in reserves in recent years.

"At the end of 2004, China had reserves totalling $610 billion, an increase of more than 50% from the year before. In India reserves jumped 28% to $125 billion. South Korea's reserves increased 28% in the same time, and Japan's were up 31% at the end of November, 2004, from a year earlier. The sheer size of reserves is drawing increased scrutiny from the public and politicians who view the caches as a form of national wealth that should be put to productive use. Another factor is the often significant cost of maintaining such large reserves.

"As some governments and central banks in Asia have moved to curb the appreciation of their currencies against the weakening dollar, they have been 'sterilizing' the reserves they are accumulating. This is generally done by issuing bonds to soak up liquidity. Central banks and governments generally must pay a higher interest rate on the money they borrow domestically than they can earn on US Treasuries and other dollar-denominated assets. And they have suffered losses as the dollar has declined relative to the local currencies.

"The Bank of Korea posted a loss last year of $147.5 million. It was the first central-bank deficit since 1994, and was largely the result of the cost of issuing so-called monetary stabilization bonds in an effort to offset foreign-capital inflows. That means that the bank made no contribution to the government treasury last year."

What is astounding about the last paragraph is that neither the South Korean central bank nor *The Wall Street Journal* seems to remember another way of monetary stabilization by having the central bank contribute earnings to the government instead of running up a deficit – simply lending the excess money to the government, at a near zero cost which would result from its ownership of the bank or seigniorage as the case may be. That money could go to improving health, education, social welfare, scientific research to strengthen South Korea's competitive position internationally and covering the immense cost of unifying the two Korea's if the two Koreas move towards union. The Seoul government has studied the costs of assimilating former Communist Germany into the united German republic and is appalled by what the equivalent burden would be if Korean union came about. But that is what the facilities of a central bank are supposed to be for. That, however, has been expunged from the memory of economists – Korean and international.

Underwhelmed with the Fruits of Globalization

Equally remarkable, it appears from the article that there is now a special craft of central bank advisors apparently to advise central banks on what they must forget of their own history: "Central banks feel 'they are both entitled to, and obliged to consider the return potential' of their reserves, says John Nugee, head of State Street Global Advisors' division providing asset-management services for central banks. State Street manages $57 billion in assets for 33 central banks. While some are more conservative than others, Mr. Nugee says, 'the great majority of our clients are looking to push their investment boundary further out along the risk spectrum' as they look for instruments that offer higher returns."

In short central banks will become more like the commercial banks that central banks were developed to bail out when their risk advisors laid too big an egg.

"Some central bankers, however, complain about a shortage of realistic choices. US Treasury returns are low; Fannie May and Freddie Mac, which buy and package US mortgages into securities for sale to investors, have been hit with scandals; all but the most highly rated corporate bonds are seen by many as too risky. Mr. Nugee says that among his clients five invest in mortgage-backed securities, compared with none in 2000.

"The South Korean legislature this year passed a law requiring the central bank and finance ministry to hand over their foreign-exchange reserves to a new, independent entity, the Korea Investment Corp. The KIC, which will focus more on maximising return, will manage $17 billion for the central bank and $3 for the finance minister." One is tempted to ask why doesn't someone simply introduce the central bank to the finance ministry instead?

William Krehm

The Intermediation of Work

The Economics of Bicycle Riding

One day while on my bike, I suddenly was overtaken by something moving very fast. It proved to be a reclining bicycle covered by a drop-formed hull. The addition of this hull, it seemed, gave the bike aerodynamic properties that enabled the rider to achieve a high level of efficacy. The hull evidently also protected the rider against rain or other vagaries of the weather. And surely the bike, if not already so, could be adapted to carry some groceries or other stuff. Clearly, this state-of-the-art bicycle was well suited to utility trips in the typical, relatively spaced – out suburban neighbourhood.

Currently, North American cities are not engineered to accommodate anything else than fast speeding cars, so safety obviously would be an issue for such bikes. But let us abstract from that for the moment and just look at the economics.

On the surface it would appear to be a win-win situation for society. The burning of fossil fuels and consequently pollution would go down, and people could get some of the exercise that they don't get in their car-only life-styles, obliterating the need for the trip in the SUV to the health club. All together, it could mean that the second car no longer would be needed.

One of the problems of modern industrialism is however that its economic system only can gauge progress if it translates into growth in variables, measurable by money. On the output side, goods and services aggregate into the GDP, while on the input side, factor payments aggregate into national income.

Thus, social benefits that do not translate into growth of the GDP and corresponding factor payments are not properly accounted for by the current system. In the market fundamentalist view, this is as it should be, because doing otherwise would be to insert fuzzy and subjective notions into the supposedly ideal workings of markets.

But the canard of the ideal workings of laissez-faire markets is overcooked. Thirty years of widening income inequalities while we have edged closer to an environmental catastrophe dispute their effectiveness by all criteria , except the one measuring the acceleration of incomes and wealth at the top.

In our societies factor payments are individualized with varying degrees of discreteness. This is, however, not a given and has indeed not been so in all societies. For instance, distributional economic systems in many tribal societies can be interpreted as systems based on non-individualized factor returns with low levels of discreteness. Modern cooperatives are an economic form in some way resembling these.

The State of Factor Payments

However, the current general pattern of individualized factor payments means that no matter how beneficial new low resource technologies otherwise might be, their implications for factor payments could be disastrous. Low resource solutions will bring on a fall in demand for existing factors, which will discontinue many existing streams of factor payments, including wages by creating unemployment. Under such circumstances it amounts to political suicide to advocate policies leading to lower resource intensities. The poster case is Gore's loss of West Virginia – and thereby the presidency – because its normally Democratic-voting mining communities already hit with high unemployment feared that his pro-environmental stand would add to their woes.

With regards to the factors level of discreteness, their state of intermediation plays an important role. For example, banks provide intermediation of money by matching people holding extra money with people who need loans. If times are hard for the banks they might raise their interest spread, but interest payments as such are not tied to the performance of any particular loans on the other side of their ledgers.

Banks thereby take the credit risk off the loans, which they can do much better than individual money holders by aggregating the risk into large loan portfolios. Furthermore, by not being tied to specific loans bank deposits are divisible into the smallest nominations of the monies in use. In a practical sense this makes bank deposits continuous, so that depositors at any time can use debit card to draw whatever sums they want from their deposits to exactly match current needs.

Discrete Wage Labour

Conversely, typical wage labour is not just individualized but discrete in one-off situations. It is either employed full-time, earning a full wage; or unemployed, earning no wage at all.

When demand for resource intense products shifts to products with lower intensities, expansion in the growing industries will not be able to absorb all the idled resources. Standard economic theory tells us that idled resources always will have a marginal price in laissez-faire markets on which they become employable again. However, it is not difficult to find cases that disprove this claim. Fixed capital can become obsolete, both for technical and market strategic reasons, in which case it can lose its value completely. Industrialization caused marginal farming lands to be abandoned as valueless in favour of jobs in the new industrial cities.

The problem is that in the case of labour, it is not just obsolete machinery or stony fields that are thrown out of the economy, but; people with families, children, friends, and hopes. Nevertheless, it quite often happens that workers are fired after having worked for many years in industries that for various reasons go into decline. If they are, say, more 50 years old when that happens, they often will find it very difficult to find placements in the job market again, since their skills are tailored to procedures no longer in demand.

In laissez-faire markets, all disruptions need time before former levels of factor employment readjust under new macro patterns. If disruptions were to be caused by the emergence of new low intensity industries, readjustments could conceivably be very protracted.

Closing factor gaps created by such shifts would require the emergence new industries with an intensity mix high in the use of labour but low in that of other resources. This could for instance be producing consumer products with higher artistic values and individual designs, which could be sold in new market forms – including internet-based ones – established for this purpose.

During the late 1960s and early 1970s, such tendencies were in fact underway. However, the corporate economy of mass-products has since hit back and almost obliterated the tendencies again. This is the mainly result of two factors. (A) The rising incomes inequalities have forced most low and middle incomes families into the sell-everything-low-price warehouses of drab and identical designs for most of their purchases. (B) The mass-assault of the new visual entertainment culture has flooded the market place with inconsequential entertainment gadgets and addictive programming, the latter often leaving people stuck in life-styles far removed from all creative activities.

Older workers dumped by declining industries might have good qualifications for entering new low intensity sectors. They often have experience and good skills at problem- solving that can be of use even outside of the settings in which they were built up. However, because of their age, the requirement to their performance would have to be less strict than what currently is the norm. Most of today's job situations are high-pressured both as a consequence of rising job insecurities caused by employers' increasingly nonchalant attitudes toward firing workers, as well as a consequence of working environments that as a hallmark of modernity often are hectic to a self-defeating degree.

Intermediating Work

At the moment, labour markets are backward and socially unjust by letting the vagaries of individual firms decide whether families can or cannot continue to enjoy the life-styles to which they are accustomed. In all modern societies it should be a human right to have employment and incomes within certain bounds.

A probable solution to the conundrum of both cyclical and demand gap unemployment would be to establish intermediating institutions in the job market. This could be done by combining and extending some functions already present in most modern economies.

Existing job placement agencies in most cases simply facilitate contacts as a service for a fee. However, some placement companies specialize in temps, whom they hire and then sell the services of to the companies actually in need of it. This comes close to performing a true intermediating function. This facet could be expanded which through legislation giving everybody in the working age population a right to be represented by an intermediating agency in the labour market.

Companies would do their hiring through the agencies and pay them. The payments that the individual workers would receive from the agencies would comprise two components: a base pay, independent of the actual employment situation, and a bonus part, dependent upon work and performance criteria. People with disabilities could be included under special arrangements that would entail lower requirements for bonus payments and probably also receive special support from general government.

Part of the payments that the firms would pay to the agencies would replace payments currently routed through the public tax-transfer systems. The agencies would have the size

and incentives to ensure smoother labour markets. They could protecting workers from arbitrary firings, by litigation based on their contractual agreements.

Upgrading skills is another function they could be involved in, and they would have the resources to arrange seminars for firms and workers on applied psychology topics such as conflict management, group interaction, et cetera. Currently, such programs, if at all implemented by firms, tend to be biased to the requirements of owners only.

Conceivably, labour intermediating agencies could be established either as public institutions, or as private-public partnerships with a certain level of competition among them. However, no matter what form labour intermediating might take, unions must be kept as an independent countervailing power, tasked with ensuring that workers right are not eroded by bureaucracy or emergence of collusive tendencies.

Finally, if comprehensive labour intermediating were to be realized a corollary would be to provide governments with a mechanism through which they could manage transitional labour demand gaps occurring in the economy. This will be of importance when we in a not too distant future will be forced to deal with the environmental file very seriously by switching to less resource intensive production modes and life-styles.

Dix Sanbeck

Darwin Can't be Blamed for our Oil-mad Economy Rushing over the Precipice

T HE OIL INDUSTRY is experiencing a period of bonanza that has left behind even the wildest hopes of its main beneficiaries even a few months back.

The Wall Street Journal ("Oil Giants Face New Competition for Future Supply" by Bhushan Bahree and Jeffrey Bail) tells the tale: "The surge in oil prices and continued high global demand are helping Big Oil reap record profits. But they are also luring a host of smaller competitors who often are beating their bigger rivals in the race for fresh fields and new exploitation-and-production contracts in places like Libya and Saudi Arabia. The interlopers undercutting the US and European oil giants, known as 'super majors,' include small Western oil producers looking to make it big, state-controlled companies from countries like China and India that are venturing beyond their borders for oil, and ambitious companies from major oil-exporting countries such as Algeria, Russia and the United Arab Emirates.

"The trend underscores a long-term problem for Big Oil: finding enough new oil and gas each year to replace what they're producing – let alone grow. The five largest publicly traded companies – ExxonMobil Corp., BP PLC, Royal Dutch/Shell Group, ChevronTexaco Corp. and Total SA – have gotten so big, so sophisticated and so beholden to shareholders that their bargaining power in the scramble for future assets is threatened."

Under these circumstances the practice of appraising corporate worth by extrapolating into the indefinite future the rate of growth already attained and incorporating that into current market price of the company shares – and by accountancy practices that are already bending under the strain – becomes a mined field. No need to search for weapons of mass-destruction: the current stock market practices and supposedly free-market gospel have set up future disasters.

But back to the *WSJ* story: "Big Oil's big profits are coming from sales of oil and gas from fields acquired on the cheap long ago, when prices were far lower. Crude-oil prices have nearly doubled since 2001. And early this month hit a record when May delivery oil rose to more than $58 a barrel on the New York Mercantile Exchange…. When adjusted for inflation, that remains well short of the price during the oil shock of the early 1980s."

But is the increase in the price level really all "inflation," i.e., due to an excess of demand for all goods and services? Is it not a fact that to run a modern urbanized high-tech society many more public services are needed than was the case thirty years ago? And is that not particularly so in major oil-producing countries that have made the transition from underdeveloped to modern lands in three decades? And that leaves out the shift for much of our exploration and production from dry land to the oceans. To ignore such details, means that even our oil economists are making forecasts blindfolded by the cop-out of orthodox economic theory.

W.K.

Getting the Economy Up and Running Again

OUR ECONOMY suffers from many losses and sequesterings, that have deprived us of the ability to learn from past policy disasters. Most of these were designed to favour speculative finance at the expense of society's producers, under lock and key with blinds drawn to exclude the slightest ray of challenging light. We must then proceed cautiously before striking out too far beyond what worked in the past. Our history, however, is one of the items that has been kept in short supply.

For at least three decades an *inverted metric* has been imposed on our economic policy-making. In our universities, the media and Parliament, almost everything that yielded positive results has been eliminated from society's recognized options.

We therefore propose respecting the immense learning backlog that voters must cope with. Whatever government emerges from the present political mess, must begin by staying within the limits of what we know proved helpful in the past. That is particularly so if the essential legislation for that is still in our law books. However, it is essential that a Royal Commission be appointed to explore the extent of the problem, and map our progress towards its solution…. Scholars of money and banking still refer to the great reports of parliamentary committees in

Britain in the mid-19th century in their efforts to understand what money and credit are about. There was a time when in Canada Royal Commissions were frequent and highly useful for protecting the free flow of vital information, without which a meaningful democracy is unthinkable

Chapter B-2, an Act respecting the Bank of Canada, in its very preamble sets out the purpose of the central bank:

"Whereas it is desirable to establish a central bank in Canada to regulate credit and currency in the best interest of the economic life of the nation, to control and protect the external value of the national monetary unit and to mitigate by its influence fluctuations in the general level of production, trade, prices and employment, so far as may be possible within the scope of monetary action, and generally to promote the economic and financial welfare of Canada."

The purpose for which the central bank was founded then was not to attain "zero inflation," although a disastrous campaign was organized at the behest of the Bank for International Settlements (BIS) to create that impression. The BIS is a purely technical body established in 1929 to handle the syndication of German reparation payments of World War I into strong currencies. The Depression of the 1930s undermined that project, and at the Bretton Woods Conference of the Allied powers in 1943, Resolution Five was passed calling for the dissolution of BIS at the earliest possible moment. Why? BIS had just about fallen over itself in surrendering to the Nazis the moment their troops marched into Prague the treasure that the Czechoslovak government had stored with it "for safekeeping."

As a result of that resolution, BIS cultivated a low profile for some years. No fake Grecian temples housed it in Basel: some of its offices were actually over a pastry shop. And that unobtrusive existence commended it as a semi-underground bunker for plotting the comeback of the banks in the Western World from the doghouse to which governments had consigned them. When Roosevelt took over in 1933, 38% of the American banks had already closed their doors. One of the first things he did was declare a bank moratorium, introduce deposit insurance and confine the banks severely to banking. Among much else they were prohibited from acquiring interests in the other "financial pillars" – the stock market, mortgage firms, and insurance. For each of these kept a liquid capital pool for the needs of its own industry. Allowing the banks to take over these reserves, and use them as a cash base for creating 10 or 12 times the credit for further acquisitions would be repeating the mistakes that brought on the Great Depression and eventually the Second World War. By 1951, however, the banks had been restored to health on the Spartan regime imposed on them, and were straining to organize a comeback.

Behind the President's Back

In his memoirs President Truman recounts how he was double-crossed by his Treasury in its negotiations with the Federal Reserve to adjust the interest rate peg. He had understood that the negotiations were to adjust the peg to the inflation brought on by the Korean war. To his astonishment, he found out – too late – that what they had agreed to was the removal of the interest rate peg entirely.

The next quarter of a century saw the constant further deregulation of the banks. The central banks laboured to hand over the management of prices and money creation to the market, even if a system of private jobbers had to be nursed into existence over some years with elaborate subsidies. The high point of the proportion of the national debt held by the Bank of Canada was reached in mid-1970s where over twenty percent of the national debt was held by the central bank. This in effect meant that over twenty-percent of the national debt was financed on an almost interest-free basis. The essential details for making that arrangement possible still remain in the *Bank of Canada Act*, if rusty with disuse.

Article 17(2) of the Act reads: "The capital shall be divided into one hundred thousand shares of the par value of fifty dollars each, which shall be issued to the Minister to be held by the Minister on behalf of Her Majesty in right of Canada."

That means that, apart from overhead and administration costs, virtually all the interest on the government bonds held by the Bank returns to the government as dividends. (Today rather than over 20% of the federal government debt, the holdings of the central bank are under 5% of it.) On the other hand interest of the bonds held by private banks remains with those banks. The interest that reverted to the government from the federal government bonds held by the central bank were an important source of revenue, which kept taxes and hence the price level lower. And the money thus saved could be applied to provide essential government services such as environmental conservation, highways, schools.

There are provisions in article 18(c) that the government may buy and sell securities issued or guaranteed by Canada or any province. "Buying and selling" implies "may hold." The Bank of Canada is thus able to lend money to the provinces with no guarantee. Note well, however, in doing so, the interest paid on BoC loans to provinces would go to its one shareholder, the federal government, not to the provinces for they own no shares of the BoC. But that opens up a new dimension for ending the constant wrangling between the federal government and the provinces, and of both with the municipalities. In return for the junior levels of government agreeing to observe federal standards in the projects financed by the Bank of Canada – with federal or provincial guarantee in the case of the municipalities – Ottawa could agree to return to the provinces or municipalities having the financing of projects provided by the BoC, all or a portion of the interest accruing to the federal government from such financing. What a difference that would make in Ottawa's relations with Quebec and the West!

Inflation — The Great Unknown that has Cast its Shadow over our Public Life for Three Decades

But would that not contribute to corruption and inflation? It calls for no small amount of cheek to suggest such a thing at a time when CEOs in the United States have been sent to prison for "cooking their books" much as our governments have done. By doing so, our successive government have ignored the advice of a whole series of Auditors General and even a Royal Commis-

sion or two. Essentially this has involved hiding or dreaming up assets where liabilities existed and vice versa.

The most systemic instance of this was the resistance to introducing capital budgeting, also known as "accrual accountancy." Instead, in their accountancy governments have treated the acquisition of a building, the building of a bridge or a highway (unless it was organized as a separate crown corporation) just as they do their acquisition of floor wax or soap for their washrooms. This set our government bookkeeping on its ear, and left the government itself clueless whether the budget was really balanced or not. Even an unsuccessful attempt to raise enough taxes to pay off the cost of a building or bridge in a single year would needlessly increase the depth of taxation that overlies the direct production costs of the private sector in our mixed economy. And conventional economics regards all increase of the price indexes as "inflation." The assumption that makes this possible is of a "pure and perfect market" – i.e., one with agents so infinitesimally small that nothing that they decide to do individually can possibly affect prices. It is 35 years since I had a paper published in the leading economic journal in France[1] making the distinction between a rising price index resulting from a real excess of aggregate demand over available supply, which is real "market inflation." and higher prices due only to the growth of the public sector within the economy to provide essential services funded by taxation. That can only turn up as a deepening layer of taxation in the price index. The goal of a flat price level in a society that is becoming ever more pluralistic, more urbanized, employing ever higher technologies requiring an increasingly educated labour force, and in a country that is ever more densely populated, is unconscionable.

When the statutory reserves were abolished in 1991 to bail out our chartered banks from the heavy losses in gas and oil, and real estate and other speculative fields incompatible with banking, it left higher interest rates as the "one blunt tool" to fight inflation. Interest rates are, of course, the very gaming dice of speculative capital. They hit everything that moves or stands still in the economy. You can flatten out prices only by flattening out society itself. Attempting to control the economy with interest rates inevitably shifts power to the financial sector. It leads to the extrapolation of the rate of growth already achieved – by fact or fiction – into the present price. Essentially that is a deal with the devil, since that rate of growth embodied into the stock price must be maintained. Its first shortfall will bring down the whole house of cards on which the capitalizations and the collateralizations of the whole financial system depend. The resulting drive to exponential growth also explains the rapid growth of the disparity between the rewards of top executives and the average wages of a skilled worker.

What the World's Central Bankers Overlooked

Hardly more reassuring is a recurrent phenomenon. Even when the abandonment of a favoured policy or some recognition of what has been ignored or actively buried has forced itself on our government, there is no open acknowledgement of the change. Our banks, further deregulated shortly after their bailout from their massive speculative losses in the 1980s, had loaded up with government bonds acquired with no down payment. But they had overlooked a crucial detail: the bond hoards acquired by the banks without a penny of their own money would drop in market value the next time same BIS called for rising interest rates "to lick inflation." For when interest move up, the market value of preexisting bonds is cut off at the knees. And under Governor John Crow, recruited as Governor of the Bank of Canada for his brilliant record in whipping lesser Latin American governments into subservience, interest rates took off as though they were headed for the moon. COMER warned our government. To no effect.[2] In December 1994, this combination of big hoards of government debt with rising interest rates imposed to lick inflation led to a massive capital flight from Mexico and sent shock-waves throughout the financial world. Only the quick intervention of President Clinton, without the backing of Congress, putting together an over $50 billion dollars standby fund with the help of the IMF and Canada, saved the world financial system – temporarily. The repercussions were a factor in the East Asian crisis of 1998 that in turn spread to Russia.

Giddy with Equilibrium Theory

The incompatibility of hoarding government bonds acquired on the cuff to make up their gambling losses, and driving up interest rates to lick inflation was certainly a major factor in the sneaking in of capital budgeting ("accrual accountancy ") by the Clinton administration in 1995. It first appeared under the misleading heading of "savings" in the statistics of the Department of Commerce in January 1996. But "savings" implies liquid cash and the $1.3 trillion of capital value retrieved by the Clinton government by bringing in capital budgeting was already invested in physical assets – bricks and mortar, and equipment. But Clinton as ever was determined to hold the political center and avoided offending the political right who held as an article of faith the view that governments cannot make worthwhile investments. That gave Clinton the isolated statistic that he needed to allow the bond rating agencies to obtain a higher rating and lower interest rates for the government debt that assured him a second term.

Canada profited richly from the lower interest rates in the US, but it failed to follow the American example. It required the refusal of the then Auditor General Denis Desautels to give unconditional approval of the government balance sheets of two years to induce Finance Minister Martin in 1999 to agree to the change, without explaining to parliament its significance. Accrual accountancy was brought in for physical investments already made, or negative capital deficits if the country's environmental undertakings under the Kyoto Protocol were not made or for the discharge of treaty obligations with the aboriginal peoples that were still not honoured. This on balance disclosed positive budgetary balances where the then Finance Minister had reported negative ones that were used to slash social programs further.

It is clear the our government still has no clear view on whether interest rates should be raised or not. It is wholly at sea where the equilibrium point that it so strongly believes in

might be. For example, with the central belief in sustaining the growth rate of the economy, or in fact an acceleration of growth rate that is projected into the distant future on the silly belief that hedging will give them a grasp on the future. The economy simply must grow at least at the rate already attained, because that has already been incorporated into the share price. Since huge subcontinental countries of immense population and ancient cultures have been brought into this game, that burst of both growth rate of demand for oil and oil prices bear a hump of purely speculative origin. And all this has resulted in oil prices – adjusted for "inflation" – reaching the historic highs of the nineteen seventies. From the standpoint of the oil-guzzling countries like the US, these are fighting words in the most literal sense of the word. But take a look at them from the point of view of oil producing countries in the Near East or Latin America. How many finished industrial products adjusted for inflation and produced in the US or Europe can still be bought at inflation-adjusted prices of the 1970s? And relate that to the nationalistic and cultural militancies that are sweeping the oil-producing emerging countries. And what could a higher interest rate possibly contribute to bringing down oil prices below its inflation-adjusted level of the 1970s?

And, there are the religious and cultural factors as well to be considered. The Koran considers the taking of interest if persisted in a mortal sin, let alone elevating it to the role of "one blunt tool for fighting inflation."

Inhuman Accountancy

The bad conscience of conventional economists on such matters does occasionally break through conventional orthodoxies. Thus a couple of years ago both the Fed and the Bank for International Settlements seemed to have abandoned the notion that the slightest amount of inflation, if tolerated, would explode into the hyperinflation that took over in Germany in 1923. Suddenly these institutions began talking of "good inflation" (variously defined as up to 2 or 3 % per year, and "bad inflation." Instead of further investigation, the model shifted from the lofty infinitesimal calculus to the humble oil-can. Good inflation was what was needed to "lubricate the economy." But alas, we have not heard of good inflation for the better part of a year by now. Apparently with naked power comes the liberty to impose and abandon models without further explanation.

Not even the Auditors General over the years have proposed depreciating investment in human, rather only in physical investments. And yet in the 1960s economists had reached the conclusion that investment in human capital is the most productive investment that a government can make. Its depreciation time spans entire generations since the children of educated, healthy parents tend to be more open to education, healthier and better adjusted to society.

But where is the money for such investment to come from? From the central bank loaned or backed with or without formal guarantee by the federal government. If the resources are available for such investments, the credit of the central government is enough to finance the project through the central bank. That is the program that must occupy the center stage in the next federal election. Alongside the suppression of the critical issues facing society not to mention the hundreds of billions of dollars of unnecessary subsidies that has gone as an annual entitlement to the private banks, the sponsorship scam was small-time pickpocketing.

William Krehm

1. *Revue Économique*, May 1970, carries the sixty-page article, "La stabilité des prix et le secteur public," which was expanded into a book, *Price in a Mixed Economy – Our Record of Disaster*, Toronto, 1975, which was most favourably reviewed in the *Economic Journal* in Cambridge and other publications. Those were years with a considerable freedom for new ideas.

2. One such early warning of the disastrous effect of the banks' totally leveraged government bond hoards and the BIS's mania for high enough interest rates to flatten prices appeared in *Economic Reform* in May, 1993, and was reproduced on page 96 of Krehm, William (Ed.) (1993), *Meltdown, Money, Debt and the Wealth of Nations*, Toronto, under the title of "The Next Trip to the Vomitorium": "The moment our central bank embarks on its next holy war to 'lick inflation,' all existing government bonds will plummet below their cost. Far from being 'risk-free,' in the world of 'zero inflation' any fixed-rate security is a bit of a long shot."

Dilemma of Analysts

THE BLINDING DAZZLE of money is such that even the best analysts in appraising the flow of ever bigger fraud cases of ever larger corporations may end up with fistfuls of statistics rather than answers. What is never pondered is how little space has been left for lessons learned in Sunday school. In our world people have become digitalized and replaced with credit-card numbers to the point that the resulting moral anonymity makes irrelevant whether society survives or goes under.

Thus in *The Globe and Mail* column of Andrew Willis, unless he means to kid us both to match the date (April 1), and the title (Street Wise), you cannot wonder whether he is writing in earnest or with a tongue simultaneously in either cheek:

"Richard Nesbitt yesterday used his first speech as chief executive officer of the Toronto Stock Exchange to take dead aim at the Montreal Stock Exchange's main line of business, derivatives trading.

"A deal between the two exchanges will keep the Toronto Stock Exchange (TSX) out of stock and bond futures and options until 2009. And it is obvious that the standstill agreement is driving Mr. Nesbitt nuts.

"Derivatives are the hot growth sector in financial markets. As CEO at the TSX, Mr. Nesbitt has promised to deliver growth. And Canada is woefully behind most mature economies when it comes to derivative trading.

"Here are the numbers. The average exchange on this planet does $1.55 in derivatives trading for every buck in cash equity trading. The Germans manage to buy and sell $5.23 of derivatives for every dollar in equities.

"In Canada, the ME does just 27 cents of derivative contracts for every dollar in cash equity deals done by the TSX. That ratio ranks near the bottom of all exchanges world-wide.

"Mr. Nesbitt's view is that the world's leading stock exchanges unite cash and derivative trading under one roof. So yesterday Mr. Nesbitt calmly announced that in four years time 'we intend to launch our own combined cash derivatives business that replicates the best global market models, building on the elements we are now putting in place.

"It's clear the ME can count on losing the monopoly hold on derivatives that began back in 2001. The TSX is already learning the ropes, by trading energy derivatives in a newly acquired Calgary subsidiary."

The conclusion: Whereas the talk is of a self-balancing market *singular*, there are in fact an indefinite number of markets at work in space, time, and the achiever's fantasy, that goose each other for the grand prize of violating one another's rules, and the laurels go to whoever on what market ends up with the most bucks. Few questions asked – above all in Canada. We are far too polite.

W.K.

Navigating for Security in a Bubble Economy

SHOULD CANADIANS be concerned about the current issue of Social Security reform in the United States? President Bush is at the forefront of a campaign to warn workers, especially younger ones, that the Social Security taxes they are paying now do not guarantee that they will receive the promised benefits if they are disabled or when they retire. They are being told in effect that the United States Government is an unreliable insurance company that plans to defraud them. Turning from fear to the temptations of greed, Bush says he will help workers put their savings (from reduced payroll taxes) into the shares of private corporations so they can join the "ownership society" and become capitalists like him. "Why be satisfied with the measly rate of return implied by the Social Security contract when you could be getting rich on capital gains in the stock market?" There has been spirited and cogent rebuttal of this rationale, but the record of the Bush team at persuading people to follow his lead on other important issues is a warning that this campaign might succeed as well. And if it does, the ripple effects on financial markets and the global economy could have a bruising impact on Canadians.

Comparing the Bush Plan with Canada's CPP

Although the Canada Pension Plan is considered to be actuarially sound since the annual contributions rate was increased a few years ago, we still note some rumbles of approval for the Bush rationale in our financial press. By that reasoning, future pensioners will be better served with a bigger direct investment in the growth of the economy through a *personal* portfolio of shares in corporate enterprises. Without even examining the pros and cons of that position, there would be an obvious and immediate benefit to the financial sector if taxes collected for the CPP were diverted through their hands. Sales pressure from that source needs to be scrutinized very carefully, therefore. Labor economists say the current CPP formula is just fine and they only wish it would be increased as a share of the retirement and rainy-day savings of Canadians.

A modest share of CPP contributions actually does get invested in the private sector as part of the adjustments to the Plan in the late '90s. There is an important distinction in this feature from the Bush proposals however. The Bush plan would reduce the payroll tax and shunt the equivalent into a personal portfolio managed by a certified fund manager of the individual's own choosing. The portion of CPP contributions that buys financial assets is managed collectively by an Investments Board under strict rules for avoiding speculative or politically oriented allocations (e.g., "ethical investments"). This reduces the cost of portfolio management enormously compared to personal accounts, for which management fees can absorb all or more of the earnings and capital gains (losses). The intensity of debate in the United States gives Canadian readers an opportunity to consolidate their understanding of the privatization issue and therefore a better sense of how to think about their own security and to plan for retirement.

Supporters of the existing Social Security system point out that stock market investing is historically risky, and there is no realistic prospect that that will change. By contrast, government power to levy taxes on any sources of wealth and income within its jurisdiction is a much more reliable constant, and the projected deficit in Social Security capacity to pay can be conveniently rectified by the solution already applied in Canada. Although administrators of the system are obviously constrained from speaking out against the policy preferences of the President, sufficient actuarial judgment of the system's general soundness was released before the privatization campaign got into full gear. The system is sound in principle; it simply needs some quite bearable adjustments to contribution and benefit rates.

The Flaws of Privately Privatized Social Security

Judging by opinion polls in early April, Americans are wary of the Bush proposal. The President nevertheless continues to maintain that substantial privatization of Social Security is the centerpiece of his domestic agenda. His insistence in the face of spirited and effective opposition has led many to wonder why he is willing to risk so much of his "political capital" on a problem that seems easy to fix with little fuss. I have observed four plausible explanations, none of which inspires confidence and all of which could be part of the answer.

1. An immediate bonanza for the financial services industry has already been noted. Critics contrast the share of an individual's savings that are absorbed by management fees to the miniscule (per capita) cost of administering the existing system. Privatization via personal accounts might therefore be simply another scheme to divert taxpayer's money into the hands of the President's already privileged peers and financial supporters of

his party. While this explanation is not out of the question, another possibility is a bit more generous in motivation, although at least as ominous in its implications.

2. The United States Government is broke, can't pay its debts and doesn't intend to try. The US system is built on the supposition that future workers will pay the benefits owing to current workers whose contributions are now supporting today's retirees. Its soundness therefore requires that the US economy will provide paying jobs in the future. To characterize the system as broken might therefore be taken as a warning that the national economy is about to collapse or that the United States is really in long-term, irremediable economic decline. President Bush reinforced that worry in early April by suggesting that the United States Government might default on its bonds. It was a pretty direct threat, for he was describing the Social Security Trust Fund as "just a bunch of IOUs." Since that Fund is held entirely in US government bonds of the same quality as are purchased by private investment funds and foreign banks and governments, the unmistakable implication is that they might soon be reduced to junk status. A deeper look at this situation leads to a third possible explanation for the privatization push.

3. The Fund has accumulated to a very large size since Social Security taxes were increased in the early 1980s to prepare for anticipated retirement of the baby boom generation. It may be conceived as a collective retirement fund for the finite period when actuaries expect the number of retirees to exceed capacity of payroll deductions from fewer workers to keep current with obligations. In effect, the payroll taxes collected as contributions to the Social Security Fund were being loaned to the US government. The current atmosphere of crisis is due to successive governments having spent the money instead of stashing it away for when the contracted payments came due. That is, they used the regressive payroll taxes, newly enhanced in quantity, to pay for ongoing operations instead of raising other taxes. They in fact reduced other taxes, under the pretext that it would stimulate technological development, economic growth, and better jobs and incomes for future workers.

Their business plan didn't work out as expected and soon the lender (the Trust Fund) will be knocking at the door demanding payment. The government has been living off the payroll taxes of workers instead of paying its own way by taxing other sources of revenue sufficiently (rents, interest, capital gains, monopoly profits). Now that the debt to workers has come due, what will the government do? Tell workers "whoops, we spent all your money. Give us some more?" Borrow even more money from some other Peter so they can pay Paul? To default on the Social Security obligations entails default on United States bonds generally, for that is what is in the Trust Fund. It's not a good option if the government plans to borrow even more. It can't really stiff Social Security claimants therefore, unless it is ready to go out of business entirely. The remaining options are to borrow even more, from somewhere else, and to collect more revenue from sources other than payroll tax. But that means that the rich who have been escaping taxes will have to pay up. The issue of reforming Social Security is inescapably a conflict between rich and poor. The American penchant for denying this reality with fancy tricks (and trickle-downs) is progressively more transparent.

4. The fourth and most sophisticated possibility entails dropping back even further in the history of the Social Security program and its relationship to other developments. Soon after its inception during the Depression, the US economy recovered strongly due to wartime production imperatives, and the pace was maintained through the forties and fifties. Laborers had bargaining power as a consequence and used it to win promises of long-term income security in the form of retirement pensions, medical, disability and survivor benefits. Simultaneously, however, the spectre of automation came onto the planning horizon and cast a shadow over the future of work. The campaign to privatize social security coincides with the hollowing out of American industry and a decline in the prospects for high-quality jobs. Uncertainty over prospects of income from paid employment may be a factor in the vulnerability of younger workers to the Bush propaganda. Why pay the tax now if the next generation won't have jobs from which to pay me back? If there are "no" jobs in the future and the real product and incomes are generated by robot, it's important to have a share in the robot. Or, if the work is being done in sweatshops overseas, let's have a share in the globalized corporations that are exploiting the slaves for our benefit. Shall we put our savings in shares of corporations (or mutual funds managers) in the belief that they are more reliable as guarantors of our future than the taxing power of governments?

Pension Fund Socialism?

In this fourth interpretation, the Government's problem with US finance is intimately linked to the fortunes of corporations. For the concessions won by labor unions in the forties required their corporate employers to set aside a portion of their revenues to make benefits payments in the future. This *Pension Fund Socialism* (after Peter Drucker) involved investment of those funds in financial assets, providing major impetus to growth of a non-industrial industry – the financial sector. Thus a specialist in the financial aspect of economic history suggests that the post-industrial economy we have been talking about for forty years is not so much a "services economy" or "information economy" as it is a *financial economy*. Michael Hudson[1] conjectures that the financial sector has grown up alongside the industrial one and has come to be a rival, or even a parasite, rather than just a supplement.

In the mid-century decades of strong growth, corporate pension fund assets earned handsomely on capital gains. As the financial economy gained strength, partly by its own churning, rising stock prices inspired corporate financial officers with the bright idea that they could boost their own bonuses and stock option values by cutting back on pension fund contributions in order to declare higher earnings. This they justified by claiming that their pension funds were fatter and earning a far higher rate of return than was needed to pay future commitments (by factoring in capital gains from inflated stock prices). Although their assumed rates of return were always overblown, the collapse of the tech bubble evaporated billions in presumed wealth and put corporations with heavy pension commitments (like GM and Ford) under serious pressure. The prospect of major corporate bankruptcies threatens the pension security of hundreds of thousands of employees. A new burst of inflation in the stock market, however, would mitigate this problem for a few years.

And that, says Hudson, explains the urgency, persistence and sheer magnitude of the campaign to privatize Social Security. It is a deliberate attempt to inflate stock market prices by government action. For comparable perfidy, says Hudson, one must look as far back as the 18th century Mississippi and South Sea Bubbles when governments solved their debt problems by inducing bondholders to accept shares in speculative ventures in exchange for promises to pay. If Bush is successful in his campaign to transfer payroll taxes from government bonds into corporate shares the impact on stock markets will go well beyond the United States. It might translate into a general acceptance of prices that are much higher relative to earnings and other measure of worth than are accepted by conservative investors. In this way, policy decisions about Social Security in the United States could make personal financial management difficult and dangerous for people well beyond its political boundaries.

Keith Wilde

1. Distinguished Research Professor of Economics, University of Missouri, Kansas City, in "The $4.7 Trillion Pyramid," *Harper's Magazine*, April 2005.

REVIEW OF A BOOK BY JOSEPH E. STIGLITZ AND BRUCE GREENWALD, CAMBRIDGE UNIVERSITY PRESS, 2003

"Towards a New Paradigm in Monetary Economics"

JOSEPH STIGLITZ, once a high official of the World Bank, has achieved renown for his independent critique within the very den of orthodoxy. However, in this imperfect world, even relative heterodoxy carries its price tag. "The material was originally presented at the Raffaele Mattioli Lectures, established by Banca Commerciale Italiana in association with Universita Commerciale Luigi Bocconi as a memorial to the cultural legacy of Raffaele Mattioli, for many years chairman of the bank. This explains the almost lyric naivete of such shrewd investigators in dealing with such delicate issues as the sifting of economic information by banks, and the headlong characterization of the statutory reserves certain countries still require the banks to redeposit with their central banks as "taxes."

But despite all that accommodation, in the preface we read: "We would be remiss not to acknowledge the vibrant intellectual atmosphere inside the World Bank, in which the ideas presented here were debated, challenged, and adopted and adapted as we confronted the most dramatic set of economic events of the last half of the twentieth century – the global financial crisis; but we would also be remiss if we did not express our sense of frustration at the attempts of the US Treasury and the IMF to suppress open discussion of these ideas. There cannot be meaningful democracy without transparency and without open public discourse of vital issues that affect the lives and livelihoods of the citizens." To which we can only add our "Amen."

At times, our reading of this in some respects rewarding book, left the impression that even while asserting these laudable principles, the authors are inclined to accept the view that transparency itself is a market and rarely a perfectly free one at that.

But first of all our applause for the substantial merits of the work. "Professional economists give money an equally mixed review. The monetarists – whose enormous popularity in the early 1980s seems subsequently to have waned – place money as a central determinant of economic activity. By contrast, in the classical dichotomy [of supply and demand], money has no *real* effects, a view which has been revived in real business cycle theory. Monetary economics has been a curious branch of economics. At times, its central tenet seems to be that it is a subject of no interest to anyone interested in real economics; at other times, it moves front and center....

"The central thesis of this chapter is that the traditional approach to monetary economics, based on the transaction demand for money, is seriously flawed [in that] it does not provide a persuasive explanation for why – or how – money matters. Rather, we argue that the key to understanding monetary economics is the demand and supply of loanable funds, which in turn is contingent on understanding the importance, and consequences of banks. We argue, in particular, that one should not think of the market for loans as identical to the market for ordinary commodities, an auction market in which the interest rate is set simply to equate the demand and supply of funds. That some loans are not repaid is central. A theory of monetary policy which pays no attention to bankruptcy and default is like *Hamlet* without the Prince of Denmark. Thus, a central function of banks is to determine who is likely to default, and in doing so, banks determine the supply of loans.... While banks are at the center of the credit system, they are also part of a broader credit 'general equilibrium' – a general equilibrium whose interdependencies are as important as those that have traditionally been discussed in goods and services markets."

The Fly in the Broth

The big fly afloat in that otherwise enticing broth, is the frequency with which banks before and during the age of Eliot Spitzer have graced the defendants' dock in celebrated cases such as Enron.

Not infrequently the enquiries disclosed our banks' part in the design and execution of derivative games that made possible a double sets of books. (Could this perhaps be excused as a derivative of double entry bookkeeping?) It certainly has done little for the information that is the special function of banks to provide according to the authors' new model.

On the other hand, though muted, there is an awareness of the obstacles that have been thrown up against their new model of openness. "Many developing countries have been placed under strong pressures to open up their financial systems – a marked change in their institutional structure. Most of the arguments for this make standard appeals to an institution-free analysis – more competition increases economic efficiency [no matter what the institutions may be]. A closer look at the impact of such reforms on the domestic banking system, and on the flow of credit to small and medium-size enterprises, suggests many circumstances in which these policy reforms have adverse consequences." That undoubtedly contributed to the displeasure of the US Treasury and the IMF.

Stiglitz is in fact a little all over the map. I quote: "Establishing a form of Say's law for government debt, Stiglitz showed that if the government reduced taxes and increased its debt, the demand for government bonds increased by an amount exactly equal to the increase in supply." The original Say's Law assured believers that there could not be such a thing as overproduction, because in this best of economic systems the very production of a commodity produced the market for its sale. We thought that the Great Depression and Keynes had knocked the wind out of Say's sails.

To add to the confusion of leaning on Say's Law, the authors adopt yet another verbal usage of the dominant financial sector: "remember the characterization of reserve requirements as a tax on borrowing by the bank." The statutory reserves require banks to redeposit with the central bank a percentage of the deposits they take in from the public – the highest in the case of deposits into their chequing and short-term accounts.

These could well be remembered in quite different connections – in their historical context as "seigniorage," a reference to the ancestral crown's monopoly in coining precious metal which has now been surrendered in large degree to our banks. Or it could be remembered as an alternative to raising interest rates to fight a rising price level which might or might not be real inflation – i.e., resulting from an excess of demand beyond what supply could fill. What practically all economists concur in is ignoring that price indexes may also rise not because of an excess of demand, but because of urbanization, population increase, and technological development that require more infrastructures and a more highly educated population. All these create the need for more public services as a proportion of total production. That leads inevitably to a deeper layer of taxation embedded into our prices. Thirty-five years ago I identified this under the name of "social lien" to distinguish it from "market inflation" that does indicate an excess of demand over market supply.

But the words we speak can smuggle in great institutional change – especially when privileged groups find these useful.

The Banks as Masters

Thus, we find on page 279, in discussing the bank crisis of the latter 1980s, the authors reach the conclusion that "lower interest rates also reduced the banks' seigniorage." That can only refer to the excess the banks lend out over the cash in their vaults. The Bank for International Settlements' *Risk-Based Capital Requirements* had in 1988 declared the debt of OECD members – the most developed countries – to be risk-free requiring no extra capital to acquire. The Statutory Reserves, unlike the case in Canada, do continue in the US on a very reduced scale, applicable only during banking hours, The interest meters in the case of government bonds that are declared risk-free tick on 24 hours a day, whether the bank doors are closed or open. And that cute innovation reduces the seigniorage regained by the state that had had the free use of the statutory reserve twenty-four hours every day – to match the uninterrupted ticking of the bond interest. In Canada the statutory reserves were abolished outright, though not very publicly, in 1991.

Significantly the term "seigniorage' harks back to when the ancestral sovereigns held a monopoly in coining gold and silver. And the significance of the bailout of the banks that the book discusses at this point is that the creation of money, once a sovereign privilege, has now been transferred to the banks. The term "seigniorage" is clearly derived from the Italian for "master" and informs us who is now master in the great counting house.

So significant a redistribution of the national income amounted to a shift in the power structure of the nation. Only that could explain how so soon after the bailout of the banks from their gambling losses in the 1980s the firewalls that the Roosevelt bank reform of 1935 that prevented banks from acquiring the other financial sectors were abolished. These other financial sectors – stock brokerages, mortgages, insurance – had their capital pools to meet the needs of their own businesses. But the banks lusted after such liquid reserves to expand their cash base on which they could exercise their growing powers of money creation given them by the end of their statutory reserves. Significantly, banks, brokerages, mortgage, and finally insurance and re-insurance conglomerates have featured as star defendants in the investigations of fraud launched by Attorney General of New York Eliot Spitzer, and the SEC.

None of these issues are spotlighted in the book. Seigniorage, of course, had always been shared by banks and the government. The BIS *Guidelines of Capital Requirements* and the decrease of the statutory reserves, merely changed the proportions of the sharing sharply to the advantage of the banks. But never before have I encountered the use of the term "seigniorage" referring to the banks' part of the take. That in itself. I suppose, should earn the authors high marks for frankness up to a point.

And that instance is not unique. For example on page 291 we read: "When [Fed Governor Alan] Greenspan seemed to support Bush's tax proposals, questions were raised not only about his economic judgment, but also his political judgment, and the arguments he gave (the notion that *eventually* the surpluses would eliminate the supply of government debt, which would have adverse effects on the conduct of monetary policy) did little to help.

"If monetary policy must rely on the credibility of the central bank and the central banker, then it is indeed a fragile instrument. For it may increasingly be the case that this particular emperor has no clothes, or is, at the very least, scantily clothed, and while such assertions are seldom made in polite circles, there is a growing suspicion that this may indeed be the case."

William Krehm

The Endless Ambiguities of the Free and Not So Free Market

SOMETIMES governments or corporations will make a special effort to appear honest to help hide manipulations of their balance sheets. Not rarely the opposite tack is adopted: they will manipulate their balance sheets to emphasize their honesty.

The future of the US dollar depends largely on the willingness of the rest of the world to accept the growing surplus of US debt as the currency in which they hold most of their foreign reserves. What has helped the strength of the US dollar is that as the world's chief guzzler of oil, and originally the greatest producer, official oil prices are quoted in its currency. That will go on as long as that is acceptable to the oil producers, a distinct advantage to the US, but an increasingly insecure one.

The case of South Korea illustrates how such a tangle of considerations may influence the future of the dollar. *The Wall Street Journal* (18/03, "Bank of Korea Sets Same Proportion of Dollar Reserves" by Hae won Choi and In Kyung Kim) reports a public statement of the South Korean central bank that could and even should be interpreted in implying the exact opposite of what it says: "SEOUL – The South Korean Central bank said it would seek to maximize profit from its big foreign-exchange holdings by investing in a broader range of assets. But bank officials said they don't plan to change the proportion of reserves held in dollars.

"The Bank of Korea roiled world markets last month by saying that it intended to 'diversify' its reserves, language that traders took to mean the bank would start selling dollars. Fears that the central bank and others in Asia would dump [that] currency sent it spiraling downward on Feb. 22.

"Accordingly, Choo Heung Sik, head of the Bank of Korea's reserve management team told an interviewer, 'We have absolutely no plans to reduce our proportion of dollar holdings. The market shouldn't interpret today's announcement like it did last month.'"

But, of course, the market would and did. The very next paragraph of the piece we are citing reports: "However, some market watchers remain skeptical. Oh Suk Tae, an economist at Citigroup in Seoul, said he believes that in the long term the Bank of Korea 'plans to shift away from dollars and purchase other currencies such as the euro or the yen.' He added: 'If they didn't have any plans to move away from the dollar, why would they need to beef up the number of the staff?' The central bank is increasing the staff managing the country's reserves to over 100 from the current 66.

We are in fact reminded of a stock anecdote of two petty traders in White Russia, when the Jewish ghetto there was a vibrant place with a special brand of wit directed at its own vulnerabilities. "On a train, Moshe runs into Jacob, his business competitor, and after warm greetings and enquiries about the health of his family, he asks where he is going. 'Minsk' came the answer. And the train ground on, and the two were lost in friendly reminiscences. Suddenly the conductor announces

Minsk as the next stop. Jacob moves to lower his baggage, and Moshe reproaches him: 'After all these years of friendship, you can't be frank with me! You told me you were going to Minsk, because you wanted me to believe that you were going to Pinsk. And here you are actually getting off at Minsk. What a way to treat a friend!'

There are other factors at work here rather than purely market considerations. In our last issue we dealt with South Korea's dissent from the Washington policy of boycotting North Korea unless it surrenders its nuclear arm project. The prospect of an economic collapse of North Korea with a flood into its country of an estimated two million refugees has led Seoul to engage the North in an extensive development program. As a country itself – like the US – economically dependent on a vastly overextended automobile industry, and with an economy vastly overdependent on consumer debt as is the US itself, any degree of frankness from South Korea about its cutting its dollar reserves would definitely place South Korea in Washington's dog house.

"Currency markets have been seesawing on sometimes-conflicting comments of officials and politicians about foreign exchange policies. Last week Japanese Prime Minister Junichoro Koizumi made the dollar reel again by telling a parliamentary committee that, in general, Japan should consider diversifying its reserves. The Japanese Ministry of Finance quickly said it doesn't plan any changes." In short, the same two-step.

W.K.

Chicken General

WE HAD BEEN ASSURED that the world was populated by natural traders whose only desire in life is to have commerce deregulated so that we can import and export enough to congest our highways' airports, railway lines and ports to the point where they become vulnerable to terrorists, and to mass unemployment. So that, should you happen to have a job today, there would be ever less assurance that you will have it to-morrow. As for the subsistence economy that allows people to raise all or part of their own food without having it hallowed by having been traded at home or preferably abroad, there should be heavy penalties for breaching the new religion. Whatever you may raise for your own consumption, and by whatever poetry you may read in private that in no way contributes to the GDP and doesn't "grow" the official economy, and must be replaced with products for body and mind produced with artificial fertilizers applied to patented hybrids.

Veterinarians Lead the Trade War

But serious cracks are turning up in this simple faith, as appears from a front-page article in *The Wall Street Journal* ("Chicken Fight – In Global Food-Trade Skirmish Safety is the Weapon of Choice" by Gregory L. White in Moscow, Scott Kilman in Springdale, Ark., and Roger Thurow in Ptitsegrad, Russia): "The gray van carrying the Russian inspector arrived at dawn outside a complex in Springdale, Ark. Uniformed Ameri-

can guards stood outside as Major General Vitaly Romansky toured the facility. He had come to verify that America was living up to an agreement reached between high-level US and Russian negotiators.

"After two hours, the poker-faced inspector came striding out of the building. The metal security gate rattled open and the van whisked him away.

"Mr. Romansky's checklist included a section on radioactive fallout. But he wasn't inspecting nuclear weapons. He is a Russian government veterinarian. The facility is a chicken-slaughtering plant. He was inspecting drumsticks.

"This cloak-and-dagger routine is more than just Cold War leftovers in the freezer section. As new food powers emerge, the drive for free trade around the world is blunting the traditional tactics governments once employed to shield their domestic industries. Now, food safety is becoming the stealth weapon of protectionism in the $522 billion market for global agricultural exports.

"'As quotas and tariffs become less important trade barriers, sanitary measures are becoming a relatively much bigger problem,' says J.B. Penn, an undersecretary of the US Agriculture Department.

"Russian veterinarians with military-style ranks – one earned the name 'Chicken Napoleon' from US executives – have blacklisted scores of US poultry plants from exporting to Russia. They are among the world's most aggressive in using their power to close off markets, trade experts say. Russian officials concede their stringent standards don't necessarily improve the meat's quality and some are blunt about the inspectors' real purpose."

"'The only tool of trade policy the Agriculture Ministry has left are our veterinarians,' then First Deputy Sergei Dankvert told an industry meeting in late 2002, according to Russian press reports. He is now head of Russia's state veterinarian agency. A spokeswoman confirmed his comments, adding: 'That's why we don't let him talk to the press any more.'

"The US-Russian 'chicken war' is the most intense example of a growing number of food-safety skirmishes. When Brazilian soybean prices soared last spring, Chinese government inspectors said they detected a deadly fungicide in some shipments. China temporarily blocked imports from Brazil, helping Chinese merchants get out of their commitments, Brazilian grain groups say. Japan has shut down imports of US apples by requiring that American growers adopt expensive measures to combat fire blight, a plant disease that US officials say isn't spread through apple shipments.

"The US, which is fast becoming one of the world's greatest importers of food, uses similar tactics. Bush administrator officials imposed a ban on Canadian cattle 19 months ago when Canada discovered its first case of mad-cow disease. Canada has now nearly identical safety measures to those in the US, but officials have been slow to complete the regulatory procedures for lifting the ban. Privately, they concede the delay is due to opposition from US ranchers who want to protect cattle prices.

"The globalization of agricultural trade, which now embraces more than 200 countries, has indeed created new food-

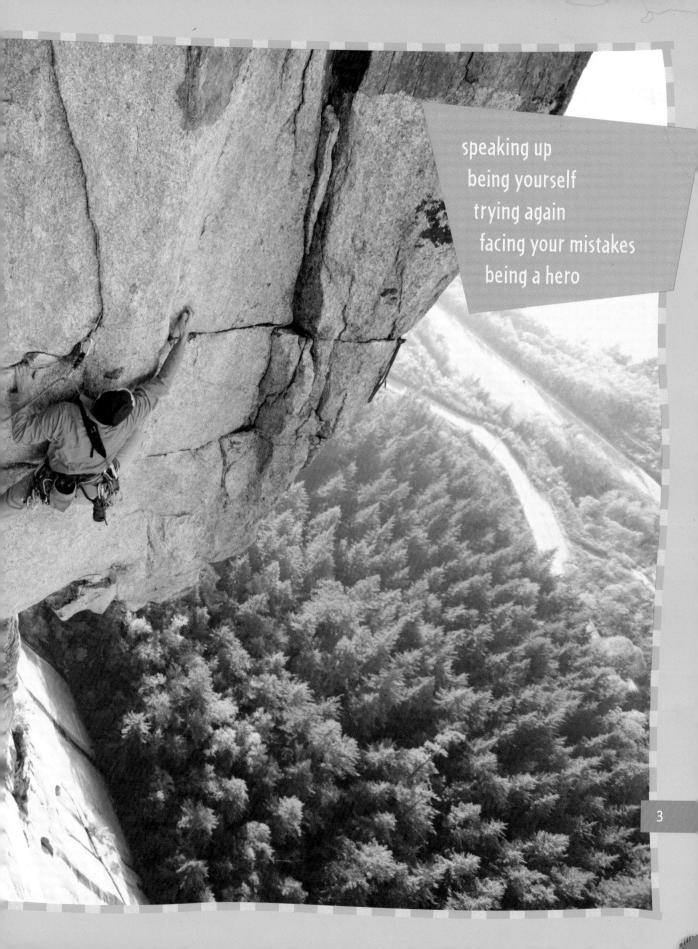

speaking up
being yourself
trying again
facing your mistakes
being a hero

3

Mia's Problem

by Sandra McLeod Humphrey

Illustrated by Diane Dawson Hearn

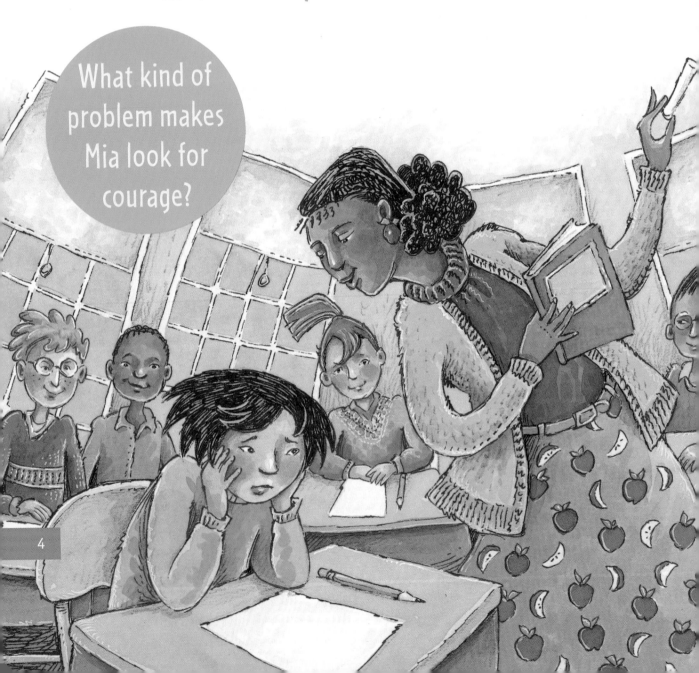

What kind of problem makes Mia look for courage?

4

My name's Mia and my problem began last Thursday. That's when Ms. Bradshaw, our language arts teacher, told our class that we had to finish up our book reports by Monday and be ready to give our oral book reports.

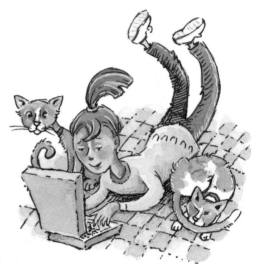

The good news is that we could choose any book. The bad news is that I don't read books.

Why should I read books when I can learn just as much from watching TV? And why should I worry about learning how to write when I can talk? If we're talking about real communication here, anyone knows that you can say a lot more and in much less time by talking than by writing.

There are a lot of things I *do* like about school— like recess and lunch and gym class and field trips and a whole bunch of other things. I just don't like to read books or write papers.

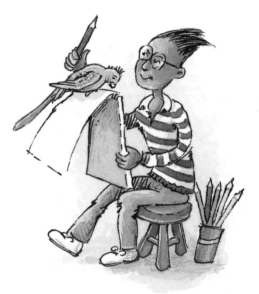

And I especially don't like to give speeches. It's not that I'm all that shy, I just don't like having to stand up there in front of the whole class and talk.

My heart starts pounding double-time, my hands get all sweaty, and my mouth is so dry that I can hardly talk.

Anyway, Ms. Bradshaw assigned us to teams, with three kids to a team. Both the kids on my team are really smart. They both read the book in one night. It took me three days to get through it.

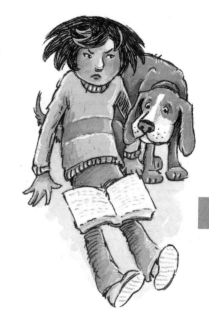

Aaron can really draw, so he did all the pictures for the book report. And Katie is a computer whiz, so she offered to type our report for us.

That left me to do the oral report! All weekend I thought about nothing else. Videos kept running through my head: twenty million different ways how I could mess up!

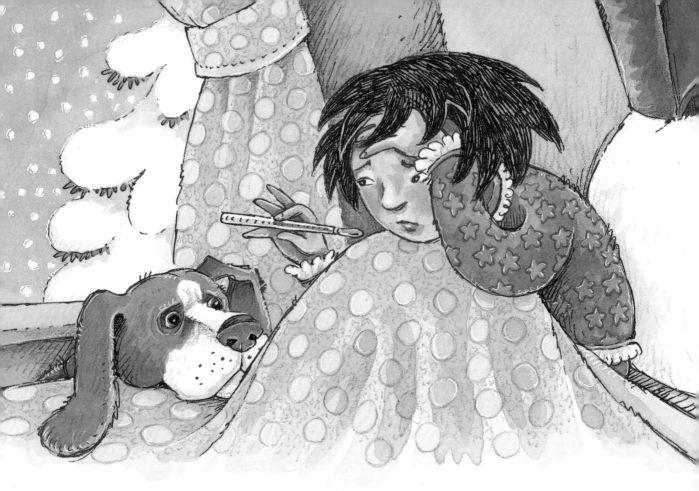

I was hoping that by Monday I could come down with some kind of weird illness that would keep me home. But no such luck!

Monday came and I didn't even have the sniffles. So that's why I'm sitting here in my math class counting the dots on the boy's shirt in front of me.

While Mrs. Marcus is talking about fractions, I'm still trying to think of ways to get out of doing the oral book report.

It's bad enough looking like a fool on my own, but this time I'm part of a team and the grades for our report will depend on *all* of us. What a bummer!

As I head to my next class, I feel like I'm walking into the doctor's office to get a flu shot.

I'm taking a last drink at the water fountain before going into class when Russell calls out to me from down the hall.

"Hey, Mia, are you ready for Ms. Bradshaw's class? You don't look too good! Are you all right?"

I'm thinking that Russell is right. I probably look as lousy as I feel, so why not head upstairs to the nurse's office? It would be easy to fake a stomach ache. Or maybe I could actually throw up.

But if I chicken out today, that just means I'll have to give the report tomorrow, and that really doesn't solve my problem.

So what do I do? Fake a natural disaster or take a deep breath and get the report over with? There's something to be said for getting it over with, even if it means letting my team down.

Meanwhile, Russell's staring at me like he's waiting for me to make up my mind. Do I go into class with him or take the easy way out and head for the nurse's office?

LET'S TALK ABOUT IT...

- What do you think Mia will do? Why? How does it take courage to deal with a problem like this?

- Role-play a time at school that made you or other students worry like Mia did. Show what courage looks and sounds like.

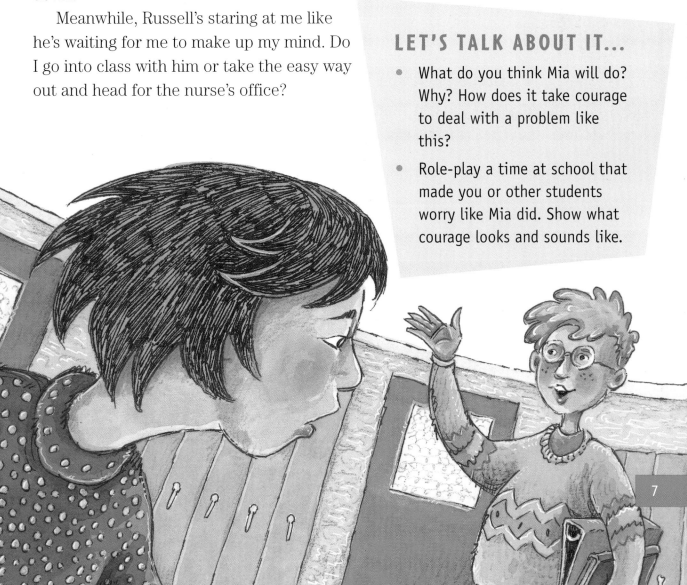

Read About Real-Life Events

Real-life events are true stories that really happened. Think about a real-life event you enjoyed reading about or watching on TV.

- What was it about?
- Why did you like it?
- How was it different from a made-up story?

TALK ABOUT IT!

- Share your real-life event with a partner or a group.
- Talk about where you can find true stories about real-life events.

  Here are some clues.

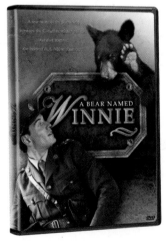

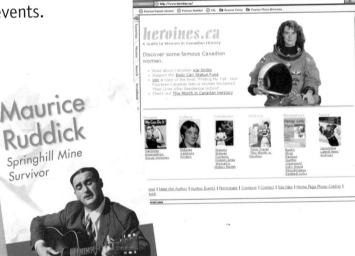

Make a chart together.

True Stories About Real-Life Events

Where you can find them	Examples

Think Like a Reader

Read with a purpose

- Why do you read about real-life events?

Crack the code

Here are some words that can help you read and write about courage. What strategies can help you read them?

▲ determination
dangerous
risking
bravery

Make meaning

Practise using these strategies when you read about real-life events:

PREDICT　　Look at the headings and pictures for clues. What do you predict will happen?

PAUSE AND CHECK　　As you read, think about your predictions. Were you right? Make new predictions about what will happen next.

CONNECT　　Think about how the story relates to what has happened to you in your own life.

Analyze what you read

- Why do you think people write about real-life events?
- Would two people writing about the same event tell the story in the same way? Why or why not?

9

Trapped in Big Beaver

The Accident

James Amell and his family live in Big Beaver, Saskatchewan. One day, James and his sister Neely were sitting in their dad's truck. They were waiting for their dad to fix a tire on a combine in the field. Suddenly, James and his sister heard their dad scream. "Get this thing off of me!" he yelled.

James and Neely ran to see what was wrong. Their dad was pinned under the combine! It had fallen on one of his legs! James and his sister tried to lift it up and free him. But they weren't strong enough. That's when James's dad told James he would have to take the truck and go find help.

James sits in the truck that he drove when he went for help.

James to the Rescue

James knew his dad was right, but he was scared. He had driven the truck in the field back home. But he had never driven the truck by himself—and never on the road.

James climbed up into the driver's seat. He couldn't even reach the pedals. He moved the driver's seat as far forward as he could. Then, he sat on the edge of the seat. Now his feet could reach the pedals.

He started the truck. His dad told him where he would find a neighbour's farmhouse. James drove eight kilometres before he found it. There was no one home! He went back to his father, who told him how to get to another farmhouse. When James found it, this time there were people there who could help him.

PAUSE AND CHECK

How will James rescue his dad?

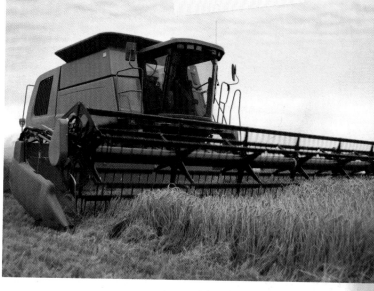

A combine is a farm machine. It is used to harvest grain.

A Hero Is Born

When James and the neighbours got back to the accident scene, they worked together to lift the combine. Then they moved his dad to safety. They also called an ambulance. His dad had a broken leg, but he would be okay.

The story of the eight-year-old who drove a truck to rescue his father was soon on the news. It was on TV, on the Internet, and in newspapers across Canada. James was a hero. His bravery saved the day.

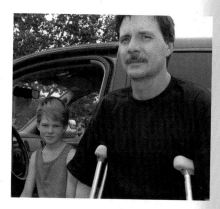

James and his dad after the rescue.

11

CONNECT

How does James's story remind you of other stories you know?

A New Beginning

PREDICT

How might a new student need courage?

Seema (left) plays with a friend in the yard at her school in Hamilton, Ontario.

A New Country, A New School

Seema Mohammad-Essa was starting another school year. How different she felt from her first day at school three years ago!

Seema and her family had escaped from war-torn Afghanistan when she was two years old. Then they lived in Pakistan for five years. She moved to Canada with her mother and brothers in 2003. She was then able to go to school for the very first time.

12

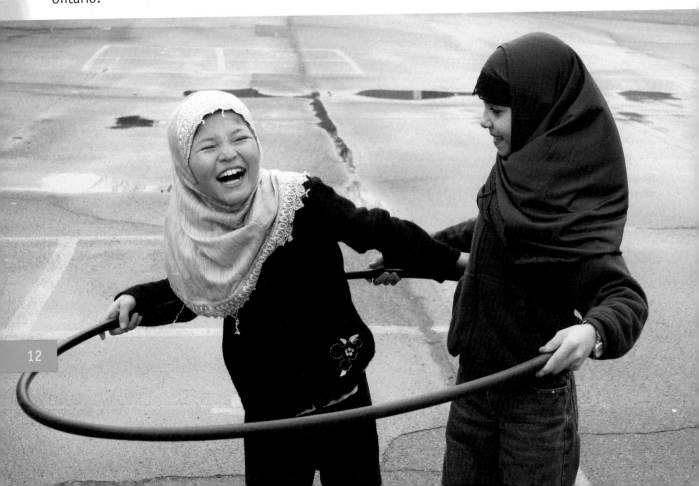

Seema remembered how scared she was on that first day. At recess, she thought that the children playing in the yard were the teachers' children. Everything she saw, did, or heard was so different from what she had known.

Ignoring Fear

The children in her class were all strangers to her. She couldn't talk to them because she didn't know how to speak English. But she decided that she would not let her fear stop her from speaking.

Slowly, Seema began to learn English. She learned the words *go* and *come* from a cartoon. She would put up her hand and say "go" and "come" to the teacher when he called her name. She was proud that she could say words in English. She felt bad, though, when some of the other students stared at her. Still, she kept practising and using new English words.

PAUSE AND CHECK

How will Seema get over being scared?

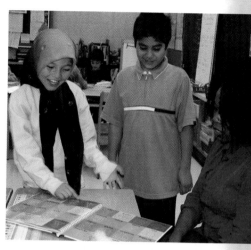

Seema translates for a student who is learning English.

Looking to the Future

Seema has never forgotten how it feels to be at school in a new country. She dreams that one day she will become a police officer. "I could help people when they don't know the language," she says. "I could help them to understand. Then they would feel less afraid as they start their new life in Canada."

Seema and her family immigrated to Canada from Pakistan on May 13, 2003.

CONNECT

How does Seema's story remind you of other stories you know?

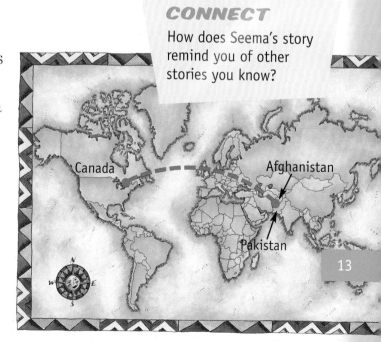

Canada

Afghanistan

Pakistan

13

As Good as Gold

PREDICT

How might an Olympic rower show courage?

Going for Gold

Silken Laumann sat in her **scull** preparing to race. Just ten weeks earlier, she had been rammed by another scull in a training accident. Her leg below the knee was broken so badly that doctors told her she would never row again. But here she was, about to row the race of her life at the Barcelona Summer Olympic Games. Would only four weeks of training before the race be enough to help her win the gold medal?

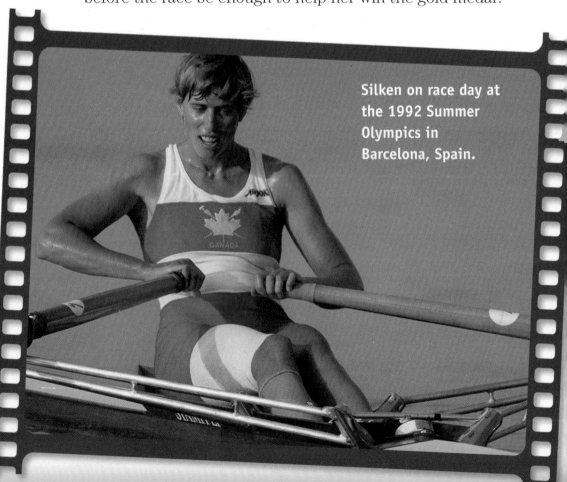

Silken on race day at the 1992 Summer Olympics in Barcelona, Spain.

14

What Is a Single Scull?

A single scull is a rowing frame designed for one person. It is 8.2 m long, and very narrow.

The boat's seat is on wheels that run on tracks. The rower faces backwards, with the seat closest to the rear of the boat.

The rower pushes the seat forward with her legs as she pulls the oars through the water. Repeating this motion makes the boat go quickly.

The Race Begins!

She waited to hear the starting gun. Every muscle in her body was ready to power her scull from the start line to the finish line. The crowd hushed. The Canadian fans watched nervously. Then the shot! All the rowers exploded from the starting gates. The race was underway!

Silken rowed the first half of the race as though she had never been injured. Then, at the halfway mark, she began to feel her lack of fitness. For a moment, she was so tired she didn't even think she could make it to the end. She fell to fourth spot.

An Amazing Comeback

What did she choose to do? Later she would describe it this way: "I went crazy. I just kind of put my oars in the water and gave it everything I could for the last 20, 30 strokes of the race." Her effort made the difference. Silken won a bronze medal.

Laumann may have finished third, but she instantly became a Canadian sporting legend. In Barcelona she showed the world what courage and determination can do.

PAUSE AND CHECK
How do you think the race will end?

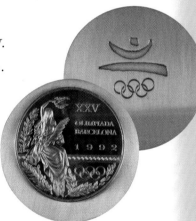

Silken received the bronze medal for single sculls at the 1992 Summer Olympics in Barcelona, Spain.

15

CONNECT
How does Silken's story remind you of other stories you know?

Reflect on Your Reading

You have . . .

- talked about courage.
- read real-life stories about courage.
- explored words and phrases that tell about courage.

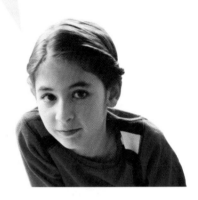

I think courage is when you are scared to do something, but you do it anyway. What do **you** think?

scared

afraid

heroism

determination

believe in yourself

bravery

risking

You have also . . .

- explored different reading strategies.

PREDICT
PAUSE AND CHECK
CONNECT

Write About Learning

Write about one of the strategies you used when you read the selection "Acts of Courage." How did the strategy help you read and understand the selection? Tell how the strategy might help you when you read other kinds of stories.

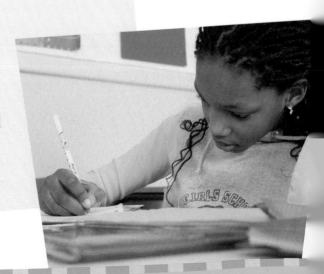

Read Like a Writer

When you were reading "Acts of Courage," you were reading *recounts*. A recount tells a series of events. It is one of the most common forms of talking, writing, and representing.

TALK ABOUT IT!

- What do you notice about the way recounts are written?

- Make a chart to show what you know about recounts. Add to the chart as you read and write more recounts of your own.

HINT!
Look at the **organization** of the information.

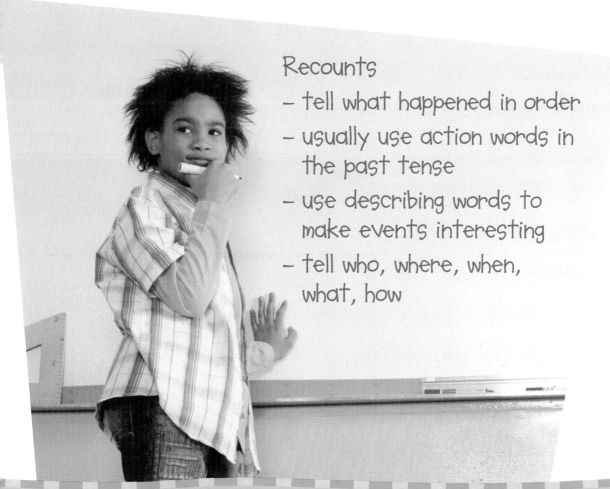

Recounts
- tell what happened in order
- usually use action words in the past tense
- use describing words to make events interesting
- tell who, where, when, what, how

Catch the Dream

by CTV news staff

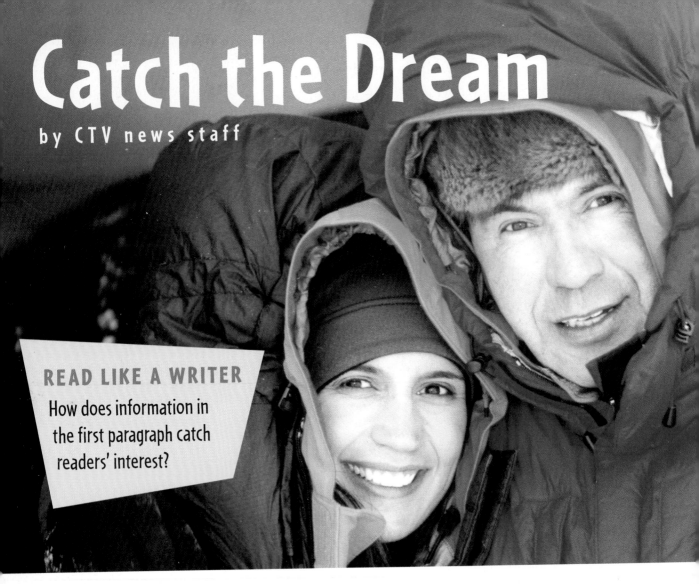

READ LIKE A WRITER

How does information in the first paragraph catch readers' interest?

How could someone catch a dream on a mountain in Africa?

18

A Dream Is Born

It's the roof of Africa. As the highest point on the African continent, Mount Kilimanjaro is considered a sacred place. Half a world away, Wendy Bigcharles and Laurie Gaucher are making plans to climb the mountain. They are Cree from Sucker Creek in northern Alberta. They want to climb the mountain for every Aboriginal child in Canada.

"I think we have to get out there as Aboriginal people and start showing each other what we're capable of doing," says Wendy.

Wendy and Laurie plan to climb the highest mountains on each of the seven continents. Their idea is called "The Ascent of the Aboriginal Spirit." In between each expedition, they will travel around to share their stories with Aboriginal children.

"We want the children to know, 'You can do whatever you want to do. Don't let anybody tell you anything different. Just believe in yourself,'" says Laurie.

Living the Dream

After raising money for the expedition, they head off on their adventure, even though Laurie is recovering from a broken ankle. It will be a gruelling 36-hour journey to the northeastern tip of Tanzania. Wendy and Laurie have two days to adjust to a new time zone, catch up on sleep, and get used to the heat.

They are excited, but still worried about Laurie's ankle. They are also worried about altitude sickness. The lack of oxygen and lower air pressure causes everything from mild headaches to death. Wendy fell ill in South America at 4900 m because of altitude sickness. If she gets sick again, will she be able to push through to the top of the mountain?

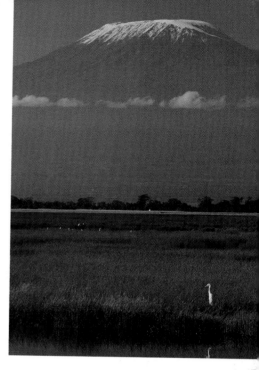

Mount Kilimanjaro's snow-capped peak is 5895 m above sea level.

Mount Kilimanjaro is in northeast Tanzania.

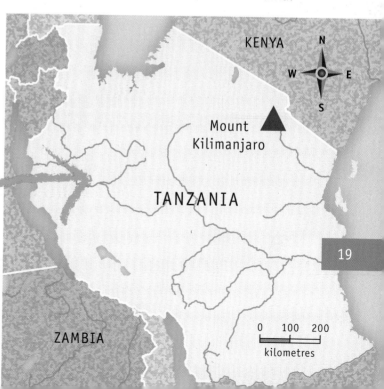

KENYA

N
W · E
S

Mount Kilimanjaro

TANZANIA

ZAMBIA

0   100   200
kilometres

Elevation	5895 m
Location	Tanzania
Latitude	3° 04' S
Longitude	37° 21' E
Best months for climbing	December, January, February, March, June, July, August

DAY ONE

It's late in the day when Wendy and Laurie begin their trip. According to their guide Tom, they have to climb for at least four hours. The temperature is over 35°C.

"I feel it, but it's not hurting. I've got a headache. The heat doesn't agree with me," says Wendy.

It's the end of the first day, which is supposed to be the easiest.

DAY TWO: 2400 m

The second day is like the first, five hours of uphill hiking. Tom decides the group is walking too fast. He will now walk in front and set a slow pace to train the group to walk at high altitude.

DAY THREE: 3400 m

It's another four or five hours of climbing for the group.

DAY FOUR: 4000 m

As the day goes on, both Wendy and Laurie begin to feel the altitude. Wendy can't keep any food or water down. Laurie is also feeling sick and his ankle is hurting. There are only 24 hours to get ready for the final climb.

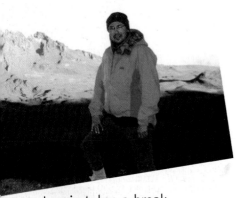

Laurie takes a break on his way up Mount Kilimanjaro.

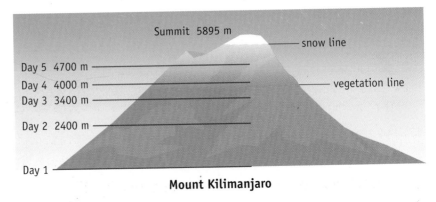

Mount Kilimanjaro

This diagram shows how high Wendy and Laurie were when they began their climb each day.

DAY FIVE: 4700 m

It's summit day on Kilimanjaro. As the day passes, Wendy and Laurie start to get their strength back. By evening, they are both feeling well enough to try and reach the summit. The final ascent begins at midnight.

Just past 5500 m, their worst fear comes true. Laurie collapses and can go no further.

Now Wendy is faced with a hard decision. Does she take Laurie down the mountain? Does she pursue the dream? Wendy doesn't have much time to decide. She's losing body heat every minute. After much soul searching, Wendy decides to go on. As Laurie is helped down, she watches him disappear into the dark.

"By the time I got to the partial summit, at around 5800 m, my lungs were just so tight. There was pain ripping my whole chest. I didn't even have the energy to talk. The last two hours to the summit were excruciating pain," she says.

Despite everything, shortly after 8 a.m. Wendy makes the summit. She can only stay ten minutes because of the altitude. It is just enough time to perform a special task. She scatters some traditional herbs, and says a prayer. The dream is now complete.

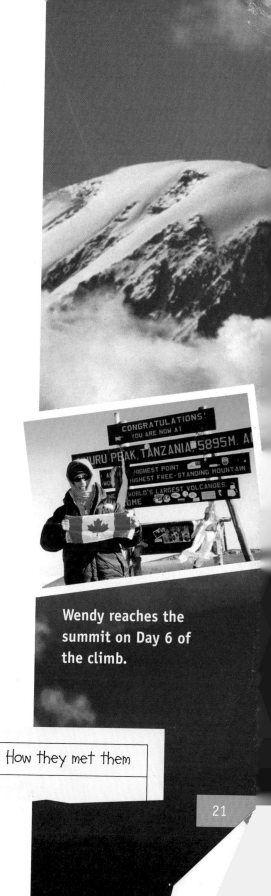

Wendy reaches the summit on Day 6 of the climb.

DIG DEEPER

1. Make a chart. List the challenges that the climbers faced and tell how they met each challenge.

Challenges	How they met them

2. Imagine that you went with the climbers. With a partner, take turns interviewing each other about your experiences and accomplishments.

21

Charlie's Story

by Charles Ecclestone

How did Charlie's courage help him win a battle?

My name is Charles Ecclestone, but I like to be called Charlie. I am ten years old and I live with my Mom and Dad, my younger brother, Steven, and my younger sister, Jennifer. I have a cat, too, called Amber. I like karate, hanging out with friends, swimming, camping, basketball, and phys. ed. class.

When I was three, right after I started Junior Kindergarten, I began to get headaches. Some days I would come home from school and flop down on the couch and not eat any lunch. My parents took me to the doctor because they knew something was wrong. We went many times, and saw many doctors. Most doctors thought I had the flu. One doctor thought I was faking it because I didn't want to go to school! While all this was going on, my brother was born. Only five days after he was born, we found out what was making me sick. I had leukemia.

LEUKEMIA IS HORRIBLE. Leukemia is a cancer of your blood. My bone marrow was making more bad cells than good cells, and the bad cells were crowding out the good ones.

I had to go into the hospital right away to start my treatment, called chemotherapy, or "chemo" for short. I don't remember much about my time in the hospital, but I remember that some of the treatments really hurt!

Chemotherapy is good because it poisons and kills the bad cells. But chemo also makes you feel really sick and it changes the way you look. I became bald, just like my Grandpa John. Once when Grandpa John was staying with me in the hospital, we both looked in the mirror. Two bald heads stared out at us!

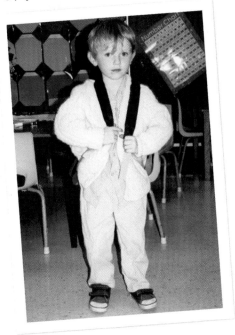

Here I am on my first day of school.

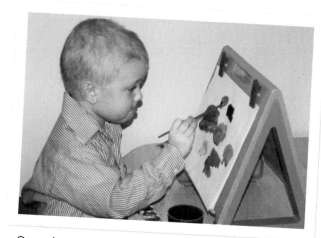

Sometimes I painted at home on the days I couldn't go to school.

23

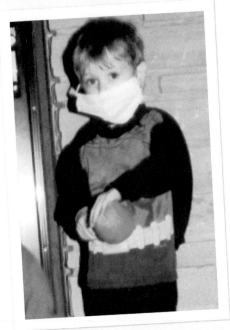

I'm wearing a mask to protect me from germs.

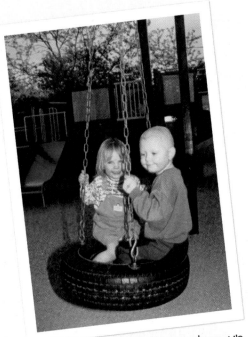

My sister often cheered me up by playing with me.

While I was having chemo, I had to be really careful that I didn't pick up germs from anyone. Sometimes I had to wear a mask if I was going to be around other people. Many days I couldn't go to school. I missed being able to see my friends. In Grade 2, I set a school record for the most days absent—43 days! I still ended up near the top of my class, though.

For almost four years, I went in and out of the hospital, having chemo, blood tests, and needles. Sometimes I just didn't want to have even one more needle! I would scream, kick, and punch. But I would have my treatment anyway. My dad says I was amazingly strong. I always tried to be brave.

I eventually became a kind of celebrity. My picture was in the paper nine times. It was even on the front page! I was interviewed on television three times and on the radio once. There was also an article in a magazine about me. One day I was walking in a parking lot and a woman recognized me from the newspaper!

The Sunshine Foundation is a group that grants wishes to kids who are seriously ill. One day we found out that the Foundation was giving our whole family a holiday at Disney World. We had special passes that meant we didn't have to wait in any line-ups to go on the rides. I even had a private photo shoot with Mickey Mouse!

Every summer, my family and I go to Camp Trillium, a summer camp for kids who have been touched by cancer and their families. Last summer my sister and I went to the camp for eleven days by ourselves. I did a lot of fun stuff like fishing, archery, and swimming. At camp I got to meet other kids from all over Ontario. Some of the kids are fighting cancer. Some of them are the brothers and sisters of kids with cancer.

It's been three years since my last chemo treatment. After my last treatment, my class at school had a huge party to celebrate. We went swimming and watched a movie. The kids in my class gave me cards and gifts. There was pizza, garbage bags stuffed with popcorn, and an amazing cake that had "Nice Going" written on it.

There were lots of fun things to do at Camp Trillium.

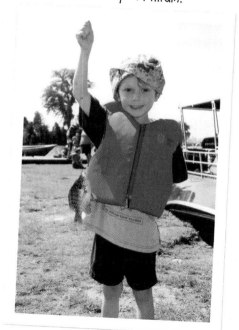

Here is the cake my friends at school gave me.

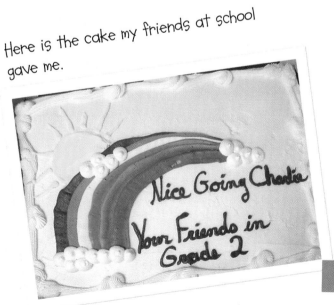

Every few months, I still need to go for blood tests to make sure that the bad cells haven't come back. When I have gone five years without needing any treatment, we are going back to Disney World. I know that in many ways I have been very lucky.

The scar on my chest from where the nurses gave me my medicine reminds me of what I had to go through when I had chemo. I think that going through chemo has made me more mature than most kids my age. I have learned that the little problems that upset some people are not really as important as they seem. I have learned what a bad day *really* is.

When I grow up, I'm going to be a lawyer. Lawyers have to fight hard to win their cases in court. With help from doctors, nurses, and my family, I fought cancer and I won. I think I will be a great lawyer!

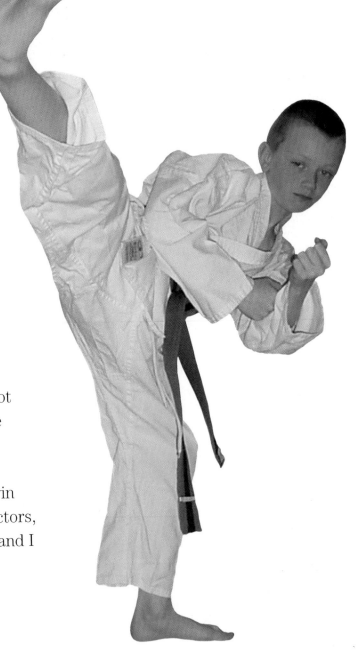

DIG DEEPER

1. Write a letter to Charlie telling him what you learned about courage from his story.

2. Why do you think people who choose stories for newspapers, radio, and TV selected Charlie's story to tell? Why is his story important? Share your ideas in a group.

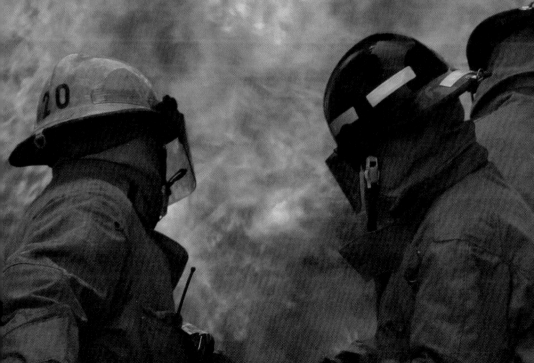

Pictures of
Courage

by Anne Bannerjee

We all have moments in
our lives when we are called
upon to show courage.

How can a photograph tell about courage?

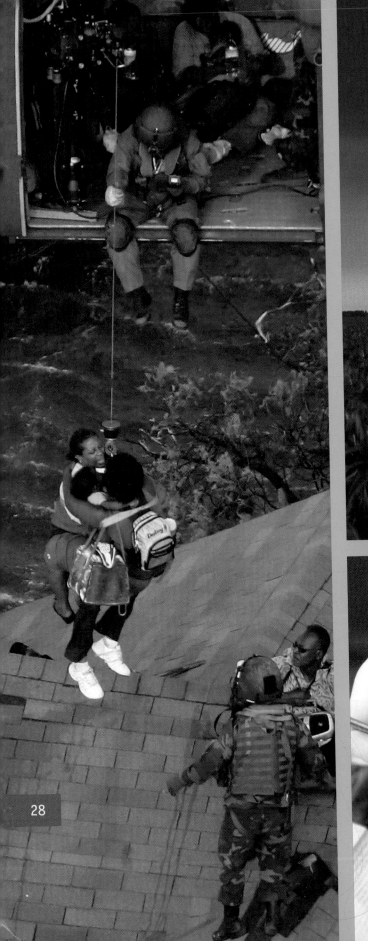

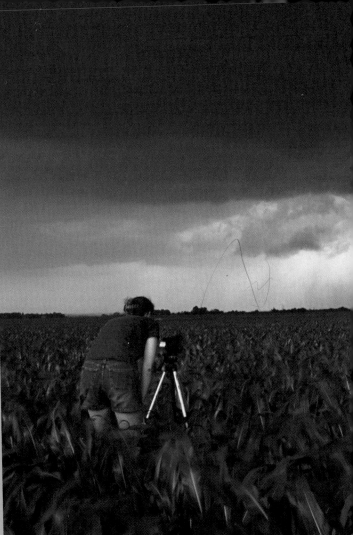

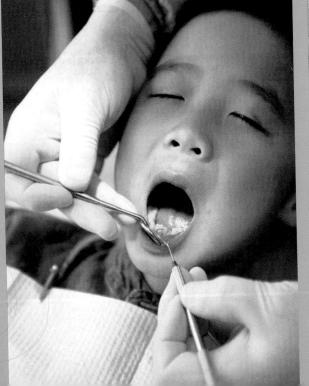

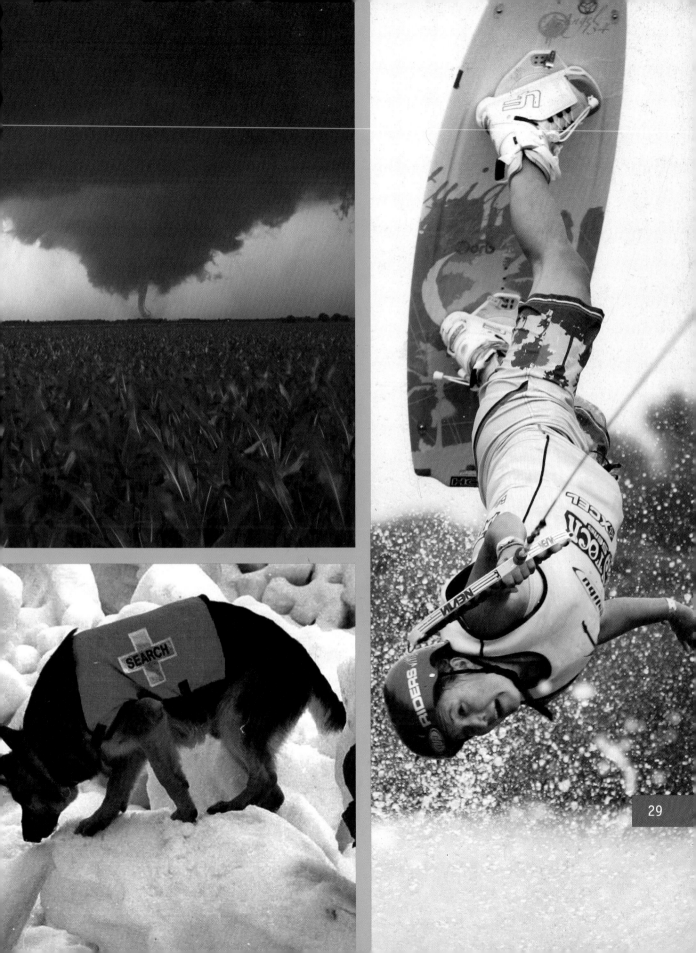

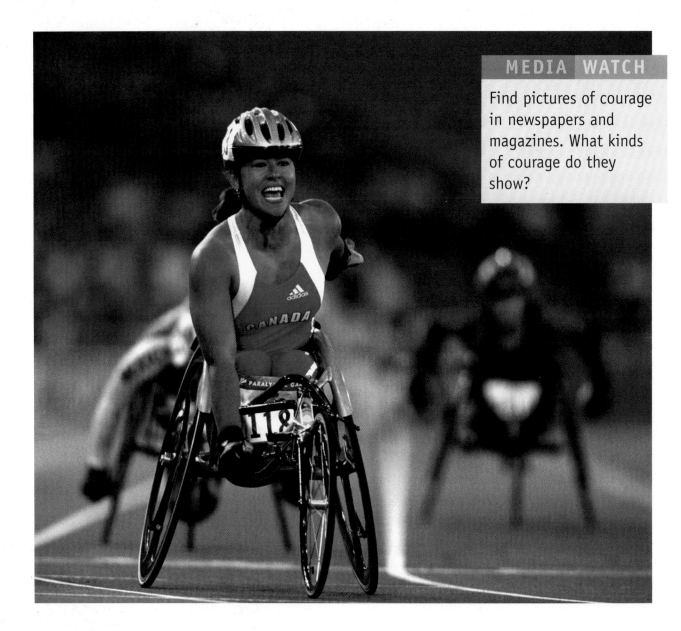

Find pictures of courage in newspapers and magazines. What kinds of courage do they show?

DIG DEEPER ·······································

1. Choose the photograph that has the strongest message about courage for you. Write about how it connects to your life and your ideas.

2. Find a photo that shows courage. The photo can be from home or from a newspaper, magazine, book, or Web site. Write a caption for your photo. Share it with a group.

"PERFECT MAN"

by Troy Wilson

Illustrated by Dean Griffiths

How can you tell
when you've met
a superhero?

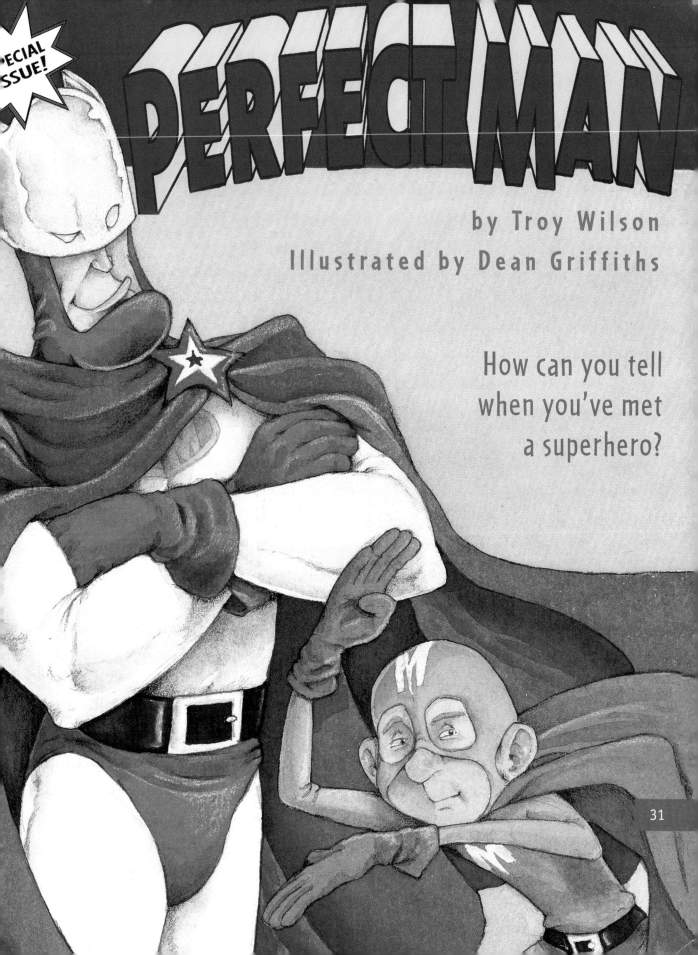

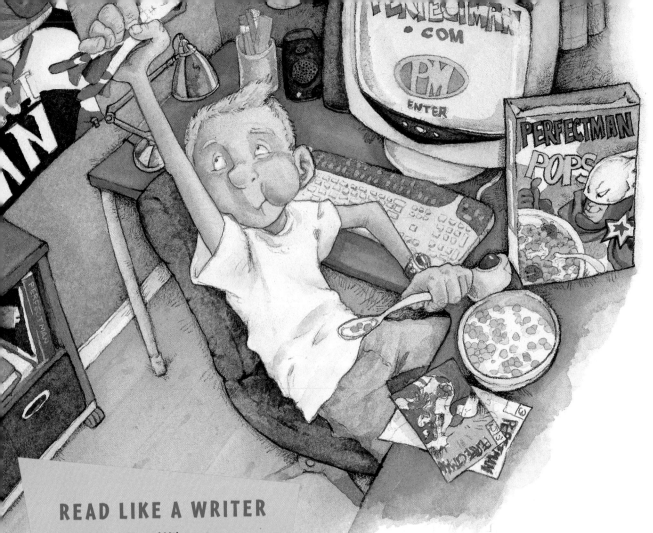

READ LIKE A WRITER

How does Troy Wilson use details to show his readers how much Michael likes Perfect Man?

Michael Maxwell McAllum was the smallest boy in his class. He lived in a small house in a small town on a small street. Sometimes he went on trips with his family.

Perfect Man was the greatest superhero of them all. He lived…well…no one knows where he lived. Sometimes he went to other dimensions.

Michael Maxwell McAllum was Perfect Man's biggest fan.

He covered his walls with Perfect Man posters. He read Perfect Man comics and played Perfect Man video games. He ate Perfect Man cereal and wore Perfect Man T-shirts.

He watched Perfect Man on the six o'clock news. He cut Perfect Man out of the newspaper. He wrote Perfect Man stories. He made a Perfect Man Web site.

Before he went to sleep each night, he turned out his
Perfect Man lamp. He dreamed about Perfect Man.

Perfect Man,

    Perfect Man,

        Perfect Man.

And then Perfect Man quit.

Just like that. He said it was time for a change. He
said it was time to start a new chapter in his life.

"Who will save the world when you're gone?" the
reporters asked.

"I used to be the only superhero around," Perfect
Man said. "These days, it's hard to keep track of them all.
They'll do just fine without me."

"What's your secret identity?"

Perfect Man smiled. "If I told you, it wouldn't be
much of a secret, would it?"

"Where will you go?"

"Someplace quiet," Perfect Man said.

"What will you do?"

"Oh, I'll find something. After
all, there's more than one way
to save the world."

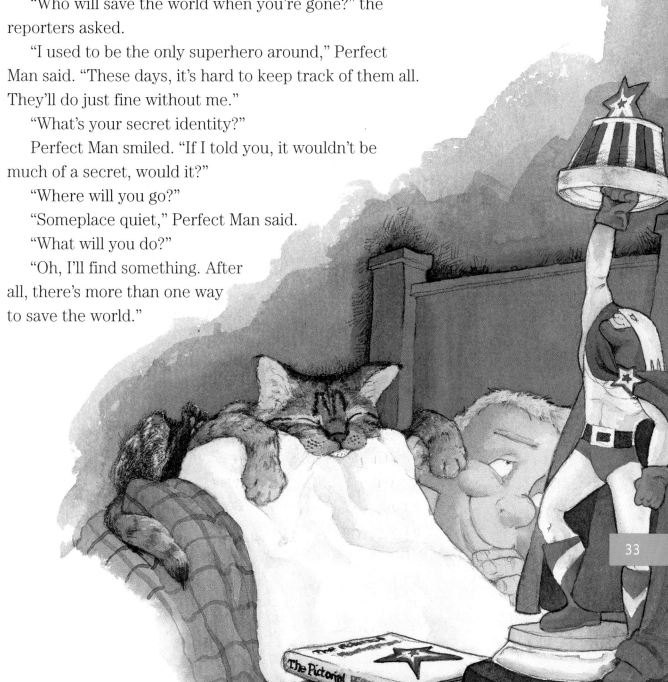

"You must be so sad," Michael's mother said. "You must feel like you've lost your best friend."

She didn't understand. She didn't know Perfect Man like he did. Perfect Man would come back. Just like the time he came back from deep space when he escaped the cosmic pirates. Just like the time he came back from Dimension Z when he beat Zrog the Unbeatable. Just like the time he came back from the dead when he...well...died. He *always* came back. Always.

That summer, Michael Maxwell McAllum watched on TV as aliens invaded New York.

They always invaded New York. They never invaded his small town. The Amazing Five teamed up with the Super Squadron to stop them.

Perfect Man will come back, he thought.

Summer ended.

Michael Maxwell McAllum went back to school.

And Perfect Man came back. Just like that. Perfect Man had changed. Michael didn't recognize him at first. He wasn't wearing his costume anymore. His hair was thinner. His stomach was rounder. He didn't even call himself Perfect Man anymore. He called himself Mr. Clark.

He was Michael Maxwell McAllum's new teacher.

Mr. Clark never broke the chalk. He never lost his temper. And he never got sick.

When Mr. Clark talked about the planets, it seemed as if he had visited them himself.

When there was trouble in the schoolyard, Mr. Clark was there. When Alexander dropped his art project, Mr. Clark was there. He was everywhere at once. At least it seemed that way.

Mr. Clark was the fastest marker in the world. And, best of all, Mr. Clark looked inside people. He saw all the good stuff and helped them bring it out. He helped them find their super powers.

Perfect Man will come back, he thought.

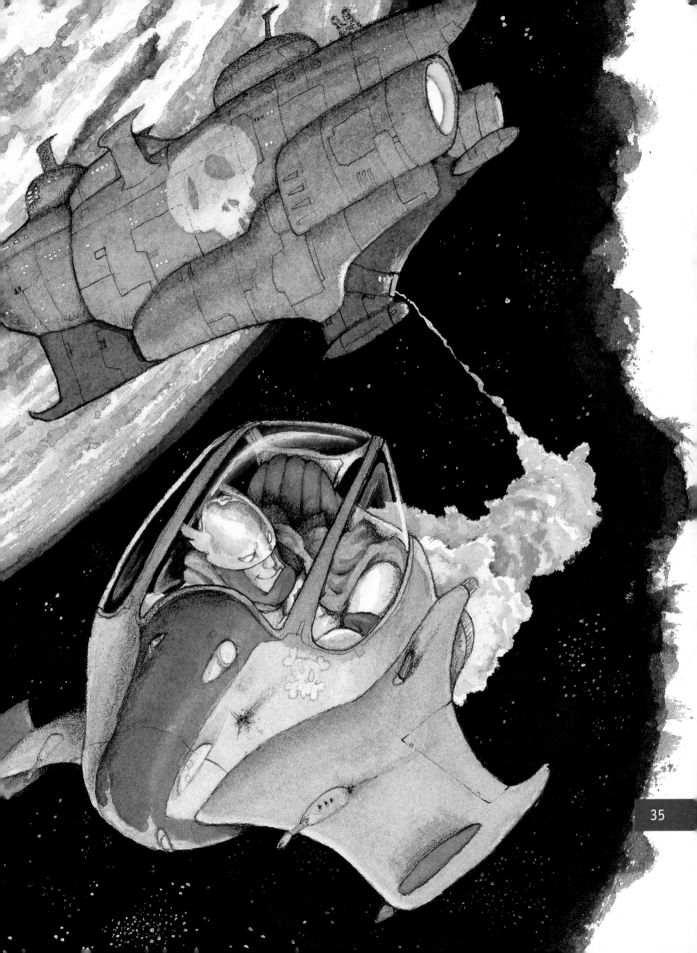

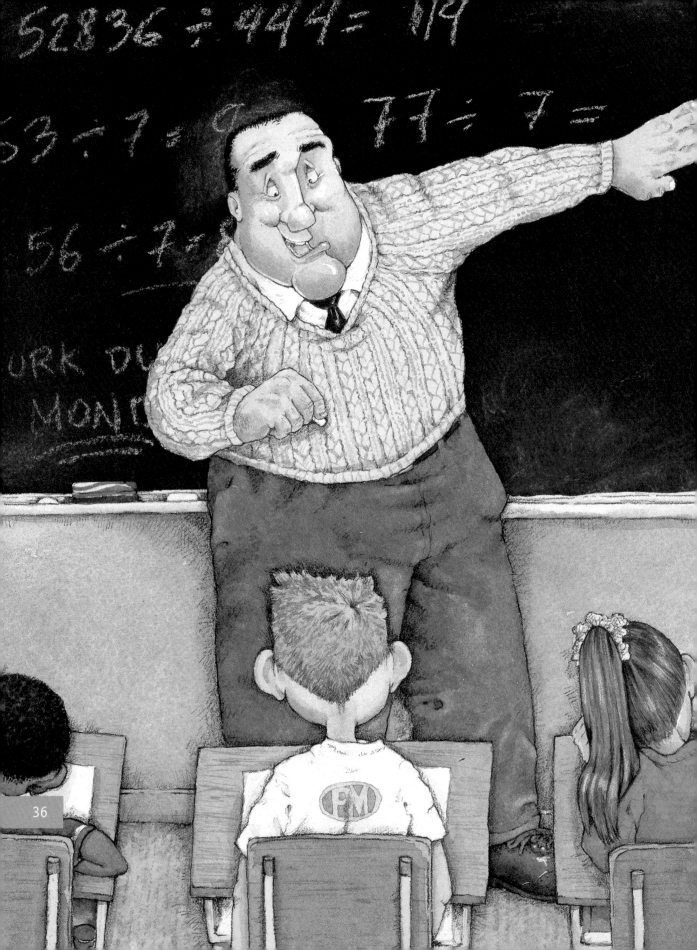

Michael Maxwell McAllum knew Mr. Clark was Perfect Man. He was sure of it. But he didn't post it on his Web site. He didn't tell Mom or Dad. He didn't tell anybody. Instead, he wrote a story about Perfect Man. In the story, Perfect Man became a teacher in a small town. Only one boy suspected his secret. When Perfect Man decided to fight crime again, he made the boy his sidekick.

Michael Maxwell McAllum gave the story to Mr. Clark.

"Well, that's an original story," Mr. Clark said. "It's the best Perfect Man story you've written yet. I think the ending could use a little work, though."

"I know you're Perfect Man," Michael said.

Mr. Clark smiled. "Do I look like Perfect Man?"

"You're disguised," Michael answered. "I remember how you kept Dr. Plasma's shape-changing machine when he went to jail. Or maybe your friend the Dark Avenger helped you out. He's a master of disguises."

"Those are good theories," said Mr. Clark.

"Am I right?" asked Michael.

Mr. Clark didn't say "yes" and he didn't say "no." He said, "If Perfect Man were here today, he'd tell you exactly what I'm telling you now. You don't need to be the sidekick, Michael. You can be the superhero."

"What do you mean?" asked Michael.

"You already have a super power," said Mr. Clark. "You have the power to write. You write very well."

"I guess I write okay…"

"No," Mr. Clark insisted. "You write very well. Do you like to write?"

Michael nodded.

"Then I hope you keep writing," said Mr. Clark. "I really do."

He paused. "Do you want to know a secret, Michael?"

Michael Maxwell McAllum leaned forward. "Yes. Yes, I do."

Only **one** boy suspected his secret.

"To be a good writer, you have to read and you have to write," said Mr. Clark. "But there's another step. A secret step."

"What?" asked Michael. "What is it?"

"You have to live," said Mr. Clark. "You have to try new things. You have to meet new people. That's what good writers do. They live. And it's all research. Every second of it."

Michael leaned back. He thought for a second. Then he said, "I have one question."

"Yes?"

"What does flying feel like?"

Mr. Clark laughed. "Don't you have another story to write?" he said.

Michael Maxwell McAllum did have another story to write. He had a lot of other stories to write. Some of them were wonderful. Some of them were awful. And most were somewhere in between.

He tried new things and met new friends. He made new mistakes.

"It's research," he told himself over and over again. "It's all research."

He grew and he wrote and he lived.

Today Mr. Clark is still a teacher. He loves what he does. Sometimes he thinks about Perfect Man and smiles.

Michael Maxwell McAllum is a best-selling author. He loves what he does.

Mr. Clark is Michael Maxwell McAllum's biggest fan.

MEDIA WATCH

Make a list of superheroes in TV and movies. What do you notice about the people on your list?

DIG DEEPER

1. Create a new secret identity for Perfect Man. Include a sketch. Share your ideas with a group.

2. How would the story be different if Perfect Man were Perfect Woman?

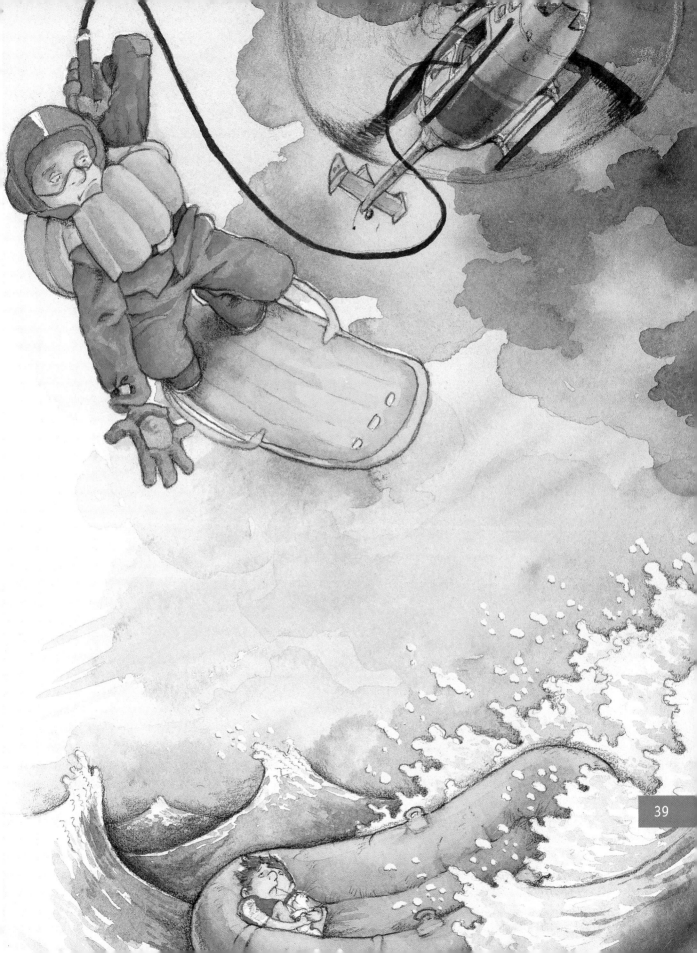

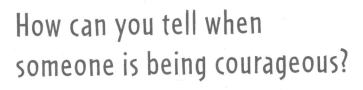

How can you tell when
someone is being courageous?

74th Street

by Myra Cohn Livingston

Hey, this little kid gets roller skates.
She puts them on.
She stands up and almost
flops over backwards.
She sticks out a foot like
she's going somewhere and
falls down and
smacks her hand. She
grabs hold of a step to get up and
sticks out the other foot and
slides about six inches and
falls and
skins her knee.

And then, you know what?

She brushes off the dirt and the
blood and puts some
spit on it and then
sticks out the other foot

again.

Courage

by Emily Hearn

Courage is when you're
allergic to cats and
your new friend says can
you come to her house to
play after school and
stay to dinner then
maybe go skating and
sleep overnight. And,
she adds, you can pet
her small kittens. Oh,
how you ache to. It
takes courage to
say 'no' to all that.

READ LIKE A WRITER

How do the poets use details to give their readers a strong picture of what's happening?

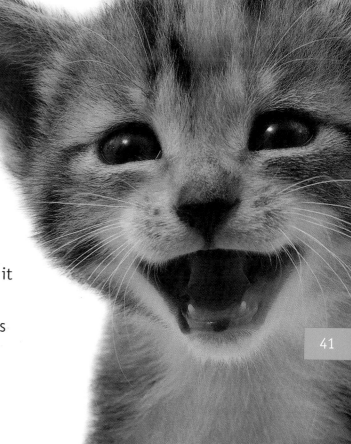

DIG DEEPER

1. With a group, practise reading and presenting one of the poems. Decide who will take each part. You can act it out, or just read the words.

2. Create a cartoon strip with four boxes that shows the story of **one** of the poems. Use speech balloons and thought bubbles.

Writers at Work!

People often get special awards for showing courage.

Think of someone you know who deserves a courage award.

> Jaleen stood up for her brother when everyone was mad at him.

Choose Someone for the Award

- Think about a time when you saw someone show courage. It might be someone in your class, a family member, or even a pet.

- Remember, courage is not always about facing danger. Often, courage is about doing what's right, even when it is hard.

Write About His or Her Courage

- Write the real-life story of his or her act of courage.

- Make a plan to organize your ideas.

- Recount what he or she did.

VOICE

- Show that you care about your topic.

- Include words or ideas that will stick in your readers' minds.

- End your recount by explaining why the person deserves an award for courage.
- Then work with a partner to improve your first draft.
- Remember to put "voice" in your writing.

Design the Award

- What kind of award will you design?
- What pictures or symbols will you use to represent courage? Your award should give people a strong message about courage.

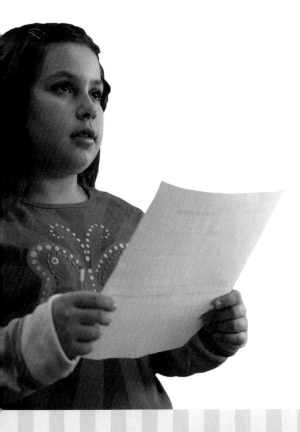

Present the Award

- Think about how you will present your award.
- You could read your writing aloud to him or her, and then present the award.
- Whatever you do, don't forget to congratulate him or her!

43

AKIAK

by Robert J. Blake

How can an
animal show
courage?

44

Day One

Akiak knew it. The other dogs knew it, too.

Some had run it many times and others had never run it at all. But not a dog wanted to be left behind.

It was Iditarod Race Day. Eighteen hundred kilometres of wind, snow, and rugged trail lay ahead, from Anchorage to Nome. Akiak had led the team through seven races and knew the trail better than any dog. She had brought them in fifth, third, and second, but had never won. She was ten years old now. This was her last chance. Now, they must win now.

Crack! The race was under way. One by one, fifty-eight teams took off for Nome.

Day Two

"Come on, old girl, show 'em how," Mick called. "Haw!"

Mick worked the sixteen-dog team through Akiak, calling "Haw!" when she needed the dogs to turn left, and "Gee!" to go right. Mick was the musher, but the team followed the lead dog. The team followed Akiak.

Through steep climbs and dangerous descents, icy waters and confusing trails, Akiak always found the safest and fastest way. She never got lost.

Day Three

Akiak and Squinty, Big Boy and Flinty, Roscoe and the rest of the team pounded across the snow for three days. The dogs were ready to break out, but Mick held them back. There was a right time—but not yet.

High in the Alaskan range they caught up to Willy Ketcham in third place. It was his team that had beaten them by just one minute last year. Following the rules, Willy pulled over and allowed Mick's team to pass.

"That old dog will never make it!" he laughed at Akiak across the biting wind.

"She'll be waiting for you at Nome!" Mick vowed.

READ LIKE A WRITER

Find a part of the story where Robert J. Blake creates strong word pictures. How does he make you see and feel what is happening?

Day Four

High in the Kuskokwim Mountains they passed Tall Tim Broonzy's team and moved into second place. Just after Takotna, Mick's team made its move. They raced by Whistlin' Perry's team to take over first place.

Ketcham made his move, too. His team clung to Mick's like a shadow.

Akiak and her team now had to break trail through deep snow. It was tough going. By the Ophir checkpoint, Akiak was limping. The deep snow had jammed up one of her pawpads and made it sore. Mick tended to her as Ketcham raced by and took first place from them.

"You can't run on that paw, old girl," Mick said to her. "With a day's rest it will heal, but the team can't wait here a day. We've got to go on without you. You'll be flown home."

Roscoe took Akiak's place at lead.

Day Five

By morning most of the other dog teams had passed through the Ophir checkpoint. The wind was building and the pilot was in a hurry to leave. Akiak tore at the leash as the volunteer brought her to the airplane.

"Get that dog in," the pilot hollered. "I want to get out of here before the storm hits!"

Akiak jumped and pulled and snapped. All she wanted was to get back on the trail. To run. To win. Then all at once, the wind gusted, the plane shifted, and Akiak twisted out of the handler's grip. By the time they turned around she was gone.

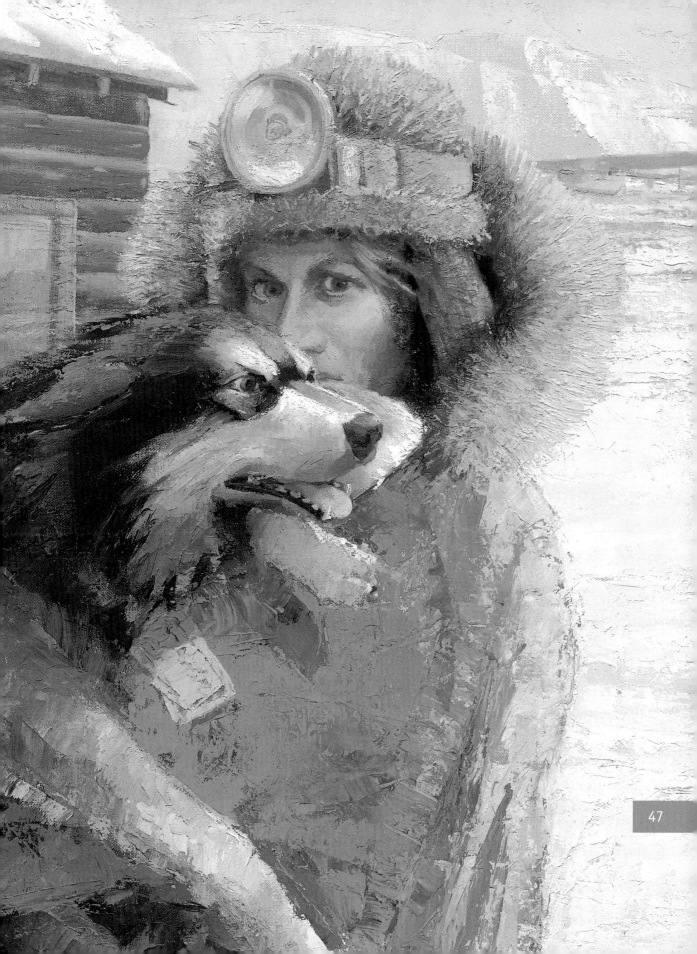

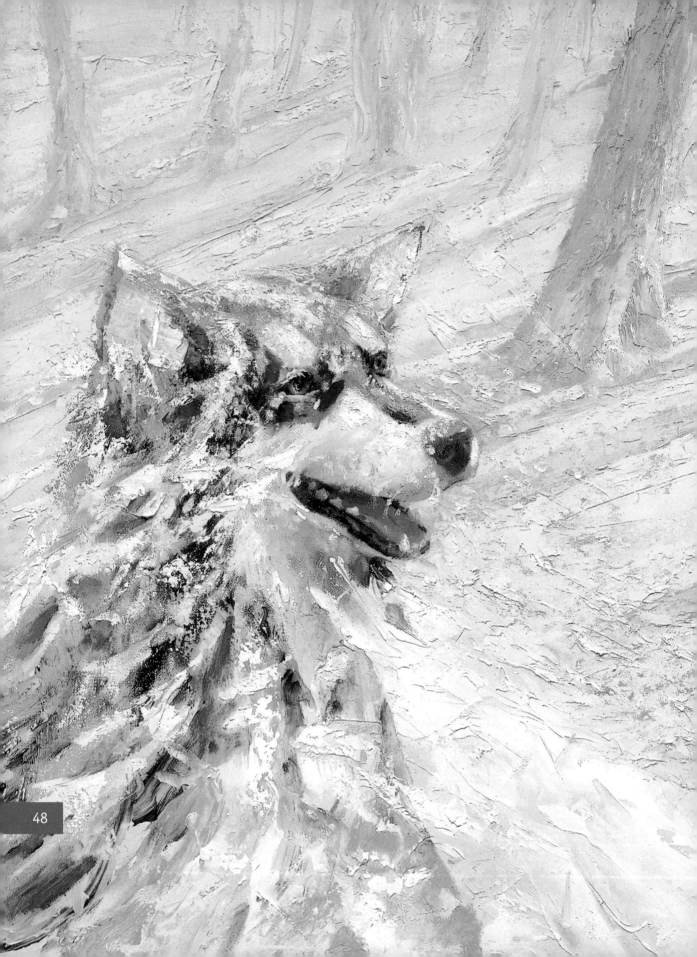

Day Six

Akiak ran while the storm became a blizzard. She knew that Mick and the team were somewhere ahead of her. The wind took away the scent and the snow took away the trail, but still she knew the way. She ran and she ran, until the blizzard became a whiteout. Then she could run no more. While Mick and the team took refuge in Galena, seven hours ahead, Akiak burrowed into a snowdrift to wait out the storm.

In the morning the mound of snow came alive, and out pushed Akiak.

Day Seven

Word had gone out that Akiak was loose. Trail volunteers knew that an experienced lead dog would stick to the trail. They knew she'd have to come through Unalakleet.

She did. Six hours after Mick and the team had left, Akiak padded softly, cautiously, into the checkpoint. Her ears alert, her wet nose sniffed the air. The team had been there, she could tell.

Suddenly, cabin doors flew open. Five volunteers fanned out and tried to grab her. Akiak zigged around their every zag and took off down the trail.

"Call ahead to Shaktoolik!" a man shouted.

Day Eight

At Shaktoolik, Mick dropped two more dogs and raced out, still six hours ahead of Akiak.

Hungry now—it had been two days since she had eaten—Akiak pounded over the packed trail. For thirst, she drank out of the streams, the ice broken through by the sled teams.

She struggled into Shaktoolik in the late afternoon. Three men spotted her and chased her right into the community hall, where some mushers were sleeping. Tables overturned and coffee went flying. Then one musher opened the back door and she escaped.

"Go find them, girl," he whispered.

At Koyuk, Akiak raided the mushers' discard pile for food. No one came after her. At Elim, people put food out for her. Almost everybody was rooting for Akiak to catch her team.

Day Nine

Mick rushed into White Mountain twenty-two minutes behind Ketcham. Here the teams had to take an eight-hour layover to rest before the final dash for Nome. Mick dropped Big Boy and put young Comet in his place. The team was down to eight dogs with 124 kilometres to go.

Akiak pushed on. When her team left White Mountain at 6 P.M., Akiak was running through Golovin, just two hours behind. A crowd lined the trail to watch her run through the town.

Day Ten

Screaming winds threw bitter cold at the team as they fought their way along the coast. Then, halfway to the checkpoint called Safety, they came upon a maze of snowmobile tracks. The lead dogs lost the trail.

Mick squinted through the snow, looking for a sign.

There. Going right. She recognized Ketcham's trail.

"Gee!" she called. Gee—go right.

But the dogs wouldn't go. They wandered about, tangling up the lines. Mick straightened them out and worked the team up the hill. At the top they stopped short. Something was blocking the trail.

"Akiak!" Mick called.

She ran to her usual spot at the harness, waiting to be hooked in.

"Sorry, old girl," Mick hugged her. "Rules say I can't put you back in harness. Get in the sled."

But instead, Akiak circled the lead dogs, pushing them and barking.

"What is it, girl?" Mick asked.

Akiak ran back down the hill.

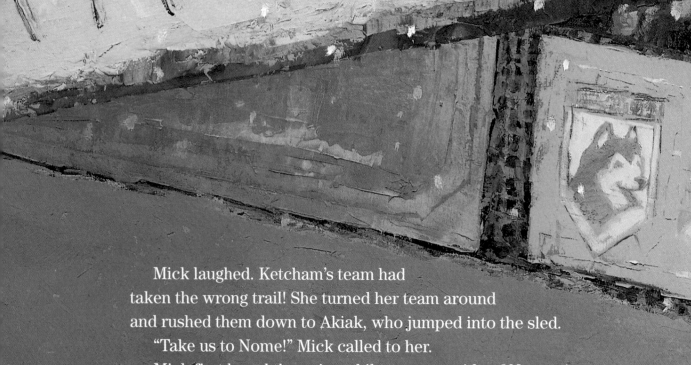

Mick laughed. Ketcham's team had
taken the wrong trail! She turned her team around
and rushed them down to Akiak, who jumped into the sled.

"Take us to Nome!" Mick called to her.

Mick first heard the noise a kilometre outside of Nome. At
first she wasn't sure what it was. It grew so loud that she
couldn't hear the dogs. It was a roar, or a rumble—she was so
tired after ten days of mushing she couldn't tell which. Then
she saw the crowd and she heard their cheers. People had
come from everywhere to see the courageous dog that had
run the Iditarod trail alone.

As sure as if she had been in the lead position, Akiak won
the Iditarod Race.

"Nothing was going to stop this dog from winning," Mick
told the crowd. Akiak knew it.

The other dogs knew it, too.

DIG DEEPER

1. Write "Akiak" in the centre of a page. Make a web of
   words and phrases describing her. Use words in the
   story and others of your own.

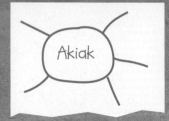

2. With a group, make a list of stories you have read,
   heard, or seen where an animal showed courage.
   Talk about which stories "Akiak" is most like.

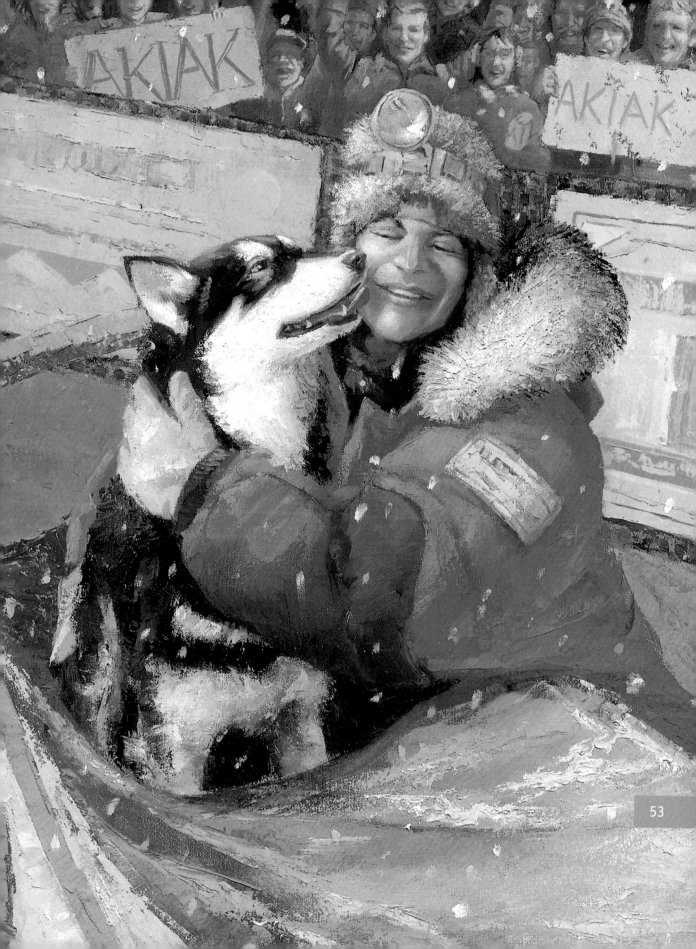

53

Connect and Share

Most people like to tell stories about courage. They share stories at home and at school.

Now it's your turn to share.

Take a story home!

- Choose a story from this unit.
- Practise telling it out loud.
- Tell it to someone you know.

Bring a story back!

- Ask family members to tell you real-life stories of courage.
- The stories can be about people they know or events that happened in the news.
- Choose one story to share with a small group at school.

PLANNING TIPS

- Get the facts right.
- Tell things in order.
- Tell the most important parts.
- Have a beginning, middle, and end.

PRESENTING TIPS

- Practise so you don't forget what to say.
- Talk so everyone can hear.
- Use expression.

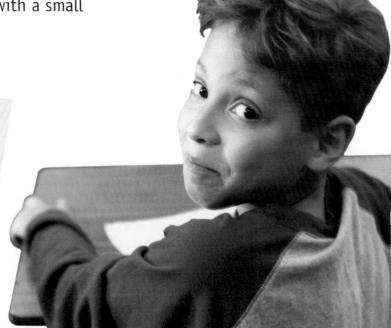

Spotlight on **Learning**

Collect

■ Gather your notebooks, charts, cartoon strip, and other work you did in this unit.

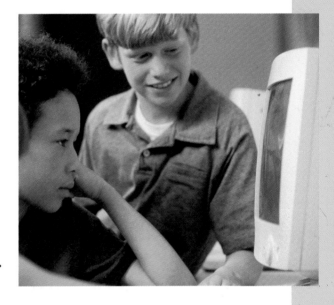

Talk and reflect

Work with a partner.

■ Together, read the Learning Goals on page 2.

■ Talk about how well you met these goals.

■ Look through your work for evidence.

My choices	I want this in my portfolio because...

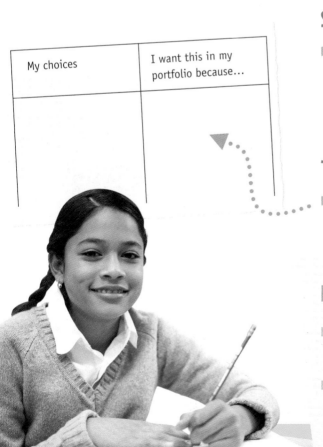

Select

■ Choose two pieces of work that show how you achieved the Learning Goals. (The same piece of work can show more than one goal.)

Tell about your choices

■ Tell what each piece shows about your learning.

Reflect

■ What have you learned about sharing real-life information?

■ What have you discovered about courage?

Get the Message!

LEARNING GOALS

In this unit you will:

- View photographs and illustrations.

- Analyze how messages can be expressed through images.

- Think critically about visual messages.

- Use text and graphics to create strong messages.

56

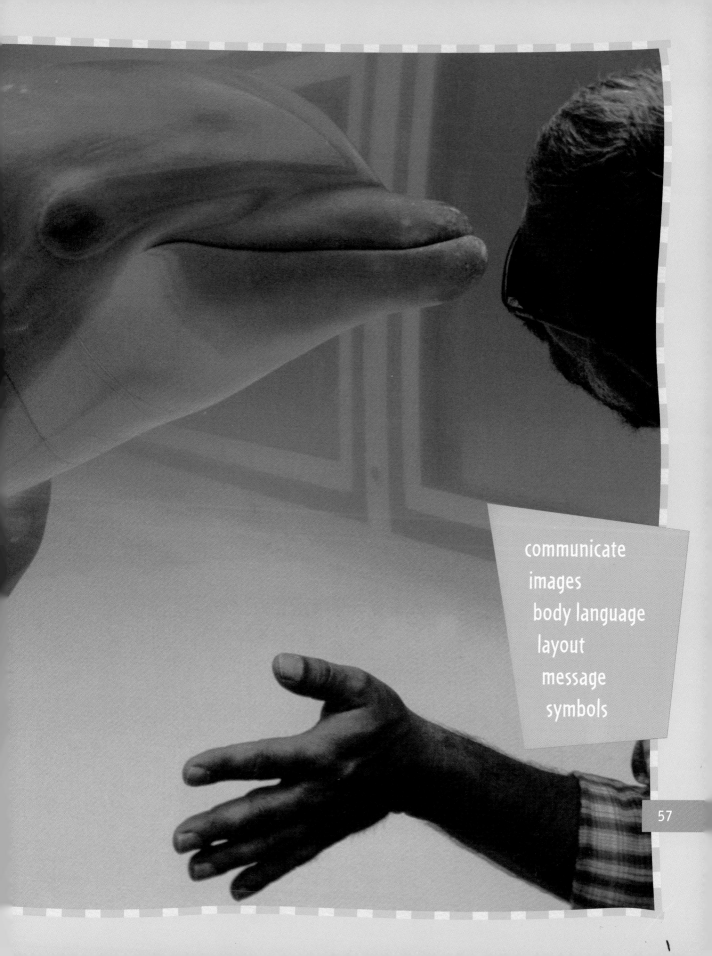

communicate
images
body language
layout
message
symbols

57

WHERE'S THE MESSAGE?

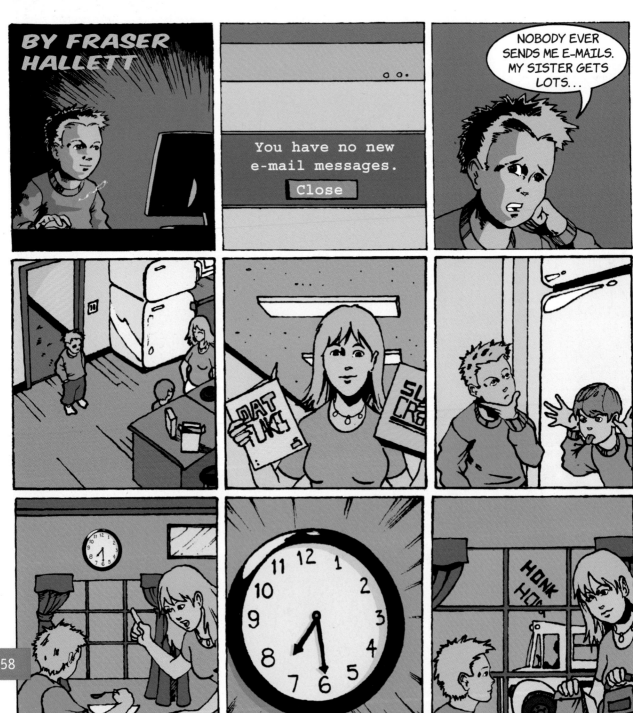

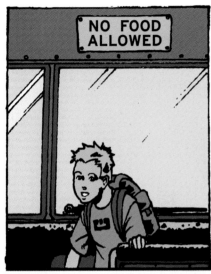

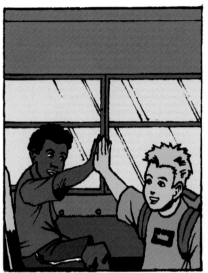

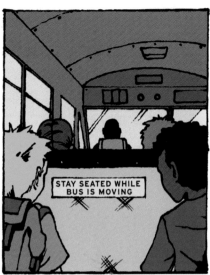

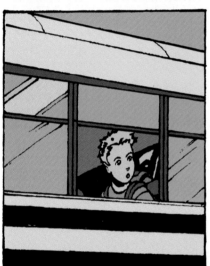

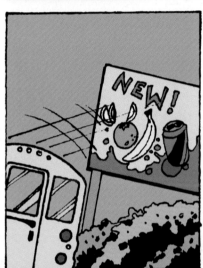

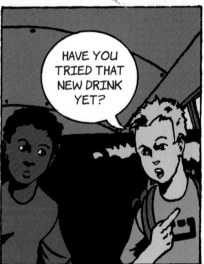

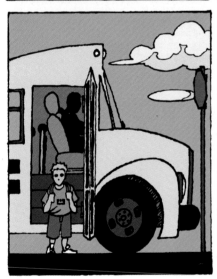

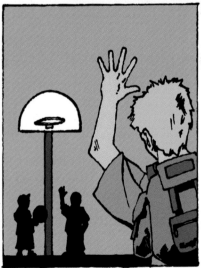

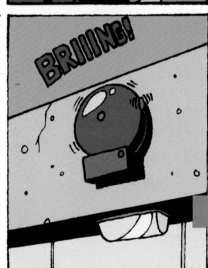

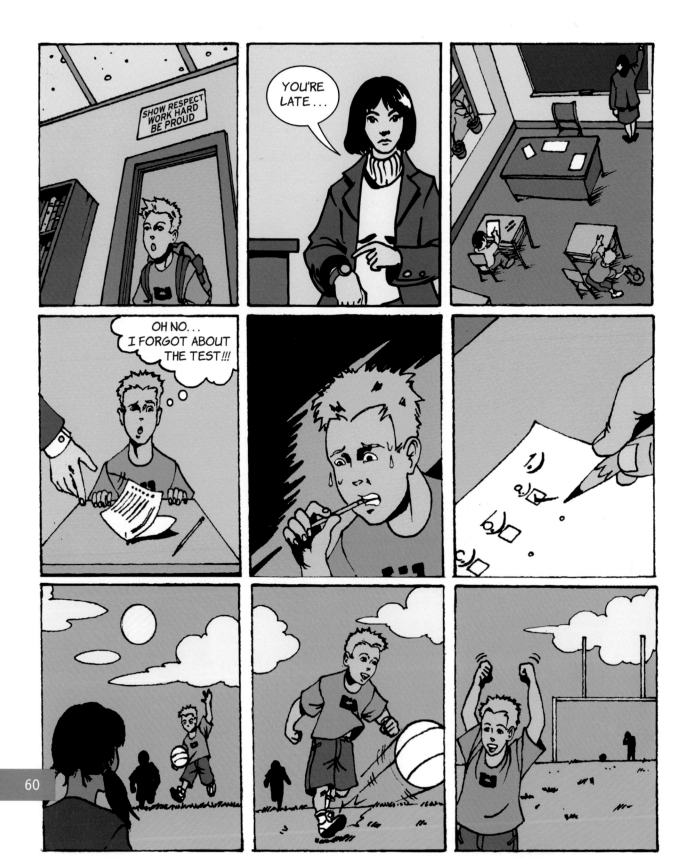

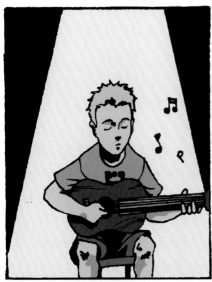

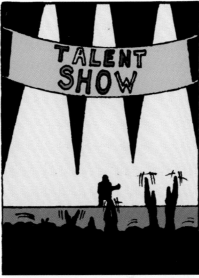

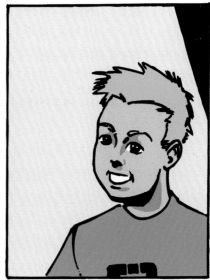

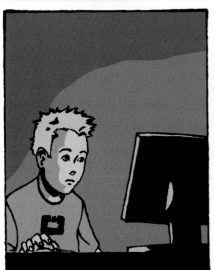

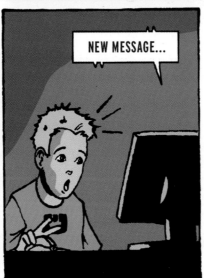

LET'S TALK ABOUT IT...

- Identify all the messages you see in the cartoon strip.

- Which of the messages you see every day are most important to you?

Viewing Messages

Many of the messages we send and receive include both words and images.

Sometimes it is mainly the image that catches our attention. Think about an ad, poster, or video game you have seen.

- What was the message?
- What were the images like?
- How did the images appeal to you?

TALK ABOUT IT!

Work with a partner.

- What kinds of messages do you see around you every day?
- Talk about all the places you find them.

  Make a chart together.

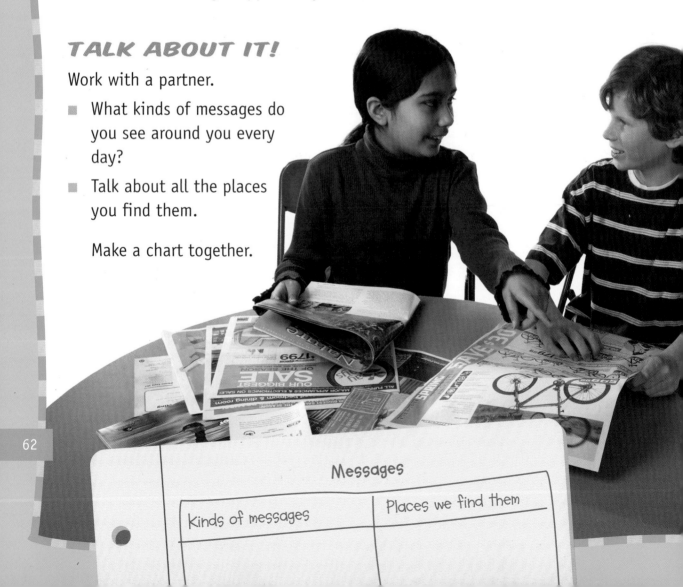

Messages	
Kinds of messages	Places we find them

Think Like a Viewer

- Why do you look at images such as photographs?

Crack the code

Here are some questions that will help you when you look at images.

- What is the first thing you notice? What does it tell you about the message?
- How did the photographers make their work interesting?

Make meaning

Practise using these strategies when you view images:

USE WHAT YOU KNOW	Ask yourself if the image reminds you of anything you have seen before.
DECIDE WHAT'S IMPORTANT	Ask yourself which parts are most important. What does the photographer want you to notice?
EVALUATE	Think about the message you see and how the photographer or artist helped you to find it.

Analyze what you see

- How do people use images to change their audience's point of view or feelings?

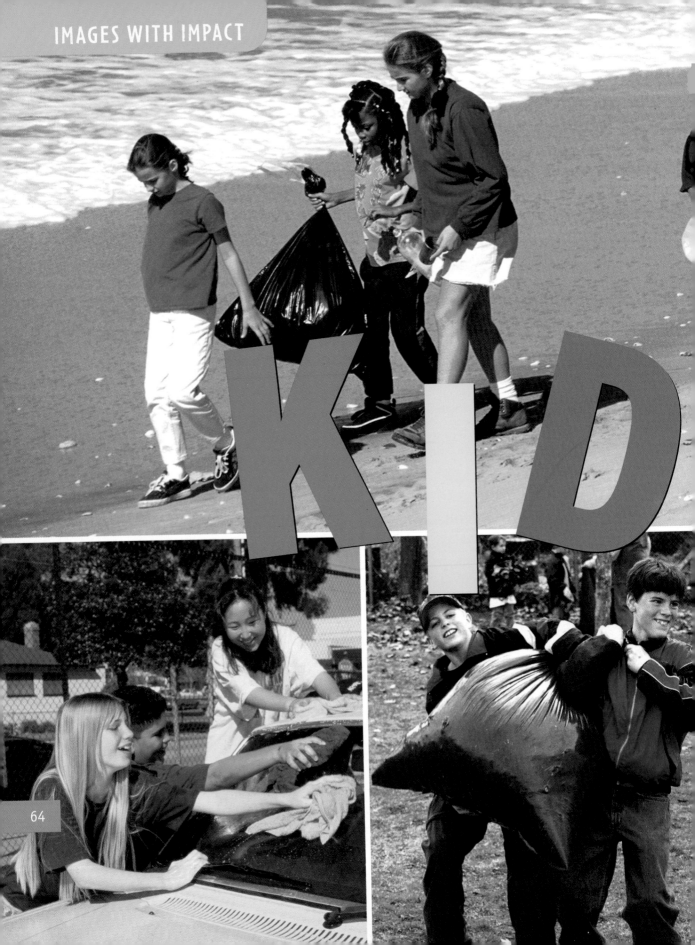

KID

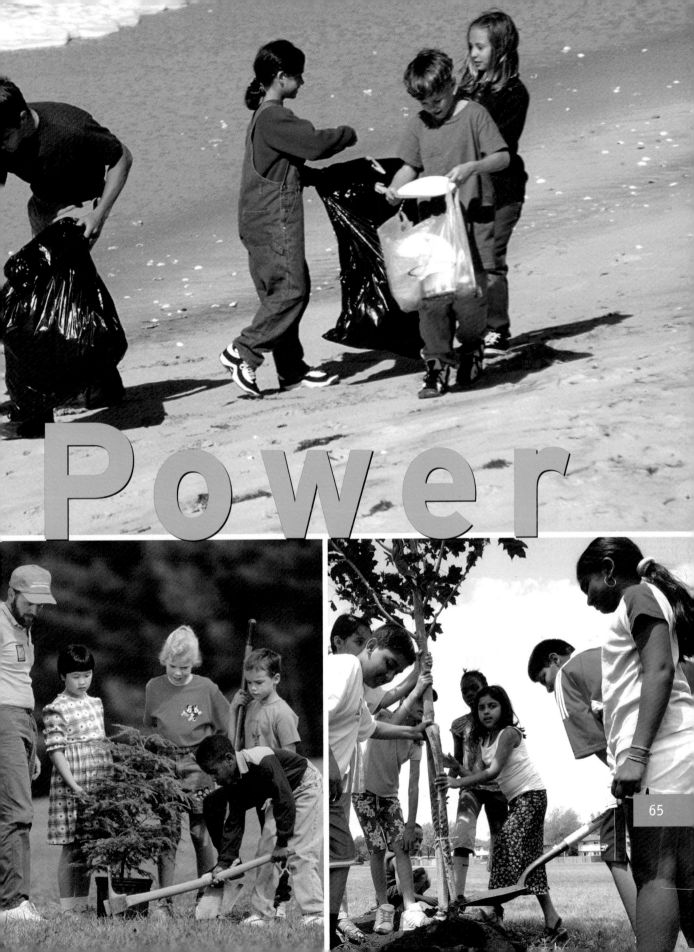

Power

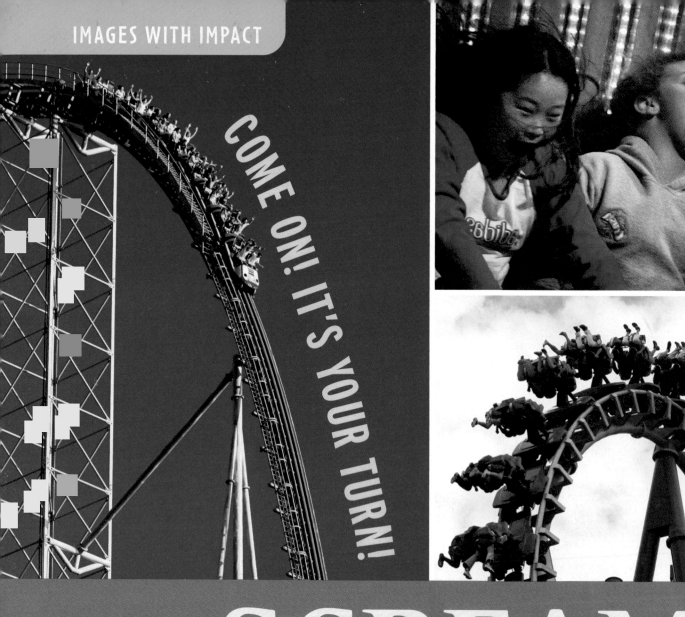

COME ON! IT'S YOUR TURN!

Canada's SCREAM

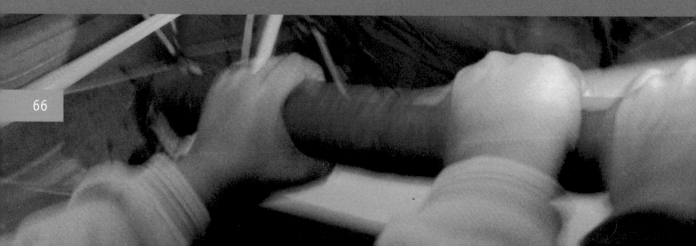

66

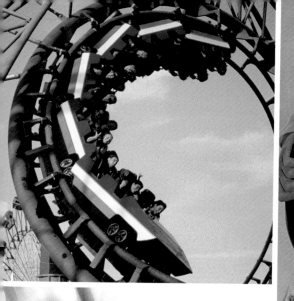
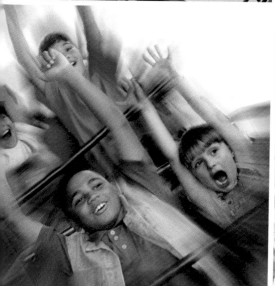
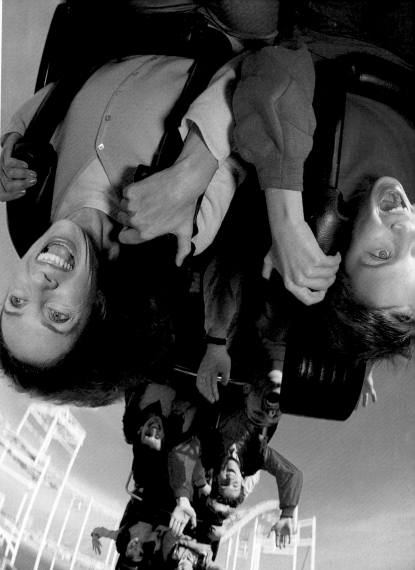

MACHINES

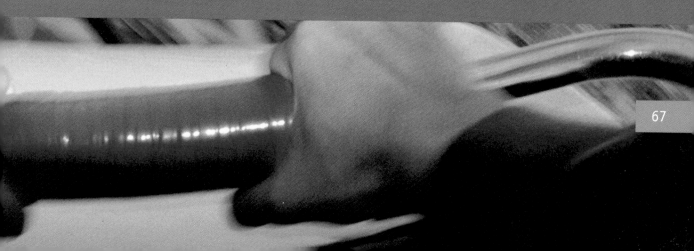

TOTAL

PLEASE
HELP US!
1-PEOPLE
1-DOG
1-CAT

68

DISASTER!

HURRICANE KATRINA HITS HARD

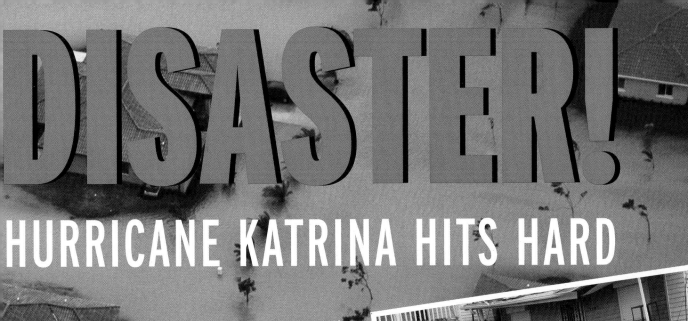

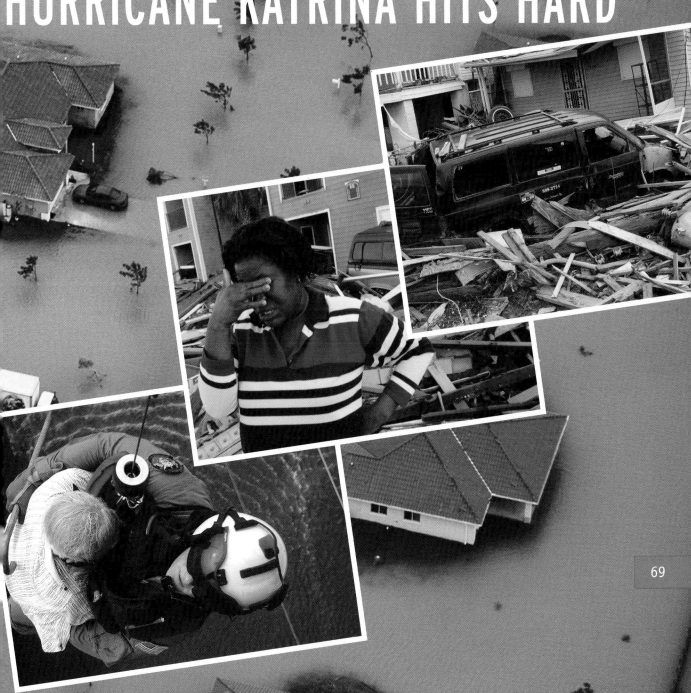

Reflect on Your Reading

You have . . .

- talked about messages.
- noticed how photographers use different kinds of camera shots.
- learned new vocabulary about viewing photographs.

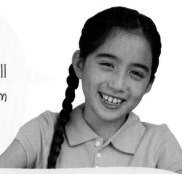

I liked the close-up of the kids in the roller coaster car. You could tell how they were feeling from the expressions on their faces.

I liked the photos that showed kids helping in their communities. Even little kids can do their part.

layout

images

message

communicate

body language

symbols

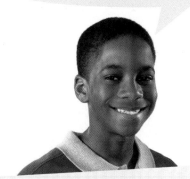

You have also . . .

- explored different viewing strategies.

USE WHAT YOU KNOW

DECIDE WHAT'S IMPORTANT

EVALUATE

Write About Learning

Write about one of the strategies you used to view and understand the poster. How did the strategy help you figure out the message? How could you use that strategy when you view other images?

View Like a Photographer

When you were looking at "Images with Impact," you were viewing posters. Posters combine pictures, shapes, and words in different ways.

TALK ABOUT IT!

- What do you notice about the way the posters are set up?
- Make a chart to show what you know about poster design.

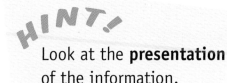

HINT!
Look at the **presentation** of the information.

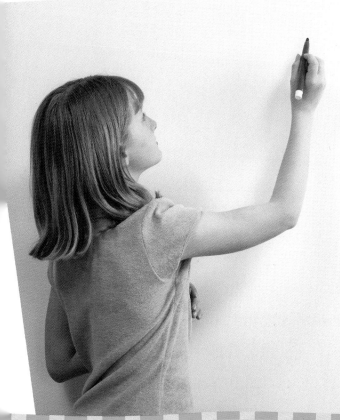

Posters
- have a large title
- have one or more photographs
- try to make you look at the most important thing first
- have some close-ups
- show parts of the message in every photograph

71

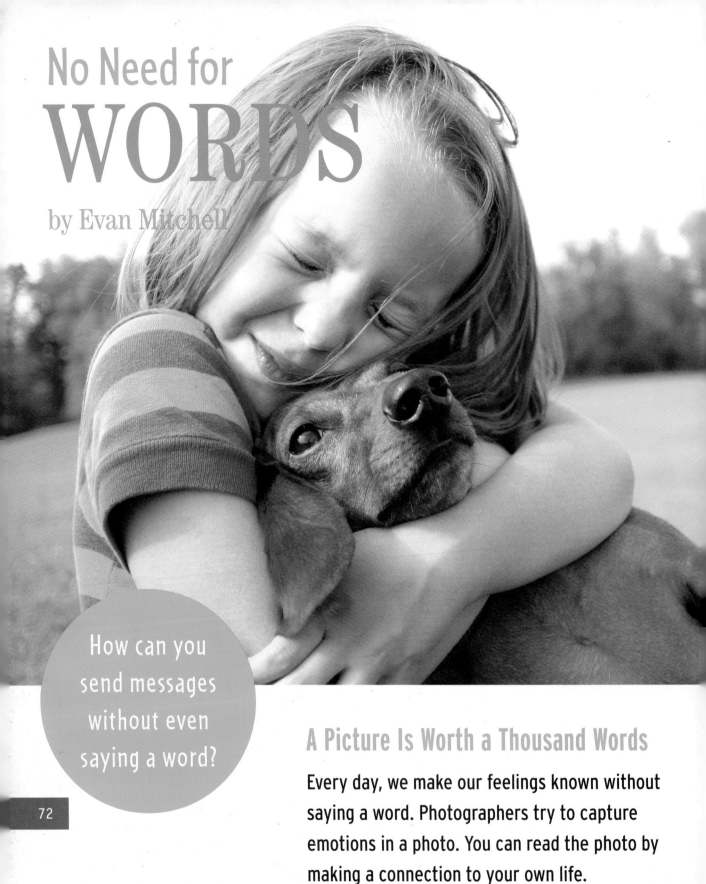

No Need for
WORDS
by Evan Mitchell

How can you send messages without even saying a word?

A Picture Is Worth a Thousand Words

Every day, we make our feelings known without saying a word. Photographers try to capture emotions in a photo. You can read the photo by making a connection to your own life.

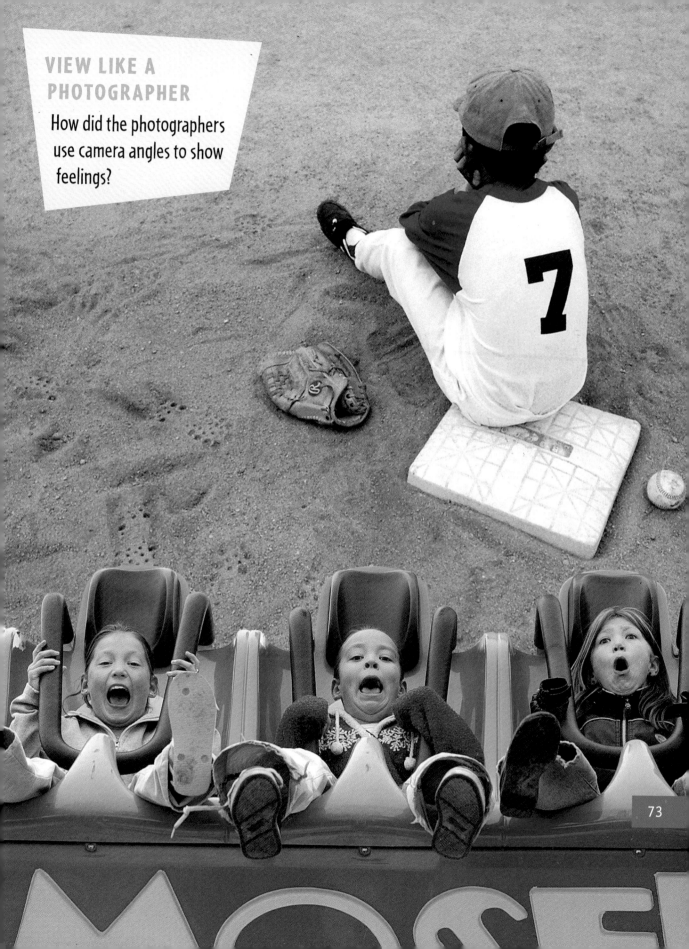

VIEW LIKE A PHOTOGRAPHER

How did the photographers use camera angles to show feelings?

73

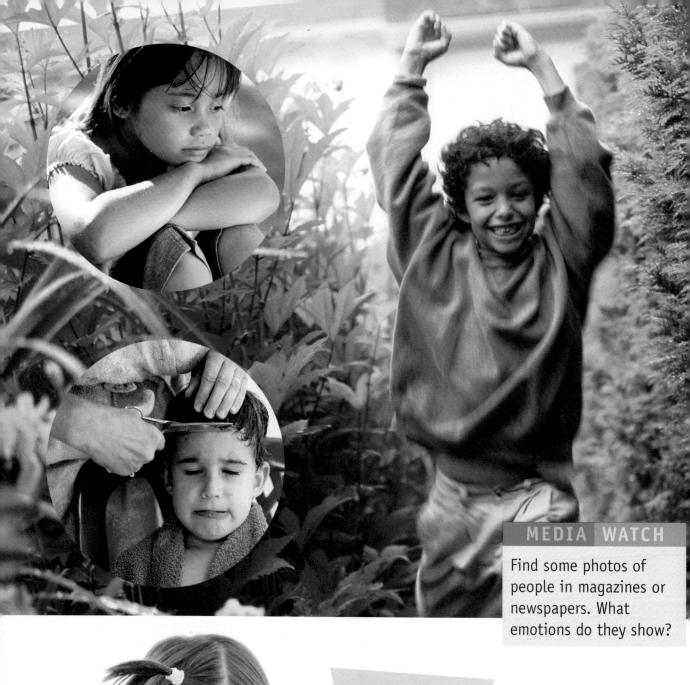

MEDIA WATCH

Find some photos of people in magazines or newspapers. What emotions do they show?

DIG DEEPER ....

1. Suggest captions for these pictures. Explain why they are good captions.

2. With a partner, take turns silently acting out (miming) one of the expressions shown in the photos. Try to guess which photo your partner is acting out.

TRICKY PICS

How can you tell if a photo has been changed?

by Jamie Kiffel

When would a cat stick out its tongue at you? When it's an April Fool joke! The secret to that funny face on the right is called *photo manipulation*.

First the artist photographed Roswell the cat many times. Then he used computer tools to place images of the cat's paws onto its body—and its mouth. (It's like how you would make a photo collage.) But the tricky part was just getting the cat to open his mouth. "We needed a cat that meowed a lot," photographer John Lund says. "Luckily Roswell is a talker!" A computer tool stretched the image of the cat's mouth even more. The result? One funny photo!

Bad to the Bone

The goggles never actually touched the real dogs' faces in this image. Photographer John Lund first took pictures of a human wearing them. Then he erased the human face using a computer and placed the goggles on the dogs.

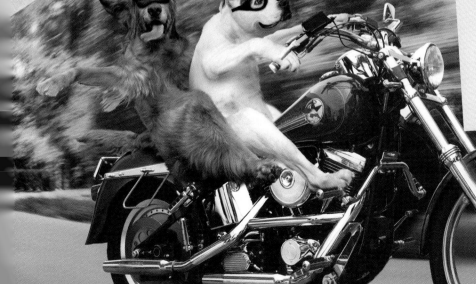

Eye DON'T Believe It

With computer programs such as Photoshop, just about anyone can change photographs. Digital artists use all sorts of tools and techniques. "Liquefying" tools help stretch smiles and bodies. A "radial zoom" effect blurs images so they look as if they are moving.

One of the most common techniques involves "cutting and pasting." Artists cut out part of one photo and paste it onto another. (That's how many of the images shown on these pages were created.)

Police use this technique to paste different hairdos on criminals to see how the bad guys may have disguised themselves. Magazine editors can even use it to alter how a model looks by changing things like eye colour.

Most manipulated photos are harmless. But sometimes people will change images to mislead you. One university digitally erased an athlete from a game photo. This player had been dropped from the team for getting into trouble. Some wondered if the school was trying to make people forget what had happened. The picture made it seem as if the athlete had never been on the team.

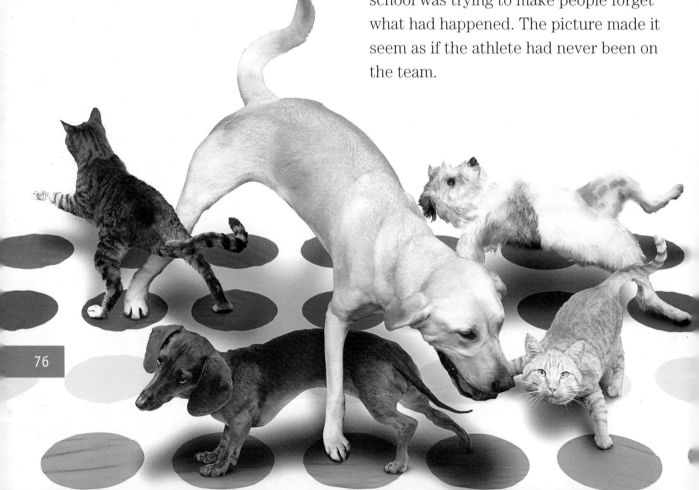

DON'T Be Fooled!

If something looks unbelievable, it probably is. Here are other clues that the picture you're looking at may not be what you think.

Out-of-Scale Images Ever seen a dog-size motorcycle? Doubtful. The dogs in the photo on page 75 had to be digitally adjusted to fit the bike.

Fuzzy Outlines "One giveaway is when some objects are fuzzy around the edges and others aren't," says digital artist Ryan Obermeyer.

Changes in Lighting Say a cat in the picture looks bright, but the background looks dim. That cat may have been pasted in.

Repeating Patterns "I was looking at a DVD cover recently," Obermeyer says. "The photo had a sidewalk made of stones, but several of the stone patterns were repeated over and over." That would not happen in real life.

Weird Shadows Are all the shadows going in different ways? Are some missing? Then the image is probably a fake.

Look for these clues—as well as some other silly secrets—in our roundup of funny photos that are not what they seem. At least in most of these cases, you *know* that seeing is not believing!

VIEW LIKE A PHOTOGRAPHER
How do the photographs help readers understand the information about tricky pics?

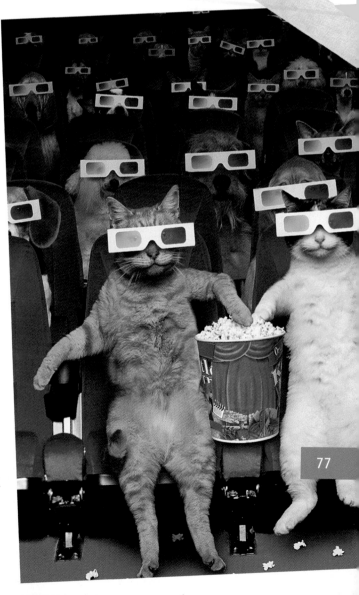

77

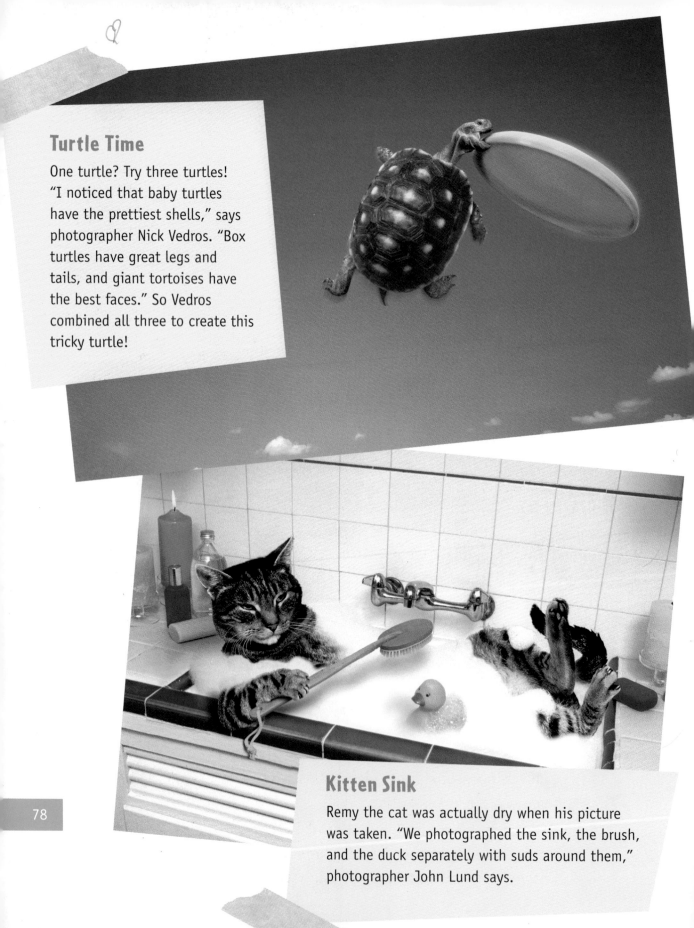

Turtle Time

One turtle? Try three turtles!
"I noticed that baby turtles
have the prettiest shells," says
photographer Nick Vedros. "Box
turtles have great legs and
tails, and giant tortoises have
the best faces." So Vedros
combined all three to create this
tricky turtle!

Kitten Sink

Remy the cat was actually dry when his picture
was taken. "We photographed the sink, the brush,
and the duck separately with suds around them,"
photographer John Lund says.

Something's Fishy!

Surprise! This photo is for real. "I was sport fishing with a man who brought his pet iguana," says photographer Bill Curtsinger. "The iguana climbed up the fishing pole to get a better view. It looked like he was fishing, so...." Curtsinger grabbed a camera for this real photo. It fools just about everyone.

Big Rig

"We sat the elephant on a circus stool at a studio where cars are usually photographed," says photographer Bob Elsdale. Why? It was the only studio with a big enough door! The car is actually a toy photographed at a beach.

DIG DEEPER

1. Choose one of the tricky pics. List the clues that tell you it is not a real picture.
2. Should the media have to tell us when they use a photo that is not real? Record your opinion. Give convincing reasons to support your view.

Designers at Work!

Designers are often inspired by images that have a message. A poster is one way to present these types of images.

Plan a Poster

Choose a message.

- Brainstorm messages you might display on a poster.
- Make a web to show your ideas.

Choose the images.

Find images that do the best job of telling your message.

- What images will catch your viewers' attention?
- Do you want images that show low angles and close-ups?

IDEAS TO TRY

- Think about what a poster could say about health, your community, or another topic or issue you care about.

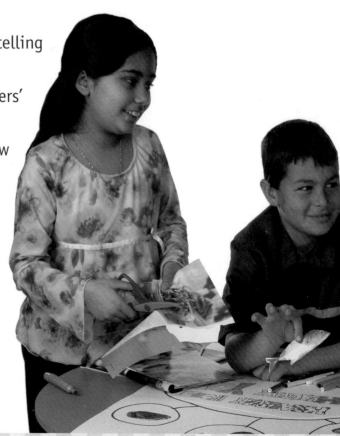

HINT!

You might want to make a sketch of how the images might be placed.

Design the layout.

- ■ Try different ways of laying out the images.
- ■ What do you want viewers to look at first?
- ■ What lettering will you use for your title?

Make the Poster

- ■ Glue the images on the poster.
- ■ Decide on a title for the poster. Think about how big the title will be and the colours you will use.

Create a Poster Gallery

- ■ Set up a class gallery of posters.
- ■ Organize a gallery walk and invite other classes to come and view the posters you have created.

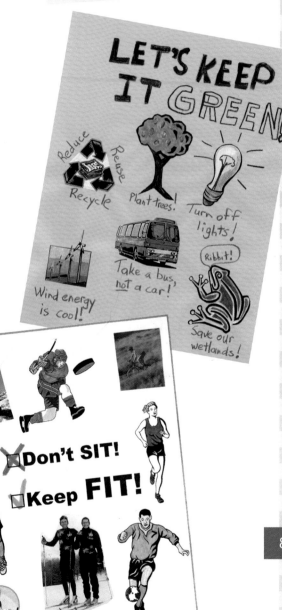

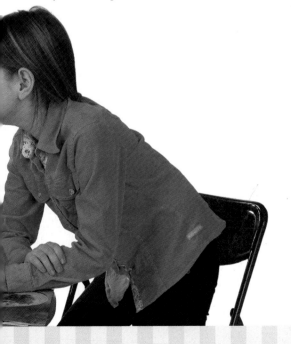

81

MESSAGES IN
STONE

by Mary Wallace

How can you make a message that will last for years to come?

An inuksuk (ee-nook-sook) is a stone marker that can give important information to an Arctic traveller. Three or more of these markers are called inuksuit (ee-nook-sweet). Inuksuit are found throughout the Arctic areas of Alaska, Arctic Canada, and Greenland. Inuksuit have been used by the Inuit to act in place of human messengers. For those who understand their forms, inuksuit can show direction, tell about a good hunting or fishing area, show where food is stored, indicate a good resting area, or act as a message centre.

Every inuksuk is unique because it is built from the stones at hand. An inuksuk is a strong connection to the land: it is built on the land, it is made of the land, and it tells about the land.

Here are some inuksuit. Their names are written in Inuktitut (Ee-nook-tee-toot), the language of the Inuit. Look on page 85 to learn what message each inuksuk is giving.

VIEW LIKE AN ARTIST

How does the artist show the beauty of the inuksuit and the vast landscape?

83

ᐃᓄᖕᓱᒡᕕᐊᖅ

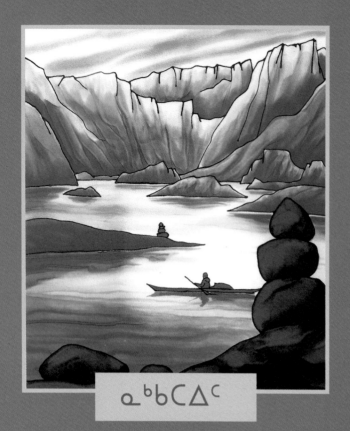

ᓇᕐᑲᑕᐃᑦ

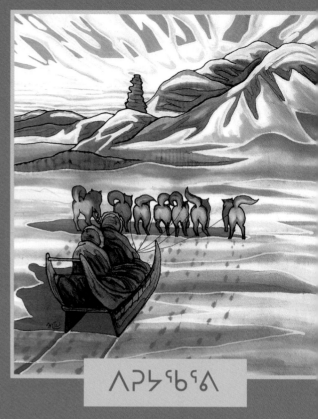

ᐱᔾᕐᑲᕐᕕ

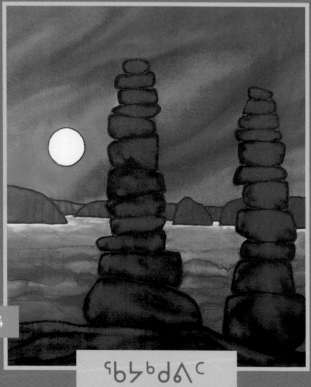

ᕐᑲᕐᑯᐱᕉ

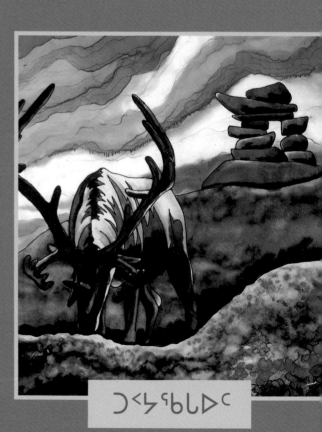

ᑐᐸᕐᑲᑲᐃᑦ

The Messages of the Inuksuit

The Inuktitut language is written in symbols that represent a combination of sounds. Below are the names of the inuksuit shown on pages 83–84. Look at the guide to pronouncing the words. The letters in upper case show which syllable you put more emphasis on when you say the word.

ᐃᓄᙳᐊᖅ	**Inunnguaq** (Ee-non-WAWK)	something that resembles a person.
ᓇᒃᑲᑕᐃᑦ	**Nakkatait** (Nah-cut-tait)	things that fell in the water. An inuksuk with this name points to a good place to fish.
ᐱᒍᔭᖃᕐᕕ	**Pirujaqarvik** (Pee-goo-yah-KHAK-vik)	where the meat supply is.
ᖃᔭᒃᑯᕖᑦ	**Qajakkuviit** (Kha-yak-koo-VEET)	place for a kayak to be stored.
ᑐᑉᔭᖃᖕᒍᐊᑦ	**Tupjakangaut** (Toob-jahk-hang-out)	footprints of game. This inuksuk steers hunters toward good places to hunt.

DIG DEEPER

1. Choose a favourite illustration from this selection. Write a journal entry telling why you like it.

2. With a partner or group, brainstorm a list of other ways people use objects to make a message. Sketch some examples.

How have messages changed over time?

FROM CAVE TO

by Anne Mackenzie

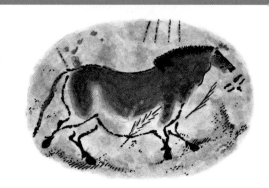

30 000– 10 000 BCE

Cave paintings or carvings record important events.
Stories of successful hunts are painted on cave walls. Today, people are still able to "read" these messages from the past.

3500–2900 BCE

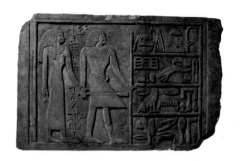

The first written languages are developed
People in Egypt and what is now Iraq develop forms of writing made up of pictures.

500 CE

The first pens in Europe are made.
Some early pens, called quills, are made from goose feathers. The writer sharpens the tip and dips it into ink.

1450s CE

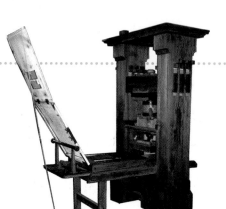

The printing press is invented in Europe.
Letters are carved backward on small blocks. The blocks can be joined to form paragraphs. They are covered with ink, then pressed on paper.

86

COMPUTER

VIEW LIKE A DESIGNER
How do the visuals help you to understand the timeline's information?

1752

The first Canadian newspaper, the **Halifax Gazette**, appears.
The paper is one sheet only. News from London, Boston, and Halifax fills the page.

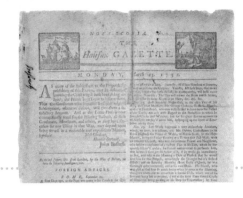

1820s

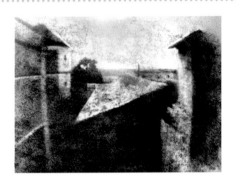

First photographs produced.
Early cameras have to be pointed at something for eight hours in order to get a photo of it.

1842

The first comic book appears.
"The Adventures of Obadiah Oldbuck" is North America's first graphic novel.

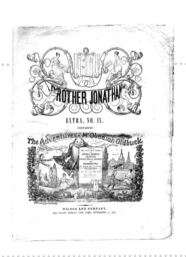

1867

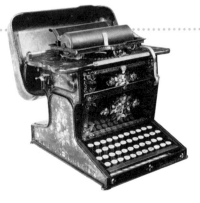

The first typewriter is produced.
The first typing machine has keys like a computer. At first, the letters jam a lot. Later, the most commonly used letters are spread out across the keyboard.

87

1927– 1950s

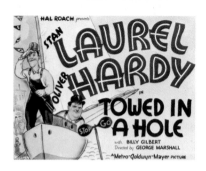

Talking motion pictures are released. Early movies are in black and white. It costs just 25 cents to watch some cartoons, see the movie, and have a drink and popcorn.

1940s– 1950s

First TV shows for children are broadcast. At first, all shows are broadcast "live." This means the audience sees everything that happens—even the bloopers!

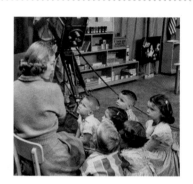

1947–1951

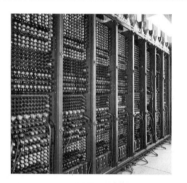

First electronic computer, ENIAC, is built. The ENIAC computer is as big as a house and weighs 30 tonnes. It performs calculations faster than any other machine.

1954

Colour TV broadcasts begin. The first RCA colour TV set costs $995. In 1954, a new car is about the same price!

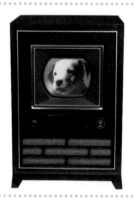

1972

Pong starts the video game craze. *Ping, Pong.* A small dot on the screen is slowly batted back and forth. Don't miss or you lose! The graphics are simple, but people play for hours.

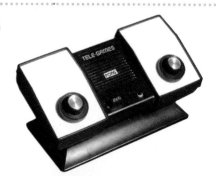

Late 1970s

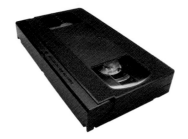

Home videos become popular.
Missed that movie at the theatre? Just rent a videocassette and watch it at home.

1980s

Computer-aided graphics appear in movies.
By the time *Jurassic Park* was made in 1993, it was getting harder and harder to tell the real thing from the special effects.

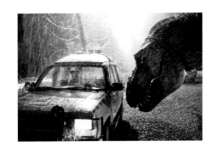

1990s

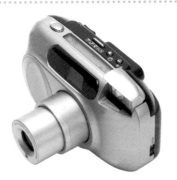

Digital cameras and scanners become popular.
People shoot and print their own pictures. Software allows images to be changed or combined. Don't believe everything you see!

2000 and beyond

Smart technology lets people stay in touch.
Cell phones allow people to make a call, send a text message, or watch TV.

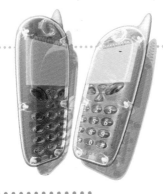

DIG DEEPER

1. Choose two inventions that are most important to you. Give reasons for your choices.

2. Think of a new way of communicating that has not been invented yet. Make an entry about it for the timeline. Include a sketch and a description.

Most important inventions	Reasons they are important

How can letters and words send a visual message?

Shrink.

h**u**g

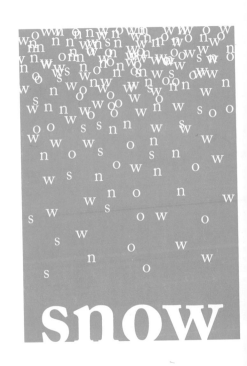

snow

STRETCH

ART

SKATEBOARD

parachute

TRIP

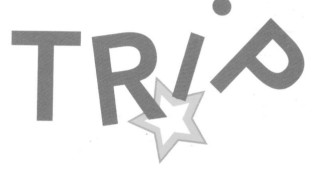

open wide

Tall

DIG DEEPER ....

1. Which word art is your favourite? Explain what you like about it.

2. With a partner, create some word art of your own. Share your words with the class.

To Each His Own

by Anna Grossnickle Hines

How can
pictures
be part of
a poem?

VIEW LIKE A POET
How do the poets create
a visual message with
their words?

When the leaves fall
   some float
       lazily
          wavily
  and taking all
         daysily
           drift
  to the ground.
Some flutter
    skuttering
       whuttering
  audibly uttering
      whispers
         of sound.
When the leaves fall
   some
     come in bunches
        swirling
      and whirling
     twisting
  and twirling
      round
       about
       round.
Some
  skip-a-dip
    bippity
      floppity
        flippity
      toppity
    tippity
  plippity
    down.
And some
  just drop
   flop.

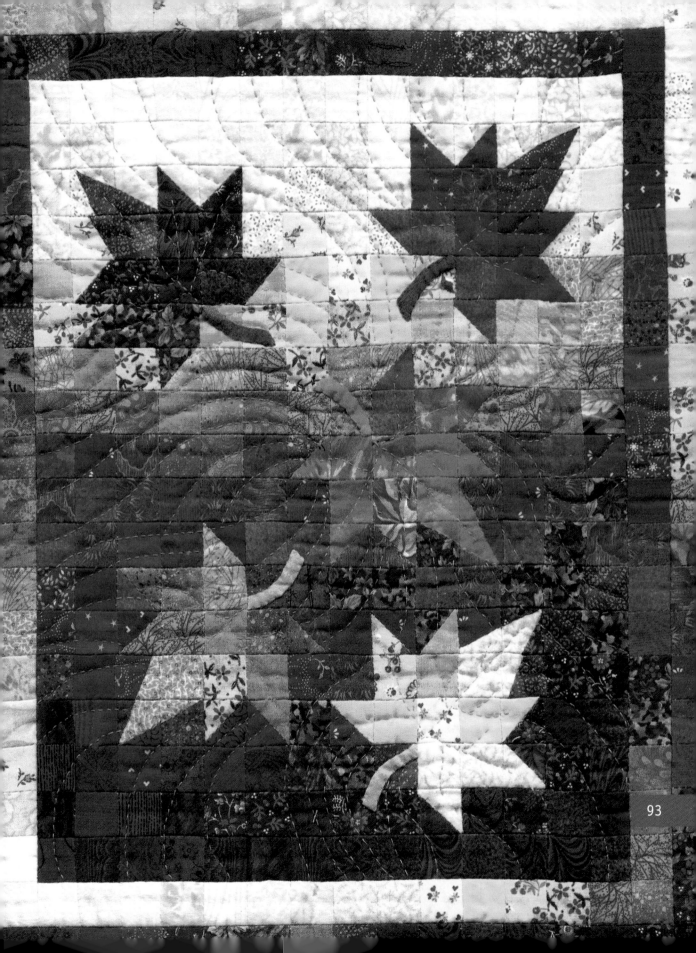

93

giraffe

by J. Patrick Lewis
Illustrated by Lisa Desimini

Tree-tall giraffe up to his neck

in brown and yellow
patchwork quilts, turns tail
and hobbles away
on wooden stilts stilts stilts stilts

94

Apple

by Cathie Peters

A
  P
    P
      L
        E

RED   RED   RED

RED   nature's ruby   RED

RED   plucked from a branch   RED

RED   polished on my sleeve   RED

RED   crisp, crunchy white flesh   RED

RED   sometimes sweet, sometimes tart   RED

RED   makes my tastebuds sing   RED

RED   juice runs down my chin   RED

RED   every bite a treat to savour   RED

RED   the taste of summer   RED

RED   and sunshine   RED

RED   RED   RED

DIG DEEPER

1. Choose one of the poems. Explain how the way the poem looks adds to its meaning.

2. Take turns reading one of the poems aloud with a partner. Make your voices interesting and consider adding gestures.

ish

by PETER H. REYNOLDS

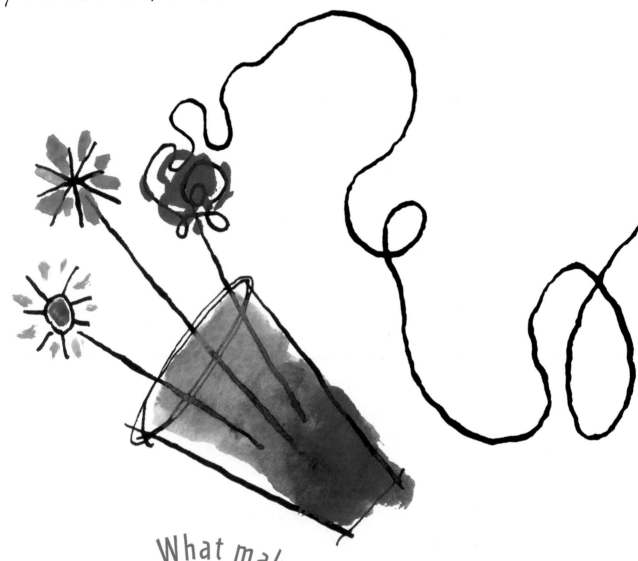

What makes art "good" art?

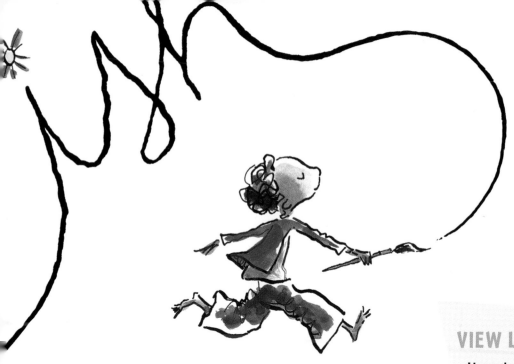

VIEW LIKE AN ARTIST
How does the art help set
the mood of the story?

Ramon loved to draw.
Anytime.
Anything.
Anywhere.

One day, Ramon was drawing
a vase of flowers.
His brother, Leon,
leaned over his shoulder.
Leon burst out laughing.
"WHAT is THAT?" he asked.

Ramon could not even answer.
He just crumpled up the drawing
and threw it across the room.

Leon's laughter haunted Ramon.
He kept trying to make his
drawings look "right,"
but they never did.

97

After many months and
many crumpled sheets of paper,
Ramon put his pencil down.
"I'm done."

Marisol, his sister, was watching him.

"What do YOU want?" he snapped.

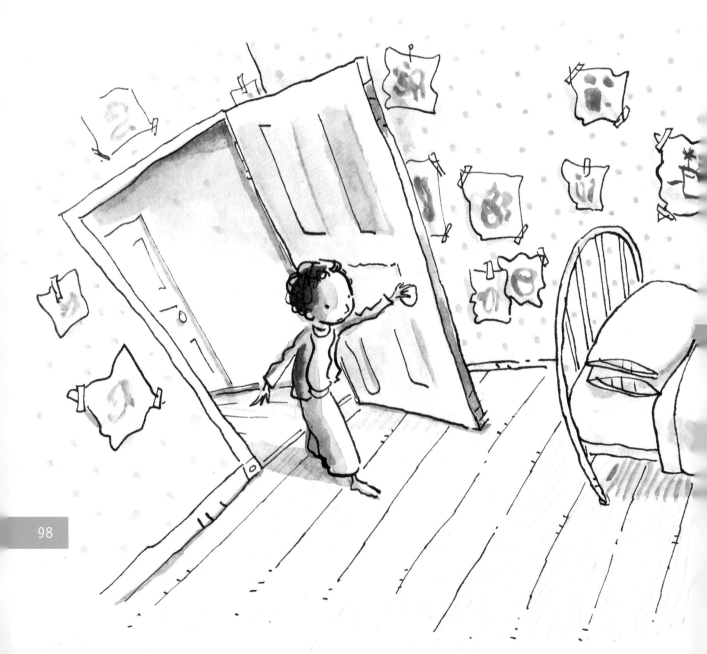

"I was watching you draw," she said.
Ramon sneered.
"I'm NOT drawing! Go away!"

Marisol ran away, but not before
picking up a crumpled sheet of paper.

"Hey! Come back here with that!"

Ramon raced after Marisol,
up the hall and into her room.

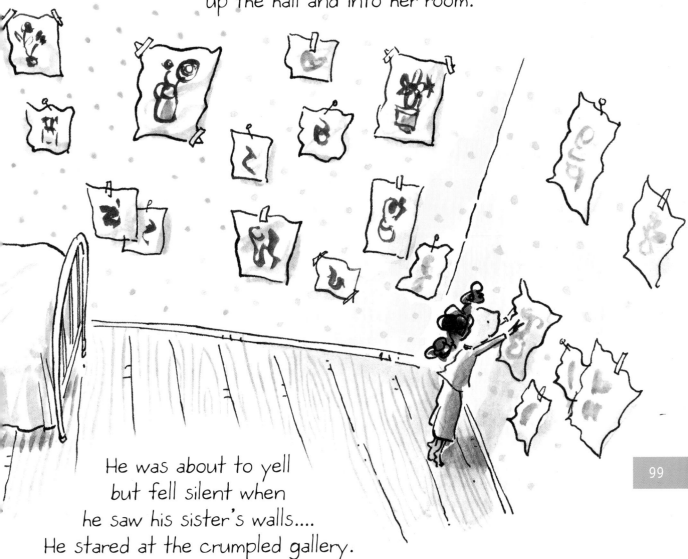

He was about to yell
but fell silent when
he saw his sister's walls....
He stared at the crumpled gallery.

"This is one of my favourites,"
Marisol said, pointing.

"That was SUPPOSED to be a
vase of flowers," Ramon said,
"but it doesn't look like one."

"Well, it looks vase-ISH!"
she exclaimed.

"Vase-ISH?"

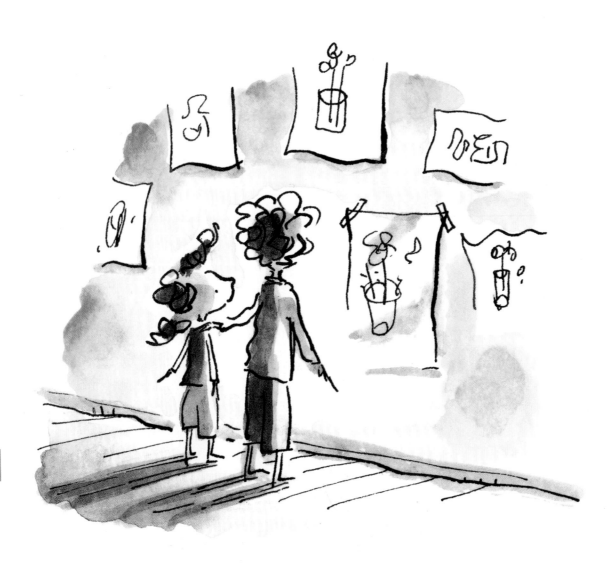

Ramon looked closer.
Then he studied all the drawings on
Marisol's walls and began to
see them in a whole new way.

"They do look...ish," he said.

Ramon felt light and energized.
Thinking ish-ly allowed
his ideas to flow freely.

He began to draw what he felt—
loose lines.
Quickly springing out.
Without worry.

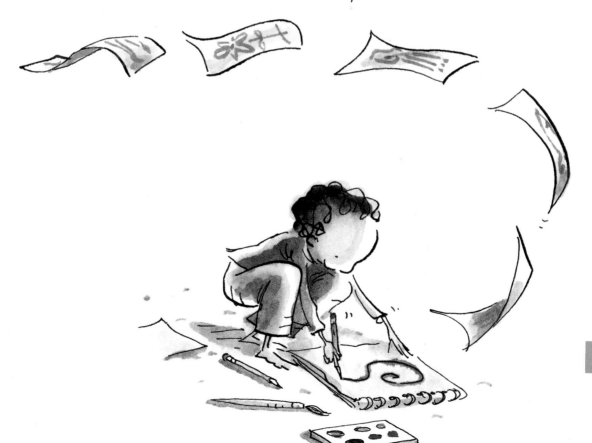

Ramon once again drew
and drew the world around him.
Making an ish drawing
felt wonderful.

He filled his journals...

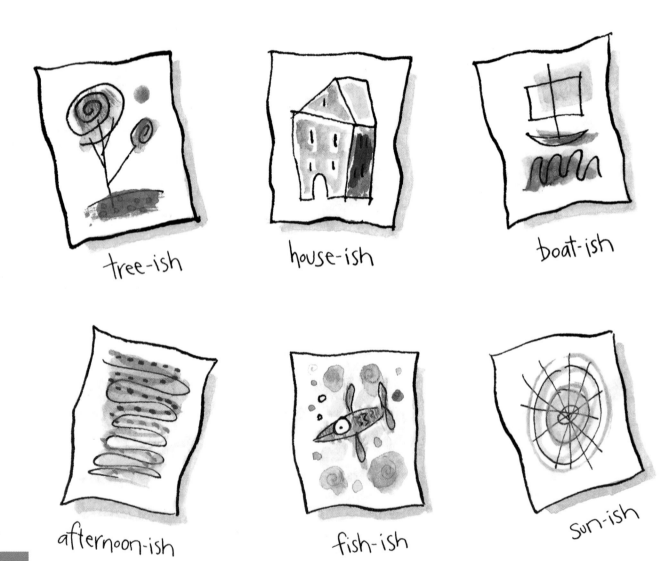

tree-ish

house-ish

boat-ish

afternoon-ish

fish-ish

sun-ish

Ramon realized he could draw ish feelings too.

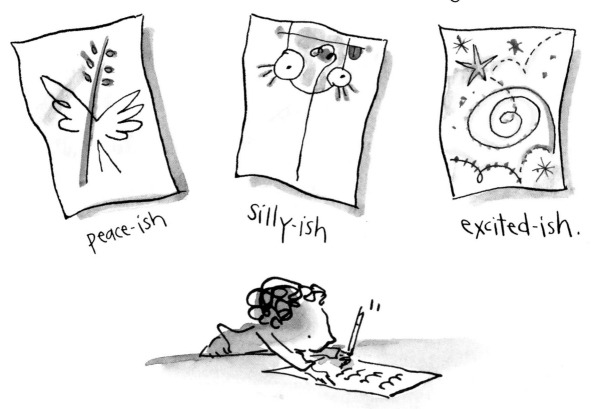

peace-ish

silly-ish

excited-ish.

His ish art inspired ish writing.
He wasn't sure if he was writing poems,
but he knew they were poem-ish.

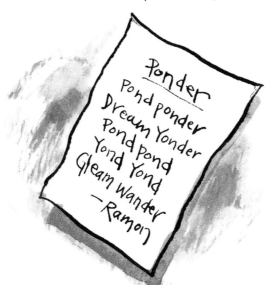

Ponder

Pond ponder
Dream Yonder
Pond Pond
Yond Yond
Gleam Wander
— Ramon

One spring morning,
Ramon had a wonderful feeling.
It was a feeling that even ish words
and ish drawings could not capture.
He decided NOT to capture it.
Instead, he simply savoured it....

And Ramon lived ishfully ever after.

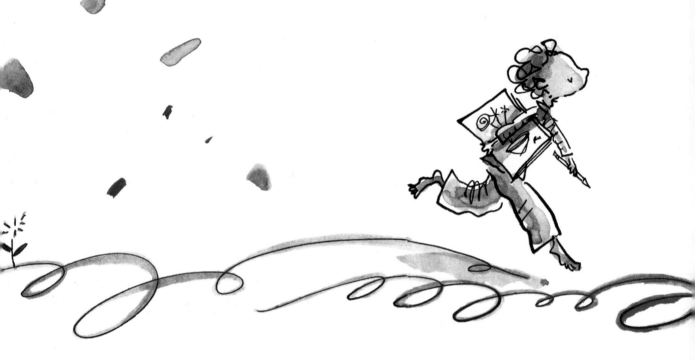

DIG DEEPER

1. What kind of person is Marisol? Tell two qualities she shows in the story. Support your ideas with evidence from the story.

Marisol's qualities	Evidence

2. Create your own piece of ish art. Show it to three other people. Ask each of them, "What kind of ish do you see?"

How can someone write a letter if they cannot see?

PRIVATE AND CONFIDENTIAL

by Marion Ripley
Illustrated by Colin Backhouse

READ LIKE A WRITER

Why did the author choose to include the letters as part of the story?

"What does PRIVATE AND CONFIDENTIAL mean?" asked Laura. "There's a letter here for Mom and it's written on the envelope in big black letters."

Joe was opening his newsletter from the local football team. "It means that no one else is allowed to read it except Mom," he said. "It's probably from the bank."

"It's not fair," said Laura. "Why doesn't anyone ever write to me?"

The next day at school, Mr. Joshi made an announcement.

"I've had a letter from a teacher in Australia," he said. "If any of you would like an Australian pen pal, come and see me."

Laura was really excited. She hurried up to Mr. Joshi's classroom.

"Can I have a girl who likes swimming, gerbils, and watching television?" she asked.

"I'm sorry, Laura," said Mr. Joshi, "all the children are boys. You can have Steve, Paul, Darren, Malcolm, or Luke."

Laura was a bit disappointed. "Never mind," she said, "I'll have Malcolm."

That night Laura sat down to write her first letter to Malcolm. It was hard to know what to say.

"Just tell him about yourself and ask him to write back. That's enough to start with," said Dad.

So that's what she did.

Dear Malcolm,

I got your address from a teacher at my school. I am ten years old and go to Hollyridge School. I like swimming and watching television and talking to my friends. Sometimes I get into trouble because I talk in class and in assembly and other times I'm not supposed to!

I would really like a letter from you. please send me a photo if you can.

What is it like living in Australia?

from
Laura O'Brien

Laura waited for the post every day and it was not long before an airmail letter arrived for her—all the way from Australia!

Dear Laura,

It was great to get your letter! I like swimming too, and there is a big pool right near where I live so I go there with my friends after school most afternoons in summer. It is too cold for swimming at the moment because it is winter here while you have summer — but I guess you knew that already!

I have a sister, Hannah, who is 16, and a brother, Sam, who is 9. My cat is called Mulberry but I can't remember how old she is!

I am sending a photo. It was taken at the pool last summer but I have grown about 10 cm since then!

Write back SOON!

From Malcolm

Laura really liked the letter and she really liked the photo. She took them to school and got told off for passing them round in Assembly.

That evening she wrote a long letter to Malcolm and sent him a photo even though he hadn't actually asked for one. At the end of the letter she wrote "Write back SOON!"

She posted it on her way to school the next morning.

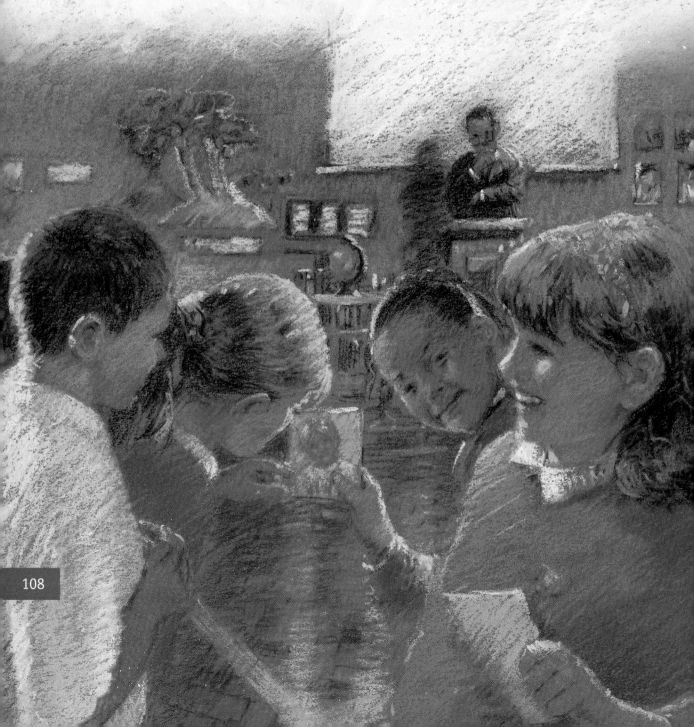

Laura waited and waited for a reply from Malcolm, and after three weeks she still hadn't heard from him. It was really disappointing.

"Perhaps he didn't like your photo," said Joe.

At last there was a letter! But it wasn't from Malcolm.

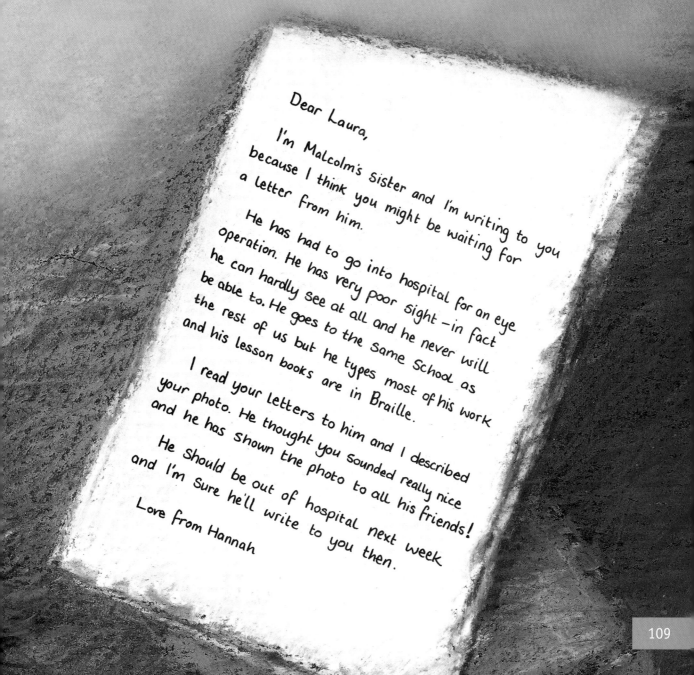

Dear Laura,

I'm Malcolm's sister and I'm writing to you because I think you might be waiting for a letter from him.

He has had to go into hospital for an eye operation. He has very poor sight — in fact he can hardly see at all and he never will be able to. He goes to the same school as the rest of us but he types most of his work and his lesson books are in Braille.

I read your letters to him and I described your photo. He thought you sounded really nice and he has shown the photo to all his friends!

He should be out of hospital next week and I'm sure he'll write to you then.

Love from Hannah

"What's up, Laura?" asked Dad as he came into the hall.

"It's Malcolm," said Laura. "He's nearly blind. He's gone into hospital for an operation but it isn't going to make him see any better. I can't believe it. Why didn't he tell me?"

"Perhaps he didn't think it was the most important thing about him," said Dad. "Maybe he wanted to talk about swimming, and his family, and the cat instead. He was probably going to tell you when you knew each other a bit better. Does it really make that much difference?"

Laura got out the photo of Malcolm. He looked so fit and happy in the picture, it was hard to imagine him being ill in hospital. Then she had an idea. She would send him a Get Well card, and she would do it in Braille!

Karen at school had an auntie who was blind. She would probably help if she was not too busy with her baby.

After school the next day, Laura went with Karen to visit her auntie.

Karen's auntie had a brailling machine, which was a bit like a typewriter but with fewer keys. She gave Laura a Braille alphabet card and showed her how to press the keys so that they made raised dots. Then she put Laura's card in the brailler and Laura brailled her message:

Get Well Soon
Love from Laura

Ten days later a letter arrived. But it wasn't a pale blue airmail envelope this time. It was a cardboard tube with a special address label on the outside. Inside the tube was a letter—IN BRAILLE! Laura sat down on the stairs with her alphabet card to find out what it said.

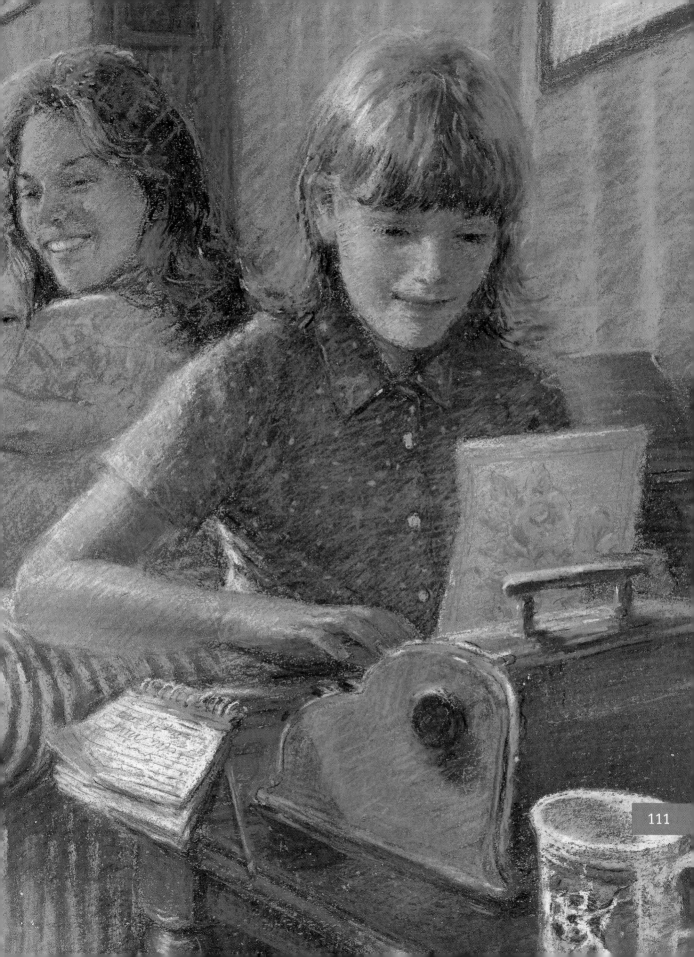

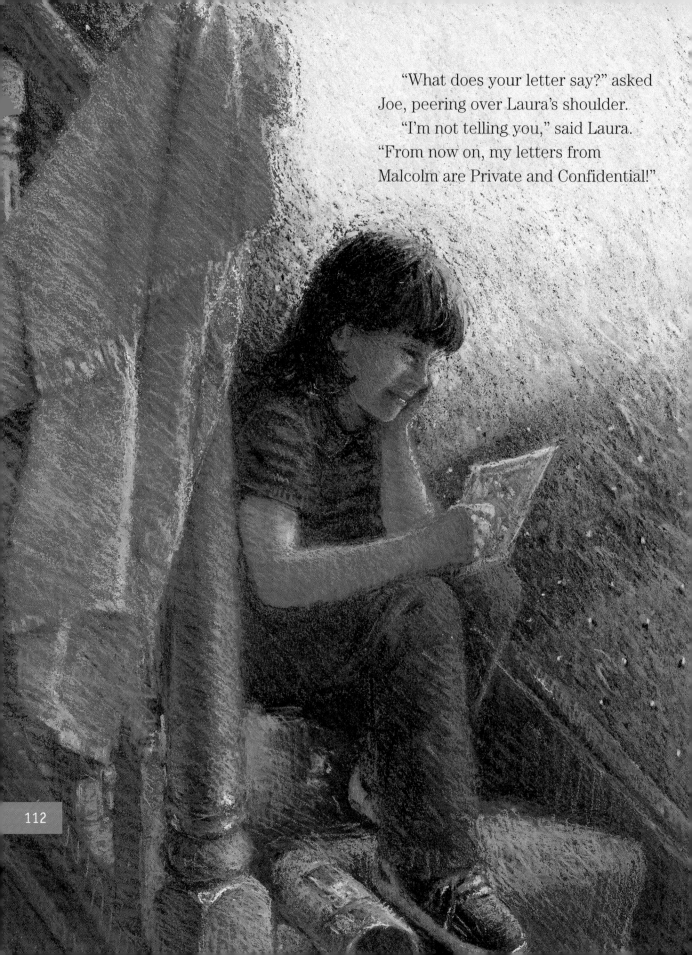

"What does your letter say?" asked
Joe, peering over Laura's shoulder.
"I'm not telling you," said Laura.
"From now on, my letters from
Malcolm are Private and Confidential!"

Here is Malcolm's braille letter. Using the alphabet card, can you find out what it says?

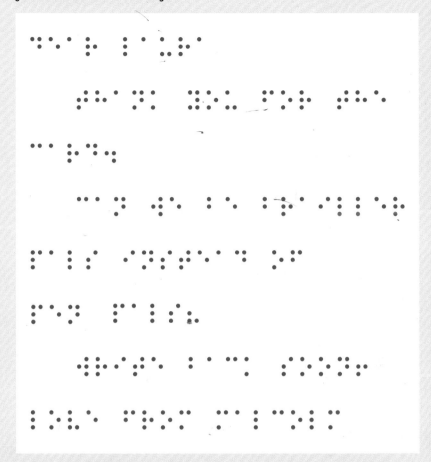

a	b	c	d	e	f
g	h	i	j	k	l	m
n	o	p	q	r	s
t	u	v	w	x	y	z

Full stop   Question mark

Exclamation mark

Here is the translation of Malcolm's letter. Did you get it right?

Dear Laura
Thank you for the card.
Can we be brailler pals instead of pen pals?
Write back soon!
Love from Malcolm

MEDIA WATCH

Ask someone to turn on the closed captioning on a TV set. How does that change the way you view a program?

DIG DEEPER

1. Imagine that Malcolm and Laura meet one day. With a partner, role-play what they might say to each other.

2. What would you say about yourself in a first letter to a pen pal? Write a letter to Laura in which you introduce yourself.

Connect and Share

Almost everyone likes to get messages!

Now it's your turn to send a message.

I could bring a picture that shows how much I love my dog.

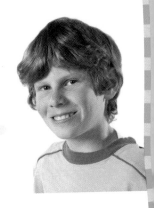

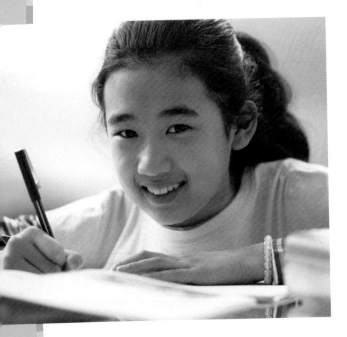

Take a postcard home!

- Choose a selection in this unit.
- Draw one of the images from that selection.
- Show it to your family and ask them to tell you the message.
- On the back of the postcard, write the message in words.

Bring a postcard back!

- Ask family members to help you choose a photo or make a picture that tells something about you.
- Work together to write a caption to describe it.
- Display the postcards in the classroom.

WRITING A CAPTION

- Don't write too much.
- Tell the key message of the image.
- Print neatly so everyone can read it.

Spotlight on **Learning**

Collect

- Gather your notebooks, poster, and other work you did in this unit.

Talk and reflect

Work with a partner.

- Together, read the Learning Goals on page 56.

- Talk about how well you met these goals.

- Look through your work for evidence.

Select

- Choose two pieces of work that show how you achieved the Learning Goals. (The same piece of work can show more than one goal.)

Tell about your choices

- Tell what each piece shows about your learning.

My choices	I want this in my portfolio because...

Reflect

- What have you learned about how to view and create visual messages?

- What have you discovered about what makes a photograph interesting?

- What have you learned about how interesting illustrations or layouts can add to a story or poem?

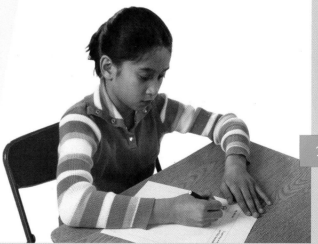

115

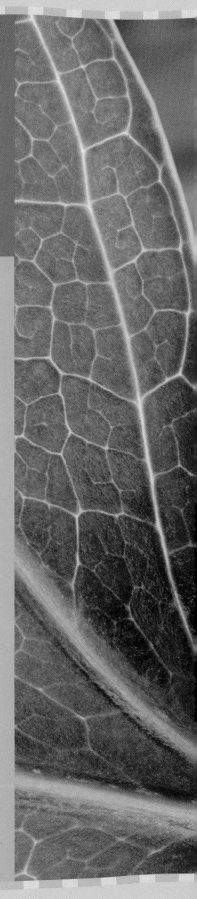

Survivors!

LEARNING GOALS

In this unit you will:

- Read and listen to non-fiction and fiction texts about plants and animals in different habitats.

- Explain how nature and people can affect habitats.

- Use science words to describe different habitats.

- Investigate and share information about a habitat using diagrams, illustrations, and headings.

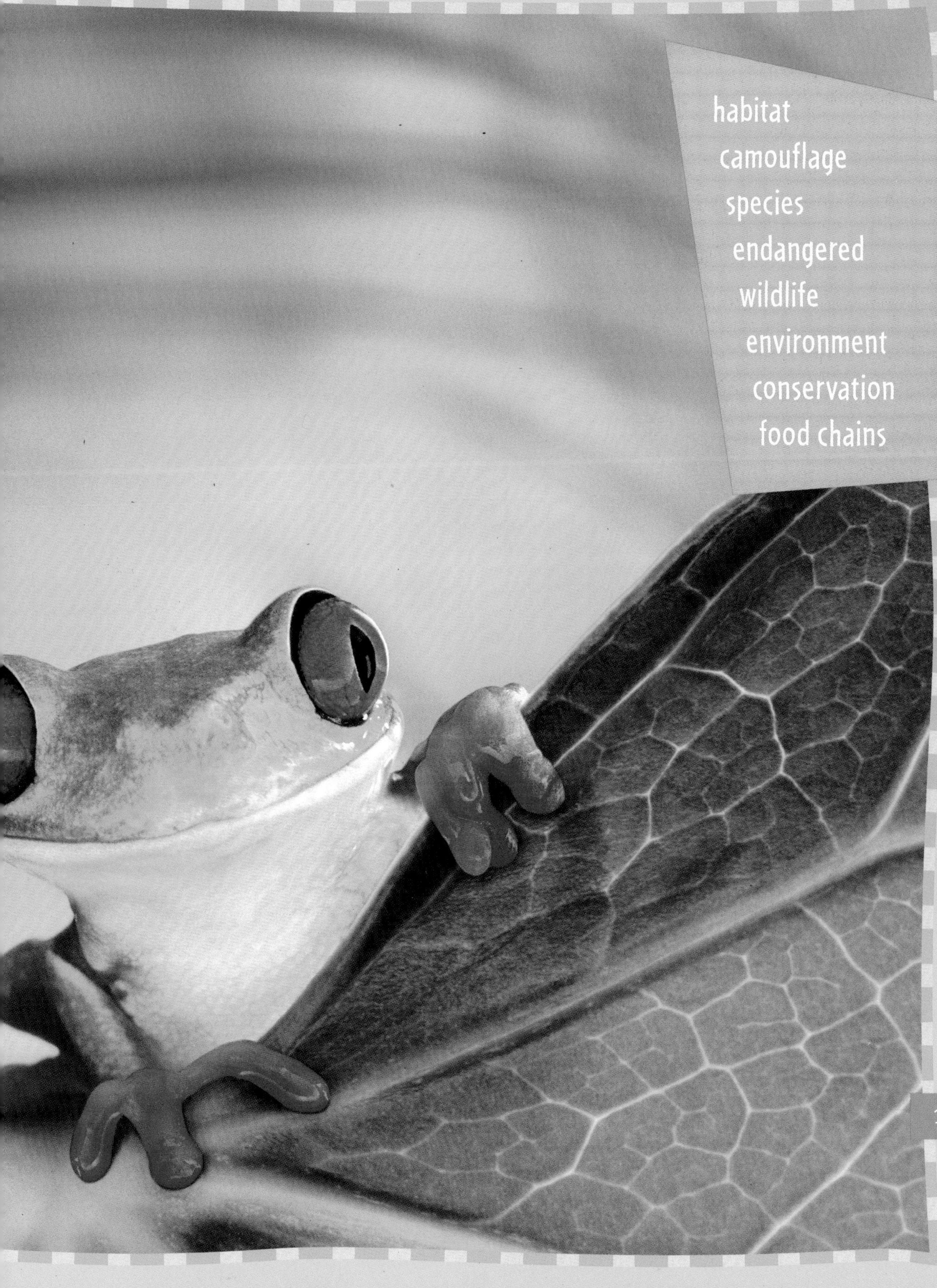

habitat
camouflage
species
endangered
wildlife
environment
conservation
food chains

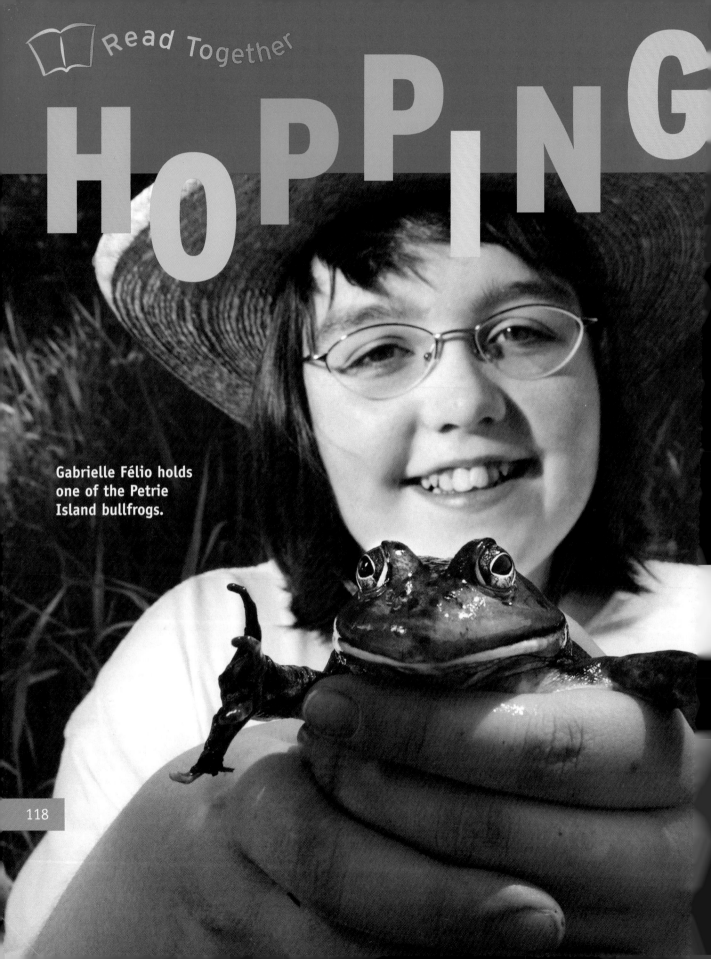

HOPPING

Gabrielle Félio holds one of the Petrie Island bullfrogs.

118

to the Rescue
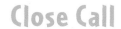
by Sydney Grant

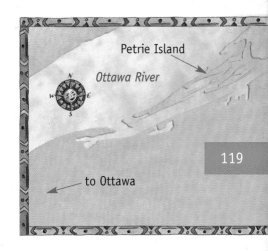

How can people show they care about saving habitats?

Close Call

When the snow started to fall last December in southern Ontario, the frogs of Petrie Island Pond were already hibernating. But they almost didn't get the chance. Only days before truckloads of sand were scheduled to fill in the frogs' pond, the Amphibian Conservation Club (ACC) came to their rescue.

The summer before, kids in the ACC learned that the pond on Petrie Island, in the Ottawa River, was destined to become a parking lot. They set to work learning everything they could about the pond, especially the wildlife that lived there.

They discovered leopard frogs, green frogs, bullfrogs, mink frogs, snapping turtles, painted turtles, and so much more—and knew that they couldn't leave them to be buried by asphalt.

Moving Day

That summer they started catching tadpoles and frogs and moved them to their new home, another pond about one kilometre away. By November, time was running out.

Petrie Island is in the Ottawa River, just north and east of Ottawa.

Petrie Island

Ottawa River

to Ottawa

119

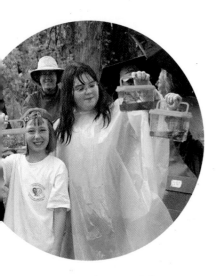

ACC members safely carry frogs to their new habitat in carrying cases.

Saturday, November 22, was their last chance. Members of the ACC leapt into action, catching frogs in nets and helping them make their trip to their new pond. The city donated two water pumps to suck the water out of the pond and into the river. Anything small enough to travel with the water got a fast water-tube ride.

As the water in the pond went down lower and lower, ACC kids just kept catching frogs. Even though it was cold, the frogs had plenty of energy to try to outrun the kids working to save them. The muck was so thick, 12-year-old ACC leader Gabrielle Félio got stuck in the mud up to her knees and needed some saving of her own!

In total, they moved 145 frogs; countless tadpoles, fish, and insects; one turtle; and a muskrat.

ACC members share information about Petrie Island's wildlife.

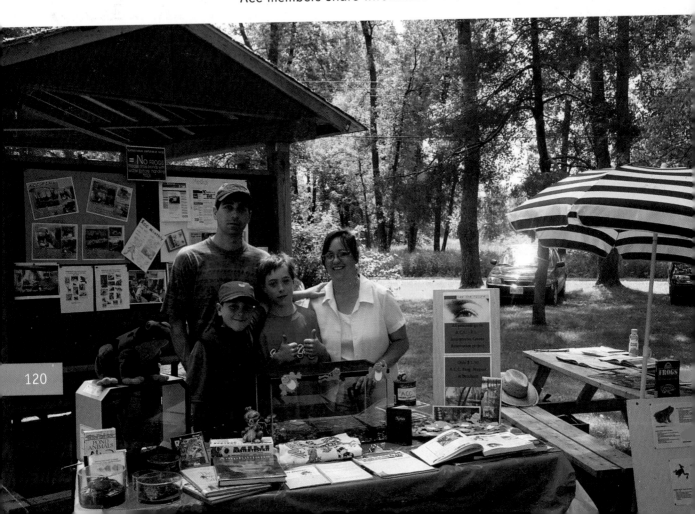

In the Spotlight

It was a moving day nobody would forget, and news of the ACC spread. Run by kids, for kids, the ACC is definitely different. Gabrielle started it two years ago.

She never imagined the club would become so popular. She found herself interested in frogs after her family built a pond in their backyard. Gabrielle wanted to learn more about pond life and went looking for other kids who wanted to join in the fun.

The club began meeting at the local community centre. They would get together to do activities, arts, and crafts and to learn more about wildlife in ponds and the environment they need to live. There are now about 30 kids in the club, and meetings are held every two months at the centre—no adults allowed!

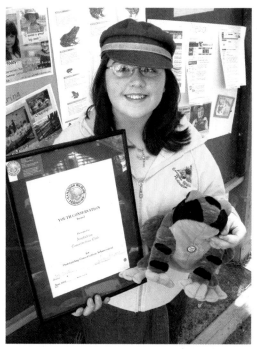

Gabrielle holds one of her awards.

Great Rewards

Gabrielle and the ACC received a Canadian Wildlife Federation Youth Conservation Award for their fab froggy feats. Gabrielle has also been awarded an Orléans Online Outstanding Youth Award and an Arbour Environmental Foundation Youth Award. For Gabrielle, however, the biggest and best reward is seeing frogs where they belong.

LET'S TALK ABOUT IT
- With a partner, think of some questions you would ask Gabrielle in an interview.
- What could you and others your age do to care for the environment where you live?

Reading in Science

Reading in science helps you learn true facts and information about the world we live in. Think about a science book or TV program you've enjoyed.

- What was it about?
- How did it capture your interest?
- How was it different from reading or viewing a story?

TALK ABOUT IT!

- Tell a partner something you learned from the book or program.
- Talk about the different places you can find science information.

Here are some clues.

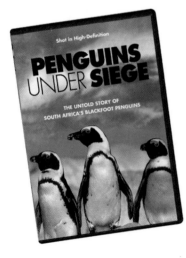

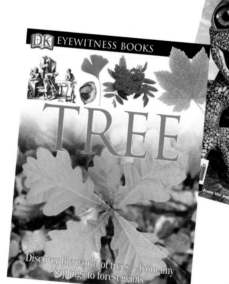

Make a chart together.

Science Information

Where you can find it	Examples

Think Like a Reader

- Why do you read about science topics?

Crack the code

When you see technical and difficult words in science, look for parts of the word you know.

scientist – science
naturalist – nature
conservation –
endangered –

Make meaning

Practise using these strategies when you are reading in science:

ASK QUESTIONS	Look at all the information in the text and visuals. Think about what you know about the topic. Ask questions about what you would like to know.
PAUSE AND CHECK	Pause at the end of each paragraph or section to check your understanding.
SUMMARIZE	Organize the information in a chart or web.

Analyze what you read

- How can you find "true" information about a science topic?
- Why might there be different points of view about a science topic?

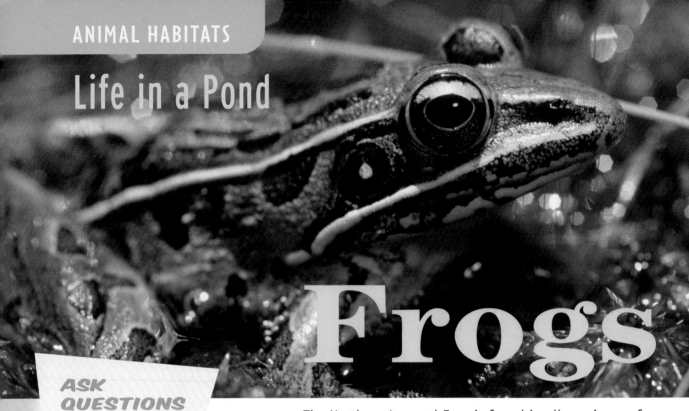

Life in a Pond

Frogs

What would you like to know about a frog's habitat?

wet skin

eyes

ear

strong legs

webbed feet

124

The Northern Leopard Frog is found in all provinces of Canada.

Long before the dinosaurs, frogs lived on earth. They belong to the amphibian family. Amphibians can live in water and on land.

There are more than 4000 kinds of frogs in the world. In Canada, there are 21 kinds.

Appearance

Most frogs in Canada are green, grey, or brown.

Frogs have smooth wet skin. They have long back legs to help them jump. Their webbed feet help them swim. Frogs' eyes bulge out from the sides of their heads. This helps them see from behind.

The bodies of most frogs are 5 to 10 cm long. Some frogs can be as long as 30 cm.

Food

Frogs eat insects, caterpillars, and earthworms. Larger frogs will even eat mice and fish. Frogs do not hunt for food but sit quietly and wait until their prey comes near. Then the frog catches its prey with its long sticky tongue.

A frog has teeth in its top jaw only. So a frog swallows its prey without chewing it.

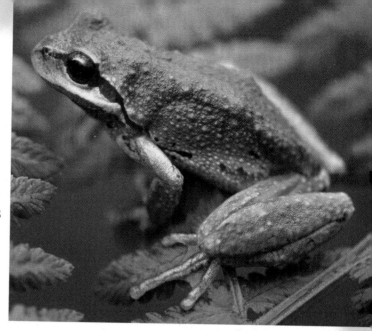

The Pacific Tree Frog lives in British Columbia. It has sticky pads on its toes that help it climb.

Habitat

Frogs live close to water. Most live in ponds or swamps, or near a lake. Some frogs live in trees. In cold places, frogs hibernate in winter.

Frogs lay their eggs in water. The eggs hatch into tadpoles that live in the water until they become adult frogs. Then they move onto land.

In many parts of Canada, frogs are losing their habitat. Builders clear the land to build houses and roads. Frogs have no place to live.

PAUSE AND CHECK

What have you learned about frogs so far? Does it make sense?

Adult frog: The tail has been reabsorbed by the body.

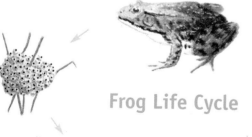

g eggs are d in water.

Frog Life Cycle

The froglet still has some of its tail but breathes using lungs.

adpoles swim in he water and reathe using gills.

125

Tadpole with legs.

SUMMARIZE

How can you organize the information in a chart or web?

Life in the Arctic
Polar Bears

Female polar bears usually give birth to twins.

ASK QUESTIONS

What would you like to know about a polar bear's habitat?

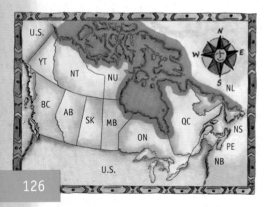

The area in dark blue shows where polar bears can be found in Canada.

126

About 15 000 polar bears live in Canada's Arctic.

The polar bear is a mammal. It is also the largest bear in the world. The polar bear is different from other bears because it does not hibernate.

Appearance

The polar bear's fur appears white. But in fact each hair is transparent—just like the colour of water. Under its fur, the polar bear's skin is black.

An adult male polar bear weighs from 350 to 650 kg. When standing, he can measure up to 3 m tall. Female polar bears weigh 150 to 250 kg. Newborn polar bears weigh less than half a kg.

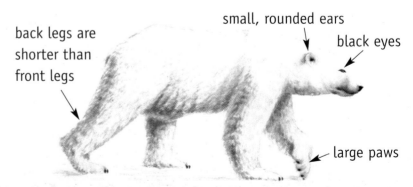

back legs are shorter than front legs

small, rounded ears

black eyes

large paws

Food

The polar bear is called a carnivore because it eats meat. Its favourite food is the ringed seal. To hunt its prey, the polar bear waits patiently by the seal's hole in the ice, until the seal comes up for air. Then the polar bear grabs it.

Polar bears do not drink water. They get all the water they need from the animals they eat.

PAUSE AND CHECK

What have you learned about polar bears so far? Does it make sense?

Habitat

The polar bear's habitat is in and around the Arctic Ocean. In winter, when it is very cold, the polar bear's fur and black skin help to keep it warm.

Polar bears travel about 24 km a day looking for food. They swim, or walk over large chunks of floating ice.

The climate of Earth is getting warmer, causing the ice in the polar bears' habitat to slowly melt. Because this habitat is slowly disappearing, scientists think that polar bears may no longer exist in a hundred years.

SUMMARIZE

How can you organize the information in a chart or web?

Polar bears are very strong swimmers.

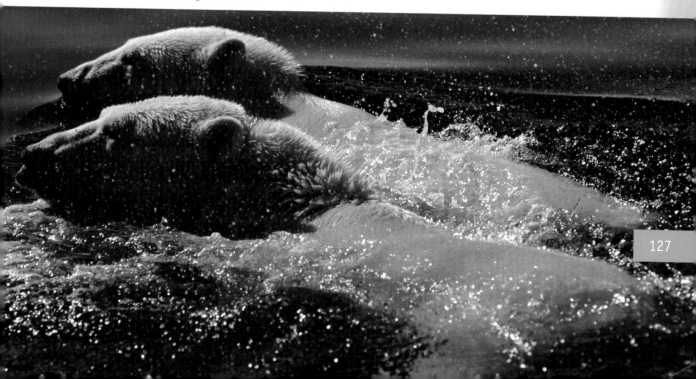

127

Life in an Ocean

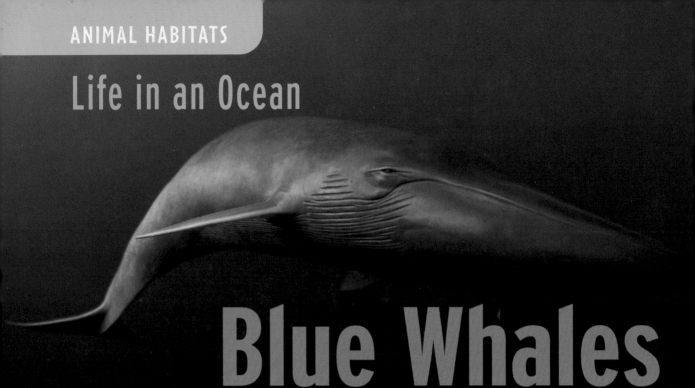

Blue Whales

The head of the blue whale forms up to a quarter of its total body length.

Blue whales live in the ocean. They are the largest mammals on Earth, and they are also the loudest! They make sounds that are louder than those of a jet plane.

There are only about 3000 blue whales left in the world today. Blue whales are often called "blues."

ASK QUESTIONS

What would you like to know about a blue whale's habitat?

Appearance

A blue whale is actually blue-grey in colour with lighter spots. Blues have two tail flukes that measure about 7.5 m from tip to tip. The blue's nostrils are the blowholes on the top of its head.

A female blue whale can measure up to 30 m in length and weigh 130 000 kg. Male blues are smaller.

dorsal fin

flukes

2 blowholes

baleen plates in mouth

128

flippers

Food

A blue whale needs to eat from 900 to 4100 kg of krill a day. Krill are small creatures like shrimp. When feeding, the blue takes in an enormous gulp of water and closes its mouth. Krill get trapped in its baleen as the whale forces the water out. Baleen are the whale's teeth and they look like large combs.

Under their skin, blues have a layer of fat called blubber. In winter, they do not eat for months, but live off their own blubber.

Habitat

Blues are found in oceans all over the world except in the far north. About 100 blues live in Canada's Gulf of St. Lawrence.

In spring and summer, blues like cool water where there is plenty of krill. In the winter, they migrate to warmer waters where their calves are born.

Blue whales have been an endangered species since 1966. In the past, whalers hunted blue whales for their oil, meat, and bones. Today, the main threats to their ocean habitat are oil spills and pollution.

Scientists can identify a blue whale by its flukes. This helps them keep track of how many whales are in an area.

PAUSE AND CHECK
What have you learned about blue whales so far? Does it make sense?

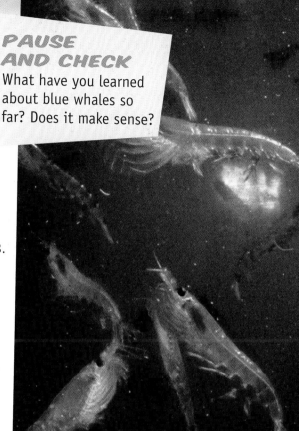

Krill are an important food for many fish and other animals that live in the sea.

SUMMARIZE
How can you organize the information in a chart or web?

Reflect on Your Reading

You have . . .

- talked about animal habitats.
- read about different animal habitats.
- learned new vocabulary that tells about animal habitats.

amphibian

hibernate

carnivore

mammal

environment

prey

You have also . . .

- explored different reading strategies.

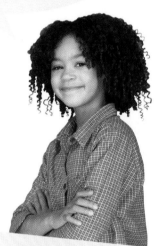

I think some animal habitats are being destroyed and it's hard for the animals to survive. What do you think?

ASK QUESTIONS

PAUSE AND CHECK

SUMMARIZE

Write About Learning

Write about one of the strategies you used when you read the selection "Animal Habitats." How did the strategy help you read and understand the selection? Tell how the strategy might help you when you read other explanations in science.

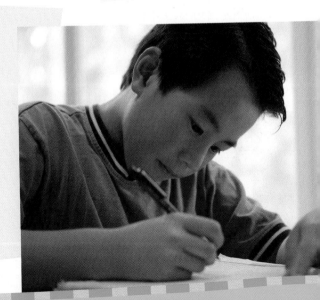

Read Like a Writer

When you were reading "Animal Habitats," you were reading some *explanations*. An explanation describes what something is like or how something works.

TALK ABOUT IT!

- What do you notice about the way explanations are written?
  Make a chart to list what you know about explanations.

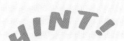

HINT!

What do you notice about the **ideas** and **details** the author uses?

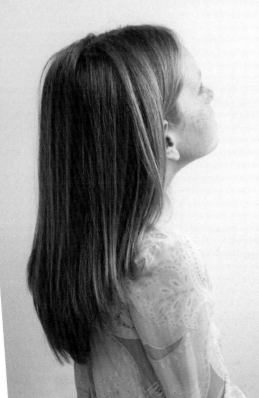

Explanations

- have a title that gives the topic
- give details so readers can understand
- have pictures or diagrams to add details

131

Canadian Habitat

by Trudee Romanek

How can ordinary people help save habitats?

For Every Child a Tree

In 1972, many countries took part in an important conference. They vowed to take care of our planet. Ten years later, though, things were no better. More forests had been cut down. Deserts were getting bigger. Mairuth Sarsfield wanted to remind countries of the vow they had made. She worked for the United Nations Environment Programme.

Mairuth suggested countries replace the trees they had cut down. She wanted children to plant the new seedlings. She thought that might help them to feel connected to nature and want to take care of it. Her team organized an event called "For Every Child a Tree."

Fourteen countries agreed to take part. Some donated extra trees for countries that couldn't afford to buy their own. Mairuth's efforts made a difference. Children planted more than 3 billion seedlings all over the world.

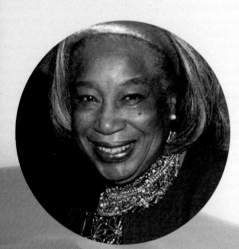

Mairuth Sarsfield

132

Mairuth knew deserts were getting bigger, especially in Asia and Africa.

Heroes

READ LIKE A WRITER

What facts and details did the author include to keep you reading?

Turtle Champion

Mike James knows a lot about leatherback turtles. He knows that some of them weigh over 450 kg. He knows that they hatch on a beach and crawl to the water. From then on, they spend most of their lives swimming. Many of these turtles swim from the warm waters of the Caribbean all the way up to the coast of Nova Scotia. Mike knows that along the way they sometimes swim into danger.

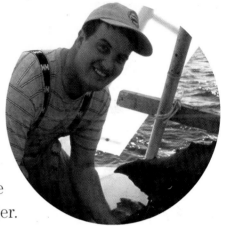

Mike James

Leatherback turtles breathe air, just like people do. They rise up and poke their heads above the water to breathe. If a turtle gets caught in a fishing net, sometimes it can't get to the water's surface. Then the turtle will drown. Mike James and his team at the Nova Scotia Leatherback Turtle Working Group want to make sure that doesn't happen.

So far, Mike's team has taught 500 volunteers how to free leatherback turtles caught in nets. Together, they are making the Nova Scotia habitat safer for the turtles.

This leatherback turtle is laying her eggs in the sand.

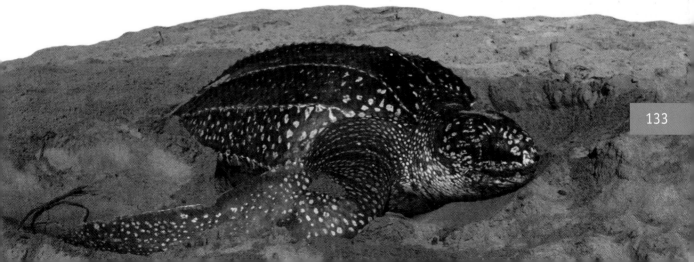

133

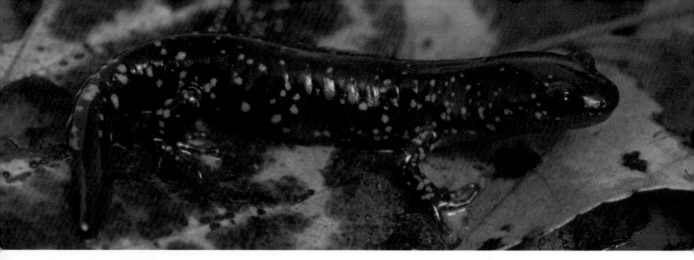

The Jefferson salamander is one species that Natalie works to protect.

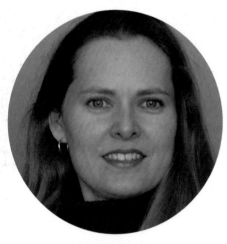

Natalie Helferty

Pathfinder

Wild animals travel a lot. Some migrate for winter. Others move around to find food. When people build a city, or even a single road, it sometimes blocks animals from getting where they need to go.

The ever-growing cities and towns in southern Ontario make it hard for animals to get from one patch of wilderness to another. So, Natalie Helferty has tried to keep some pathways open.

Natalie is a biologist. She lives on a long ridge of land called the Oak Ridges Moraine. In this moraine there are towns and cities as well as woods, lakes, bogs, and other animal habitats. Many frogs, salamanders, turtles, snakes, and even deer and foxes live there.

Natalie helps developers plan before they build so that the wilderness pathways do not get blocked. She also suggests new pathways be made to help animals avoid roads already in their way. Because of her work, local governments have built tunnels under roadways. Natalie has even suggested a special wildlife bridge for large animals like deer and coyotes.

Natalie believes that, in most cases, animals just need people to stay out of their way. If we do that, we may get to keep these wild creatures as neighbours.

134

Friend of the Arctic

Andy Carpenter has spent his whole life in Arctic Canada. The land and its creatures are very important to him. Andy is a very skillful hunter and trapper, but he follows the code of the Inuvialuit people. He takes only as many animals as his family needs.

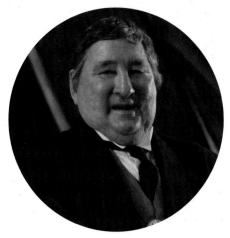

Andy Carpenter

Andy noticed that oil companies had started to explore and drill in the Arctic. He also noticed that more hunters were coming north. He worried that these changes might not be good for the land. So Andy decided to make sure the people of the Arctic would have animals to hunt in the future.

Andy helped to establish Aulavik National Park, home to a large group of muskoxen and the endangered Peary caribou. He also helped to create Ivvavik National Park. Then Andy and his people joined with other Arctic groups to create an action plan to protect polar bears.

Andy Carpenter has worked hard to do what's right for Arctic Canada. That way, he hopes, the animals he respects will always be there.

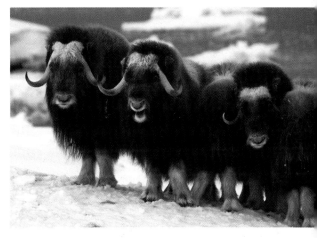

Muskoxen

DIG DEEPER

1. Make a three-column chart to summarize what you learned about each habitat hero.

   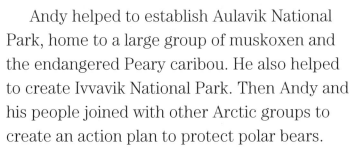

Hero	Problem	Solution

2. Create a sign or slogan for a habitat that is at risk.

MEDIA WATCH

Look for stories about other habitat heroes in newspapers and magazines.

135

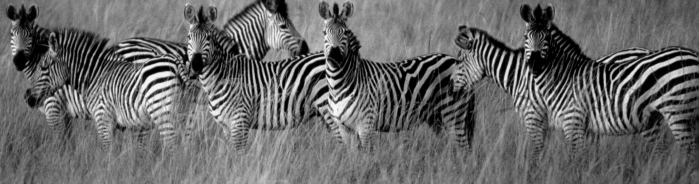

Food Chains by Peter Riley

How are food chains and habitats closely connected?

The way plants and animals are linked together by feeding is called a food chain. Most food chains start with energy from the sun. Plants use this energy to grow. In turn, the plants may be eaten by animals, and these animals by other animals.

Grasslands

The grasslands of North America, Africa, and Australia each have their own unique food chains.

North America

The meadows of North America and Europe are home to field mice. These animals eat the lower part of grass stems. Field mice make tunnels through the grass to hide from predators like hawks and owls. A predator is an animal that kills and eats other animals.

136

On the plains, prairie dogs make burrows in which to hide from predators such as coyotes and hawks. They eat the grass around their home so they can see any approaching attackers.

sun

grass   prairie dog   hawk

In this food chain, the grass uses energy from the sun to grow. The prairie dog eats the grass, then the hawk feeds on the prairie dog.

Black-tailed prairie dog. In Canada, they are found only in southern Saskatchewan.

The African Plains

Large numbers of zebras, gnus, and Thomson's gazelles graze on the African plains. Zebras eat the tops of the grass first, then gnus eat the middle part of the grass. Thomson's gazelles eat the young shoots that are left behind. All these animals are herbivores, which means they eat only plants. They may become prey to lions, hyenas, and other carnivores.

The Australian Outback

In Australia, grasses are eaten by kangaroos and wallabies. These herbivores may be eaten by packs of wild dogs called dingoes. Grass seeds are eaten by diamond firetail finches, which in turn are eaten by the peregrine falcon. The falcon dives out of the sky to attack and feed on the finches.

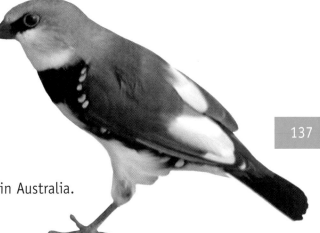

The diamond firetail finch is found in the wild only in Australia.

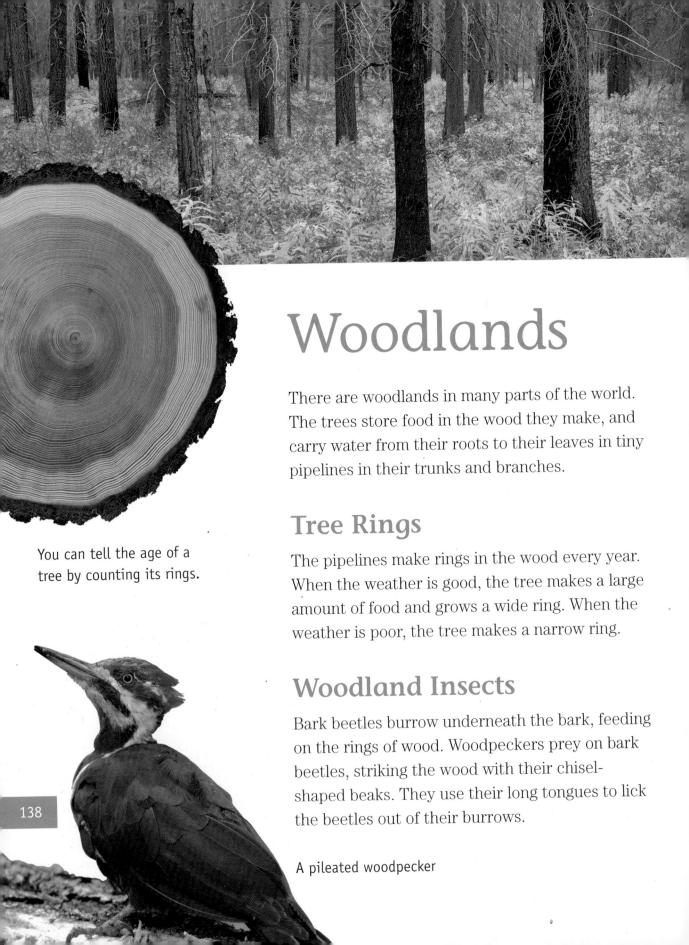

You can tell the age of a tree by counting its rings.

Woodlands

There are woodlands in many parts of the world. The trees store food in the wood they make, and carry water from their roots to their leaves in tiny pipelines in their trunks and branches.

Tree Rings

The pipelines make rings in the wood every year. When the weather is good, the tree makes a large amount of food and grows a wide ring. When the weather is poor, the tree makes a narrow ring.

Woodland Insects

Bark beetles burrow underneath the bark, feeding on the rings of wood. Woodpeckers prey on bark beetles, striking the wood with their chisel-shaped beaks. They use their long tongues to lick the beetles out of their burrows.

A pileated woodpecker

Some spiders spin webs between twigs. They hide on a twig, waiting for an insect to fly into the web and become stuck on its threads. As the insect struggles, the spider rushes up to it and gives it a poisonous bite.

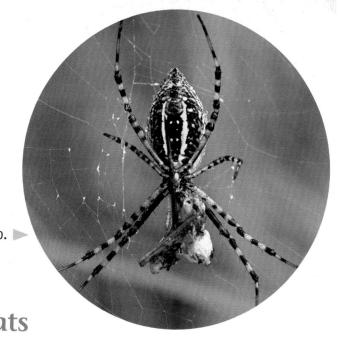

This orb weaver spider has trapped prey in its web. ▶

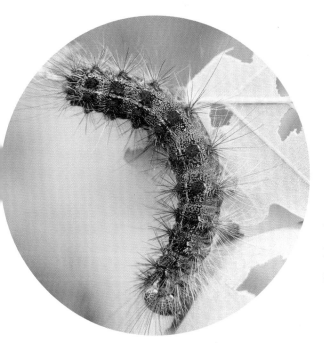

Bats

Moth caterpillars feed on leaves. They are camouflaged, so many of them escape predators. When they become moths, they fly at night, trying to avoid bats. These predators roost in tree holes during the day and fly through the woodland at night, feeding on moths and other insects such as gnats and beetles.

Each gypsy moth caterpillar can eat an average of one square metre of leaves. This can damage or kill a tree.

Woodland Birds

The tree creeper bird feeds on insects and spiders, using its hooked beak to pull them out of their hiding places.

This tree creeper bird is found throughout southern Canada, but its camouflage makes it difficult to spot.

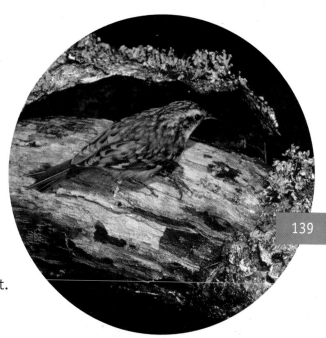

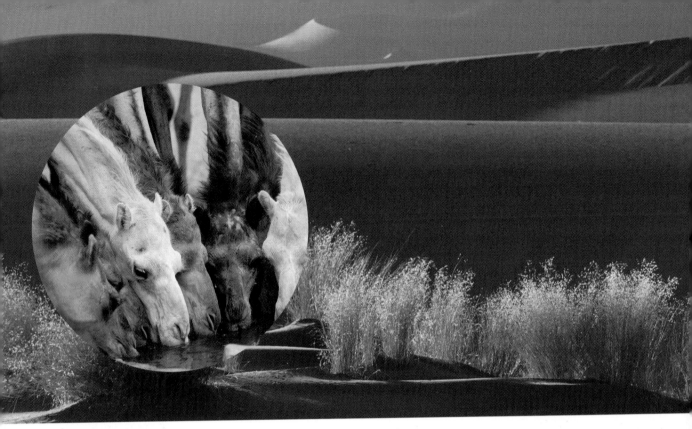

A thirsty camel can drink up to 100 litres in 10 minutes.

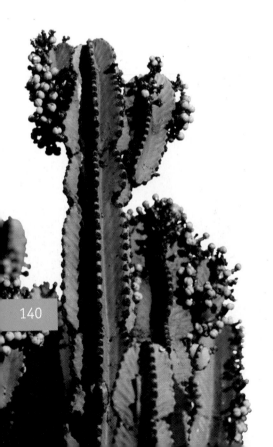

Desert

All life needs water. In a desert it may rain for only a very short time in a year, so the plants here have adapted to survive. Their long roots collect as much water from the ground as possible.

Surviving Without Rain

Since plants lose water through their leaves, desert plants have only small leaves. Some plants have only spines. Some plants survive the dry conditions by remaining as seeds while it is dry. When it rains, they germinate and grow quickly into plants.

Desert plants have long roots and small leaves or spines.

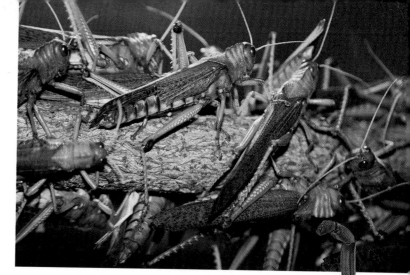

Desert animals are also able to survive without much water. One of the best known, the camel, lives in the Sahara Desert. It can manage for weeks without drinking any water—as long as it can find succulent desert plants to eat. These are plants that store water in their leaves and stems.

Swarms of locusts can devour a plant's leaves in a matter of seconds.

Desert Plants and Food Chains

Because of their stores of water, desert plants provide the basis for many desert food chains. Insects that eat desert plants include locusts, grasshoppers, and crickets. These animals, in turn, provide food for lizards, birds, and scorpions.

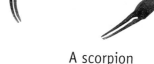

A scorpion

In cold deserts, lichen and moss grow on rocks and on the ground. Here, an Arctic tern chick nestles between lichen-covered rocks.

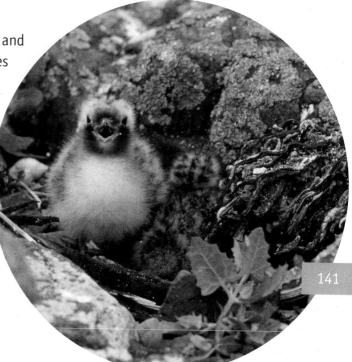

DIG DEEPER ....

1. How is a food chain affected when the habitat is changed by lack of rain?
2. Investigate a food chain in a rainforest, pond, or on a mountain. Draw a diagram to explain your food chain and habitat.

141

Researchers at Work!

Scientists investigate topics that interest them. They share what they find out in different ways.

A brochure is one way to explain what you have learned, so that others can learn about the topic too.

Choose a Habitat to Research

- Think about the animal and plant habitats you have read about.
- What question about habitats would you like to explore?
- Brainstorm ideas with a partner or in a group.

Plan Your Research

- Choose a research question.
- List different resources you can use to help you find the answer.
- Decide how you will record the information.

RESEARCH TIPS

- Look for information in books, magazines, and on CD-ROMs.
- Browse Web sites, like the site for the Canadian Wildlife Federation.
- Interview an expert about your habitat.
- View science videos and TV programs.

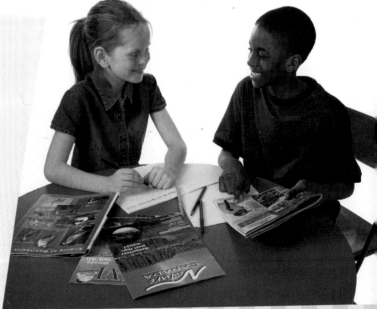

Create a Brochure

Make a brochure to share what you learned.

Here are some important things to think about:

- your audience
- how you will organize the information
- what you will put on the front of the brochure
- what visuals you will use
- how you will make the brochure

Display the Brochure

- Think of how you can share your brochure in different ways.
- You could place the brochure in the library resource centre or create a classroom display.

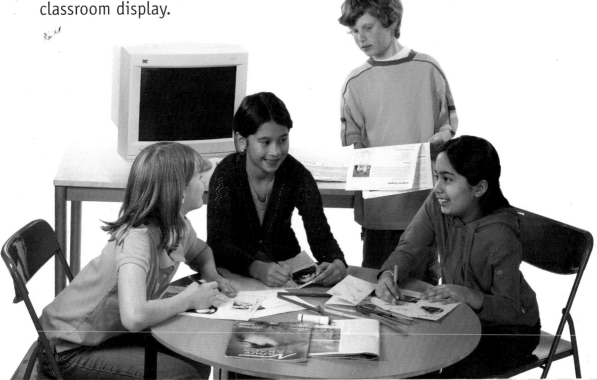

143

ART Underfoot

by Jeff Siamon

How can art help people think about the natural world?

Drain covers usually look something like this.

The city of Vancouver uses art to remind people to care about the environment. Recently, the city held a competition called Art Underfoot. The winning designs in the competition will be cast in iron on city drain covers. If you've noticed drain covers before, they are usually round, made of metal, and cover the openings to underground sewers. Drain covers are usually grimy and dirty—*not* works of art.

This is the winning entry by Susan Point and Kelly Cannell.

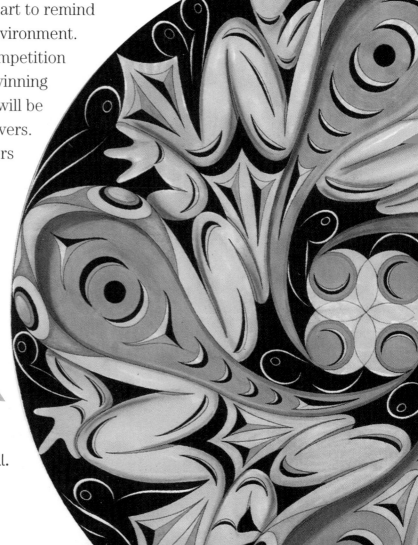

One of the winning designs was by the team of Susan Point and Kelly Cannell. Susan and Kelly are from the Musqueam First Nation in Vancouver. They are also mother and daughter. Much of their work is based on traditional Coast Salish art and designs.

Their drain cover shows the life cycle of a frog. The design will remind people to not put harmful chemicals down their drains. When people dump chemicals, they can travel to the bodies of water where frogs live and breed.

You can also see that the winning design forms a circle of images. The eggs in the centre swirl out into tadpoles, then into frogs. Susan Point often presents images in a circle pattern. This helps viewers understand that all things in nature are somehow connected, with no end and no beginning, just like a circle.

So, the next time you are out for a walk, look down at your feet. You might see something that is both beautiful *and* makes you think!

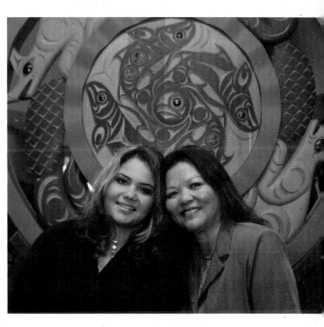

Kelly Cannell (left) and Susan Point are Coast Salish artists. They have also worked together on silkscreen prints, paintings, and wood carvings.

DIG DEEPER

1. In what ways could the water that goes down a drain hurt a habitat?
2. Design a drain cover that will remind people to respect the environment.

Friends of the
BLUE PLANET

How Children Feel About Our Environment

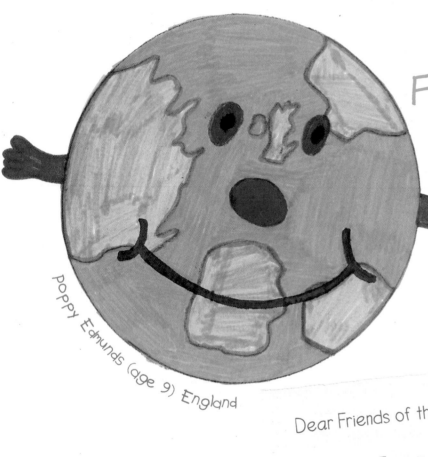

Poppy Edmunds (age 9) England

How can children share ideas about our planet?

Dear Friends of the Blue Planet,

When I am in the middle of nature I feel that it is part of my family. If any child breaks a branch off a tree, I feel sorrow, as if they had broken a part of my soul.

If every leaf, every blade of grass, every tree, every flower were to disappear, I would feel like I was losing my family.

Your friend,
Lurubaru Mihaela (age 12)
Romania

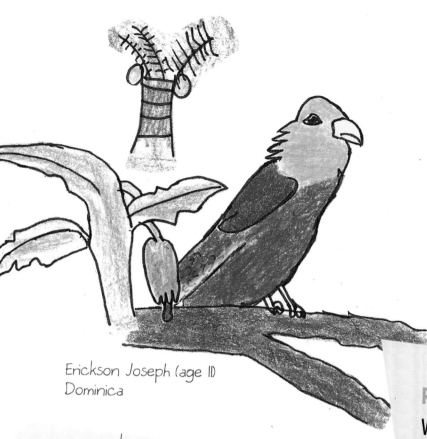

Erickson Joseph (age 11)
Dominica

Without
Our
Respect
our
Land
will be
Destroyed

Your friend,
Megan O'Keeffe (age 12)
Australia

READ LIKE A WRITER

Why did the children use "feelings" words and phrases to express their views about the environment?

My favourite part of nature is to be with the Sisserou parrots. I would like to play and talk with the Sisserou, and help them make a huge family so that they may show the world that they are special.

My dream is that man may not destroy everything of Dominica but will see the wonders and I want this dream to come true. My children in time to come will continue my dream. And they will do the same thing that I did.

Ricard St. John (age 10)
Dominica

147

I am happy to see the trees. The trees give us medicines. If you cut the trees down the dryness will come. When you cut the trees down the rain carries the topsoil away. In my opinion, if there are no trees everyone will die.

Badra Plea (age 13)
Mali

Dear World,

I live in the country and most of the trees are dead. You can take a walk through there and some of the trees, if you touch them, they may fall or break. A lot of it is the acid rain. There is a creek there and the deer drink that water. The water is orange and it is mainly from acid rain.

Your friend,
Jennifer Stroud (age 10)
Canada

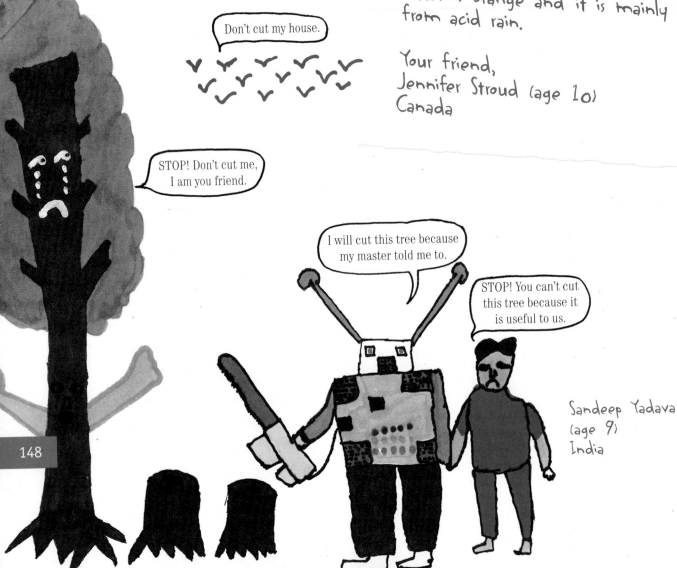

Sandeep Yadava
(age 9)
India

148

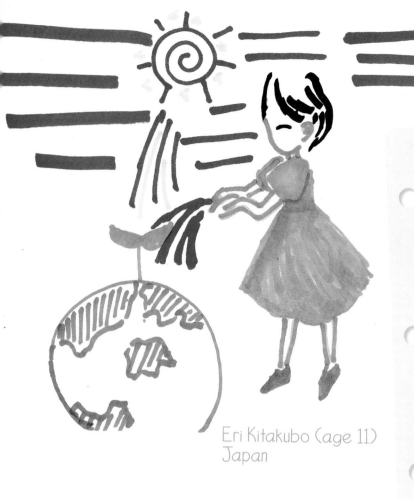

Eri Kitakubo (age 11)
Japan

My Friends,

    I dream that people will not throw everything into the environment, and that people will understand that they are only harming themselves. One can only hope.

Stefan Wieland (age 9)
Germany

Dear people all over the globe!

I want all the people on earth to gather as one united family and clear nature of pollution. Also I want every person on earth to do some good deed for the preservation of nature! Take care of nature!

Marina Semyonova (age 10)
Russia

DIG DEEPER

1. Choose your favourite letter or poem. What would you say to the author about their work?

2. Create your own letter, poem, or drawing to show how you feel about the environment.

149

How Does a Possum Cross the Road?

by Andrew Charman

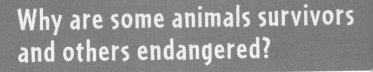

Why are some animals survivors and others endangered?

Q How does a possum cross the road?

A Today the rare mountain pygmy possums of Australia use an underpass! When a road was built through their reserve, many males were hit by cars when they went to visit the females. A tunnel was built for them to cross the road safely.

For many years, people thought mountain pygmy possums were extinct. Then, in 1966, a live possum was discovered.

Q Which endangered animal is the most shy?

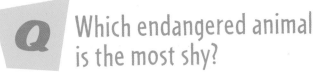

A The shy okapi is so hard to find that scientists didn't even know it existed until 1901. Today there are fewer okapis than ever, because their rain forest home is being cut down.

150

It looks much like a zebra, but the okapi is actually a relative of the giraffe.

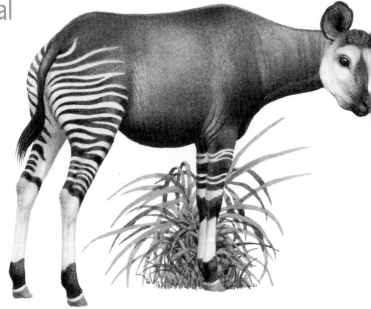

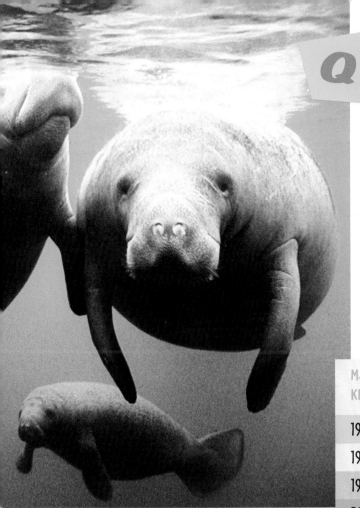

Why are boats bad for manatees?

A Manatees are gentle animals—they spend their life swimming along, grazing on sea grass. Unfortunately, they share their waterways with fast-moving boats, and many manatees are injured by propeller blades. This means the animals are getting rarer.

Manatees killed in Florida by watercraft KEY: 🐋 = 10 manatees		
1975	🐋	6
1985	🐋🐋🐋🐋	33
1995	🐋🐋🐋🐋🐋	42
2005	🐋🐋🐋🐋🐋🐋🐋🐋	80

The largest population of manatees is found in Florida.

Q Which "extinct" animal returned to the wild?

A Père David's deer were once extinct in the wild. The only ones left lived in zoos and parks. Luckily they were bred so successfully that now they are being returned to their grassland homes in northern China.

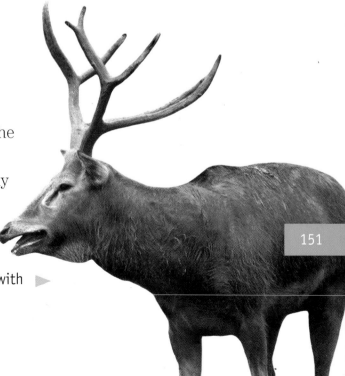

Adult deer have summer coats that are bright red with a dark stripe. They have dark grey coats in winter. ▶

151

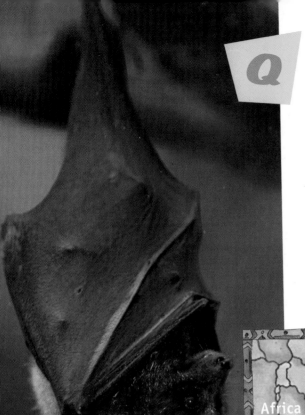

Which fox flies to its food?

A The Rodrigues flying fox isn't a fox—it's a bat that lives on Rodrigues Island. It eats fruit, so it needs lots of fruit trees. Sadly, most of its forest home has been cut down and there are now only about 400 of these bats left.

The body of the Rodrigues flying fox is quite small, but its wing span can be up to 90 cm across.

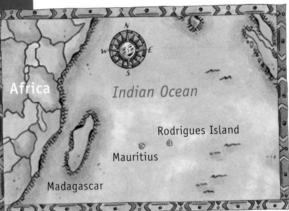

Rodrigues Island is in the Indian Ocean, about 550 km northeast of the island of Mauritius.

Q Which endangered whale has a unicorn's horn?

A The narwhal is a kind of whale that lives in the Arctic seas. The male is hunted for its spiralled tusk, which looks just like a unicorn's horn. If too many narwhals are taken, they may one day become extinct.

The tusk is really a narwhal's left tooth that has grown outward in a spiral. Narwhal tusks can grow to be 2 to 3 m long.

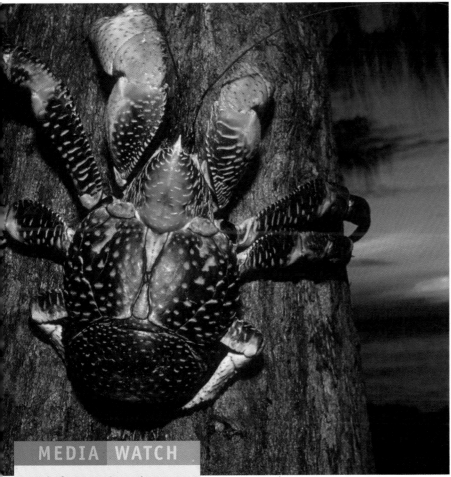

A Robber crabs live on islands in the Pacific and Indian Oceans. Some grow up to nearly a metre across. They are hunted for food and made into souvenirs for tourists.

Robber crabs climb trees, such as coconut trees, and snip off fruit with their giant pincers. They then climb down the tree, gather the fruit, and pound it until they get it open to eat.

MEDIA WATCH

Look for stories about endangered animals or habitats.

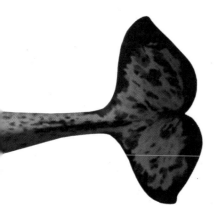

DIG DEEPER ························

1. How can endangered animals and their habitats be brought to people's attention? Discuss with a partner some ways to raise people's awareness of habitat loss.

2. Locate some interesting facts about an endangered animal habitat. Create your own Question and Answer card to share the information with others.

153

Dare to Care...

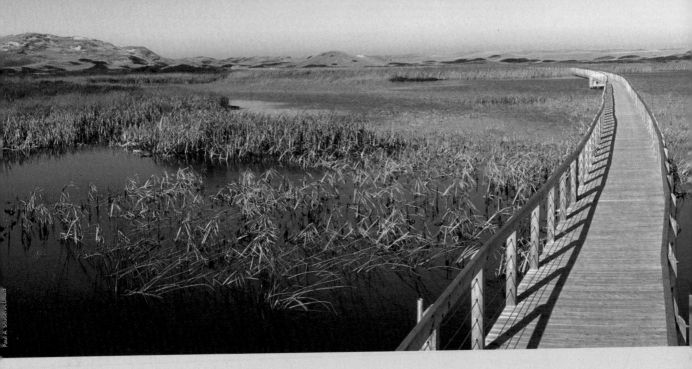

© 2005 www.cwf-fcf.org

Sponsored by the Canadian Association of Principals, Canadian Museum of Nature, Canadian Wildlife Federation,
Coastal Zone Canada Association, Environment Canada (Biodiversity Convention Office and Marine Environment Branch),
Fisheries and Oceans Canada, Parks Canada, and Scouts Canada.

154

How can a poster create interest in a natural habitat?

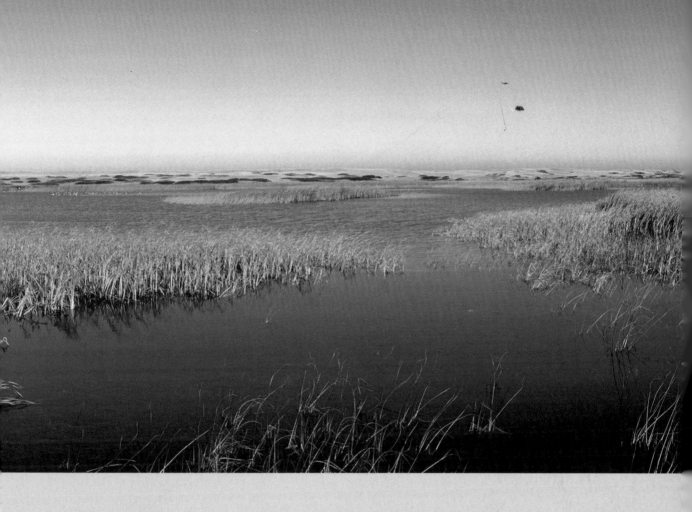

becial Marine Places...Get to Know One

Celebrate Oceans Day June 8

DIG DEEPER ·····················

1. What can you learn about this natural habitat by looking closely at the images and words?

2. In a small group, brainstorm some different ways that Oceans Day could be promoted across Canada.

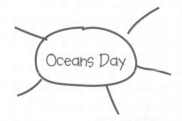

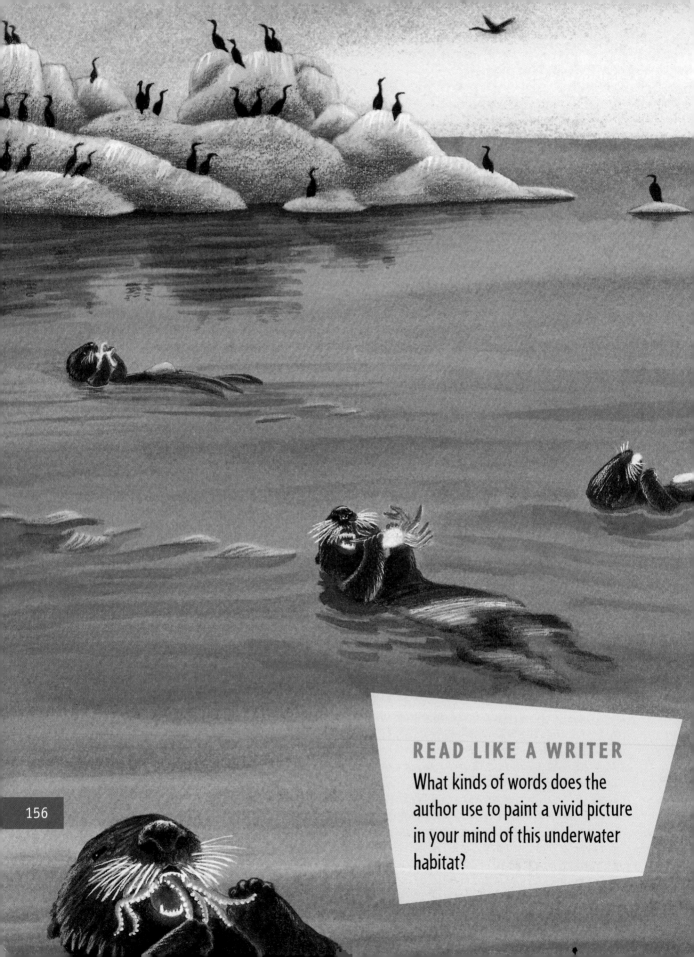

156

READ LIKE A WRITER
What kinds of words does the author use to paint a vivid picture in your mind of this underwater habitat?

Sea Otter Inlet
by Celia Godkin

How can people affect habitats in both positive and negative ways?

In a long arm of the sea,
hemmed in by land on either side,
lived a colony of sea otters.

The sea otters lived their whole lives
in the waters of this inlet.
They dived in the deep
seaweedy forests of kelp,
looking for good things to eat.
They dined on crabs and shellfish,
on sea stars and octopi,
but their favourite food of all
was the spiny purple sea urchin.

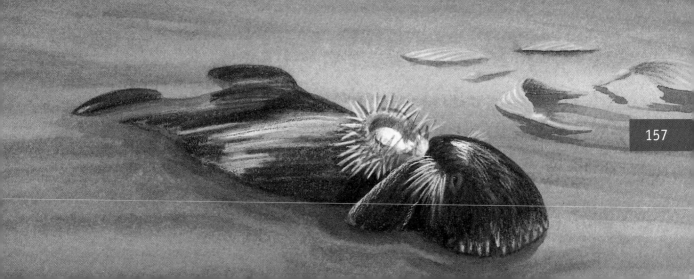

157

After a meal of these delicacies,
the otters groomed themselves with great care.
When they were as clean as they could be,
they wrapped themselves in a frond of kelp
and went to sleep.
The kelp anchored them gently in place
so they could not drift away.

One day the otters awoke from their nap
to find hunters all around.
The hunters hurled harpoons at them
or shot them with guns.

The otters dived to escape the hunters.
But they could not stay below the water for ever.
The hunters waited patiently
for the otters to come up for air.

One by one,
the otters were hunted and killed
for their soft, warm fur.
When there were no more otters left,
the hunters sailed away,
and life in the kelp forest went on.

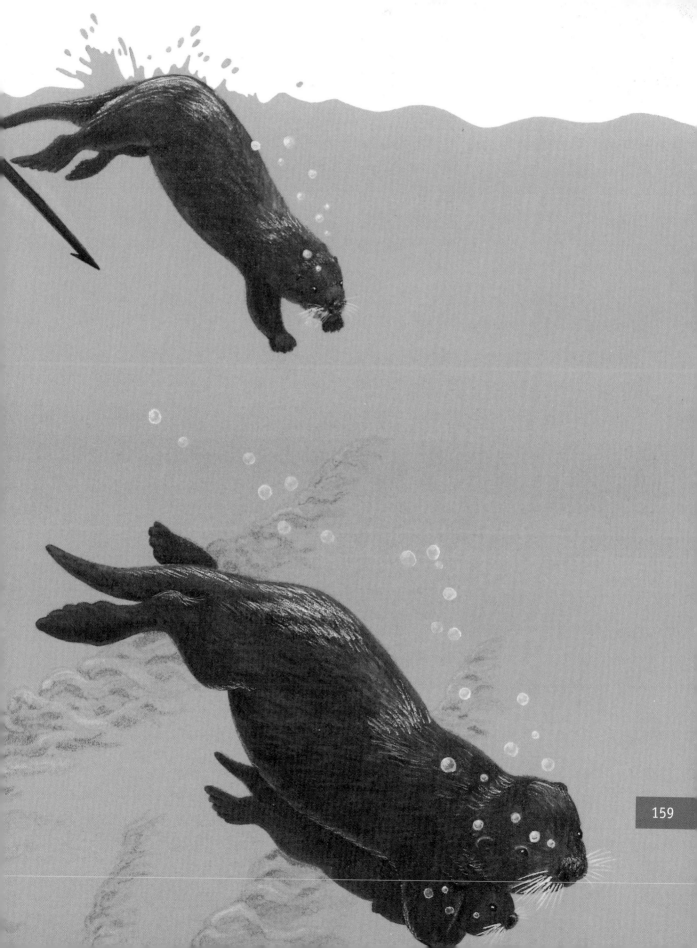

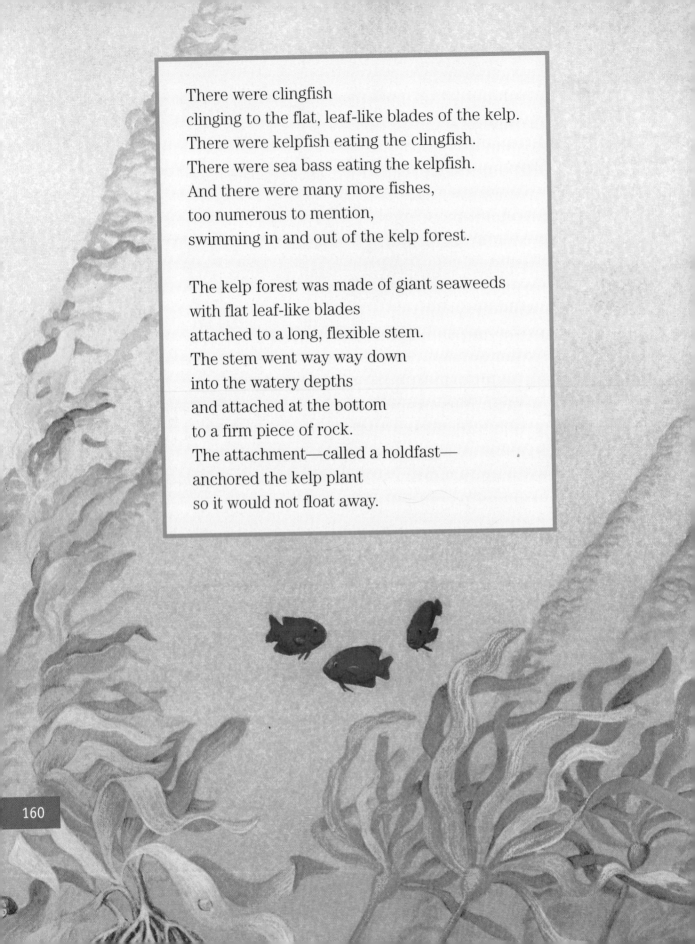

There were clingfish
clinging to the flat, leaf-like blades of the kelp.
There were kelpfish eating the clingfish.
There were sea bass eating the kelpfish.
And there were many more fishes,
too numerous to mention,
swimming in and out of the kelp forest.

The kelp forest was made of giant seaweeds
with flat leaf-like blades
attached to a long, flexible stem.
The stem went way way down
into the watery depths
and attached at the bottom
to a firm piece of rock.
The attachment—called a holdfast—
anchored the kelp plant
so it would not float away.

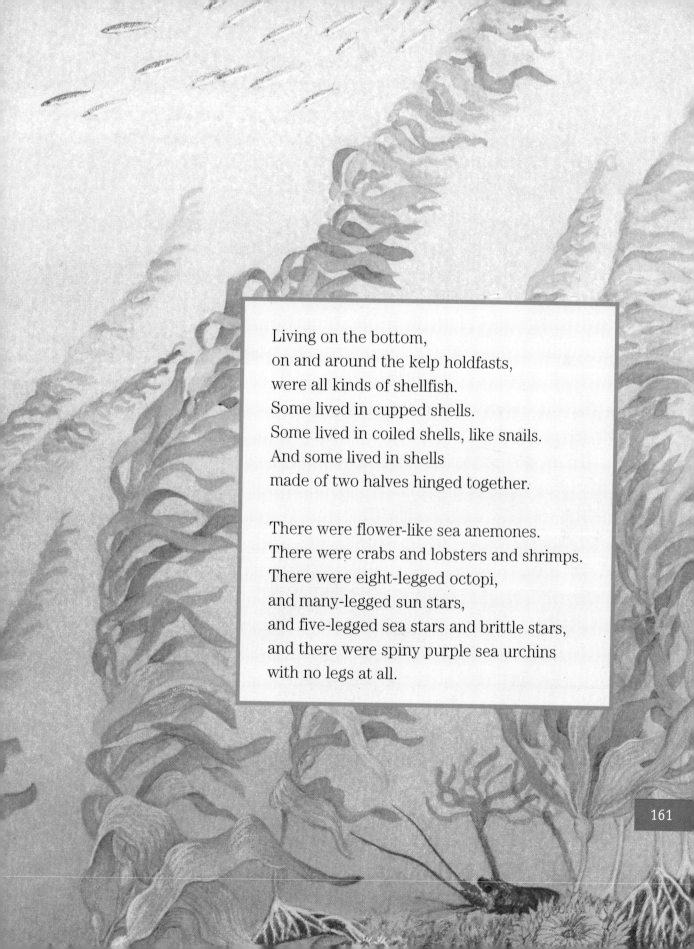

Living on the bottom,
on and around the kelp holdfasts,
were all kinds of shellfish.
Some lived in cupped shells.
Some lived in coiled shells, like snails.
And some lived in shells
made of two halves hinged together.

There were flower-like sea anemones.
There were crabs and lobsters and shrimps.
There were eight-legged octopi,
and many-legged sun stars,
and five-legged sea stars and brittle stars,
and there were spiny purple sea urchins
with no legs at all.

161

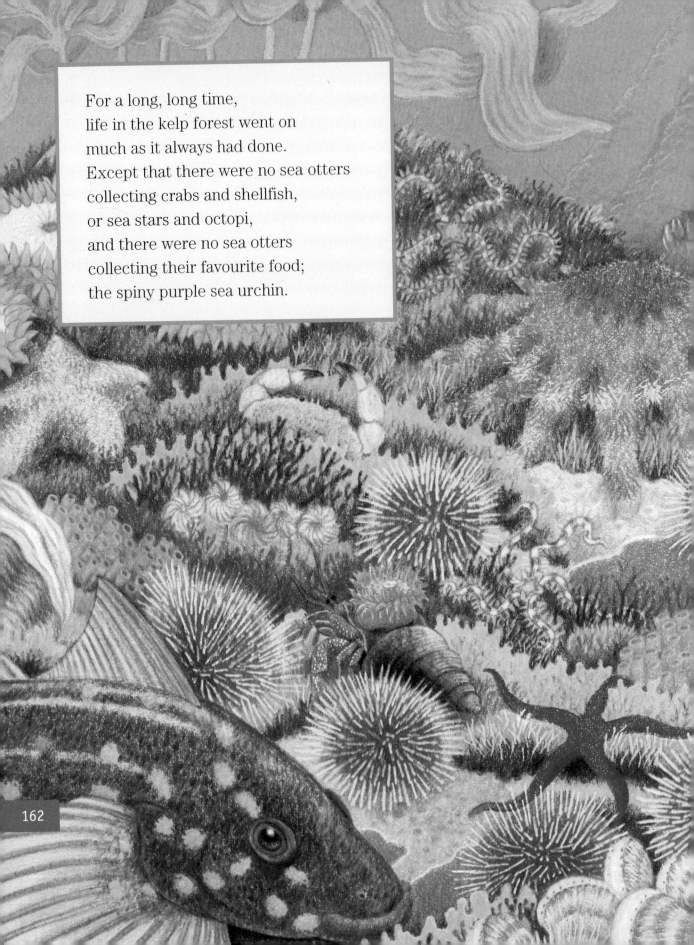

For a long, long time,
life in the kelp forest went on
much as it always had done.
Except that there were no sea otters
collecting crabs and shellfish,
or sea stars and octopi,
and there were no sea otters
collecting their favourite food;
the spiny purple sea urchin.

162

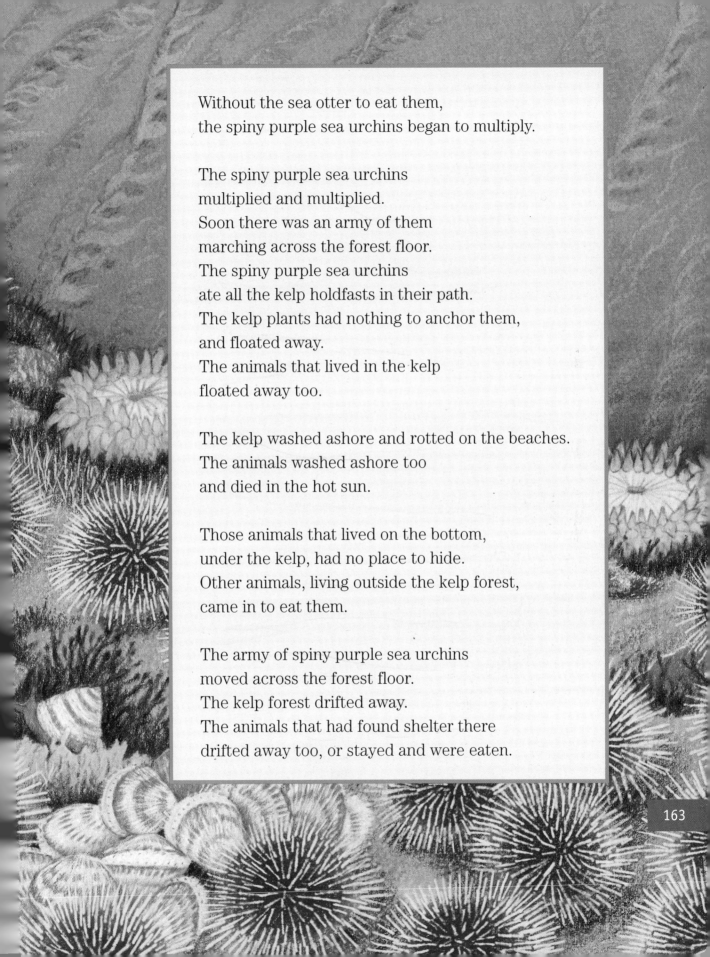

Without the sea otter to eat them,
the spiny purple sea urchins began to multiply.

The spiny purple sea urchins
multiplied and multiplied.
Soon there was an army of them
marching across the forest floor.
The spiny purple sea urchins
ate all the kelp holdfasts in their path.
The kelp plants had nothing to anchor them,
and floated away.
The animals that lived in the kelp
floated away too.

The kelp washed ashore and rotted on the beaches.
The animals washed ashore too
and died in the hot sun.

Those animals that lived on the bottom,
under the kelp, had no place to hide.
Other animals, living outside the kelp forest,
came in to eat them.

The army of spiny purple sea urchins
moved across the forest floor.
The kelp forest drifted away.
The animals that had found shelter there
drifted away too, or stayed and were eaten.

Then, one day, a wonderful thing happened.
Some sea otters swam into the inlet.

Some otters had survived in places
which the hunters had not found.
No one was hunting them anymore.
There were now enough otters
that some could come back
to live again in their old home.

The otters dived in the waters of the inlet.
They found plenty of spiny purple sea urchins.
Their favourite food!
Soon, other otters joined them.

Gradually, very gradually,
as the otters ate more and more
spiny purple sea urchins,
the kelp began to grow back again.
Gradually, very gradually, the animals
that had lived in the kelp forest returned.

Once again, there were clingfish
and kelpfish and sea bass,
and many more fishes,
too numerous to mention.

There were all kinds of shellfish.
There were flower-like sea anemones,
and crabs and lobsters and shrimps.
There were eight-legged octopi
and many-legged sun stars
and five-legged sea stars and brittle stars.

There were even
some spiny purple sea urchins,
with no legs at all.
But not too many.

DIG DEEPER

1. How did people change this natural habitat?
2. In a small group, choose two or three parts of this story for choral reading. Practise reading the selection before performing for an audience.

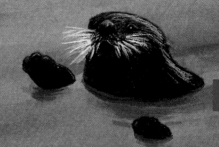

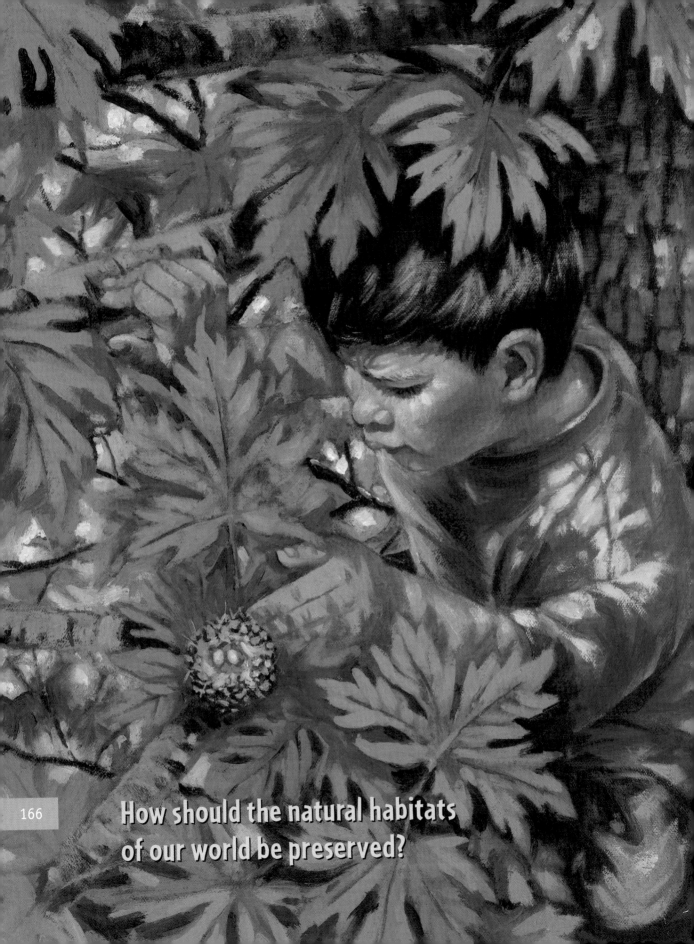

How should the natural habitats of our world be preserved?

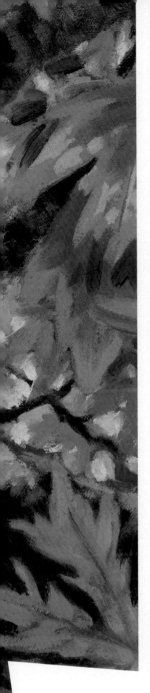

Solomon's Tree

by ANDREA SPALDING
Illustrated by JANET WILSON

The cedar trees around Solomon's house were special. They shaded in summer and sheltered in winter and whispered secrets to each other on the breath of the wind.

But the big old maple was very special. This was the tree that shared its secrets with Solomon. Every day Solomon climbed its knobby trunk and curled up in his favourite notch.

"Hello, tree," he whispered and stroked the rough bark.

"Hello, Solomon," the tree rustled back. Its branches cradled his body.

In spring the maple showed him a hummingbird nest. Solomon gazed in astonishment at the fragment of woven lichen clinging to a forked twig and marvelled at the tiny eggs, smaller than his little fingernail.

"You mustn't tell," whispered the tree.

"I promise," Solomon whispered back.

In summer the maple showed Solomon where the chrysalis hung, hidden in a crack of bark.

"Watch carefully," whispered the tree.

"I will," Solomon whispered back.

He watched with wonder as the chrysalis cracked open, and bit by bit a brand-new butterfly unfolded its wings and danced away on the breeze.

READ LIKE A WRITER

The author uses the senses (sight, touch, smell, sound, taste) to show Solomon's relationship to the tree. How does this help the reader understand how he feels?

167

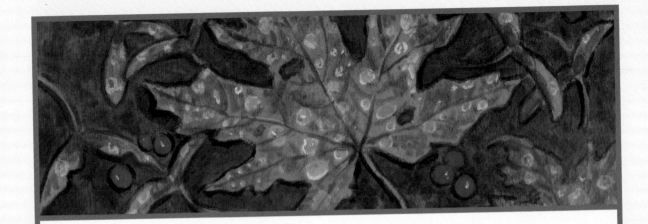

In fall the maple shed its golden leaves and winged seeds and rustled and chuckled as it showered Solomon. Solomon chased the dancing propellers and gathered together piles of leaves.

"Winter's coming," whispered the tree.

"I know," Solomon answered softly from under his leafy blanket.

With the winter came wind and rain. The cedars surrounding Solomon's house tossed their branches and chanted winter songs. The big old maple creaked out lullabies to comfort Solomon's sleep.

Then came a midwinter storm. The wind howled and shrieked. Inside Solomon's house only the voice of the wind could be heard.

"This storm is too big," said Solomon. "I'm scared." He burrowed under his quilt and pulled the pillow around his ears.

The storm raged for hours, whipping the treetops back and forth and playing a fearsome tug-of-war with their branches. The old maple creaked in protest and writhed and wriggled but couldn't loosen the wind's grip.

CRAAACK.

The maple gave a last despairing cry, crashed over the woodshed, and fell silent.

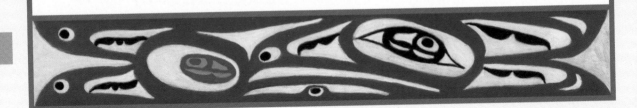

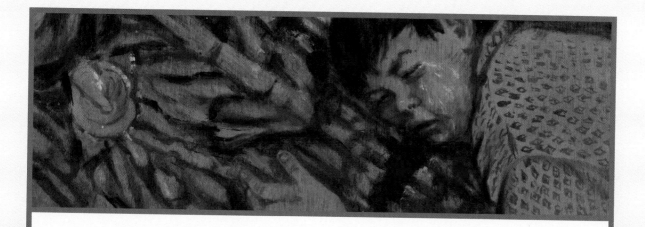

"My tree," sobbed Solomon the next morning. He ran through the rain and hugged the fallen trunk. "She was my friend…now she's gone…and I never said goodbye."

All that day Solomon's family worked. Father used the chainsaw to buck up the fallen trunk. Uncle burnt the branches scattered over the driveway and fixed the woodshed. Mother and Solomon stacked the maple logs inside.

Father handed the last log to Solomon and took him to stand in front of Uncle.

"Would you like to see the spirit of your special tree?" Uncle asked.

Solomon nodded.

"Tomorrow we'll start a mask together."

The next day Solomon carried the log to Uncle's workshop. Uncle swung the axe and split it straight down the middle. Solomon clutched half the log to his chest. He closed his eyes and thought about his tree. Uncle picked up his drum and began to dance and sing.

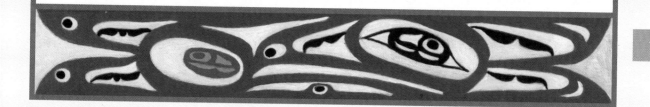

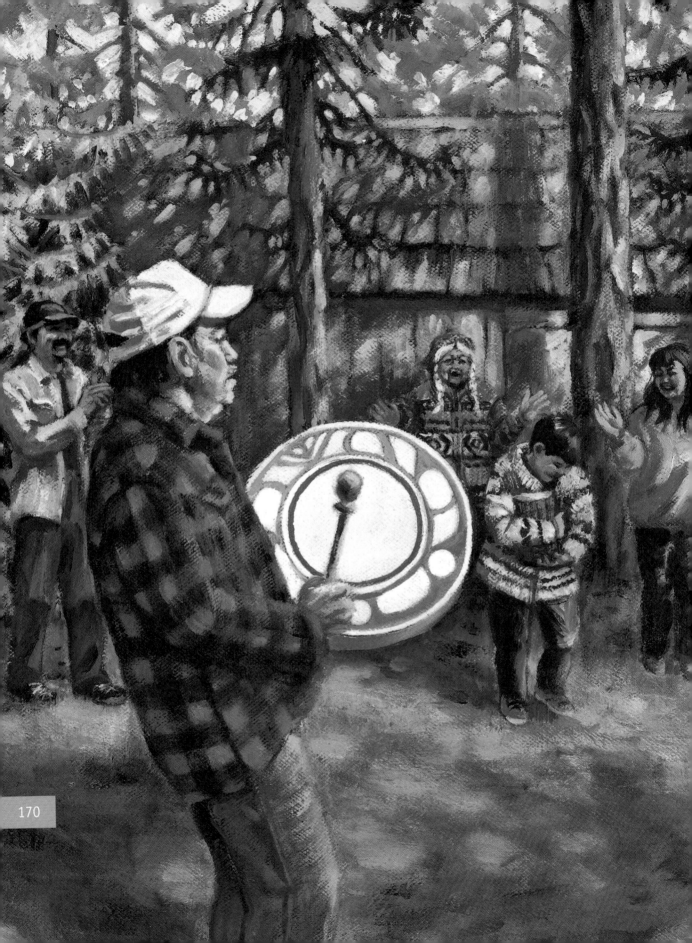

Gwā eee dim haoou,
Here is what I have to say:
Today we begin a carving.
We invite our ancestors to guide us,
To show my nephew the spirit of this special tree.
We honour our ancestors and thank them for their help.

Uncle's voice rang out. His drumming filled the clearing and rose to the sky.

Solomon's voice was small and his feet sad and heavy, but as his Uncle drummed, Solomon grew braver. He sang his own song.

Gwā eee dim haoou,
Here is what I have to say:
Tree, let your spirit guide Uncle's fingers,
Let those fingers show your face,
Let your face help my memory,
Let my memory always honour you.

Solomon took the pencil and marked the centre ring at each end of his log. Uncle drew a line through the middle and measured on each side.

The chainsaw whirred and sawdust flew as Uncle made the first cuts. Day by day the log transformed.

"Tell me about your tree," said Uncle as he planed the angles of the face. "What did you see among the branches?"

Solomon described the hummingbird nest and the antics of the baby birds. Uncle rounded the brow with the adze, chipped the hollows of the eyes, and told the hummingbird story.

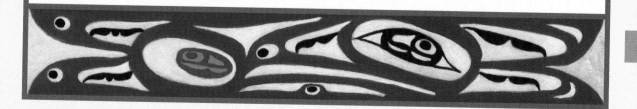

"Did your tree smell nice?" asked Uncle as he used the hook knife to carve the nose.

Solomon remembered the sweet spring smell of sap and the pungent fall odour of crushed leaves. Uncle told of fall mushroom gathering in his grandmother's village.

"Did your tree have a voice?" asked Uncle as he showed how to carve the mouth.

Solomon told of whispered secrets and nightly lullabies. Uncle taught Solomon a family song.

"Is my mask finished now?" asked Solomon.

"Not yet. A mask needs to be worn. We must make room for your face. Careful…stand back," warned Uncle. He thinned out the back of the mask with the tip of the chainsaw. Then he showed Solomon how to hollow the nose and cheeks. Solomon helped scrape and chip. Shavings curled and the mask became thin and beautiful, a face to wear over a face.

Solomon was in charge of drying the mask. He stood on a chair and placed it in the microwave.

"Three times, at three minutes," he said, "with lots of turns."

They smoothed and sanded and rubbed and stroked until the face glowed under their fingers and began to look alive.

"Now what?" asked Solomon.

Uncle drew a hummingbird design across the smooth wooden forehead. Next he chose a tiny brush and began to paint. First the beak, then an eye and a face, finally a wing feathering across the brow. Last he painted the outline of the mask's lips and eyeballs, and very, very carefully Solomon filled them in.

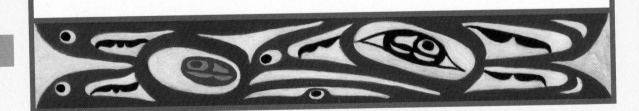

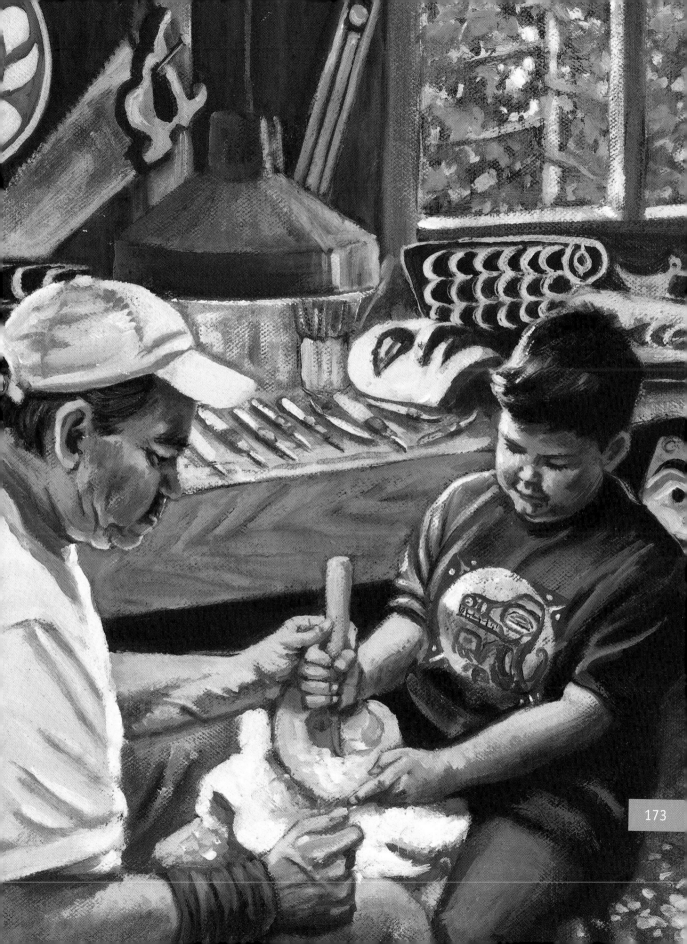

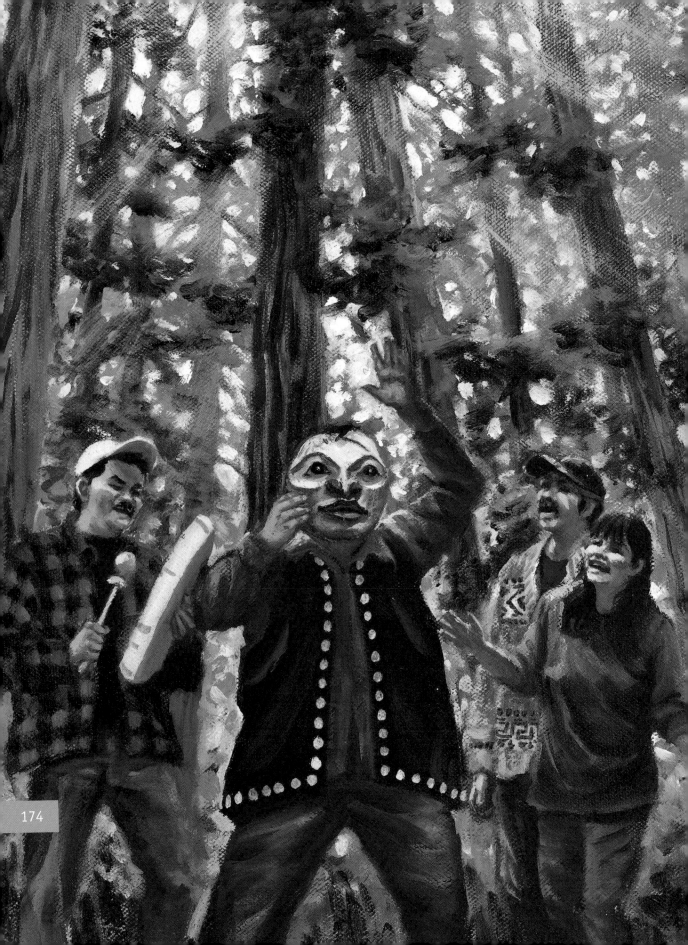